Clinical Intensive Care Medicine

Introductory Series in Medicine Vol. 1

Series Editor: **Nadey Hakim**

Clinical Intensive Care Medicine

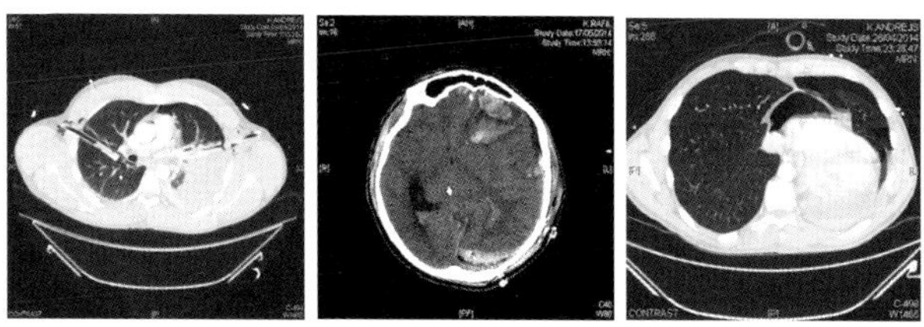

Editor

Carlos M H Gómez

St Mary's Hospital and Hammersmith Hospital, UK

ICP Imperial College Press

Published by

Imperial College Press
57 Shelton Street
Covent Garden
London WC2H 9HE

Distributed by

World Scientific Publishing Co. Pte. Ltd.
5 Toh Tuck Link, Singapore 596224
USA office: 27 Warren Street, Suite 401-402, Hackensack, NJ 07601
UK office: 57 Shelton Street, Covent Garden, London WC2H 9HE

Library of Congress Cataloging-in-Publication Data
Clinical intensive care medicine / edited by Carlos M.H. Gómez.
p. ; cm. -- (Introductory series in medicine ; volume 1)
Includes bibliographical references and index.
ISBN 978-1-84816-388-1 (hardcover : alk. paper) -- ISBN 978-1-84816-389-8 (electronic)
I. Gómez, Carlos M. H., editor. II. Series: Introductory series in medicine ; v. 1.
[DNLM: 1. Intensive Care. 2. Clinical Medicine. 3. Critical Illness--therapy. WX 218]
RC86.7
616.02'8--dc23
2014026685

British Library Cataloguing-in-Publication Data
A catalogue record for this book is available from the British Library.

Typeset by Stallion Press
Email: enquiries@stallionpress.com

Printed in Singapore by Mainland Press Pte Ltd.

To Carlos, Luis and Tomás
Wonderful, glorious boys: my soul, my spirit, my life

Contents

Foreword from the Series Editor

My collaboration with Imperial College Press dates back to 1995 when I was commissioned to write a book on transplantation entitled *Introduction to Organ Transplantation*. I have since edited several textbooks on different surgical fields including a second edition of *Introduction to Organ Transplantation* in 2012. Collating a series of textbooks introducing different specialties is a challenge I have undertaken with the hope that the knowledge and expertise presented will spur the next generation on to even greater knowledge. I envisage the series to be useful to physicians and surgeons at all levels of training and experience, extending the tradition of textbook excellence and leadership.

I have invited experts to put together volumes to ensure a full display of the state-of-the-art of several surgical and associated specialties in order to provide a complete coverage of current practice as well as a glimpse of the future.

This first volume, selected and brought together by Dr Carlos Gómez, explores the latest in current intensive care practice in a broad range of areas. Intensive care is a specialty which has evolved and progressed exponentially over the last few years, and this timely volume will be an important guide for current and future doctors.

Professor Nadey Hakim, MD, PhD
Imperial College London
Honorary Secretary Royal Society of Medicine
Past President International College of Surgeons
June 2014

Foreword

It is a great pleasure for me to write the foreword to *Clinical Intensive Care Medicine* and to congratulate Carlos Gómez and colleagues — all of whom are hands-on, practicing clinicians — on this outstanding achievement. As a vascular surgeon with an interest in complex aortic disease, I have plenty of reasons to thank the current generation of expert intensivists. This book enshrines today's approach to the management of the critically ill patient and as such it demonstrates the authors' desire to spread best current practice as well as a commitment to teaching the next generation. Dr Gómez believes this book is relevant to everyone from medical student to intensive care unit chief. I would add that it is useful also for those working in the most technologically advanced hospitals to those in field or temporary establishments.

Critical care has come of age in the last two decades and the specialty continues to expand its role. It does not take too much imagination to see the hospitals of the future as one where expensive in-patient real-estate can only be justified for patients with critical care needs. That patients are getting ever older and ever more sick with ever more multi-system disease only adds to this vision. It means that developed societies are likely to need more people with critical care skills. As well as continuing to improve outcomes, the challenges for intensive care unit practitioners now are to optimise training of the next generation — it surely cannot all be done on the job — and to develop an evidence base to underpin each of the massive range of pharmacological, interventional, monitoring and supportive strategies now available. To me both of these make the case for the promotion of academic intensive care unit medicine throughout the developed world.

A final word about governance and resource allocation; in the future — consistent with the rising role of intensive care unit medicine — intensivists must become more involved in the running of the hospitals in which they work. Only by doing this will they be able to appropriately direct and understand intensive care unit care, its costs and the context of funding in an increasingly competitive health care world.

I am happy to see that most of my questions are addressed in this excellent book. Good luck to all who read it, especially those about to embark on a career in clinical medicine. I suggest you learn from Dr Gómez and his colleagues. The time for intensive care medicine is now.

N. J. Cheshire MD FRCS
Professor of Vascular Surgery
Head of Circulation & Renal Sciences
Imperial College Healthcare
London
June 2014

Preface

The book is intended as an authoritative guide to practical intensive care medicine written by acknowledged specialist practitioners from the UK, Europe and North America, most of whom are also internationally acclaimed authors. Target audiences are medical students, trainees in intensive care medicine and other acute specialties, consultants wishing to remain up to date on all branches of this vast specialty and other allied professionals practising in intensive care, including nurses and physiotherapists. The book therefore has a practical and educational common thread rather than an encyclopaedic approach.

Intensive care patients are the sickest and most challenging in any hospital and use up a disproportionate amount of resources. The specialty is relatively young, only about 40 years old, and expanding worldwide as patients grow older, harbour greater expectations and present increased demands on already stretched health systems.

The older generation of intensivists is approaching retirement. The middle generation trained in various medical and surgical specialties and then subspecialised in intensive care. These doctors now lead the way in clinical practice, research, management and training. The younger generation of intensivists includes an ever increasing number of doctors who, for the first time, enjoy a structured training programme with clinical rotations, courses and exam qualifications.

This book is aimed at this younger generation. My vision is for this book to become a useful resource for those wishing to study, practice and excel in intensive care medicine.

While conceiving this book I have reflected on the true challenges which face the intensive care clinician. They are of three types: clinical, managerial and life challenges.

On the clinical front there are several crucial decisions to be made and revisited for every patient, every day. What is acceptable physiology, what is achievable and at what price? The clinician may, for example, decide that intravascular volume is the priority. He/she must therefore be prepared to accept as a trade-off an increase in unwanted fluid in the form of pulmonary (capillary), peripheral and cerebral oedema. Equally, given a different scenario — or a different clinician — perfusion pressure may become the prime goal. This will of necessity be at the expense of increased cardiac work and also of peripheral vasoconstriction, the combination of these two potentially giving rise to tissue hypoxia and acidaemia. Finally, normalisation of acid-base chemistry may be the utmost priority. Strategies targeted to achieve this can lead to raised intrathoracic pressure (through increased ventilatory settings), increased cardiac work and peripheral oedema.

Also worth reflecting upon is the challenge of blending in with other intensive care colleagues who might have somewhat different clinical philosophies. Changing treatment plans for the sake of change or in order to prove a point seldom benefits the patient, often has a negative effect on team morale and frequently causes undesirable confusion. When taking over the care of a human being who is making satisfactory clinical progress but is perhaps being weaned differently, on inotropes which one would not necessarily have chosen or on antibiotics not amongst one's favourites, the challenge facing the clinician is this: is it really necessary to change these when they are being effective? Some of us refer to this phenomenon as the 'Monday syndrome'.

Perhaps the most important decision facing the intensive care team is to decide which patient requires immediate intervention and which patient can and will benefit from masterful inactivity and close observation. Which patient should be left alone? When should resident doctors be encouraged to do nothing but just observe? One of the eminent contributors to this book once told me that it is just as important to do something which causes benefit as it is to stop others from doing something which may cause harm.

On a philosophical note the reader will agree with me that there is always the possibility of being wrong. The problem here is not necessarily the wrong itself but the consequence of not realising it. The wise, humble clinician is mindful of the possibility of being wrong, however knowledgeable and experienced, and therefore is likely to recognise a wrong decision early and thereby be better positioned to rectify it. The less wise and perhaps less humble intensivist displays an inability to entertain being wrong, which can lead to catastrophe.

The managerial front requires quite a different mind-set. Gifted administrators have an almost innate ability to get the most out of the resources available to them. Perhaps the greatest resource is time and I am always admiring of colleagues who excel in time management. The ability, desire and vision to delegate the right task to the right individual seems inextricably linked to that of successful time management. One of the hallmarks of good management is the creation of efficient and robust systems to ensure clinical safety and governance. The ideal system practically runs itself, accepts newcomers, is understood and appreciated by all and can be modified as new standards develop. For any system to function to a high standard there must be good communication within its members as well as with other clinical groups.

Intensive care specialists are of course members of the human race with a multitude of complex personal, professional and family interactions which clearly are constantly undergoing evolution. We bring children, partners, wives, husbands, holidays, parties, funerals, weddings, deaths, illness, injuries, rota difficulties and an endless list of life events to the table of intensive care medicine. The management of these individually and collectively and the support we give to but also draw from our colleagues constitutes an important challenge in our life as a member of an intensive care department.

Life has thrown a couple of curve balls in my direction while editing this book and I must forever thank Neville, David, Robert and Claire. They know how much they have helped.

An endeavour of this kind requires a lot of activity behind the stage. My wonderful colleagues have challenged, criticised, amused, assisted and supported me throughout. Our nurses, physiotherapists and all members of the wider team make it possible for care to be administered and have over the years provided much clinical advice and feedback; many regularly provide support and some have become friends. Our residents no longer live in the hospital but provide constant care and vigilance, vibrant energy, an inquisitive and stimulating approach as well as a valuable source of criticism and advice; with the nurses, they are an important gateway to the outside world.

My talented, dedicated and incredibly knowledgeable contributors deserve enormous admiration. It is right that they receive my most profound gratitude. If this book finds success then they will deserve immense credit. The faults, misgivings, errors and omissions are, however, exclusively mine. I am grateful to Nadey Hakim for inviting me to contribute this book to his series *Introductory Series in Medicine* and for guiding me through its various stages.

Susanne, Annie, Patricia and now Robyn have been looking after me and my affairs, and without them I would not be where I am today.

The various publishing editors at Imperial College Press have displayed an unquantifiable amount of patience with me and have provided invaluable advice and support throughout the various stages, delivered with great professionalism. Thank you Tasha D'Cruz, Sarah Haynes, Lizzie Bennet and Lance Sucharov.

Finally our patients and their families have my most heartfelt sympathy and respect, especially those who did not survive the journey. I wish them all well and although it has been a privilege to care for them I am sorry we had to meet in the circumstances that we did.

Carlos M Gómez
London
June 2014

List of Authors

Kanupriya Agrawal MBBS MD DNB FRCR
Consultant Radiologist
Mid Essex Hospitals NHS Trust
Chelmsford, Essex, UK

Lena C. Andersson MD
Medical Director
Anelca Clinic for Aesthetic and Reconstructive Plastic Surgery
London, UK

Amisha V. Barochia MBBS
Staff Clinician
Laboratory of Asthma and Lung Inflammation
Cardiovascular and Pulmonary Branch/NHLBI
National Institutes of Health
Bethesda, MD, USA

Allen Bashour MD
Department of Cardiothoracic Anesthesiology
Cleveland Clinic
Cleveland, OH, USA

David Brealey BSc PhD MRCP FRCA FFICM
Consultant in Anaesthesia and Intensive Care Medicine
University College Hospital
London, UK

Borja G. Cosío MD PhD
Consultant in Respiratory Medicine
Hospital Universitario Son Espases
Palma de Mallorca, Spain

José M. Echave Sustaeta MD
Head of Department
Respiratory Medicine
Hospital Universitario Quirón
Madrid, Spain

Peter Q. Eichacker MD
Critical Care Medicine Department
National Institutes of Health
Bethesda, MD, USA

Carlos M. H. Gómez LMS FRCA MD EDICM FFICM
Consultant and Honorary Senior Lecturer in Intensive Care and Anaesthesia
St Mary's and Hammersmith Hospitals
Imperial College Healthcare NHS Trust
Clinical Director of Intensive Care
Harley Street Clinic
London, UK

Marius Gota MD
Physical Medication and Rehabilitation
Cleveland Clinic
Cleveland, OH, USA

Dr Mark J. D. Griffiths
Reader in Critical Care Medicine
National Heart and Lung Institute
Imperial College London
South Kensington Campus
London, UK

A. B. Johan Groeneveld MD PhD FCCP FCCM
Internist Intensivist
VU Medical Centre
Amsterdam, Netherlands

Sunil Grover MBBS MD FRCA.
Registrar
Department of Anaesthesia and Intensive Care
Hammersmith Hospital
London, UK

Andrew Hartle MB ChB FRCA FFICM
Consultant Intensivist and Anaesthetist
Chairman, Clinical Risk Committee
Trust Lead for Mental Capacity
Imperial College Healthcare NHS Trust
London, UK

Nicholas Hirsch FRCA FRCP
Consultant in Neuroanaesthesia and Neurocritical Care
Honorary Senior Lecturer
The National Hospital for Neurology and Neurosurgery
University College London Hospitals
London, UK

Paul Holloway PhD BM BCh FRCPath EurClinChem
Consultant Chemical Pathologist and Honorary Senior Lecturer in Metabolic Medicine Imperial College Healthcare NHS Trust
Medical School, St Mary's Hospital,
London, UK

David Howell BSc (Hons) MBBS (Hons) PhD FFICM FRCP
Divisional Clinical Director, Critical Care
University College London Hospitals
London, UK

Susan Jain BSc MBBS MRCP FRCA
Locum Consultant Anaesthetist
University College London Hospitals NHS Trust
London, UK

Annette Jepson MA MSc PhD FRCPE FRCPath
Consultant Medical Microbiologist
Imperial College Healthcare NHS Trust
London, UK

Jennifer Jones MBBS FRCP FRCA
Consultant Anaesthetist
St Mary's Hospital
Imperial College Healthcare NHS Trust
London, UK

Lesley Kay FRCP FRCPath
Consultant Haematologist and Physician
The Princess Grace Hospital
London, UK

Nicholas Lees MBChB FRCA EDIC FFICM
Consultant Anaesthetist
Royal Brompton and Harefield NHS Foundation Trust
London, UK

Richard Leonard FRCP FRCA FANZCA FCICM FFICM
Consultant and Honorary Senior Lecturer in Intensive Care and Anaesthesia
St Mary's Hospital
Imperial College Healthcare NHS Trust
London, UK

Surbi Malhotra MBBS FRCA
Consultant Anaesthetist
St Mary's Hospital
Imperial College Healthcare NHS Trust
London, UK

S. Ramani Moonesinghe BSc (Hons) MBBS MRCP FRCA FFICM
Consultant
Anaesthesia and Critical Care Medicine
University College Hospital
Honorary Senior Lecturer
Anaesthesia and Critical Care Medicine
University College London
Director
UCL/UCLH Surgical Outcomes Research Centre
London, UK

Simon Munk MBBS FRCA
Specialist Registrar
Department of Anaesthesia and Intensive Care
St Mary's Hospital
Imperial College Healthcare NHS Trust
London, UK

Michael G. Mythen MBBS MD FRCA FFICM FCAI
Smiths Medical Professor of Anaesthesia and Critical Care
University College London
Director of Research and Development
University College London Hospitals
Research Support Centre
National Clinical Lead
Department of Health
Enhanced Recovery Partnership
London, UK

Simon Nadel MBBS FRCP
Consultant and Honorary Reader in Paediatric Intensive Care
St Mary's Hospital
Imperial College Healthcare NHS Trust
London, UK

Charles Natanson MD
Senior Investigator and Head
Anaesthesia Section
The National Institute of Health Clinical Center
Bethesda, MD, USA

Hans C. Nettelblad MD
Department of Hand Surgery, Plastic Surgery and Burns
University Hospital Linköping
Linköping, Sweden

Shaikh A. Nurmohamed MD
Internist Nephrologist
VU Medical Centre
Amsterdam, Netherlands

Michael O'Connor DO MPH
Chairman, Cleveland Clinic Anesthesia Institute
Department of Cardiothoracic Anesthesia
Cleveland Clinic Foundation
Cleveland, OH, USA

Mark G. A. Palazzo MB ChB FRCA FRCP FFICM MD
Clinical Program Director – Specialist Services
Imperial College Healthcare NHS Trust
London, UK

Parind Patel MBBS FRCA DMS EDICM FFICM
Consultant in Intensive Care Medicine
Honorary Clinical Senior Lecturer
Hammersmith Hospital
Imperial College Healthcare NHS Trust
Harley Street Clinic
Bupa Cromwell Hospital
London, UK
Andrew Rhodes FICM FRCA FRCP
Consultant in Intensive Care Medicine and Anaesthesia
Department of Intensive Care Medicine
St George's Healthcare NHS Trust
London, UK

Gayathri Satkurunath FRCA MRCP
Specialist Registrar
Royal National Orthopaedic Hospital
Stanmore, UK

Peter J. Shirley FRCA FIMC RCS (ed) EDIC
Consultant in Intensive Care and Anaesthesia
Royal London Hospital
London, UK

Virinder S Sidhu MB BCh FRCP FRCA.
Consultant and Honorary Clinical Senior Lecturer in Anaesthesia and Intensive Care
Imperial College Healthcare NHS Trust
Harley Street Clinic
London, UK

Folke Sjoeberg MD
Department of Hand Surgery, Plastic Surgery and Burns
University Hospital Linköping
Linköping, Sweden

Martin Smith FRCA
Consultant in Neuroanaesthesia and Neurocritical Care
Honorary Reader in Anaesthesia and Critical Care
The National Hospital for Neurology and Neurosurgery
University College London Hospitals
London, UK

Neil Soni MB ChB FANZA MD
Consultant and Honorary Senior Lecturer in Intensive Care and Anaesthesia
Chelsea and Westminster NHS Trust
London, UK

Sarah L. Stirling MRCP FRCA
Consultant in Intensive Care & Anaesthesia
Harefield Hospital
London, UK

Richard Stümpfle MRCP FRCA EDIC FFICM
Consultant in Intensive Care and Anaesthesia
Hammersmith Hospital
Imperial Healthcare NHS Trust
London, UK

Christopher Taylor MRCP FRCA
Consultant in Neuroanaesthesia and Neurocritical Care
Honorary Senior Lecturer
The National Hospital for Neurology and Neurosurgery
University College London Hospitals
London, UK

David Treacher MA FRCP
Department of Intensive Care
St Thomas' Hospital
Guy's & St Thomas' NHS Foundation Trust
London, UK

Marc G. Vervloet MD
Internist Nephrologist
VU Medical Centre
Amsterdam, Netherlands

David J. Watson BSc (Hons) MBBS FRCA FFICM
Honorary Professor of Intensive Care Education
Homerton University Hospital NHS Foundation Trust and Barts
The London School of Medicine and Dentistry
Queen Mary University of London
London, UK

Umeer Waheed FRCA EDICM FFICM
Consultant in Intensive Care
Department of Anaesthesia and Intensive Care
Hammersmith Hospital
Imperial Healthcare NHS Trust
London, UK

Patrick A. Ward MB ChB BSc FRCA
Specialist Registrar in Anaesthetics
Imperial School of Anaesthesia, London
London, UK

Andrew R. Webb MD FRCP
VP Medicine, Fraser Health Authority
Clinical Professor, UBC Faculty of Medicine
Vancouver, Canada

Ian Webb PhD MA MRCP
Cardiac Research Registrar
Rayne Institute
St Thomas' Hospital
King's College School of Medicine
King's Health Partners
London, UK

Julia Wendon FRCP
Consultant in Liver Intensive Care
Professor of Hepatology
King's College NHS Trust
London, UK

Raha Rahman West MD
Department of Intensive Care Medicine
St George's Healthcare NHS Trust
London, UK

Harriet Wordsworth BM BCh MSc
Specialist Registrar
Oxford Radcliffe NHS Trust
Oxford, UK

Andrew R. Wright MA MBBS FRCP FRCR
Consultant Radiologist and Honorary Senior Lecturer
Imperial College Healthcare NHS Trust
London, UK

1

History of Intensive Care

Jennifer Jones

When the first World Congress of Intensive Care was held in London in June 1974, it was attended by more than 2,000 delegates from all parts of the globe and the astonished organisers had to hire extra space to accommodate them all. The success of the event illustrated the fact that, over the previous decade, the provision of care for critically ill patients in units separate from general wards had been accepted as an essential feature of hospitals throughout the world.

How did this acceptance come about and what changes have taken place since?

It had been recognised for many years that there were advantages in treating patients with the greatest need for care in one place. In the Crimean War, Florence Nightingale's insistence on keeping the sickest patients closest to the central nursing station may be regarded as an early example of the practice. Before the Second World War recovery rooms adjacent to operating theatres were introduced. 'Shock wards' were established during the war to treat the most severely injured casualties, and coronary care units after the war demonstrated that mortality from acute myocardial ischemia could be reduced by treating the victims in a single area.

Mechanical ventilation of the lungs was introduced to treat victims of poliomyelitis and tetanus. It was originally believed that negative pressure ventilation (NPV) was the 'physiological' way to ventilate the lungs, and machines were designed to enclose the patient from the neck down in a box from which air was rhythmically pumped in and out to mimic expiration and inspiration. The first electrically driven device was the 'iron lung' devised in the USA by Drinker and Shaw and introduced into clinical practice in 1928 [1]. In the USA, four large poliomyelitis units were set up to meet the country's needs for artificial respiration.

Intermittent positive pressure ventilation (IPPV) combined with tracheostomy (which is very difficult to manage in combination with a tank respirator) was introduced during the poliomyelitis epidemic in Copenhagen in 1952. Lassen, who was in charge of the hospital for infectious diseases, which lacked enough tank respirators to deal with the influx of patients, asked an anaesthetist, Ibsen, if techniques used in the operating theatre could be applied to the management of patients with respiratory failure on the wards. To begin with, positive pressure ventilation was provided manually, using a to-and-fro breathing system, by relays of medical students [2].

Later, the students were superseded by the Engstrom ventilator.

During the course of the Copenhagen epidemic, Astrup's work on blood gas analysis made it possible to assess the adequacy of alveolar ventilation and established the superiority of IPPV over NPV in this regard [3]. It also became clear that another — and perhaps the greatest — advantage of IPPV was the ease of access to the patient that it offered to nursing staff. Lassen's account of the epidemic stresses the need for humidification of inspired gas in preventing encrustation of respiratory secretions in a patient with a trachcostomy and physiotherapy in airway management, although both were improved in later years.

The importance of the poliomyelitis epidemic in Copenhagen in the development of intensive care was, therefore, profound. It not only demonstrated the superiority of IPPV over NPV in respiratory support, but introduced the concept of a multidisciplinary approach to the management of very sick patients and involved anaesthetists in the provision of their care. Some intensive care specialists today might not consider the latter an advantage.

The introduction of the Salk vaccine in 1955, which consists of injected inactivated poliomyelitis virus, and of the oral Sabin vaccine in 1957, which uses an attenuated live virus, has eradicated poliomyelitis from most countries in the world [4]. However, the demand for respiratory support continued to increase, driven by the needs of patients with tetanus and chest injuries and, perhaps most importantly, by the proliferation of cardiac surgery. As mechanical ventilators were increasingly used to support patients with acute pulmonary disease, their design became more sophisticated and more subtle modes of IPPV were introduced (see Chapters 7 and 8).

Awareness of the dangers of IPPV grew at the same time. The introduction of positive end-expiratory pressure (PEEP) to improve arterial oxygenation rapidly showed that excessive intrathoracic pressures could be associated with barotrauma in the shape of pneumothorax or mediastinal emphysema or with a reduction in cardiac output, which could be overcome by expanding the circulating volume to improve venous return [5]. Methods of assessing 'best PEEP' for optimising oxygen delivery to the tissues were explored [6].

More recently, it has been recognised that over-distension of the alveoli during IPPV with excessive tidal volumes may result in pulmonary damage, and lower than traditional tidal volumes have gained acceptance [7]. Ventilator-associated pneumonia is a common nosocomial infection which has been shown to be associated with prolonged intensive care stay and a marked increase in mortality [8].

The intensive care units set up in the 1960s and 1970s were, for the most part, small. A report from the British Medical Association [9], which confined itself to recommendations, envisaged that only 1% of acute hospital beds would need to be set aside for intensive care, although it clearly saw that such beds would need huge amounts of space, staff and services. Most of these intensive care units were run by anaesthetists, the majority of whom regarded intensive care as a hobby in addition to their sessions in the operating theatre and almost all of whom learned on the job. There was no recognition of intensive care as a specialty, no supervised training programmes and no literature.

One of the most important sequels to the first World Congress of Intensive Care is that these points have been addressed. Intensive care is now recognised internationally as a specialty, training programmes are ubiquitous and there are a huge number of journals of critical care. Standards for space and facilities exist at national and international levels. The question of whether intensive care units should be 'open' or 'closed' has been settled in favour of the trained specialist intensivist, who is today running a much larger unit than those of the 20th century.

Intensive care is expensive. No one — least of all the paymasters — wants to see it profligately dispensed to patients who cannot benefit. Numerous scoring systems have been devised to assess the severity of a patient's illness (of which Knaus' Acute Physiology and Chronic Health Evaluation II (APACHE II) [10], is perhaps the most widely used) but, so far, none of them can be used to predict outcome in an individual case. The incorporation of APACHE II into the Intensive Care National Audit and Research Centre (ICNARC) system of audit in the UK [11] has made it possible to assess the performance of individual intensive care units, and has provided a useful monitor of standards of care.

At the turn of the 20th and 21st centuries, a new approach to the management of sick patients, which has come to be known as outreach, was taken in Australia. In certain hospitals the cardiac arrest team was replaced by a medical emergency team of intensive care doctors and nurses who could be summoned by ward staff to attend patients who showed marked physiological abnormalities which might lead to a cardiac arrest [12]. When a paper published in the UK suggested that the care provided for sick patients in general wards was often inadequate [13], a similar concept, with modified call-out criteria, was introduced with support from the Department of Health and guidance from the Intensive Care Society [14]. Outreach schemes are based on the premise that early intervention in the development of critical illness can improve outcome. By nipping such illnesses in the bud, it might also obviate the need for a number of admissions to the intensive care unit. Outreach might, it was hoped, save lives and perhaps even money. The evidence collected so far is disappointing: outreach has not as yet fulfilled its promises of improved outcome or reduced costs [15].

In terms of organisation, then, the history of intensive care may be seen as one of steady progress and growing professionalism. Clinical progress is also evident in the development of respiratory support and in the understanding and management of the acute respiratory distress syndrome (ARDS) first described in 1967 [16]. With the introduction of haemofiltration, early recourse to renal replacement therapy in acute renal failure (ARF) has supplanted the practice of squeezing a urine output from failing kidneys with diuretics and dopamine infusions.

It is also possible to trace 'fashions' in the waxing and waning popularity of various treatment methods. To give an example, in the 1970s many intensivists believed that human albumin was the solution of choice in fluid resuscitation, and that furthermore, it was important to maintain a patient's serum albumin within the normal range as far as possible. A number of small comparative studies in North America, however, suggested that albumin conferred no advantage over (the much cheaper) Hartman's solution [17]. It was further demonstrated in a randomised prospective study of patients in an intensive care unit that outcomes were similar whether gelatine or albumin solution were employed. A meta-analysis of the small North American studies was interpreted as showing that patients were more likely to die if they received albumin during resuscitation, which discouraged many intensivists from using it at all [18].

The controversy seems to have been settled by a large randomised trial of albumin and balanced salt solution, which found that, for most patients, the use of albumin offers neither benefit nor harm [19].

Red blood cell transfusion has become less fashionable. Since the demonstration that oxygen delivery to the tissues in acute normovolaemic anaemia was optimal at haemoglobin (Hb) concentrations of 10 g/dl [20], most intensive care patients were transferred to maintain their Hb concentrations at this level. Since a large randomised Canadian study demonstrated that intensive care patients transfused to a Hb level of 8 g/dl enjoyed an outcome at least as good as those transfused to a level of 10 g/dl [21], most intensive care specialists have pursued a more conservative transfusion policy.

The pulmonary artery catheter has also been a bone of contention. Introduced in 1970 by Swan and Ganz [22], its use became widespread after Shoemaker advocated the goal of 'supra-normal' oxygen delivery in intensive care patients as a means of improving their chances of survival [23]. Enthusiasm for such 'goal-directed' therapy was tempered after studies showed that in the acutely critically ill, seeking to raise oxygen delivery beyond normal limits was not helpful [24]. 'Optimisation' of oxygen delivery, however, does seem to be of benefit in patients undergoing high-risk elective surgery [25].

The use of pulmonary artery catheters was further discouraged when a non-randomised cohort study suggested that their use was associated with increased patient mortality and length (and cost) of hospital stay [26]. An editorial published in the same journal demanded a moratorium on the use of pulmonary artery catheters and a prospective multicentre trial [27]. Further studies have yielded conflicting results [28] and, whilst pulmonary artery catheters continue to be employed in intensive care units, less invasive methods of assessing cardiac output have become more popular.

Intravenous feeding is another example of a treatment that has been over-enthusiastically pursued, then denounced and finally reinstated with caution. There is good reason to believe that patients in intensive care units should be fed within 24 hours of admission (see Chapter 9), but enteral feeding is simpler and cheaper than intravenous, and may be associated with fewer infective complications. Parenteral feeding is now something to fall back on if attempts to establish enteral feeding fail.

Clinical practice in intensive care has, then, not been without controversy. It is encouraging that, as large randomised trials have been published, intensive care has gradually become based more upon evidence than conjecture.

The history of intensive care may be regarded as a story of the successful developments of a new and challenging medical specialty. In a recent critical review [29] Soni complained that its *raison d'être* of providing support for failing organs has led the specialty to focus on syndromes — such as ARDS and ARF — and give them 'real disease status', regardless of the disparity of their causes. He argues that more attention should be paid to the causes of organ failure and suggests that it might be beneficial if the abbreviations and acronyms of intensive care — ARDS, sepsis, systemic inflammatory response syndrome (SIRS), amongst others — were 'relegated to history'. Whatever happens, the future of intensive care will bring change.

References

[1] Drinker, P. and Shaw, L.A. (1929). An apparatus for the prolonged administration of artificial respiration I. A design for adults and children, *J Clin Invest*, **7**, 229–247.

[2] Lassen, H.C.A. (1953). A preliminary report on the 1952 epidemic of poliomyelitis in Copenhagen, with special reference to the treatment of acute respiratory insufficiency, *Lancet*, **1**, 37–40.

[3] Astrup, P., Gotzche, H. and Neulukirch, F. (1954). Laboratory investigations during treatment of patients with poliomyelitis and respiratory paralysis, *BMJ*, **4865**, 780–785.

[4] Aylward, R.B. (2006). Eradicating polio; today's challenges and tomorrow's legacy, *Ann Trop Med Parasitol*, **100**, 401–413.

[5] Sykes, M.K., Adams, A.P., Finley, W.E.I. *et al.* (1970). The effects of variations in end-expiratory inflation pressure on cardiorespiratory function in normo-, hypo- and hypervolemic dogs, *Brit J Anaesth*, **42**, 669–677.

[6] Suter, P.M., Fairley, H.B. and Isenbery, M.D. (1975). Optimum end-expiratory airways pressure in patients with acute pulmonary failure, *N Engl J Med*, **292**, 284–289

[7] The Acute Respiratory Distress Syndrome Network (2000). Ventilation with lower tidal volumes as compared with traditional volumes for acute lung injury and the acute respiratory distress syndrome, *N Engl J Med*, **342**, 1301–1308

[8] Safdav, N., Desfulian, C., Collard, H.R. *et al.* (2005). Clinical and economic consequences of ventilator — associated pneumonia, a systematic review, *Crit Care Med*, **33**, 2184–2193.

[9] British Medical Association (1967). *Intensive care, BMA Planning UNIT Report No1*, British Medical Association, London.

[10] Knaus, W.A., Draper, E.A., Wagner, D.P. *et al.* (1985). APACHE II; a severity of disease classifications system, *Crit Care Med*, **13**, 818–829.

[11] Rowan, K.M., Kerr, J.H., Major, E. *et al.* (1993). Intensive Care Society's APACHE II study in Britain and Ireland — II: Outcome comparisons of intensive care units after adjustments for case mix by the American APACHE II method, *BMJ*, **307**, 977–981.

[12] Lee, A., Bishop, G., Hillman, K.M. *et al.* (1995). The medical emergency team, *Anaesth Intens Care*, **23**, 183–186.

[13] McQuillan, P., Pilkington, S., Allan, A. *et al.* (1998). Confidential inquiry into quality of care before admission to intensive care, *BMJ*, **316**, 1853–1858.

[14] The Intensive Care Society (2002). *Guidelines for the Introduction of Outreach Services*, The Intensive Care Society, London.

[15] Fletcher, S.J. and Cuthbertsen, B.H. (2010). Outreach, epistemology and the evolution of critical care, *Anaesthesia*, **65**, 115–118.

[16] Ashbaugh, D.G., Bigelow, D.B., Petty, T.L. *et al.* (1967). Acute respiratory distress in adults, *Lancet*, **2**, 319–323.

[17] Cochrane Injuries Group Albumin Reviewers (1998). Human albumin administration in critically ill patients; systematic review of randomised clinical trials, *BMJ*, **317**, 235–240.

[18] Stockwell, M., Soni, N. and Riley, B. (1992). Colloid solutions in the critically ill. A randomized comparison of albumin and polygeline 1. Outcome and duration of stay in the intensive care unit, *Anaesthesia*, **47**, 3–6.

[19] The SAFE Study Investigators (2004). A comparison of albumin and saline for fluid resuscitation in the intensive care unit, *N Engl J Med*, **350**, 2247–2256.

[20] Mesmer, K., Lewis, D.H., Sunder-Plassman, L. *et al.* (1972). Acute normovolemic hemodilution, *Europ Surg Res*, **4**, 55–70.

[21] Hébert, P.C., Wells, G., Blajchman, M.A. *et al.* (1999). A multicenter, randomized, controlled clinical trial of transfusion requirements in critical care, *N Engl J Med*, **340**, 409–417.

[22] Swan, H.J., Ganz, W., Forrester, J. *et al.* (1970). Catheterization of the heart in man with use of a flow-directed balloon-tipped catheter, *N Engl J Med*, **283**, 447–451.

[23] Shoemaker, W.C., Appel, P.L., Kram, H.B. *et al.* (1988). Prospective trial of supranormal values of survivors as therapeutic goals in high-risk surgical patients, *Chest*, **94**, 1176–1186.

[24] Hayes, M.A., Tinemins, A.C., Yau, E.H. *et al.* (1994). Elevation of systemic oxygen delivery in the treatment of critically ill patients, *N Engl J Med*, **330**, 1717–1722.

[25] Boyd, O., Grounds, R.M. and Bennett, E.D. (1993). A randomized clinical trial of the effect of deliberate peri operative increase of oxygen delivery on mortality in high — risk surgical patients, *JAMA*, **270**, 2699–2707.

[26] Connors Jr, A.F., Speroff, D., Dawson, N.V. *et al.* (1996). The effectiveness of right heart catheterization in the initial care of critically ill patients, *JAMA*, **276**, 889–897.

[27] Dalen, J.F. and Bobe, R.C. (1996). Is it time to pull the pulmonary artery catheter? *JAMA*, **276**, 916–918.

[28] Harvey, S., Young, D., Brampton, W. *et al.* (2006). Pulmonary artery catheters for adult patients in intensive care, *Cochrane Database Syst Rev*, C0003408.

[29] Soni, N. (2010). ARDS, acronyms and the Pinocchio effect, *Anaesthesia*, **65**, 976–979.

2

Cardiovascular Physiology

Ian Webb and David Treacher

2.1 Introduction

The central role of the heart within circulation has long been understood. Galen (129–200 AD) first implicated the heart in setting blood in motion but did not understand the concept of the circulation. Servetus (1511–1553) later described the right and left heart circulations (and paid for his ideas with his life) and, together with contemporaneous dissections by the Paduan anatomist Vesalius (1514–1564), provided highly detailed anatomical information on the entire cardiovascular system. In 1628 William Harvey (1578–1657) published *De Motu Cordis*, his treatise on the mammalian circulation which demonstrated that the blood circulated around the body and which is now acknowledged to be the basis of modern cardiovascular physiology [1].

The normal adult heart (weight 250–400 g) may be considered as two pumps in series. The right heart pumps blood through the pulmonary circulation, returning de-oxygenated venous blood to the lungs, whilst the left heart receives oxygenated blood for systemic arterial distribution via the systemic circulation. Flow within the heart is pulsatile and unidirectional, with retrograde flow being prevented by the atrioventricular and semilunar valves. The systemic or left ventricle is approximately three times larger than the right ventricle and semi-conical in shape. Inner and outer longitudinal muscle fibre layers are interspersed with central circumferential fibres contributing to the torsion effect during systolic contraction. There is little shortening of the base-to-apex axis. The right ventricle wraps itself around the left ventricle forming an elliptical cavity.

Systolic contraction involves free-wall shortening with downward displacement of the tricuspid valve and lateral compression of the chamber. The atria act mainly as passive conduits for blood passing to the ventricles, although they do contribute to active diastolic filling in sinus rhythm and this contribution is particularly relevant in certain pathological states.

Except at the insertion and exit sites of the great vessels, the heart is entirely encompassed within the fibrous pericardium. The inner visceral and outer parietal layers of this are separated by a thin layer of fluid (10–15 ml) which serves to reduce friction during cardiac motion. The left and the right coronary arteries take their origin from the sinuses of Valsalva just above the aortic valve leaflets and course over the epicardial surface of the ventricles beneath the visceral pericardium towards the apex of the heart, giving off myocardial branches that penetrate through the myocardium to the endocardium.

The rhythmical contraction of the heart is dictated and modified by the intrinsic pacemaker network within the heart. This specialised system of conducting cells propagates autonomous electrical impulses, normally initiated within the sino-atrial node (SAN) of the right atrium and passed sequentially to the atria and ventricles via the atrioventricular node (AVN), the bundle of His and Purkinje fibre network. Normally the greater excitability and therefore the higher depolarisation frequency of the SAN dominates the hierarchy of automaticity within the cardiac myocytes, although occasionally alternative sites may dominate as a primary pathology or provide life-saving escape rhythms in the event of higher conduction block.

2.2 The Cardiac Cycle

The cardiac cycle consists of a highly coordinated sequence of electrical and mechanical events that result in a controlled cardiac contraction with anterograde flow of blood during systole followed by cardiac relaxation and filling during diastole.

All cardiac cells exhibit a negative resting membrane potential (−90 to −60 mV) determined by a combination of active and passive ion exchange processes. With the exception of SAN cells, this potential is largely stable and determined principally by the membrane conductance to potassium. Signal propagation and electromechanical coupling both depend upon cell depolarisation, and this is triggered once the resting membrane potential achieves a certain threshold. In the case of the cardiac myocytes this stimulation is from adjacent cell depolarisation, whilst in SAN pacemaker cells it is determined by the rate of spontaneous diastolic depolarisation, mediated primarily by the Na^+–K^+ dual inward current (I_f current).

The resulting action potential, recorded at the cellular level, is divided into five phases (Fig. 2.1) according to ion currents and membrane potential. Two principal types of action potential (AP) exist: (i) the

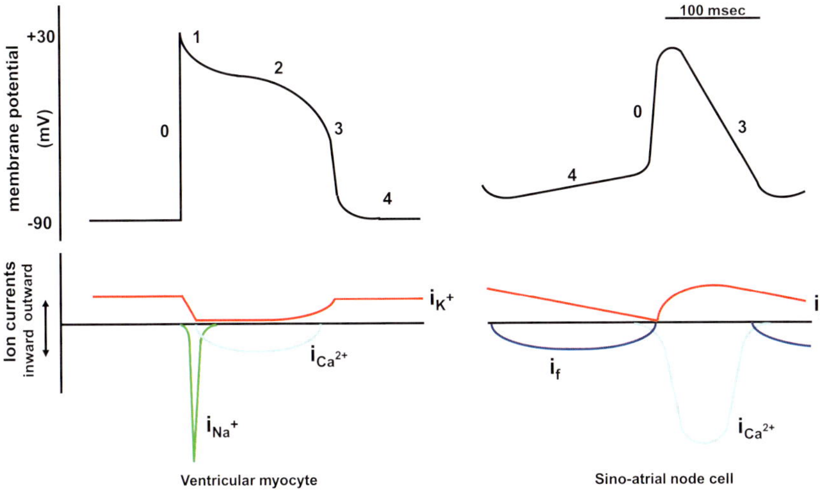

(A) (B)

Figure 2.1. Rapid (A) and slow (B) cardiac action potential profiles with associated major ion currents. (A) Depolarisation in ventricular myocytes (Phase 0) is rapid and mediated by fast I_{Na} currents. This is followed by a prompt but limited repolarisation (Phase 1) as a result of a transient outward K^+ current. The plateau phase (Phase 2) is determined by the balance of $I_{Ca}{}^{2+}$ and $I_K{}^+$. Eventually, this balance falls in favour of outward K^+ conductance as $I_{Ca}{}^{2+}$ diminishes and the cell begins to repolarise (Phase 3). Resting diastolic membrane potential (Phase 4) is determined principally by K^+ conductance. (B) In the SAN cell, the resting membrane potential (Phase 4) is less negative and there is a slow autonomous depolarisation determined principally by the I_f (Na^+–K^+ dual inward) current. When threshold is eventually reached, depolarisation proceeds (Phase 0) with a comparatively slower upstroke and peak amplitude, mediated by $I_{Ca}{}^{2+}$. Repolarisation is dependent upon the balance of diminishing calcium conductance and outward repolarising $I_K{}^+$ current (Phase 3). I_f is re-activated by hyperpolarisation and begins the cycle again.

fast-response AP is seen in atrial and ventricular myocytes and the specialised Purkinje fibres (Fig. 2.1A). This rapid depolarisation is mediated by fast Na^+ channels and the cell regains normal excitability (post-refractory phase) as soon as fully repolarised; (ii) the slow-response AP recorded from SAN and AVN conducting cells generally has a less-negative resting potential and an action potential with slower upstroke and peak amplitude. This is mediated predominantly by Ca^{2+} channels and cells remain in a refractory state for longer. The familiar P-QRS-T complexes of the electrocardiogram represent an amalgamation of all cardiac signals recorded at the body surface and chart the progressive depolarisation–repolarisation sequence of the cardiac cycle [2]. The P-wave and QRS complexes correspond to atrial and ventricular depolarisation respectively while the T-wave represents ventricular repolarisation. Ventricular potentials dominate the surface signal due to the larger currents generated by their greater muscle mass. Consequently the atrial repolarisation signal is hidden within the QRS complex during normal conduction (Fig. 2.2).

Myocardial contraction results from electrical stimulation of myocardial fibres in the presence of competent electromechanical coupling. The atria and ventricles both exhibit systolic and diastolic phases:

- During atrial diastole blood flows passively through to the ventricles (early rapid filling phase), which accounts for the majority of ventricular filling.
- Atrial systole, which occurs only in sinus rhythm, contributes up to 15% ventricular filling (late filling phase), but this varies with venous return, atrial compliance, atrioventricular valve integrity and heart rate. It accounts for the 'a'-wave seen in the jugular venous pressure.
- Ventricular systole is divided into three phases (Fig. 2.3):

  (i) *Isovolumic contraction* is defined by the period of earliest rise in ventricular pressure after atrial systole to the point of opening of the semilunar valve: ventricular volume is constant during this period.

  (ii) *Rapid ejection* begins with the opening of the semilunar valves when intraventricular pressure exceeds aortic/pulmonary pressures. There is a quick upstroke to both ventricular and arterial pressures, coincident with greater aortic blood flow and reduced ventricular volume. This contrasts with

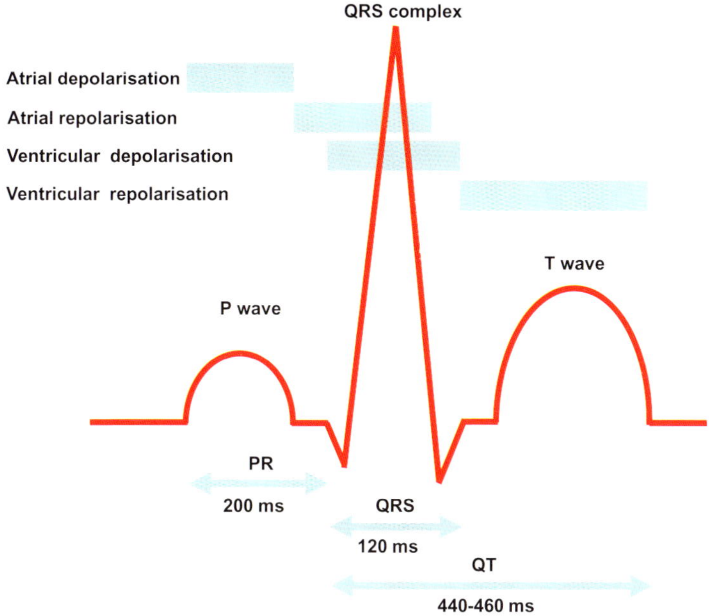

Figure 2.2. The electrocardiogram. This is a surface amalgamation of all cardiac potentials within the heart. The P, QRS and T-wave components of each cycle represent specific depolarisation–repolarisation sequences within the different chambers of the heart. Changes in amplitude, axis and duration of any one of these may reflect normal variation (e.g. lead–lead differences) or alternatively indicate intrinsic myocardial disease (e.g. ischaemia) or extrinsic systemic abnormalities (e.g. hyperkalaemia).

(iii) *Reduced ejection* phase, during which time ventricular stroke volume diminishes and aortic flow tails off rapidly as blood is distributed to the periphery.

- Ventricular diastole is also divided into three phases (Fig. 2.3):

  (i) *Isovolumic relaxation* begins with closure of the semilunar valves when ventricular pressure falls below that of the distal arterial pressure and ends with the opening of the atrioventricular valves. The volume of blood within the ventricle is again constant during this period.

  (ii) *Rapid filling* occurs when the atrial pressure exceeds the ventricular pressure as a result of venous return (preload effect), but the elastic recoil of the relaxing ventricle may also contribute (afterload effect).

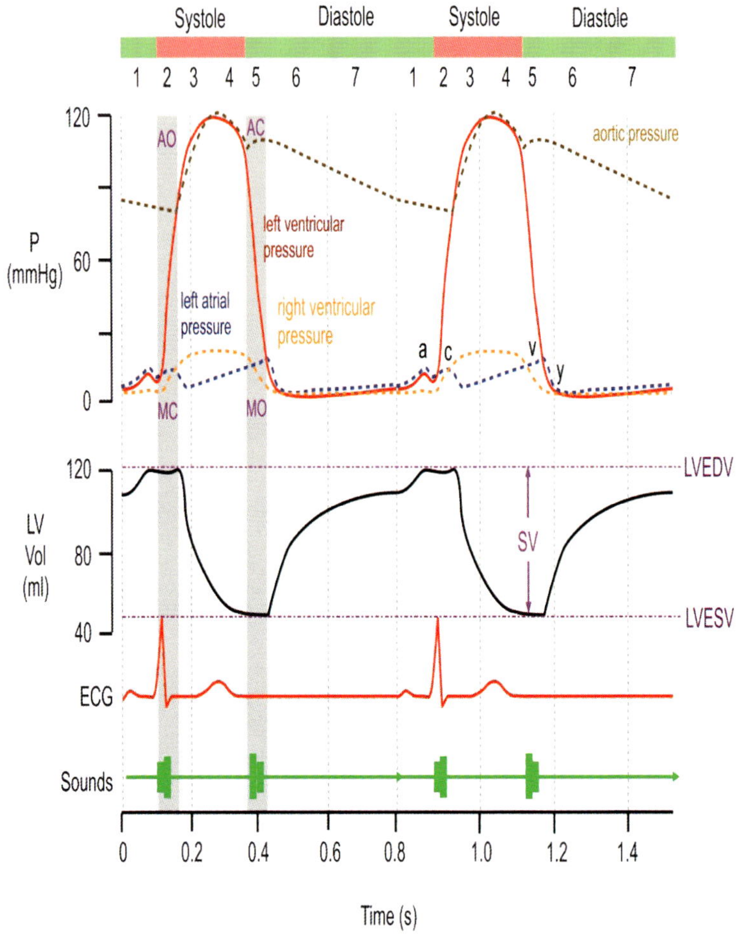

Figure 2.3. The cardiac cycle. Active filling (1) in sinus rhythm gives rise to the a-wave in both left and right atrial waveforms. Isovolumic ventricular contraction (2) occurs between closure of the mitral valve (MC) and opening of the aortic valve (AO). Blood is then expelled into the systemic circulation during the rapid (3) and reduced (4) ejection phases. Right ventricular and pulmonary pressures are normally less than a quarter that of the systemic circulation. The stroke volume (SV) is the amount of blood ejected from the ventricle during one cardiac cycle. Expressed as a percentage of the end-diastolic volume (EF = left ventricular end-diastolic volume (LVEDV)-left ventricular end-systolic volume (LVESV)/LVEDV), this gives the ejection fraction. The aortic valve closes once the mean systemic pressure exceeds the intraventricular pressure (AC). This coincides with the isovolumic relaxation phase of ventricular diastole (5). A dicrotic notch is usually seen in the pressure waveform in the aorta and proximal large arteries as a result of arterial elastance

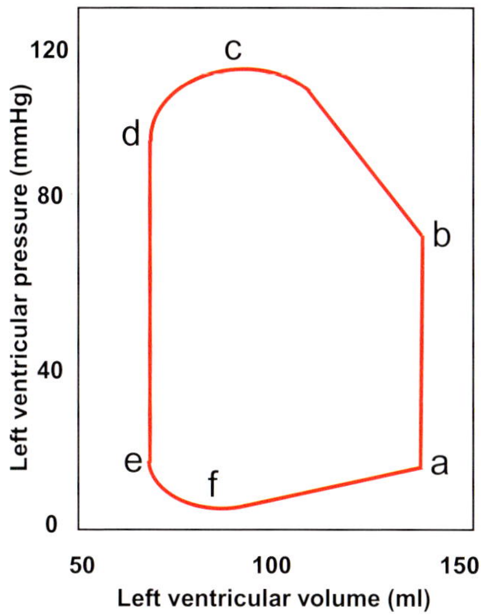

Figure 2.4. Normal pressure–volume (P–V) relationship of the left ventricle. Systole begins with isovolumic contraction (a–b), which rapidly increases intraventricular pressure until it exceeds aortic pressure and opens the aortic valve (b). Blood is ejected from the ventricle into the aorta during the rapid (b–c) and reduced (c–d) ejection phases. Diastole begins with closure of the aortic valve (d) and onset of isovolumic relaxation (d–e). The mitral valve opens (e) once the left atrial pressure exceeds left ventricular pressure and the ventricle fills during the rapid (e–f) and reduced (f–a) filling phases.

(iii) *Reduced filling (diastasis)* follows up to the point of atrial systole and describes the slower period of ventricular filling coincident with a more gradual elevation of atrial, ventricular and venous pressures.

The haemodynamic changes of the ventricle may alternatively be considered as a time-independent pressure–volume (P–V) relation (Fig. 2.4). The contour of the P–V loop is dependent not only on the anatomical and

---

Figure 2.3. (*Continued*) and recoil. This phenomenon serves to maintain blood pressure and flow in the peripheries for as long as possible into the (pulsatile) cardiac cycle, but also ameliorates the afterload resistance against which the ventricle has to contract. The mitral valve opens (MO) once the left atrial pressure exceeds the ventricular pressure. Diastolic filling is predominantly passive during the rapid (6) and reduced (7) filling phases. a-wave = atrial systole; c-wave = closure of the mitral valve; c–v wave corresponds to ventricular contraction; y-descent corresponds to early rapid ventricular filling.

functional integrity of the heart but also on changes in preload and afterload, which are discussed in more detail in the following section.

2.3 Ventricular Performance and the Determinants of Cardiac Output

The principal function of the heart is to generate the work necessary to provide a cardiac output and blood pressure that both perfuses the lungs to re-oxygenate the venous blood and propels the oxygenated arterial blood through the systemic circulation so that the fluctuating metabolic requirements of all the organs are met at rest and during exercise. Maintenance of oxygen delivery (the product of cardiac output and the arterial oxygen content) that meets the oxygen requirements of the tissues (global oxygen consumption) is crucial for survival since there is no storage system for oxygen within the body. Typically oxygen consumption for a normal 75 kg person in an office environment would be 200 ml/min and their systemic oxygen delivery would be around 950 ml/min resulting in an oxygen extraction ratio (OER) of just over 20%. Most tissues can increase their OER three-fold which meets any increase in oxygen demand in the short term and thus allows aerobic metabolism to continue, pending an increase in oxygen delivery [3].

Ventricular function may be defined in terms of the preload, the afterload and the resulting flow or cardiac output which is determined by the ventricular contractility. This requires the measurement of six variables: the right and left atrial pressures (RAP, LAP: the preload), the mean systemic and pulmonary arterial pressures (MAP, PAP: the afterload) and the stroke volume and heart rate [4].

2.3.1 *Ventricular preload*

The predominant determinant of preload is the venous return, which is dependent on the intravascular volume, and the venous 'tone', which is influenced by the sympathetic nervous system, circulating catecholamines and local factors, particularly pH, lactate and nitric oxide. Although traditionally assessed as the *pressure* preload of the ventricles (right and left atrial pressures), when applying the Frank–Starling law of the heart, one should consider the *volume* preload since in a three-dimensional setting this relates more closely to the myocardial end-diastolic fibre length [5].

On the general ward, the RAP or jugular venous pressure (JVP) or the central venous pressure (CVP) is measured from the sternal angle but, in critical care, vascular pressures are measured from the mid-axillary line in the fifth intercostal space. From this reference point, with the patient in the semi-supine position, the normal RAP is between +4 and +8 mmHg and the LAP, or pulmonary artery occlusion or 'wedge' pressure is between +8 and +12 mmHg. Relative changes in either the contractility of the two ventricles or the respective vascular resistances will change the relationship between the atrial pressures, which must then be independently assessed. Normal values for pulmonary artery and systemic pressures would be 20/12 (mean 15 mmHg) and 120/75 (mean 90 mmHg).

The systemic venous bed is the major intravascular capacitance or reservoir of the circulation with a compliance that can vary from 30 to over 300 ml/mmHg and which provides the main buffer against the effects of intravascular volume loss. It also explains the response observed in major haemorrhage and subsequent transfusion. Figure 2.5 shows the different lines of constant venous 'tone' or compliance (isophlebs) relating venous pressure to the volume of the systemic venous capacity bed: as

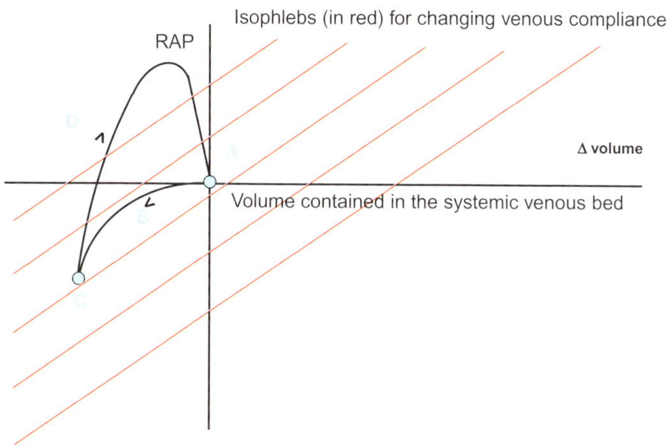

Figure 2.5. Relationship between RAP and the volume contained by the systemic venous capacity bed.

volume is lost, venous tone increases preventing the large falls in atrial filling pressures and cardiac output that would otherwise occur (A→B→C). If the equivalent volume is returned over the subsequent few hours, the RAP gradually returns to normal as the intravascular volume is restored and the reflex increase in sympathetic tone abates (C→B→A). However, rapid re-infusion of the same volume will not allow sufficient time for the venous and arteriolar tone to fall and in certain patients may result in the RAP rising to a level that precipitates pulmonary oedema (C→D) although the intravascular volume has only been returned to the pre-haemorrhage level [6].

The intrathoracic blood volume or the left ventricular volume preload can be assessed using the Valsalva manoeuvre. This involves taking a maximum inspiration and then attempting to exhale against a closed glottis or an external pressure of at least 30 mmHg thereby increasing the intrathoracic pressure. Figure 2.6 shows the classic Valsalva responses in a normal subject and a patient with a high intrathoracic blood volume [7]. If a 'normal' type trace is observed on the monitor, further volume is indicated, whereas a 'square wave' response (Fig. 2.7) indicates a high left

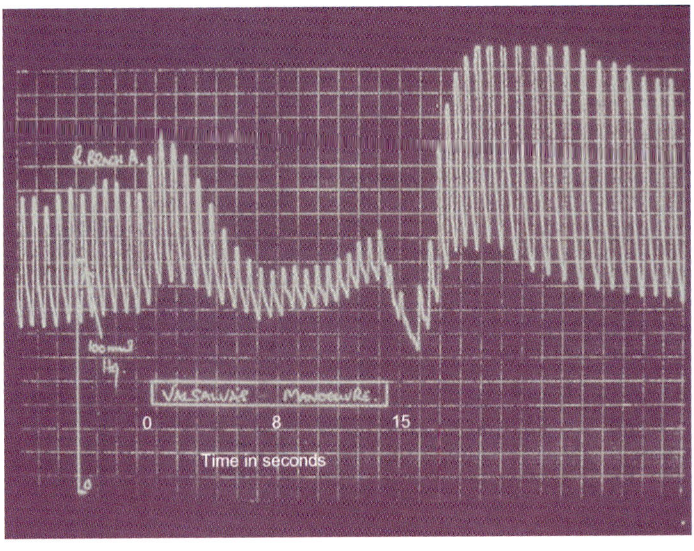

Figure 2.6. Valsalva in normal subject or patient with normal to low LV volume preload.

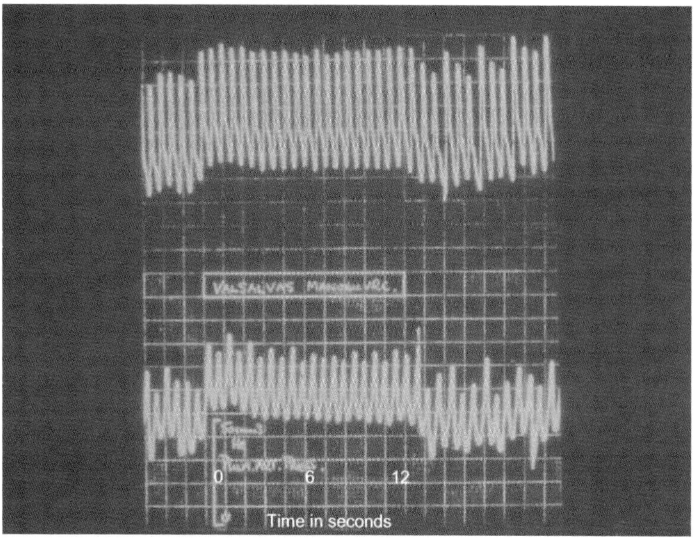

Figure 2.7. Square wave Valsalva in patient with high LV end-diastolic volume.

ventricular volume preload. This response can be quantified by calculating the ratio of the pulse pressure during Phase 2 of the manoeuvre to the baseline value. This correlates with measurements of pulmonary artery 'wedge' pressure and can be applied at the bedside in ventilated patients.

If the preload is low and either blood pressure or cardiac output is inadequate, the priority is volume loading to restore intravascular volume and venous return.

Raised preload pressures reflect either (i) increased intravascular volume, (ii) impaired myocardial contractility or (iii) increased afterload pressures which includes raised intrathoracic or pericardial pressures.

Preload may be reduced by either:

(i) Removing volume from the circulation (diuretics, venesection, haemofiltration).
(ii) Increasing the capacity of the vascular bed with venodilator therapy (glyceryl trinitrate, morphine).
(iii) Increasing contractility.
(iv) Reducing afterload.

When interpreting atrial pressures as measures of preload, two points must be remembered:

- The heart lies within the thoracic cavity and therefore operates as 'a pump within a pump'. Consequently, intravascular pressure (P_v) measurements are misleading if the intrathoracic pressure (P_{it}) is raised, since the true distending pressure that determines ventricular end-diastolic volume is the transmural pressure (P_v–P_{it}) [8]. This is particularly relevant when there is significant alveolar gas trapping as in asthma, with positive-pressure ventilation when high positive end-expiratory pressure levels or an inverse inspiratory to expiratory time ratio are used or when there is a significant intrapleural fluid collection or a raised intra-abdominal pressure.
- Although in the healthy heart there is a fairly linear relationship between atrial pressures and ventricular end-diastolic pressure and volume, in disease states when the ventricle is dilated and poorly compliant, the end-diastolic pressure–volume relationship is not necessarily linear and pressure will no longer reflect the volume preload.

2.3.2 *Ventricular afterload*

The ventricular afterload is the arterial pressure against which each ventricle has to eject the stroke volume during each systole and the major determinant of the arterial pressure is the vascular resistance or 'tone' in each arteriolar 'bed'. Circulatory management requires a clear understanding of this relationship between pressure, flow and resistance. The vascular resistance is traditionally calculated, by analogy with Ohm's law of electrical currents, as the pressure gradient across the vascular bed divided by the cardiac output (Table 2.1, Equation 1). Pressure gradients in cardiovascular physiology may refer to differences within a single arterial conduit [proximal pressure (P_{prox}) — distal pressure (P_{dist})], across a heart valve [e.g. left ventricular pressure (P_{LV}) — pressure in the aorta (P_{aorta})] or across an entire vascular bed [arterial pressure (P_a) — venous pressure (P_v)].

Flow and velocity are distinct but linearly-related entities (Table 2.1, Equation 2). Intraluminal diameter dramatically affects flow and is inversely proportional to resistance. This is a key feature of tissue

Table 2.1. Haemodynamic equations.

Equation 1	Ohm's law	$V = iR$	V = voltage (pressure gradient) i = current (flow) R = resistance
Hence, systemic vascular resistance = (MAP – RAP)/Qt			MAP = mean systemic arterial pressure, RAP = Right arterial pressure Qt = cardiac output or flow
Equation 2		$Q = VA$	Q = blood flow V = blood velocity A = intraluminal area
Equation 3	Poiseille's law	$Q = \frac{\pi(P_i - P_o)r^4}{8\eta l}$	Q = blood flow l = artery length [from (i) inflow to (o) outflow] $(P_i - P_o)$ = pressure gradient along artery r = artery radius $\pi/8$ = constant of proportionality η = blood viscosity
Equation 4	LVSW = SV × (MAP – LVEDP) × 0.0136 g RVSW = SV × (PAP – RVEDP) × 0.0136 g		VSW = ventricular stroke work SV = stroke volume MAP = mean systemic arterial pressure PAP = mean pulmonary artery pressure EDP = end diastolic pressure or preload
Equation 5	Reynold's number	$Re = VD\rho/\eta$	V = velocity D = diameter ρ = blood density η = blood viscosity
Equation 6	LaPlace's law	$T = \frac{Pr}{W}$	T = wall tension P = transmural pressure r = artery radius W = arterial wall thickness

autoregulation, in which organs are protected (acutely or chronically) against changes in perfusion pressure through a modulation in resistance vessel diameter. A more detailed relationship between pressure and flow within an artery is given by Poiseuille's law (Table 2.1, Equation 3), although this incorrectly assumes laminar flow of a Newtonian fluid (e.g. water) along straight indistensible blood vessels.

If ventricular work is constant, an increase in vascular resistances produce higher pressures but with a lower cardiac output. A systemic dilator such as sodium nitroprusside will reduce systemic resistance and blood pressure and increase cardiac output. Although such manipulation is attractive in increasing cardiac output for the same cardiac work, it is important to maintain a blood pressure that ensures appropriate distribution of blood flow and a diastolic pressure sufficient to maintain coronary artery perfusion, particularly in patients with known ischaemic heart disease or pre-existing hypertension.

2.3.3 *Venticular contractility and stroke work*

The work that the ventricle performs for a given preload defines contractility. The efficiency of each ventricle is the external, 'useful', work generated expressed as a percentage of the total work performed and typically for the normal left ventricle this is, somewhat surprisingly, rather low at around 25–30%. Most of the work performed is dissipated as heat is lost into the cardiac veins, mainly the coronary sinus, and from the epicardial surface of the heart into the mediastinum. The external work performed by each ventricle with each heart beat is the stroke work (LVSW/RVSW) and this represents the energy required to propel in a pulsatile fashion a volume of blood into the systemic/pulmonary circulations which at the given heart rate generates an adequate flow (cardiac output) and arterial pressure to perfuse all the organs according to their metabolic needs.

Assuming that the circulation operates as a linear, constant flow, fixed compliance system, the 'useful' external work of the left and right ventricles may be calculated for each heart beat as the product of the stroke volume (SV) and the pressure increase from end-diastole to end-systole (Table 2.1, Equation 4). This ventricular stroke work is determined by

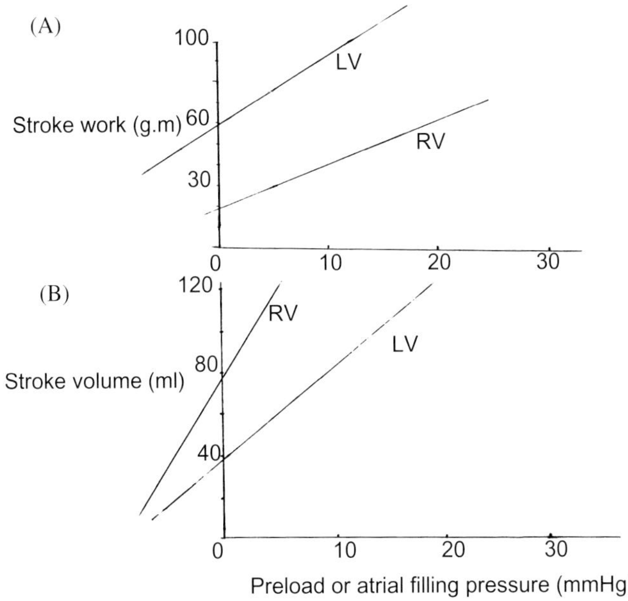

Figure 2.8. Graphs of (A) stroke work (B) stroke volume against preload/atrial filling pressure.

the myocardial contractility and the preload or 'stretch' of each ventricle at end diastole according to the Frank–Starling law of the heart [5]. The relationship between the stroke work and stroke volume and ventricular preload or atrial filling/ventricular end-diastolic pressure is shown in Fig. 2.8 [5].

However, in reality the additional energy needed to generate pulsatile flow should be included; this pulsatile energy is 'stored' by the elastic elements in the proximal arterial tree, particularly the aorta, and is important in maintaining flow during diastole. Cardiovascular haemodynamics should additionally consider the effects of turbulence, and blood viscosity, which also adversely affect the linear relationship between flow and pressure. Turbulence, for example, is typically seen at points of stenosis or arterial branching. Disruption of laminar parabolic flow occurs at a critical threshold defined by the Reynolds number (Table 2.1, Equation 5) and this has the effect of reducing blood flow for a given pressure gradient (Fig. 2.9).

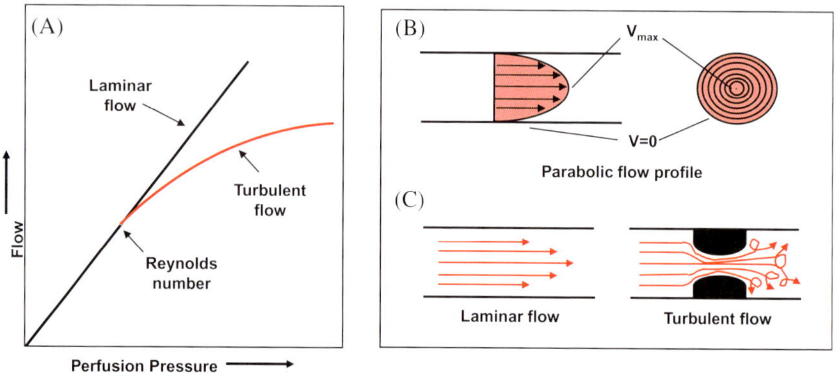

Figure 2.9. Effect of turbulence on blood flow. (A) Blood flow becomes turbulent in conditions defined by the Reynold's number (see Table 2.1). Beyond this point, turbulence results in a greater perfusion pressure required for a given flow. (B) Blood flow in a cylindrical vessel results in a parabolic flow profile; maximal velocity is within the centre of flow (V_{max}) whereas friction and drag at the endothelial-blood surface interface result in slower velocities ($V = 0$). (C) Turbulence disrupts laminar parabolic flow, reducing V_{max} and slowing mean blood flow.

If circulatory failure is due to impaired myocardial contractility as defined by a 'flattened' stroke work/filling pressure equation, the atrial pressures are often already raised. Provided this accurately reflects volume preload, further volume challenges to increase the atrial filling pressures are not helpful since the ventricle becomes increasingly distended with high wall tension as predicted by Laplace's law (Table 2.1, Equation 6). An increased wall tension compromises myocardial blood supply, particularly epicardial to endocardial blood flow, resulting in endocardial ischaemia, further impairing ventricular contractility and increasing atrial pressures.

Ventricular contractility can be increased either by removing negatively inotropic influences (acidaemia, hyperkalaemia, drugs, e.g. β-blockers) or by using a positive inotrope, which may be defined as an agent that increases the gradient of the stroke work to filling pressure relationship resulting in a larger stroke volume for the same pre- and afterload pressures. When considering the use of an inotropic agent, the adverse effects of vasoactive agents on ventricular efficiency, metabolic rate and regional distribution of flow should be considered [9].

2.3.4 *Stroke volume*

The volume of blood ejected by each ventricle with each heart beat (the stroke volume) is determined by the individual ventricular contractility, the preload and the afterload against which the ventricle is pumping i.e. the systemic or pulmonary artery pressures. In this sense the ventricles may be assessed independently but, although there is some variation in the stroke volume generated between the two ventricles, such as during the respiratory cycle, over any significant period of time the mean stroke volume from the right ventricle must equal that from the left. The ventricles are also 'interdependent' since they are physically united by the pericardium, have a shared interventricular septum and have the same heart rate.

The resulting stroke volume varies with the resistance of the vascular bed into which the ventricle is ejecting. Although the right ventricle generates a much smaller amount of stroke work than the left, the afterload (pulmonary vascular resistance (PVR)) against which it ejects is correspondingly lower since the right and left ventricular stroke volumes must necessarily be the same over time.

2.3.5 *Heart rate*

In sinus rhythm, atrial systole contributes an extra 10–15% to end-diastolic ventricular volume and this change in ventricular preload increases stroke work. For heart rates of up to approximately 100 beats/min, ventricular preload is not affected by the reduction in diastolic filling time and therefore stroke volume is rate independent but cardiac output increases linearly with the heart rate. This explains the markedly beneficial effect of ventricular pacing in complete heart block, when increasing the rate from 30 beats/min to 90 beats/min will approximately treble the cardiac output. At rates above 100 beats/min, the reduction in diastolic filling time causes a progressive reduction in preload.

2.3.6 *Ventricular interdependence*

Although the left and right sides of the heart are frequently assumed to be independent and to function as two pumps in series, they are of course anatomically closely linked, sharing the interventricular septum and both being wrapped in a single fibrous membrane, the pericardium, the properties of which relate to the elastic and collagenous fibres from which it is made. As a result the distension of one ventricle alters the distensibility/compliance of the other ventricle and the associated filling pressures. This is the phenomenon of ventricular interdependence. In the healthy heart this is most apparent in the respiratory and postural changes that occur in ventricular volume and in the contribution that left ventricular contraction makes to right ventricular systolic pressure and flow, estimated to be as much as one-third [10]. The extent of this interdependence is related to the relative compliances of the left and right ventricular free walls, the septum and the pericardium. However, the pericardium is responsible for many of the features of ventricular interdependence. It limits the degree of acute cardiac dilatation to no more than 10–15% at which point the elastic fibres are fully stretched and the tense collagenous fibres with low compliance prevent further expansion acutely. At this point further dilatation of one chamber must result in a reduction of volume and also distortion of the other. Therefore any changes in right ventricular volume preload, due to giving or removing volume or changes in afterload due to new pathology or drug administration will cause either a leftward or rightward shift of the interventricular septum and influence the left ventricular compliance and hence the LV pressure–volume relationship. Thus an infusion of glyceryl trinitrate will reduce RV preload, causing a rightward shift of the septum thereby increasing LV compliance and reducing LV preload, at least partly, due to ventricular interdependence. However a massive pulmonary embolus causes not only an increase in pulmonary outflow obstruction but also a leftward shift of the interventricular septum, which reduces left ventricular diastolic compliance, leading to a profound fall in left ventricular volume preload and hence in stroke volume and cardiac output.

2.4 Coronary Blood Flow

The heart has a very high basal oxygen consumption (8–10 ml O_2/min/100g) and at rest receives approximately 5% of the cardiac output (approximately 250 ml/min). This equates to 60–90 ml blood/100 g heart weight/minute. The left and right coronary arteries originate from their respective sinus recesses above the aortic valve leaflets. They divide horizontally to supply the entire epicardial surface of the heart on which they lie, and give off smaller branches, which penetrate vertically deep down as far as the endocardium. Flow rate is determined by Poiseuille's law (Table 2.1, Equation 3), but assuming the majority of Poiseuille's components to be constant, the two key practical determinants of coronary flow in a given cardiac cycle are (i) aortic pressure (P_i) and (ii) arterial radius (r), which allows for both the effects of extrinsic extravascular compression and intrinsic neurohormonal vasoreactivity or fixed atherosclerosis.

Changes in aortic pressure (P_i) induce parallel changes in coronary perfusion. Ventricular systole contributes significantly to this driving aortic perfusion pressure, but uniquely exerts a potent extravascular compression effect on the epicardial arteries, resulting in a phasic coronary flow profile (Fig. 2.10). This is particularly true of the left ventricle,

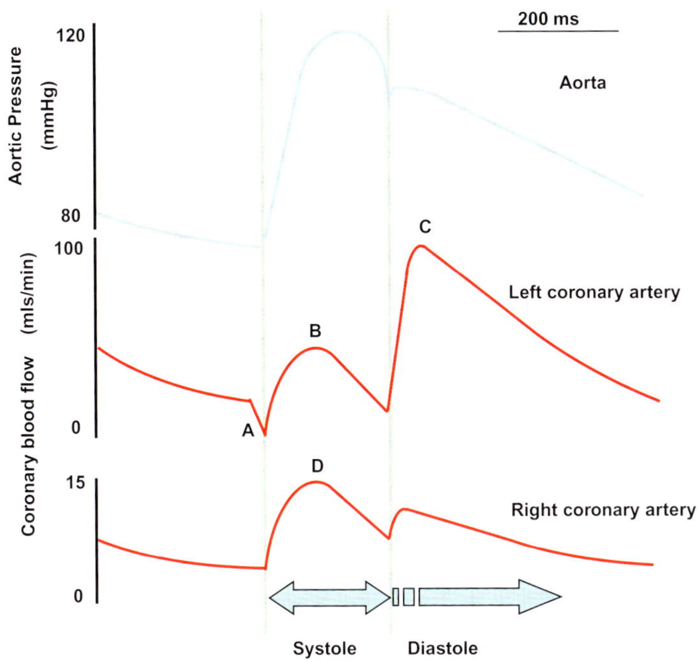

Figure 2.10. Phasic coronary blood flow. Isovolumic contraction of the left ventricle transiently halts coronary flow down the left coronary artery (A). This extravascular compression effect persists through systole, attenuating epicardial perfusion (B) until ventricular relaxation in diastole (C). The right ventricle is far less constrictive and peak coronary flow in the right coronary artery is during systole (D) in parallel with the rise in aortic pressure.

in which isovolumic contraction transiently halts coronary flow down the left coronary system, followed by a muted increase during ventricular ejection and then rapid increase at diastole as the ventricle relaxes. Flow slowly declines during this period in parallel with aortic pressure. The phasic effect in the right coronary artery is less pronounced due to the lower developed pressure within the thinner right ventricular wall. Systolic blood flow therefore contributes a greater proportion of total flow compared with the left artery.

Coronary flow, whilst critically dependent upon aortic and coronary perfusion pressures, is protected over a wide physiological range (approximately 60–200 mmHg) as a result of autoregulation (Fig. 2.11). This describes the intrinsic neurohormonal modulation of the coronary resistance vessels to maintain the (P_i–P_o) gradient and, thus, flow. Vagal and sympathetic stimulation of the heart both result in increased coronary flow. Alpha-adrenergic and vagal stimulation cause a small but direct vasoconstrictor response, whilst beta-1 adrenergic stimulation results in positive inotropic and chronotropic effects which, in turn, release local

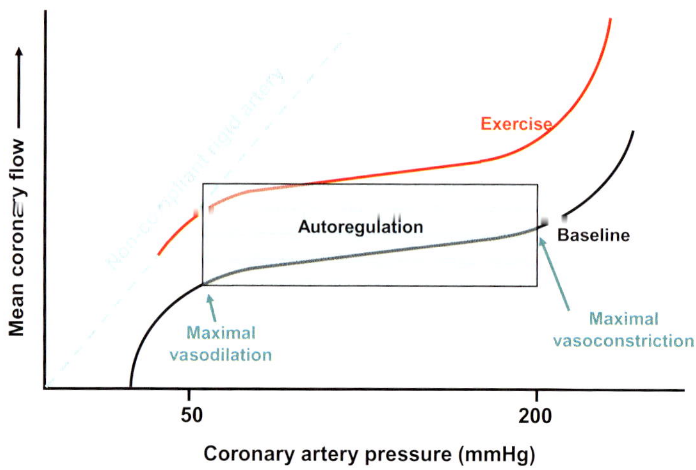

Figure 2.11. Autoregulation in the coronary vasculature. Coronary flow is preserved over a wide-range of perfusion pressures (60–200 mmHg) as a result of modulation in arterial diameter (vasoconstriction and vasodilation). Exercise and exogenous vasodilators shift the autoregulation plateau upwards, increasing flow for any given pressure. This is referred to as the coronary reserve. Re-drawn from [11].

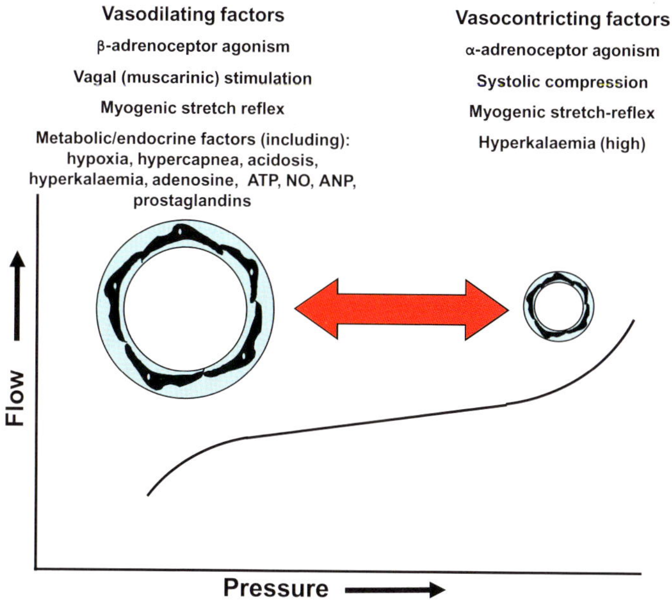

Figure 2.12 Vasoactive factors which influence coronary resistance and mediate autoregulation. A variety of mediators and physiological processes have been implicated, including neuro-hormonal activation, local paracrine mediators and an intrinsic smooth-muscle cell myogenic reflex in response to wall tension.

paracrine metabolites with potent vasodilatory properties. Autonomic stimulation forms the efferent limb of baroreceptor- and chemoreceptor-mediated reflexes and a direct response to circulating hormones. It is not, however, considered the major determinant of coronary resistance.

The proportional relationship between myocardial oxygen consumption and coronary flow has long been recognised. The causative link between the two, however, remains to be fully characterised. Several mediators have been proposed, including potassium, lactate, adenosine, nitric oxide and altered oxygen partial pressures (Fig. 2.12). Finally, an intrinsic myogenic reflex also exists, whereby resistance arterioles constrict in direct response to elevations in transmural pressure and vice versa. This has been demonstrated in various tissues in addition to the heart and is likely to involve both endothelial-dependent nitric oxide and independent signalling mechanisms.

2.5 Peripheral Circulation

The haemodynamics of the peripheral circulation are dominated by two important interacting principles: (i) blood flow from the heart is intermittent, and (ii) the arterial conduits are distensible (compliant). The perfect pump system would provide continuous flow and pressure to the body, but evolution has created the heart as an intermittent pump. This is estimated to add 10% and 35% additional workload to the left and right ventricles respectively compared with steady-state flow. Furthermore, in order to maintain distal perfusion pressure during the latter stages of the cardiac cycle, energy from the systolic pulse wave is taken up by the large compliant proximal arteries and delivered back (recoil) during diastole (Windkessel function); this is perhaps demonstrated best in the dicrotic notch (incisura dicrota) of the central aortic pressure waveform (Fig. 2.13).

Arterial elasticity is determined by the relative collagen and elastin content of conduit vessels. Proximal arteries have higher amounts of

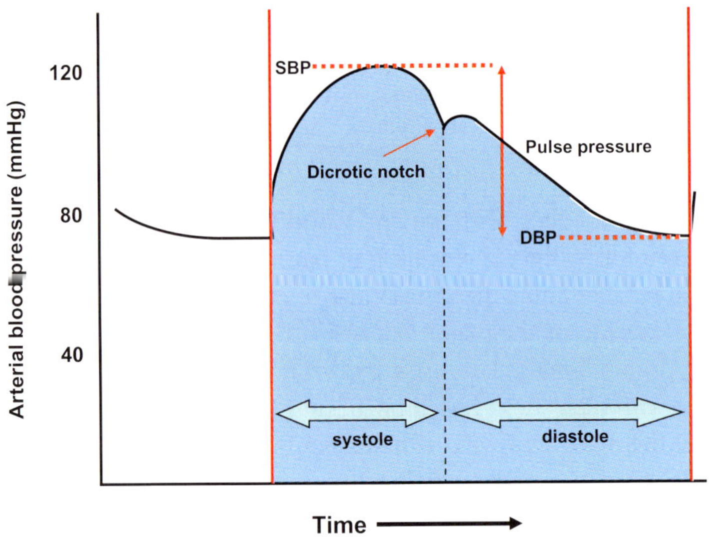

Figure 2.13. Arterial pressure tracing for a single cardiac cycle. Pulse pressure is defined as the peak pressure (systole (SBP)) — trough pressure (diastole (DBP)). Mean arterial pressure can be calculated from the area under the curve throughout the entire cycle; an estimate is often derived as the diastolic pressure +1/3 pulse pressure; this reflects the greater contribution of diastole to the cardiac cycle length. Re-drawn from [12].

elastin and are more compliant. This reduces with age as a result of progressive changes to the tunica intima and media. Pulsatile flow results in a pressure waveform with systolic (peak) and diastolic (trough) pressure components. Pulse pressure represents the difference between the two measurements, and mean arterial pressure calculated over the entire cardiac cycle. The pressure wave propagates rapidly through the arterial tree in advance of blood flow itself. Velocity is inversely proportional to vascular compliance and, accordingly, is generally faster in older individuals and also becomes faster towards the peripheries in all age-groups. Pulse wave morphology also changes more distally (Fig. 2.14). Three principal findings have been described:

1. The systolic upstroke becomes quicker and peak amplitude increases.
2. Dampening of the dicrotic notch (and other higher-frequency signal components).
3. A later diastolic pressure wave is occasionally apparent.

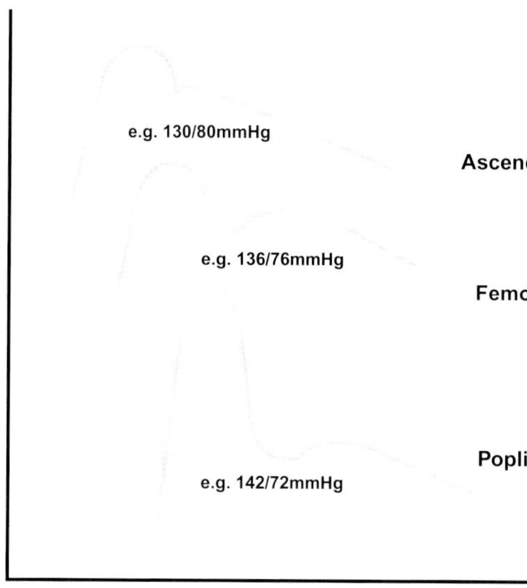

Figure 2.14. Representative changes in pressure-waveform along the arterial tree. The characteristic findings of the more distal waveform are (i) a faster and higher-amplitude peak pressure, (ii) a dampening of higher-frequency signal components (including the dicrotic notch), and (iii) the occasional presence of a later diastolic pressure wave.

These characteristics result in part from the visco-elastic properties of the arterial wall, but also reflect more complex components of fluid dynamics, including reflection, resonance and tapering.

Mean arterial pressure is calculated from an invasive arterial tracing as the total area beneath the waveform divided by the time interval. Approximations from non-invasive assessment can be made as the diastolic pressure plus a third of the pulse pressure, reflecting the longer diastolic timeframe of the cardiac cycle. Systemic blood pressure is determined by a combination of interacting physiological and physical components: (i) cardiac output, (ii) peripheral resistance, (iii) blood volume and (iv) arterial compliance.

Under steady-state conditions cardiac output (Q_{co}) equals the peripheral run-off (Q_{pr}). The dependence of arterial pressure on cardiac output and peripheral resistance is best considered using the modification of Ohm's law:

$$Q_{co} = \frac{(P_a - P_v)}{R} = Q_{pr},$$

where Qco = cardiac output, Qpr = peripheral run-off, Pa = mean arterial pressure, Pv = mean right atrial pressure and R = resistance.

Assuming Pv is negligible:

$$Q_{co} = \frac{(P_a)}{R} = Q_{pr}.$$

Acute changes in either cardiac output or resistance result in temporary imbalances between Q_{co} and Q_{pr}, which are tempered, in the first instance, by reciprocal changes in P_a proportional to the magnitude of shift. Another important mediator of the rate of blood pressure change is arterial compliance (C_a). Longer term, Q_{co} and R will be affected by autonomic reflexes and other physiological processes which ameliorate the chronic changes in mean arterial pressure.

The effect of volume changes on arterial pressure is best explained considering the systemic pressure–volume relationship and pulse-pressure during the cardiac cycle (Fig. 2.15). Blood ejected during systole will cause total arterial volume to increase (V_1 to V_2) and results in transient Q_{co}:Q_{pr}

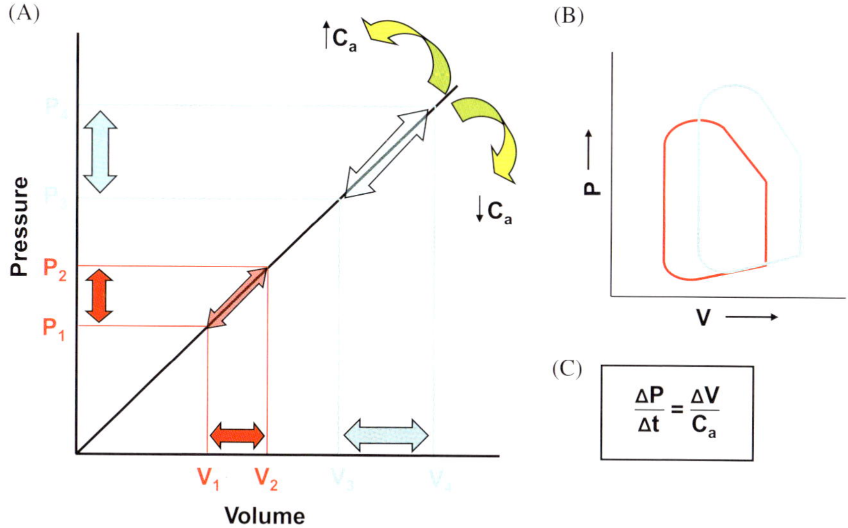

Figure 2.15. The effect of volume on arterial pressure. (A) Arterial pressure–volume (P–V) relation. (B) Corresponding left ventricular P–V loop. (C) Equation of compliance (C_a). Ventricular systole results in a transient rise in arterial volume, V_1 to V_2 (the arterial volume increment), which causes a corresponding increase in arterial pressure, P_1 to P_2 (the pulse pressure). As blood flow filters rapidly through to the peripheries, volume and pressure fall back to baseline. Increases in arterial volume (V3 and V4) result in a parallel shifts in pressure (P3 and P4), in the presence of stable heart rate and peripheral resistance. In a rigid arterial system, the P–V relationship is linear. However, *in vivo* arterial compliance will modify this gradient and linearity. A simple calculation of compliance is given by equation (C). Furthermore, arterial pressure changes in response to volume shift do not occur in isolation, and will be modified by heart rate and peripheral resistance, which are influenced by autonomic and other physiological processes. Modified from [12].

mismatch (i.e. $Q_{co} > Q_{pr}$). Under normal circumstances, this volume (also known as the arterial volume increment) represents approximately 20% of the stroke volume only, as the remaining 80% passes directly to the peripheral circulation during the rapid ejection phase. The corresponding pressure rise along the linear P–V relation (P_1 to P_2) is the pulse pressure. Peripheral run off then exceeds cardiac output during the remainder of the cardiac cycle ($Q_{co} < Q_{pr}$) and pressure and volume return back to diastolic baseline P_1 and V_1, respectively. Changes in stroke volume (V3–4), in the presence of constant heart rate and peripheral resistance, will result in proportional changes in arterial pressure (P3–4) (Fig. 2.15). In reality, arterial compliance renders the P–V relation curvilinear and is, accordingly, an important contributor to the rate and change of blood pressure response to changes in cardiac output. Furthermore, autonomic and other physiological processes again need to be considered in determining the longer-term effect on mean arterial pressure.

2.6 The Microcirculation

The arterial system delivers nutrient-rich blood to tissue beds via an extensive network of arterioles (diameter range 5–100 μm), metarterioles (10–20 μm) and capillaries (5–10 μm), which are estimated to cover between 50,000 and 60,000 miles in length! This is depicted in Fig. 2.16. This provides a high-surface exchange area for active and passive diffusion of nutrients and waste products (nutritional flow). Muscular arterioles are the major resistance vessels determining capillary flow and, in some cases,

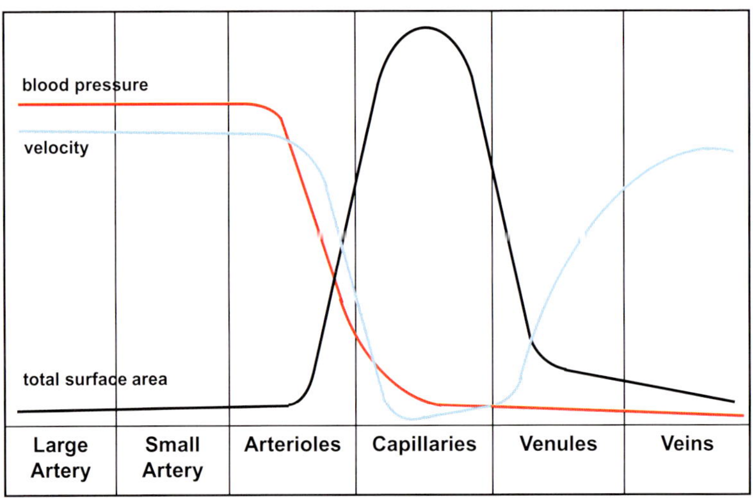

Figure 2.16. Proportional plot of cross-sectional area and haemodynamics of the vasculature. The arterial tree sub-divides and multiplies to give an extensive capillary network within the body. This dramatically increases vascular total cross-sectional area and reduces blood velocity, encouraging active and passive diffusion processes within tissues. The large capacitance vessels of the venous system hold approximately 70% of the circulating volume.

Table 2.2. Circulation dimensions: redrawn from [13].

	Diameter	Wall thickness	Wall tension (dynes/cm)
Aorta	25 mm	2 mm	170,000
Artery	4 mm	1 mm	60,000
Arteriole	30 μm	20 μm	1200–1500
Terminal arteriole	35 μm	30 μm	—
Capillary	8 μm	1 μm	16
Venule	20 μm	2 μm	26
Vein	0.5 mm	0.5 mm	400
Vena cava	30 mm	1.5 mm	21,000

may result in blood bypassing the capillary bed altogether (non-nutritional or shunt flow). The distribution of interconnecting endothelium-lined capillaries varies between tissues, with a higher concentration in metabolically-active organs such as cardiac and skeletal muscle. Blood flow in capillaries is not uniform and depends largely on the upstream arteriole resistance and the effect of extrinsic compression. Average blood velocity in these terminal vessels may range between 1 and 10 mm/s.

Arteriolar tone and microvascular perfusion are dependent upon a combination of endothelium-dependent (predominantly mediated by nitric oxide) and endothelium-independent factors, as outlined in Fig. 2.13. This serves a primary autoregulatory function in afferent nutritional blood supply to a tissue, but additionally may play an important role in other physiological processes, such as thermoregulation in the skin or hypoxic pulmonary vasoconstriction in the lungs in the event of ventilation–perfusion mismatch.

Microvascular function can be assessed by perfusion imaging (e.g. contrast ultrasonography, magnetic resonance imaging or radio-isotope perfusion) or through invasive physiological interrogation of flow-reserve (e.g. Doppler-ultrasonography, pressure-interrogation, thermodilution measurements), defined by the ratio of baseline pressure/velocity or flow to that achieved with maximal arteriolar dilatation in the absence of fixed obstruction to flow in larger upstream arteries (e.g. epicardial coronary artery stenosis). Although the clinical application of this is relatively limited at the current time, assessment may provide useful information regarding the integrity of tissue perfusion, metabolism and organ function.

2.7 Clinical Case

A 52-year-old man is admitted to the intensive care unit with severe pancreatitis and a history of heavy alcohol consumption. He has a smoking history of 25 years but denies any specific cardiac symptoms.

Examination revealed cool peripheries; heart rate 100 beats/min; MAP 69 mmHg; RAP/JVP assessed clinically at <0 cm H_2O from sternal angle; breathing spontaneously with good gas exchange; urine output 40 ml over the past 2 hours; diffuse abdominal tenderness with some epigastric guarding; ascites positive; absent bowel sounds; CNS alert and oriented.

Electrocardiogram (ECG) showed sinus rhythm with partial right bundle branch block (RBBB); chest X ray (CXR) was normal; partial pressure of oxygen in arterial blood (PaO_2)10.5 kPa at fraction of inspired oxygen (FiO_2) 0.7; amylase was markedly raised; liver function tests (LFTs) showed a mildly raised gamma-glutamyltransferase and alkaline phosphatase; international normalised ratio (INR) 1.5; platelets 168; haemoglobin (Hb) 10.8 g%.

An attempted line insertion into the right subclavian vein failed and central access was established via the right internal jugular vein. The patient was thought to be intravascularly deplete (RAP +4 from mid axillary line) and he was therefore filled with Hartman's and also given 500 ml of gelofusine. He responded well, warmed peripherally, MAP increased to 74 mmHg and his urine output increased.

However, over the next hour his condition deteriorated with his RAP rising to +14 mmHg and MAP falling to 55 mmHg. Norepinephrine was started and rapidly increased to 0.8 μg/kg/min to achieve a MAP of 60 mmHg.

2.7.1 *What is the diagnosis?*

His abdomen was not obviously more acute although the ascites seemed rather more tense. He was not in hyperdynamic 'shock' since his peripheries were cold and he had a weak 'thready' pulse. An abdominal ultrasound was requested but showed nothing markedly different from the one performed six hours earlier which had shown a moderate amount of ascites and a somewhat swollen pancreas. There was no evidence of an obstructed biliary tree.

2.7.2 *What next?*

An ECG was performed and still showed RBBB with a sinus tachycardia of 125/min but nothing to suggest cardiac ischaemia. A CXR was ordered.

His gas exchange deteriorated and it was decided to intubate him and he was started on pressure support ventilation with positive end-expiratory pressure (PEEP) +10 cmH_2O. His condition further deteriorated: he was now requiring norepinephrine at over 1 µg/kg/min and an epinephrine infusion to achieve a MAP of 54 mmHg, RAP was +22 mmHg. PaO_2 6.8 kPa on FiO_2 0.8.

A pulmonary artery catheter was inserted and showed a pulmonary artery occlusion pressure (PAOP) of +26 mmHg, a cardiac index of 1.4 l/min/m^2 and a mixed venous oxygen saturation of 45%. An echocardiogram was requested but could not be performed within the next two hours.

The repeat CXR was reviewed — see Fig. 2.17.

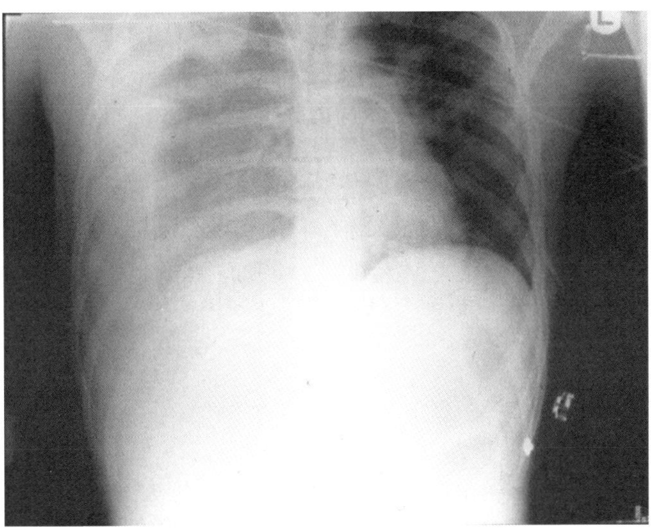

Figure 2.17. Repeat CXR image.

This showed a large right pleural effusion and a shift of the mediastinum to the left. A Valsalva manoeuvre was performed and demonstrated a markedly 'empty' circulation with virtual obliteration of the arterial blood pressure after ten seconds.

A chest drain was inserted and two litres of fresh blood was drained over the next hour with the result that the RAP fell to +6 mmHg, the PAOP fell to 13 mmHg and the MAP increased to 85 mmHg. The epinephrine had been stopped and the norepinephrine was reduced to 0.05 μg/kg/min. He was given fresh frozen plasma (FFP) to correct an INR of 1.7. The bleeding from the subclavian artery punctured at the attempted R subclavian line insertion stopped and the chest drain drained only a further 100 ml of blood over the next six hours by which time he was warm and well perfused peripherally, off all vasopressors with a MAP of 78 mmHg and a mixed venous oxygen saturation (SvO_2) of 75%.

2.7.3 *Lessons to learn*

- Always consider the intrapleural pressure and think of the transmural distending pressure of the left ventricle particularly in patients (i) who are on positive pressure ventilation and receiving PEEP, (ii) who have significant pleural fluid/gas collections and (iii) who have high intra-abdominal pressure from ascites or ileus.
- The high filling pressures did not indicate that he was adequately filled. Although not measured, as a result of the bleed he had sustained from the right subclavian artery, his intrapleural pressure would have risen to > +15 mmHg and therefore the true, transmural distending pressure of the left atrium would have been <10 mmHg and he was therefore severely volume depleted.
- The Valsalva manoeuvre revealed the true situation as would have done an echocardiogram if that had been available.

References

[1] Harvey, W. (1628). *Exercitatio Anatomica de Motu Cordis et Sanguinis in Animalibus (An Anatomical Exercise on the Motion of the Heart and Blood*

in Living Beings), Frankfurt. For translation see: http://www.fordham.edu/halsall/mod/1628harvey-blood.html [Accessed 5 February 2013].

[2] Murgatroyd, F.D., Krahn, A.D., Klein, D.J. *et al.* (2002). *Handbook of Cardiac Electrophysiology: A Practical Guide to Invasive EP Studies and Catheter Ablation*, ReMedica Publishing, London.

[3] Leach, R.M. and Treacher, D.F. (2002). Oxygen delivery and consumption in the critically ill, *Thorax*, **57**, 170–177.

[4] Ross, J.J. (1976). Afterload mismatch and preload reserve: a conceptual framework for the analysis of ventricular function, *Prog Cardiovasc Dis*, **18**, 255–264.

[5] Sarnov, S.J. and Bergland, E. (1954). Ventricular function 1. Starling's law of the heart studied by means of simultaneous right and left ventricular function curves in the dog, *Circulation*, **9**, 706–718.

[6] Bradley, R.D. (1977). *Studies in Acute Heart Failure*, Edward Arnold Ltd, London.

[7] Sharpey-Schafer, E.P. (1955). Effects of Valsalva's manoeuvre on the normal and failing circulation, *BMJ*, **1**, 693–695.

[8] Buda, A.J., Pinsky, M.R., Ingels, N.B. *et al.* (1979). Effect of intrathoracic pressure on left ventricular performance, *N Engl J Med*, **301**, 453–459.

[9] Mueller, H., Ayers, S.M., Gianelli, S. *et al.* (1972). Effect of isoproterenol, L-norepinephrine and intra-aortic counterpulsation on haemodynamics and myocardial metabolism in shock following acute myocardial infarction, *Circulation*, **45**, 335–351.

[10] Santamore, W.P. and Dell'Italia, L.J. (1998). Ventricular interdependence: significant left ventricular contributions to right ventricular systolic function, *Prog Cardiovasc Dis*, **40**, 289–308.

[11] Opie, L. (2003). *Heart Physiology. From Cell to Circulation*, fourth edition, Lippincott Williams and Wilkins, Baltimore, MD.

[12] Berne, R.M. and Levy, M.N. (eds) (1993). *Physiology*, third edition, Mosby Publishing, St Louis.

[13] Burton, A.C. (1954). Relation of structure to function of the tissues of the wall of blood vessels, *Physiol Rev*, **34**, 619–642.

3

Respiratory Physiology

Nicholas Lees and Neil Soni

3.1 Introduction

The origins of intensive care practice as we now know it and respiratory physiology are inextricably entwined. The polio epidemic produced the immediate need for ventilation on a large scale and impressive survival results demonstrating a modality of treatment that had massive benefits [1]. The lack of adequate monitoring of blood gases and the awareness of a massive void of knowledge as regards ventilation physiology produced the emergence of respiratory physiology as we know it today, while the negative cardiovascular effects of ventilation generated new interest in cardiovascular physiology. Applied integrated physiology became an entity. Equipment design improved and development increased drastically.

As critical care has diversified, ventilation has become less predominant as the key feature of management but it is still a significant and unavoidable part of critical care and will remain so.

3.2 Regulation of Respiration

Breathing is carefully controlled by the central nervous system. The brainstem contains a respiratory centre producing spontaneous rhythmic, automatic breathing activity. This is regulated by a multitude of connections from higher centres and the periphery including chemoreceptors, mechanoreceptors and reflexes within and outside of the lungs and airways (Fig. 3.1). Furthermore it may be overridden voluntarily or

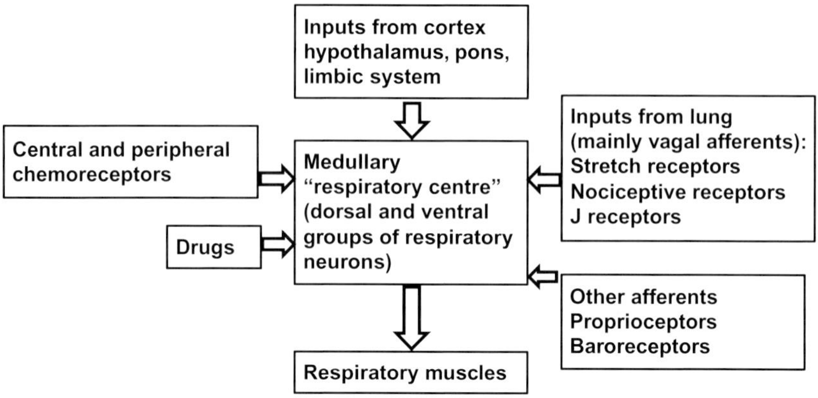

Figure 3.1. Control of respiration.

involuntarily and to facilitate activities such as speech, swallowing and coughing. Impulses are sent via motor neurons to the effectors, the respiratory muscles, and in health this integration allows close control of partial pressure of oxygen (PO_2), partial pressure of carbon dioxide (PCO_2) and pH.

The respiratory centre consists of several distinct groups of neurons within the medulla: the dorsal group, located near the nucleus tractus solitarius associated mainly with timing and control of inspiration, and the ventral group in the ventrolateral medulla, comprising four nuclei with inspiratory, expiratory and laryngeal and pharyngeal dilator functions. Neurotransmitters involved include glutamate (excitatory) and gamma-aminobutyric acid (GABA) and glycine (inhibitory) [2].

The automatic pattern of respiration is generated from the dorsal group of neurons and other adjacent groups within the medulla. The inspiratory signal transmitted to the respiratory muscles and airway dilators builds up like a ramp then ceases; allowing steady ventilation and preventing gasps. Expiration is passive during quiet breathing resulting from elastic recoil of the lungs and chest wall and most expiratory neurons are quiet but become active at times when minute volume is increased.

Respiration is regulated by inputs from chemical and non-chemical stimuli. Chemical control is via the chemoreceptors. The central chemoreceptors are involved in the response to CO_2 while the peripheral chemoreceptors respond to oxygen. The central chemoreceptors are found in the ventral surface of the medulla and respond quickly to changes in [H^+] via the rapid diffusion of CO_2 from the blood into the cerebrospinal fluid (CSF) which is then hydrated and dissociates giving H^+ ions. An increase in [H^+] stimulates respiration; a decrease in [H^+] inhibits it. This response is rapid and fairly linear but variable and affected by disease and drugs. It is augmented by hypoxia, implying interaction with the peripheral chemoreceptors.

The peripheral chemoreceptors are the carotid and aortic bodies found at the carotid bifurcation and aortic arch (of which the carotid bodies are the most influential) and send signals to the medulla in response to decreases of oxygen or pH or increases in H^+ and CO_2 concentrations in arterial blood. Afferents are via the glossopharyngeal nerves or vagi (in the case of the aortic bodies). Due to their exceptional blood supply, they are exposed to arterial blood at all times and respond quickly to changes in arterial PO_2. They also respond to hypoperfusion, temperature elevation and drugs. The response to oxygen is non-linear (Fig. 3.2),

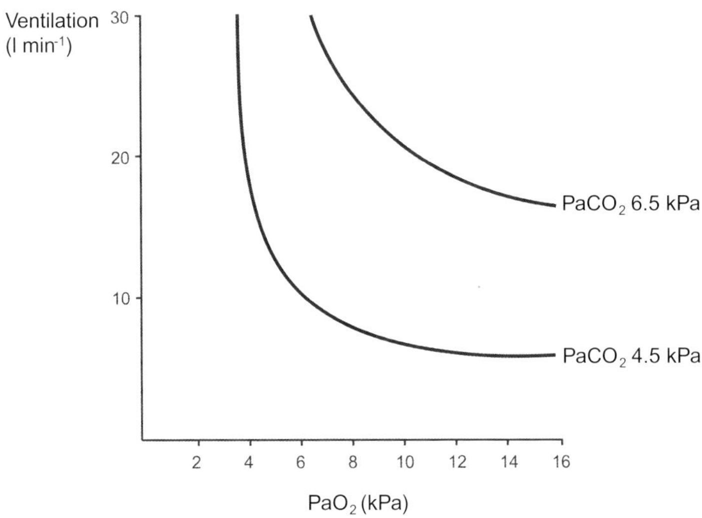

Figure 3.2. Ventilation-response curve to hypoxia. Pulmonary ventilation is increased by progressive hypoxia in response to the central chemoreceptors. Note how the curve, a rectangular hyperbola, is displaced upwards by hypercapnia. Hypocapnia displaces the curve downwards.

becoming particularly sensitive at levels of around 7 kPa and below, causing increased rate and depth of breathing. The response is affected by arterial PCO_2 ($PaCO_2$) whereby the response is augmented by hypercapnia and depressed by hypocapnia [3–5].

In metabolic acidaemia, there is compensatory hyperventilation, thereby reducing alveolar PCO_2 and causing a fall in blood [H^+]. In metabolic alkalaemia, ventilation is depressed, allowing the opposite to happen. Any rise in $PaCO_2$ stimulates ventilation thereby increasing its pulmonary excretion. The response to this is roughly linear, however it depends on the alveolar PO_2 (P_AO_2) in that hypoxia increases the sensitivity to increases in $PaCO_2$. The response to oxygen is non-linear where minute volume is not increased up to levels of around 7 kPa or less, assuming a normal $PaCO_2$. At higher $PaCO_2$ levels minute volume is increased in general and will increase further at P_AO_2 levels greater than 7 kPa [6].

Much of the non-chemical regulation of breathing is via vagal afferents to the medulla through myelinated and unmyelinated fibres. 'Slowly adapting' stretch receptors in the airway smooth muscle are responsible for the inflation reflex limiting inspiration and shortening the expiratory time, known as the Hering–Breuer reflex. 'Rapidly adapting' nociceptive receptors found amongst respiratory epithelial cells are responsible for hyperpnoea, cough, bronchoconstriction and mucus production. Juxtacapillary or J receptors found close to blood vessels respond to lung hyperinflation and exogenous or endogenous chemicals such as serotonin to cause apnoea, bronchospasm and rapid breathing. Their role is unclear but probably important in pathological states such as pulmonary oedema and pulmonary embolism.

Signals from higher centres including the cortex, hypothalamus and limbic system affect respiration at times such as anxiety, pain, sneezing, coughing and yawning. The cortex can override brainstem centres to an extent, sending signals directly to the respiratory muscles via the corticospinal tracts bypassing the medulla. The brainstem receives inputs from the pneumotaxic centre in the dorsolateral pons which itself receives many afferents and influences the rate and depth of inspiration. Other inputs to the medulla are from proprioceptors in muscles and joints, stimulating respiration with muscular activity; arterial baroreceptors (that have a very weak effect) and pain and temperature receptors in the upper airway. Drugs also affect the respiratory centre, mainly depressing it, in particular opioids and other sedatives. Doxapram is a respiratory stimulant that acts on the peripheral chemoreceptors to increase minute ventilation.

3.3 Mechanics of Ventilation

In mammals the lungs and chest wall are a low-pressure system designed to pull air into the proximity of the pulmonary capillaries. The ventilatory unit comprises the rigid but mobile chest wall, the diaphragm and the intercostal and accessory muscles as the 'pump'. This acts on the lungs contained in the pleura. Air is then entrained through the mouth and lower airways to the alveoli. On inspiration the effective expansion of the chest as the ribs move and the contraction of the diaphragm increase the chest volume. This generates a negative pressure in the pleural space and expands the lungs, which produces a negative pressure in the interstitium and in the alveoli and airways and allows air entrainment. The negative pressure within the chest cavity reduces venous pressure in the great veins and enhances venous return to the heart [7].

Potentially opposing these events will be the resistance to airflow in the airways whether from closed glottis, large-airway obstruction, small-airway disease, consolidation, collapse or just the surface tension that exists between two wet surfaces in collapsed alveoli. The pleural space may also impede these effects if filled with air or fluid as it is a potential space rather than real and the 'adhesion' properties between the parietal and somatic pleura are important. On expiration intrapleural pressure returns towards normal, but remains negative while interstitial and alveolar pressures return to either neutral (atmospheric) or slightly positive pressure on expiration.

This is in direct contrast to positive-pressure ventilation where the cycle is reversed. Pressure is exerted down the airways, generating high intrathoracic pressures on inspiration. This pressure is transmitted, depending on compliance, to the alveoli and the interstitial tissues. These are now pushed open with gas following the path of least resistance. The airway, interstitial pressures and intra-alveolar pressures remain positive throughout inspiration as do the intrapleural pressures. All will tend to return towards atmospheric pressure on expiration. Add positive end-expiratory pressure (PEEP) and this may remain positive throughout. These pressures will be high enough to affect capillary flow in inspiration adversely but may also reduce flow during expiration, particularly if intrathoracic pressure is maintained with PEEP [8,9].

These same pressures will influence the hydrostatic gradient between capillary and interstitium, as described in Frank–Starling's equation. Positive pressure in alveoli and in the interstitium will influence fluid movement. The transcapillary gradients will be significantly affected, especially if there is also raised venous capillary pressure commensurate with raised intrathoracic pressure [10–12].

Under some circumstances this may be beneficial if, for example, it helps push fluid from the alveoli and increases the alveolar surface available for gas exchange which explains the rationale for continuous positive airway pressure (CPAP)/PEEP in management of pulmonary oedema, but this effect may be balanced by other effects elsewhere in the lung. Clearly the higher the pressures exerted by ventilation, the greater the effect.

3.4 Work of Breathing

Work is performed by the respiratory muscles to move the chest wall and lungs. Work is defined as the product of force and distance moved ($N \times m = J$), which has the same dimensions as pressure multiplied by volume and can be calculated from a pressure–volume curve. The ease with which the lung volume responds to pressure change is the compliance ($\Delta V/\Delta P$). High compliance is good while low compliance requires more work. Compliance and resistance vary regionally and more so in lung disease (Fig. 3.3).

The ability of gas to flow through the air passages is determined by the resistance. Narrowing or blockage will increase resistance, hence bronchodilators, which increase the lumen, and helium, which is of low density, reduce resistance and augment flow. The work of breathing (WOB) comprises elastic work required to overcome the elastic forces of the lung parenchyma and chest wall and the resistive work required to move viscous or inelastic tissues and overcome airway resistance to move air into the lungs. In healthy adults, about two-thirds of the WOB can be attributed to elastic forces opposing ventilation, the remaining third being due to frictional resistance to gas and tissue movement. In disease, the WOB can

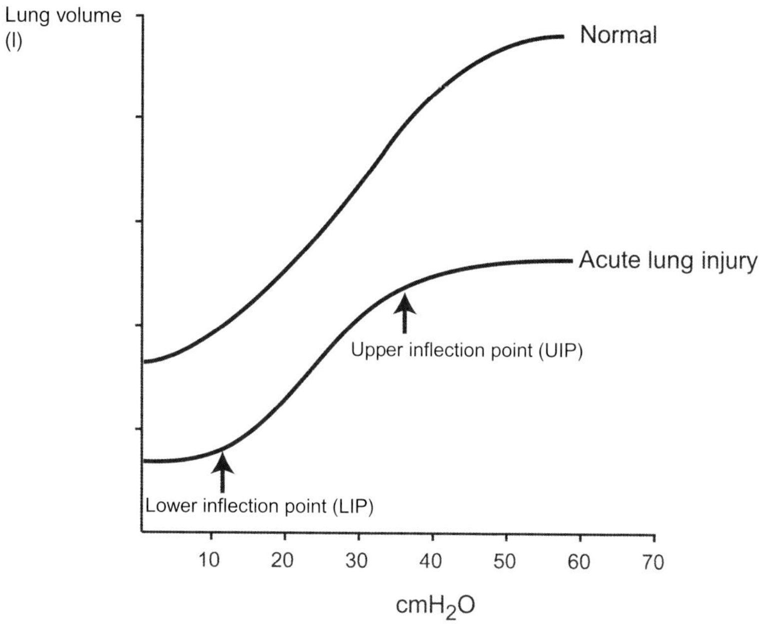

Figure 3.3. Pressure–volume curve demonstrating inflation of a normal lung and the reduced compliance seen in acute lung injury (ALI). The lower inflection point (LIP) is thought to represent the point at which smaller airways and alveoli reopen, corresponding to closing volume. The upper inflection point (UIP) possibly represents encroachment on total lung capacity; inflation beyond this may cause barotrauma.

increase dramatically. Increased elastic resistance may be seen in diseases such as pulmonary fibrosis and increased airflow resistance in asthma and other obstructive diseases. Normal physiological WOB per l in adults is around 0.3 to 0.6 J, which represents only about 1–3% of total oxygen consumption; however in severe disease this figure can reach 20%.

The pressure–volume curve is taken from static measurements of distending pressures at different lung volumes during inspiration and expiration and demonstrates the work of breathing. Intrapleural pressure is estimated by measuring oesophageal pressure. When plotted, the two curves for inspiration and expiration produce a hysteresis loop. This is due to the collapse of small airways and from the surface tension within alveoli that must be overcome to inflate the lungs. The slope of each curve is equal to the static compliance of the lungs and thorax ($C=\Delta V/\Delta P$). In quiet breathing, expiration is a passive process, as during inspiration work is stored as potential energy in the elastic tissues which is greater than the work required to overcome frictional resistance on expiration. Heat is dissipated during inspiration and expiration in overcoming these resistive forces. In forced expiration, expiratory work is greater than elastic work, therefore the process becomes active and respiratory and accessory muscles are required, thereby increasing the WOB. In disease these muscles can fatigue, leading to inadequate ventilation and hypercapnic respiratory failure. Increased WOB manifests clinically as respiratory distress: tachypnoea, accessory and expiratory muscle recruitment, intercostal recession, tracheal tug and other well-recognised signs. Patients may need to be mechanically ventilated to reduce their WOB by assisting and unloading the respiratory muscles. A further consideration is the efficiency with which the lungs are working. The rate and pattern of breathing will determine the amount of work per breath. Small-volume breaths may mean less work but as there will be a higher rate the workload will accrue. During spontaneous breathing a range of factors will influence the work of breathing (Table 3.1).

Table 3.1. Factors influencing work of breathing.

Driving forces	Muscle tone — stretch receptors Carbon dioxide elimination Oxygenation Central nervous system — 'voluntary' or induced Irritability / toxic factors
Physical considerations during inspiration	Elastic and other forces resisting chest expansion, e.g. eschar in burns Pleural space e.g. air or fluid will impede expansion. Chest wall shape and size may make breathing inefficient, e.g. the barrel chest Impaired muscle function, e.g. phrenic nerve palsy Resistance to airflow in the respiratory passages, e.g. narrowed airways, sputum inspisation Tissue deformation — consolidation, pneumothorax Inertia of gas movement
Physical considerations during expiration	Air trapping may make it difficult Airway narrowing may impede flow External pressure such as CPAP may resist exhalation

In mechanical ventilation muscular work is largely removed as air is pushed down the airways. The simple equation V=IR can be used. In inspiration, flow will be determined by the amount of pressure exerted and the resistance to flow which may be at any point in the airway, the interstitium, the pleura, the pleural space and the chest wall itself. The gas density will also influence flow. The ventilator, whether a simple bag or a sophisticated device, generates a pressure waveform pattern over a period of time. All of the factors discussed above will influence distribution of gas through the different regions of the lung. Expiration will be largely passive with the elastic forces trying to regain its original state.

Mechanically ventilated patients have an additional flow resistance workload on top of the physiological WOB, an imposed work required to breathe through the endotracheal tube, ventilator circuit and demand valve. This additional work can be offset by using techniques such as pressure support ventilation.

Intrinsic PEEP (PEEPi) also affects the WOB. PEEPi is positive pressure in the alveoli during expiration as a result of dynamic airways collapse or insufficient expiratory time. As in patients with chronic obstructive pulmonary disease (COPD), this increased load on the respiratory muscles significantly increases the WOB, for before the lung volume can increase on inspiration the respiratory muscles must overcome the level of PEEPi before any pressure gradient and thus flow can occur [13–16].

Studies have in the past looked at measuring WOB as a bedside predictive factor of weaning success but demonstrated only moderate predictive value. WOB measurements have been very helpful in the advancement of ventilator technology [17].

3.5 Ventilation–Perfusion

The key part of breathing is the apposition of gas in the alveolus with the capillary blood. This allows oxygen uptake and carbon dioxide removal. In an ideal lung unit comprising an alveolus and surrounding capillaries, ventilation (V) and perfusion (Q) would be matched such that sufficient alveolar gas is transported by an adequate blood flow in the pulmonary capillaries. Ventilation and perfusion are not equal in the lung, with significant differences in ventilation and perfusion occurring throughout the lung, depending on position, gravity, disease and mechanical ventilation. Most diseases causing hypoxaemia and impaired gas exchange can be thought of in terms of differences in ventilation and perfusion.

Ventilation and perfusion is described as a ratio (V:Q) which varies regionally in the normal upright lung. There are regional variation in gas volume distribution in normally breathing volunteers and the distribution of ventilation and perfusion has been well delineated by West and subsequently by others [18,19]. Lung pathology amplifies aberrant distribution of both blood and gas. If there is insufficient ventilation, for example as a result of obstruction as in COPD or consolidation from pneumonia then alveolar PO_2 will fall as less oxygen is delivered and alveolar PCO_2 will rise as less CO_2 is expired. In cases such as this where there is adequate perfusion but inadequate ventilation, V:Q is <1 which increases the shunt fraction. The converse will occur in cases of reduced perfusion as seen in pulmonary embolism. Here the alveolar PO_2 will rise as it is not transported by the blood and alveolar CO_2 will decrease as less is being delivered to the alveolus. V:Q is >1 which will increase alveolar dead space. Physiological shunt and dead space can therefore be thought of as the two extremes of V:Q mismatching. If those lung units are also considered where V and Q are equal then this gives three distinct hypothetical regions of alveolar gas exchange, those with no Q (dead space), those with no V (shunt) and those with matched V:Q (ideal) (Fig. 3.4).

In spontaneous breathing the chest wall and diaphragm pull the lung open and the negative pressure generated entrains air into the respiratory tree. The negative pressure in any region will be influenced by the state of the alveoli, interstitium and airways in that region. Gas distribution is passive, following a pressure gradient.

The alveoli are pulled open easily due to surfactant, which modifies considerably most of the effects of Laplace's law at these low pressures. Consequently, small alveoli are relatively easy to inflate, and the tendency for small alveoli to collapse on expiration is reduced. The effect of different V:Q ratios in different lung regions will affect the overall arterial PO_2 and PCO_2 [21].

Arterial blood comprises blood from each alveolar region and blood that bypasses the alveoli (shunt). This is what accounts for the difference in alveolar and arterial oxygen tensions, the A–a gradient, which in good

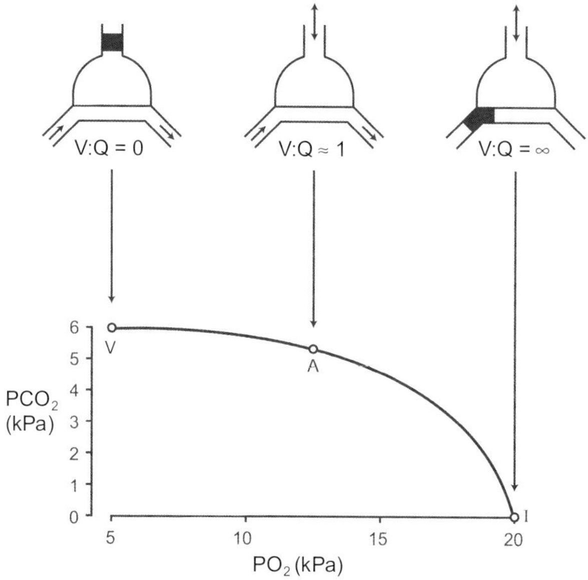

Figure 3.4. The effects of V:Q mismatch on gas exchange (adapted from [20]). The PO_2–PCO_2 diagram shows changes in alveolar gas composition according to ventilation:perfusion ratios for a lung unit. V:Q increases along the line from 0 in mixed venous blood (V) to a normal V:Q ratio at the alveolar point of alveolar end capillary blood (A) to the inspired gas point (I).

health is very small (PaO_2 about 2 kPa less than P_AO_2). The lung units at the base, with their lower V:Q ratios than at the apex, make the greatest contribution to lowering arterial oxygen tension below alveolar as they have more flow with a lower PO_2. The opposite effect occurs at the apex where a higher P_AO_2 is not enough to compensate for the venous admixture at the lung base because there is much less flow and haemoglobin is already almost fully saturated. In disease the A–a gradient can be considerable. Estimating the A–a gradient using the alveolar gas equation and arterial PO_2 (PaO_2) from a blood gas gives an indication of the extent of ventilation–perfusion mismatching (Eq. 3.1). V:Q inequalities cause both hypoxaemia (from shunt) and hypercapnia (from dead space ventilation) although the hypercapnia may not be seen as the chemoreceptors lead to an increase in minute ventilation as a result.

$$P_AO_2 = P_IO_2 - \frac{P_ACO_2}{R}$$

Equation 3.1. The alveolar gas equation

P_AO_2 = partial pressure of alveolar oxygen, P_IO_2 = partial pressure of inspired oxygen, P_ACO_2 = partial pressure of alveolar CO_2 (almost equivalent to arterial CO_2) and R = respiratory exchange ratio.

Positive-pressure ventilation forces air down the airways and is influenced by airway resistance and alveolar compliance. Highly compliant areas are ventilated preferentially at the expense of stiffer less compliant alveoli and there may be over-distension of normal alveoli (Fig. 3.5).

The ease and speed with which alveoli open is determined by time constants. Different alveoli exhibit very different time constants; hence the pattern of ventilation will result in a diverse distribution of gas determined by the local characteristic of airways and alveoli. Obstructed airways will not allow flow and collapsed alveoli will be hard or impossible to inflate. The aim of lung recruitment is to open and keep open under-ventilated areas to increase alveolar surface area and therefore gas exchange, however regional differences in compliance in the normal and diseased lung will affect this (Fig. 3.6).

The efficacy of gas exchange is dependent on the blood flow through the pulmonary capillaries, the alveolar ventilation and the proximity of those capillaries to the alveoli which are ventilated. Flow and pressure are

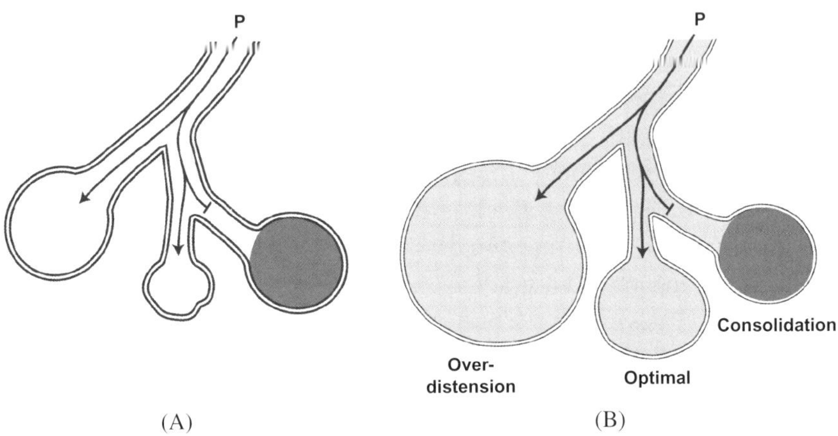

Figure. 3.5. Alveolar inflation: (A) start of inspiration (B) end of inspiration.

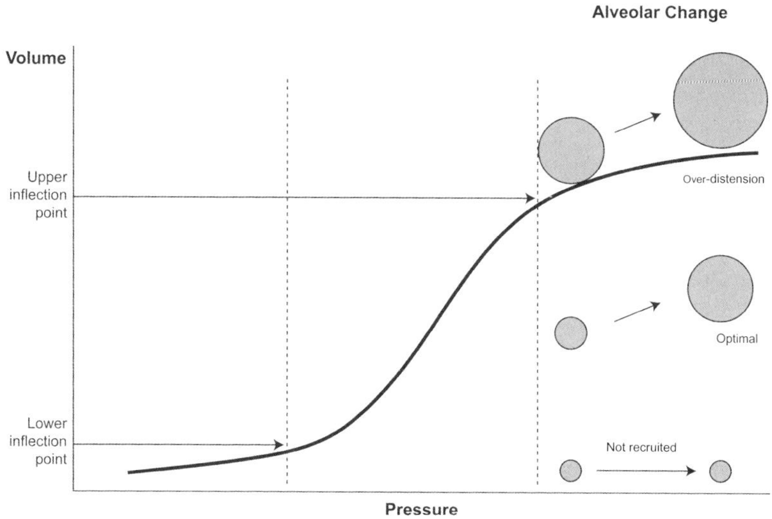

Figure 3.6. Pressure–volume curve and the effects on alveoli (adapted from [22], with permission). Below the lower inflection point there is no change as the alveoli fail to inflate. Above the upper infection point over-inflation ensues. In the midzones and healthy lung there is appropriate inflation. As inflation pressures rise, more of the lung moves above the upper inflection point. The same is not necessarily the case in diseased lung below the lower inflection point.

related and it is generally believed that the mean capillary pressure is somewhere between 7 and 10 mmHg. The driving pressure across the pulmonary capillary will be the gradient between the pulmonary artery pressure and the venous outflow pressure to the left atrium, and both are influenced equally by increased intrathoracic pressure. Under most circumstances capillary pressures are low and it is a low-pressure system. Local pressure from the alveoli will act on the interstitium and push on the capillary walls. In compliant lung pressure, transmission will be effective so that with high airway pressures capillary, flow will be impaired. Paradoxically, if the lung is consolidated and transmits airway pressures poorly, flow may be normal.

Local effects, such as hypoxic vasoconstriction, which may be highly effective in a low-pressure environment may be overwhelmed by the pressures being delivered, although there is very little information available on how they respond in positive pressure ventilation.

Air flow distribution has been investigated by a wide range of techniques but recently computed tomography (CT) scanning and electrical impedance tomography (EIT) have revolutionised the ability to 'see' what actually happens [23–25]. EIT has been used to try to identify the lower and upper inflection points [26,27]. The lower inflection point is thought to represent recruitment while the upper inflection point represents over-distension. This methodology suggests that there is both recruitment and over-distension in the same lung exposed to the same pressure waveform. CT scanning has also been used in particular to try to evaluate the effects of recruitment [26]. The fundamental concept behind recruitment is to use the physics of inflation judiciously to increase the number of alveoli and hence alveolar surface area involved in gas exchange. The central tenet is that with better aeration oxygenation should be improved. The range of strategies aiming to 'recruit' alveoli all involve a combination of pressure and time which are employed under different guises [28–31]. While far from conclusive, available evidence suggests that in severely injured lungs these techniques are relatively ineffective. They demonstrate the futility of trying to predict an optimal value for pressure and time that will suit all regions, each lung or both lungs. Furthermore whole-lung inflection points do not represent individual areas [27, 32–34].

It is important to note that PEEP is used not only to recruit but also to prevent collapse and derecruitment. In this it may be more effective [35,36].

In summary the physics of the lung with variable regional compliance dictates that a single pressure waveform will result in unpredictable gas distribution. This will be determined by airway resistance and individual alveolar compliance, which in part will be determined by alveolar size. The likely result is over-distension of normal alveoli and failure to recruit significantly collapsed areas. High intrathoracic pressures far in excess of the 7–10 mmHg of the capillary will influence blood flow adversely. The physiological consequences are alteration of the pattern of alveolar ventilation associated with variable alterations in capillary flow.

V and Q can be altered clinically to improve gas exchange. Mechanical ventilation, clearance of airway secretions, recruitment manoeuvres and judicial use of PEEP and CPAP can improve V. Q can be improved by increasing cardiac output and the use of vasodilators. Inhaled vasodilators such as prostacyclin and nitric oxide will have the benefit of only increasing Q in ventilated areas, so as to not exacerbate intrapulmonary shunt, as can be the case with intravenous agents. A high A–a gradient is characteristic of ARDS. Here there is marked V:Q mismatching with substantial areas of lung being perfused but inadequately ventilated. When these patients are mechanically ventilated the preferential ventilation of areas with high V:Q ratios will lead to reduced alveolar perfusion owing to the consequent high airway pressures, which reduces Q and exacerbates the V:Q inequality.

3.6 Carbon Dioxide and Interpretation of Expired Alveolar Gas

Ventilation and perfusion is of particular relevance for oxygen uptake. The apposition of haemoglobin in capillary blood and alveolar oxygen is crucial for oxygen uptake. Carbon dioxide is far more soluble and the equilibration between capillary interstitium and alveolus is rapid. Carbon dioxide delivery to the lungs is dependent on cardiac output, hence it falls with pulmonary embolism, but once delivered it equilibrates rapidly. Its removal from the lungs is a direct function of ventilation. To be removed, the alveoli in which it resides need to be ventilated. Therefore carbon dioxide can be issued as a marker of alveolar ventilation (Equations 3.2–3.4).

$$[CO_2] = VCO_2/VA$$

Equation 3.2. The concentration of carbon dioxide will be determined by the production of CO_2, and by the alveolar ventilation.

$$VA = VE - VD$$

Equation 3.3. Alveolar ventilation is that part of total ventilation that is not dead space.

$$VA = \frac{VCO_2}{P_ACO_2} \times K$$

Equation 3.4. The alveolar ventilation equation.

(VCO_2 = volume of CO_2 exhaled per unit time, VA = volume of alveolar gas in the tidal volume, VE = expired total ventilation, and VD = dead space ventilation and P_ACO_2 partial pressure alveolar CO_2).

So it is easy to see that in a situation where carbon dioxide production is constant then the dead space will influence CO_2 removal. Hence the efficiency with which ventilation controls carbon dioxide is determined by the dead space.

This can now be estimated. Under normal circumstances minute ventilation in the order of 100 ml will produce normocapnia. In ventilatory disorders a change in dead space will necessitate an increase in minute ventilation to avoid a commensurate rise in carbon dioxide.

3.7 Blood Gases

This section shall only deal with the blood gas implications of ventilation. The fundamental principles of homeostasis in acid–base depend on the balance between respiratory and metabolic influences on the acid–base balance. In spontaneous breathing, metabolic derangements causing acidosis result in respiratory compensation with hyperventilation. Metabolic alkalosis results in a rising carbon dioxide to compensate. Conversely, respiratory acidosis brings about metabolic compensation with rising bicarbonate and respiratory alkalosis results in slow metabolic compensation. This is seen in acclimatisation to altitude.

In ventilated patients carbon dioxide is determined by the ventilator and the other mechanisms remain intact, so the balance of the two major mechanisms is disrupted. Carbon dioxide is controlled independently of afferent signals arriving at the respiratory centre and the resultant acid–base equilibrium is the signal to which the metabolic compensation responds. In severe acidosis the drive to ventilate often has to be suppressed with sedation and muscle paralysis.

Permissive hypercapnia over a long period of time can result in a significant compensatory metabolic alkalosis which has two effects. Firstly it maintains the pH close to normal unless the carbon dioxide is blown off, which may then impair respiratory drive and weaning. Secondly it can take a long time to return to normal, and rapid resetting of the ventilation to force the carbon dioxide down may result in significant acid–base disequilibrium.

3.8 Physiological Effects of Positive-Pressure Ventilation

Physiological effects of positive-pressure ventilation are summarised in Fig. 3.7.

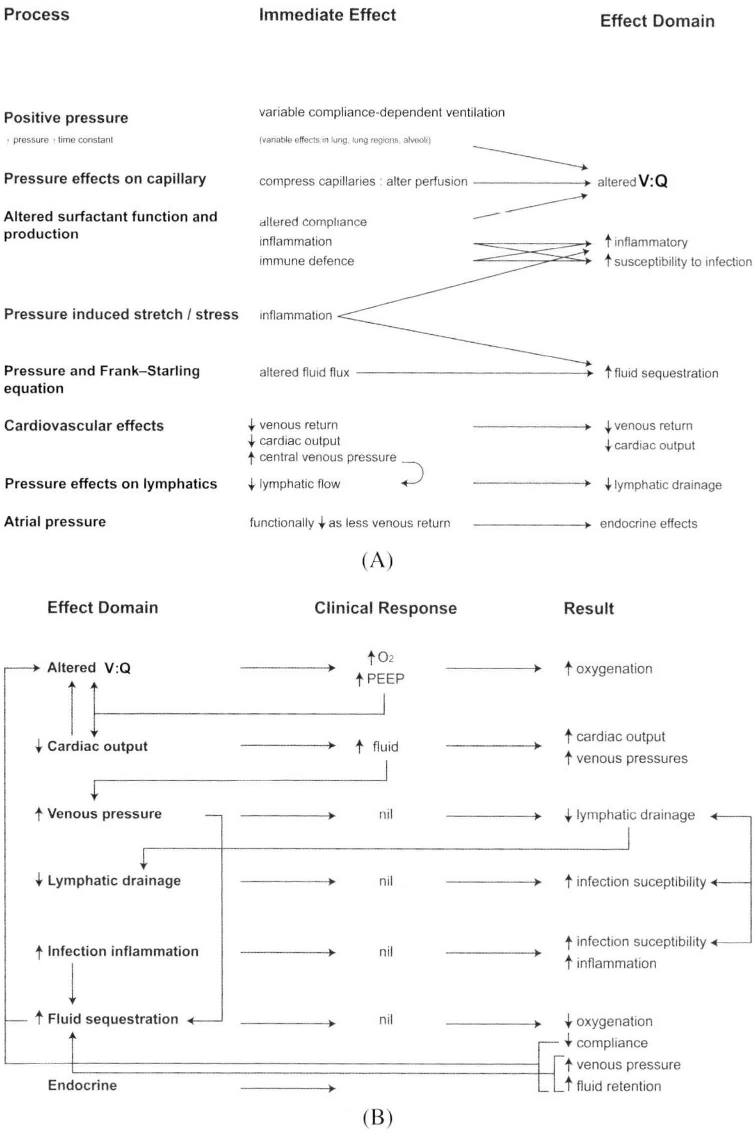

Figure 3.7. The effects of positive pressure ventilation. A leads to B leads to C (adapted from [22], with permission).

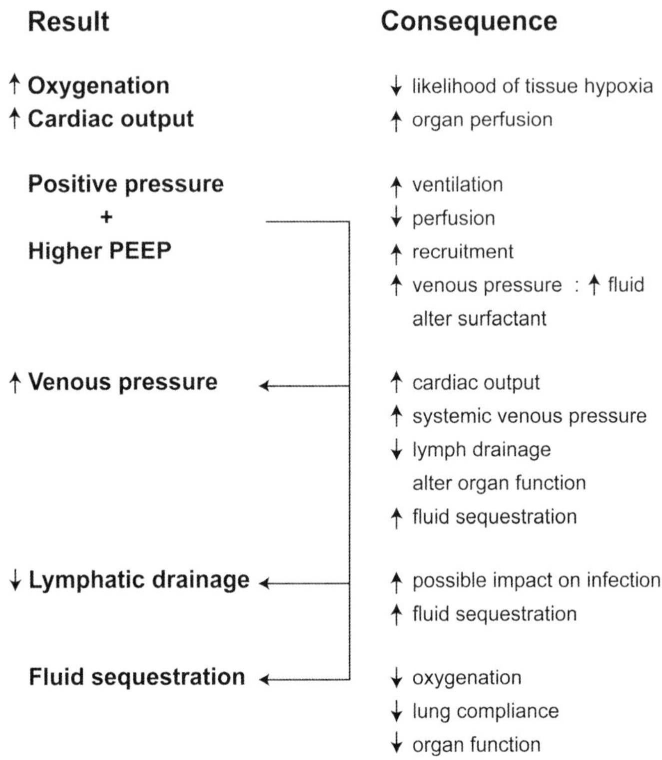

(C)

Figure 3.7. (*Continued*)

3.8.1 *Effects on the lungs*

Positive pressure applied to the lung was considered relatively benign unless excessive but it is now clearly recognised that several aspects of inflation may create problems [37–39]. The acute respiratory distress syndrome (ARDS) net study clearly indicated a reduction in mortality with use of less aggressive ventilation. This created huge interest in potential mechanisms of ventilator-induced lung injury. In addition to the high peak pressures, the shear forces that occur with positive pressure, particularly in initiating inflation, can cause lung damage [40–50].

In keeping with elements of Laplace's law the force required to inflate from small to large radius is far greater than that for inflation from large to larger radius. Stress and shear forces exerted during the cyclic opening and closing of alveoli result in increased cytokine production, as seen on bronchoalveolar lavage (BAL), as does distension of alveoli [51]. A range of potentially injurious ventilatory patterns have been evaluated and all cause increased cytokine production [39,48,51–54]. They may also predispose to infection [54,55]. A further aspect of this phenomenon is that regular distension of the lungs exerts different shear forces to those in ventilation modes where both volume and duration are varied. This is seen as reduced impairment in gas exchange during anaesthesia [57,58]. The effects in the lung may have repercussions on other organs [59–63].

For these reasons, if recruitment manoeuvres are to be used, it is advisable to use a lower peak pressure (to reduce the shear forces) but a higher PEEP (to hold alveoli open) than previously thought. The net result is peak pressures of 30 mmHg, often sustained for a greater portion of the respiratory cycle, together with higher levels of PEEP [36]. Nevertheless, although this reduces stretch and shear forces it increases mean intrathoracic pressure and can also create over-distension.

3.8.2 *Effects on surfactant*

Surfactants have multiple roles [64–66]. They modify the surface tension and hence Laplace's law, but also have an immunological function [67,68]. The mechanical effects of surfactant are highly efficient during normal negative pressure spontaneous breathing. The efficacy of the densely packed molecules reduces as they thin out during alveolar inflation.

This neat and effective mechanism may be altered by positive pressure [69]. Little is known of the wave mechanics of surfactant with positive pressure but it is highly likely that forced redistribution and distortion of surfactant molecules occurs. The production and functionality of surfactant are altered. If there is injury or infection damage type II pneumocytes then production will be reduced. The ability of the surfactant to form surface structures will be affected by fluid or inflammatory mediators mixing with the surface layers, a common feature in patients requiring ventilation. Fluid will dilute surfactant while polymerising fibrin released in injury adsorbs these surface-active compounds, effectively removing them. Infections are thought to alter surfactant function and the mechanics of positive pressure ventilation may also disrupt surface molecules and alter function [70,71]. Lavage, BAL and suctioning all tend to remove surfactant. The dysfunction that results will alter compliance and hence regional lung inflation and is unlikely to be uniform across the lung. As lungs become less compliant, altered ventilation may aggravate this problem. The immune defences of the lung are also surfactant-dependent. Surfactants have activity as collectins — molecules that bind to foreign particles such as bacteria, fungi and viruses and assist in their phagocytosis [72,73].

3.8.3 *Effect on the cardiovascular system*

In normal breathing the negative-pressure phase of inspiration improves venous return. The negative pressure through the interstitium alleviates pressure on the pulmonary capillaries and encourages flow.

In positive-pressure ventilation intrathoracic pressure rises during inspiration reducing venous return. The pressure is transmitted through the lung interstitium and influences capillary flow. If the pressure exceeds 7–10 mmHg it will impede capillary flow. The distribution of pressure through the interstitium will be influenced by regional lung compliance so the more compliant and therefore better aerated areas will have more pressure transmission and therefore more effect on capillary flow. In inspiration, reduced venous return reduces right ventricular output and drops pulmonary blood flow.

Paradoxically there may be a reduction in right ventricular impedance but whether this offsets the fall in venous return is unknown [74]. There is some evidence to show that as PEEP increases, right ventricular outflow tends to decrease [10,75] with consequent reduced left ventricular return. This effect may be partially offset by the raised intrathoracic pressure increasing the intrathoracic–extrathoracic gradient and assisting left ventricular output. The latter may be beneficial in cardiac failure but is not usually relevant in other circumstances where raised intrathoracic pressure reduces output [76].

In expiration the intrathoracic pressure returns towards zero so that venous return will increase. PEEP maintains positive intrathoracic pressure and continues to inhibit venous return throughout the cycle.

Manoeuvres to obviate this phenomenon may include increased fluid administration to increase venous return. While this will help correct atrial filling and hence cardiac output, it will also raise end-capillary pressures in the lungs and other organs. This in turn will have an effect on capillary flow. In many situations these effects are reversible by increased fluid administration but the effects of high end-capillary pressure on organ function have never been fully evaluated [77,78].

In positive pressure ventilation with PEEP the inferior vena cava is less collapsible throughout the respiratory cycle, indicating a degree of venous stasis [10].

3.8.4 *Effect on lymphatics*

Positive pressure also affects the flow of lymph. The lymphatics are important in immune defence, draining fluid from the interstitium to a collection and filtration system via the reticuloendothelial system; this removes extraneous material before it reaches the circulation. The application of pressure to what is a very efficient low-pressure drainage system may significantly influence the efficacy of the system and impair drainage. It is postulated that this phenomenon predisposes to infection. Most importantly, however, it is chronic venous and lymphatic obstruction that leads to infection [79–81].

With positive-pressure ventilation four effects will influence the mechanics of the system. At the alveolus, positive pressure will push fluid from the alveoli towards the interstitium and potentially towards the lymphatics. The gradient will push fluid into the lymphatics. Positive pressure on the interstitium will compress some peripheral lymphatics aiding flow, but others more medially which are larger collecting ducts may be easily compressed by relatively low pressures, inhibiting forward flow. Positive pressure may therefore assist and inhibit lymph flow [82]. The thin walls with one way valves assist ongoing flow especially in the larger lymphatics. The increased pressure in the central veins due to the increased intravascular volume needed to maintain cardiac output will form a hydrostatic gradient of some magnitude (Fig. 3.8) [83–86].

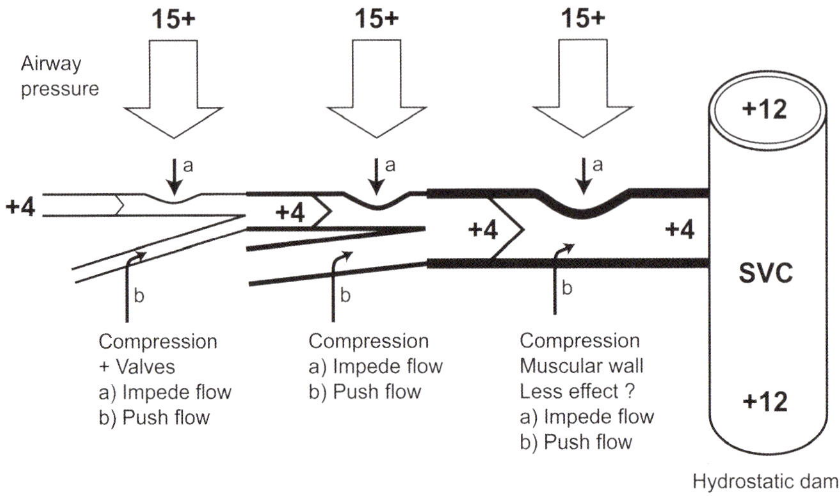

Figure 3.8. The effect of positive pressure on lymph flow in the lymphatics (adapted from [22], with permission). SVC = superior vena cava.

In expiration the central venous pressures will drop and so will intrinsic pressure on the interstitium. Flow can potentially return and the cyclical nature of pressure ventilation may be helpful. Unfortunately the application of PEEP, especially high PEEP, may obviate this, as may persistently high venous pressures. The net effect of PEEP and high central venous pressure will be a hydrostatic dam to lymphatic drainage. Several studies have demonstrated that positive-pressure ventilation is associated with increased lung water, as is the application of PEEP [87–94]. That PEEP helps remove fluid from alveoli has never been in doubt but where the fluid goes after that has never been demonstrated.

3.8.5 *Effects on fluid balance*

Positive-pressure ventilation is associated with salt and water retention [95]. Classically this is due to increased secretion of antidiuretic hormone (ADH), secondary to reduced venous return and reduced atrial distension due to the influence of positive pressure on cardiac function. Recently there has been a suggestion that the changes in ADH are not adequate to explain this effect and atrial natriuretic peptide (ANP) may also be involved, probably also mediated through the reduced atrial distension seen with positive pressure ventilation. The net effect is fluid retention [22].

References

[1] Lassen, H.C. (1954). Poliomyelitis in Copenhagen 1952, *Dan Med Bull*, **1**, 7–9.

[2] Iizuka, M. (2003). $GABA_A$ and glycine receptors in regulation of intercostal and abdominal expiratory activity *in vitro* in neonatal rat, *J Physiol*, **551**, 617–633.

[3] Bristow, J.D., Brown Jr, E.B., Cunningham, D.J. *et al.* (1971). The effects of hypercapnia, hypoxia and ventilation on the baroreflex regulation of the pulse interval, *J Physiol*, **216**, 281–302.

[4] Sandek, K., Bratel, T., Hellstrom, G. *et al.* (2001). Ventilation–perfusion inequality and carbon dioxide sensitivity in hypoxaemic chronic obstructive pulmonary disease (COPD) and effects of 6 months of long-term oxygen treatment (LTOT), *Clin Physiol*, **21**, 584–593.

[5] Ursino, M., Magosso, E. and Avanzolini, G. (2001). An integrated model of the human ventilatory control system: the response to hypercapnia, *Clin Physiol*, **21**, 447–464.

[6] Kara, T., Narkiewicz, K. and Somers, V.K. (2003). Chemoreflexes — physiology and clinical implications, *Acta Physiol Scand*, **177**, 377–384.

[7] Pinsky, M.R. (1990). The effects of mechanical ventilation on the cardiovascular system, *Crit Care Clin*, **6**, 663–678.

[8] Mergoni, M. and Rossi, A. (2001). Physiopathology of acute respiratory failure in COPD and asthma, *Minerva Anestesiol*, **67**, 198–205.

[9] Nieman, G.F., Paskanik, A.M. and Bredenberg, C.E. (1988). Effect of positive end-expiratory pressure on alveolar capillary perfusion, *J Thorac Cardiovasc Surg*, **95**, 712–716.

[10] Mitaka, C., Nagura T., Sakanishi, N. *et al.* (1989). Two-dimensional echocardiographic evaluation of inferior vena cava, right ventricle, and left ventricle during positive-pressure ventilation with varying levels of positive end-expiratory pressure, *Crit Care Med*, **17**, 205–210.

[11] Cope, D.K., Parker, J.C., Taylor, M.D. *et al.* (1989). Pulmonary capillary pressures during hypoxia and hypoxemia: experimental and clinical studies, *Crit Care Med*, **17**, 853–857.

[12] Siegel, L.C., Pearl, R.G. and August, D.A. (1993). Pulmonary capillary pressure measurement during global hypoxia in sheep, *Anesth Analg*, **76**, 149–155.

[13] Ranieri, V.M., Giuliani, R., Cinnella, G. *et al.* (1993). Physiologic effects of positive end-expiratory pressure in patients with chronic obstructive pulmonary disease during acute ventilatory failure and controlled mechanical ventilation, *Am Rev Respir Dis*, **147**, 5–13.

[14] Milic-Emili, J. (1990). Dynamic pulmonary hyperinflation and intrinsic PEEP: consequences and management in patients with chronic obstructive pulmonary disease, *Recent Prog Med*, **81**, 733–737.

[15] Fernandez, R., Benito, S., Blanch, L. *et al.* (1988). Intrinsic PEEP: a cause of inspiratory muscle ineffectivity, *Intens Care Med*, **15**, 51–52.

[16] O'Donoghue, F.J., Catcheside, P.G., Jordan, A.S. *et al.* (2002). Effect of CPAP on intrinsic PEEP, inspiratory effort, and lung volume in severe stable COPD, *Thorax*, **57**, 533–539.

[17] Marini, J.J. (1990). Strategies to minimize breathing effort during mechanical ventilation, *Crit Care Clin*, **6**, 635–661.

[18] West, J.B. and Dollery, C.T. (1960). Distribution of blood flow and ventilation-perfusion ratio in the lung, measured with radioactive carbon dioxide. *J Appl Physiol*, **15**, 405–410.

[19] Milic-Emili, J., Henderson, J.A., Dolovich, M.B. *et al.* (1966). Regional distribution of inspired gas in the lung, *J Appl Physiol*, **21**, 749–759.

[20] Farhi, L.E. (1966). 'Ventilation–perfusion relationship and its role in alveolar gas exchange', in Caro, C.G. (ed.), *Advances in Respiratory Physiology*, Arnold, London, pp. 148–197.

[21] Nicholas, T.E. (1996). Pulmonary surfactant: no mere paint on the alveolar wall, *Respirology*, **1**, 247–257.

[22] Soni, N. and Williams, P. (2008). Positive pressure ventilation: what is the real cost? *Br J Anaesth*, **101**, 446–457.

[23] Hinz, J., Moerer, O., Neumann, P. *et al.* (2006). Regional pulmonary pressure volume curves in mechanically ventilated patients with acute respiratory failure measured by electrical impedance tomography, *Acta Anaesthesiol Scand*, **50**, 331–339.

[24] Gattinoni, L., Agostoni, A., Damia, G. *et al.* (1980). Hemodynamics and renal function during low frequency positive pressure ventilation with extracorporeal CO_2 removal. A comparison with continuous positive pressure ventilation, *Intens Care Med*, **6**, 155–161.

[25] Kallet, R.H. and Katz, J.A. (2003). Respiratory system mechanics in acute respiratory distress syndrome, *Respir Care Clin N Am*, **9**, 297–319.

[26] Albaiceta, G.M., Taboada, F., Parra, D. *et al.* (2004). Tomographic study of the inflection points of the pressure–volume curve in acute lung injury, *Am J Respir Crit Care Med*, **170**, 1066–1072.

[27] Pestana, D., Hernandez-Gancedo, C., Royo, C. *et al.* (2005). Pressure–volume curve variations after a recruitment manoeuvre in acute lung injury/ARDS patients: implications for the understanding of the inflection points of the curve, *Eur J Anaesthesiol*, **22**, 175–180.
[28] Barbas, C.S., de Matos, G.F., Okamoto, V. *et al.* (2003). Lung recruitment maneuvers in acute respiratory distress syndrome, *Respir Care Clin N Am*, **9**, 401–418, vii.
[29] Hinz, J., Gehoff, A., Moerer, O. *et al.* (2007). Regional filling characteristics of the lungs in mechanically ventilated patients with acute lung injury, *Eur J Anaesthesiol*, **24**, 414–424.
[30] Meier, T., Luepschen, H., Karsten, J. *et al.* (2008). Assessment of regional lung recruitment and derecruitment during a PEEP trial based on electrical impedance tomography, *Intens Care Med*, **34**, 543–550.
[31] Valente Barbas, C.S. (2003). Lung recruitment maneuvers in acute respiratory distress syndrome and facilitating resolution, *Crit Care Med*, **31**(Suppl. 4), S265–S271.
[32] Bayle, F., Guerin, C., Viale, J.P. *et al.* (2004). Effects of positive end-expiratory pressure on the sigmoid equation in experimental acute lung injury, *Intens Care Med*, **30**, 2121–2125.
[33] Gattinoni, L., D'Andrea, L., Pelosi, P. *et al.* (1993). Regional effects and mechanism of positive end-expiratory pressure in early adult respiratory distress syndrome, *JAMA*, **269**, 2122–2127.
[34] Hickling, K.G. (2002). Reinterpreting the pressure–volume curve in patients with acute respiratory distress syndrome, *Curr Opin Crit Care*, **8**, 32–38.
[35] De Robertis, E., Servillo, G., Pezza, M. *et al.* (2003). Derecruitment of the lung induced by stepwise lowering of positive end-expiratory pressure in patients with adult respiratory distress syndrome, *Eur J Anaesthesiol*, **20**, 794–799.
[36] Lapinsky, S.E. and Mehta, S. (2005). Bench-to-bedside review: Recruitment and recruiting maneuvers, *Crit Care*, **9**, 60–65.
[37] The Acute Respiratory Distress Syndrome Network (2000). Ventilation with lower tidal volumes as compared with traditional tidal volumes for acute lung injury and the acute respiratory distress syndrome, *N Engl J Med*, **342**, 1301–1308.
[38] dos Santos, C.C. and Slutsky, A.S. (2006). The contribution of biophysical lung injury to the development of biotrauma, *Annu Rev Physiol*, **68**, 585–618.
[39] Slutsky, A.S. and Imai, Y. (2003). Ventilator-induced lung injury, cytokines, PEEP, and mortality: implications for practice and for clinical trials, *Intens Care Med*, **29**, 1218–1221.

[40] Simbruner, G., Mittal, R.A., Smith, J. *et al.* (2007). Effects of duration and amount of lung stretch at biophysical, biochemical, histological, and transcriptional levels in an in vivo rabbit model of mild lung injury, *Am J Perinatol*, **24**, 149–159.

[41] Copland, I.B., Reynaud, D., Pace-Asciak, C. *et al.* (2006). Mechanotransduction of stretch-induced prostanoid release by fetal lung epithelial cells, *Am J Physiol Lung Cell Mol Physiol*, **291**, L487–L495.

[42] Marini, J.J. (2004). Relative importance of stretch and shear in ventilator-induced lung injury, *Crit Care Med*, **32**, 302–304.

[43] Chu, E.K., Whitehead, T. and Slutsky, A.S. (2004). Effects of cyclic opening and closing at low- and high-volume ventilation on bronchoalveolar lavage cytokines, *Crit Care Med*, **32**, 168–174.

[44] Gattinoni, L., Vagginelli, F., Chiumello, D. *et al.* (2003). Physiologic rationale for ventilator setting in acute lung injury/acute respiratory distress syndrome patients, *Crit Care Med*, **31**(Suppl. 4), S300–S304.

[45] Zhang, H., Downey, G.P., Suter, P.M. *et al.* (2002). Conventional mechanical ventilation is associated with bronchoalveolar lavage-induced activation of polymorphonuclear leukocytes: a possible mechanism to explain the systemic consequences of ventilator-induced lung injury in patients with ARDS, *Anesthesiology*, **97**, 1426–1433.

[46] Suter, P.M. (2006). Reducing ventilator-induced lung injury and other organ injury by the prone position, *Crit Care*, **10**, 139.

[47] Dreyfuss, D. and Saumon, G. (1998). From ventilator-induced lung injury to multiple organ dysfunction? *Intens Care Med*, **24**, 102–104.

[48] Dos Santos, C.C. and Slutsky, A.S. (2000). Invited review: mechanisms of ventilator-induced lung injury: a perspective, *J Appl Physiol*, **89**, 1645–1655.

[49] Gattinoni, L., Chiumello, D. and Russo, R. (2002). Reduced tidal volumes and lung protective ventilatory strategies: where do we go from here? *Curr Opin Crit Care*, **8**, 45–50.

[50] MacIntyre, N.R. (2005). Current issues in mechanical ventilation for respiratory failure, *Chest*, **128**(5, Suppl. 2), 561S–567S.

[51] Gattinoni, L., Carlesso, E., Cadringher, P. *et al.* (2003). Physical and biological triggers of ventilator-induced lung injury and its prevention, *Eur Respir J Suppl*, **47**, 15s–25s.

[52] Halbertsma, F.J., Vaneker, M., Scheffer, G.J. *et al.* (2005). Cytokines and biotrauma in ventilator-induced lung injury: a critical review of the literature, *Neth J Med*, **63**, 382–392.

[53] Ranieri, V.M., Suter, P.M., Tortorella, C. *et al.* (1999). Effect of mechanical ventilation on inflammatory mediators in patients with acute respiratory distress syndrome: a randomized controlled trial, *JAMA*, **282**, 54–61.

[54] Ricard, J.D., Dreyfuss, D. and Saumon, G. (2003). Ventilator-induced lung injury, *Eur Respir J Suppl*, **42**, 2s–9s.

[55] Lin, CY., Zhang, H., Cheng, K.C. *et al.* (2003). Mechanical ventilation may increase susceptibility to the development of bacteremia, *Crit Care Med*, **31**, 1429–1434.

[56] Tremblay, L.N., Miatto, D., Hamid, Q. *et al.* (2002). Injurious ventilation induces widespread pulmonary epithelial expression of tumor necrosis factor-α and interleukin-6 messenger RNA, *Crit Care Med*, **30**, 1693–700.

[57] Mutch, W.A., Eschun, G.M., Kowalski, S.E. *et al.* (2000). Biologically variable ventilation prevents deterioration of gas exchange during prolonged anaesthesia, *Br J Anaesth*, **84**, 197–203.

[58] Boker, A., Haberman, C.J., Girling, L. *et al.* (2004). Variable ventilation improves perioperative lung function in patients undergoing abdominal aortic aneurysmectomy, *Anesthesiology*, **100**, 608–616.

[59] Kredel, M., Muellenbach, R.M., Brock, R.W. *et al.* (2007). Liver dysfunction after lung recruitment manoeuvres during pressure-controlled ventilation in experimental acute respiratory distress, *Crit Care*, **11**, R13.

[60] Edibam, C. (2000). Ventilator-induced lung injury and implications for clinical management, *Crit Care Resusc*, **2**, 269–277.

[61] Moloney, E.D. and Griffiths, M.J. (2004). Protective ventilation of patients with acute respiratory distress syndrome, *Br J Anaesth*, **92**, 261–270.

[62] Mandava, S., Kolobow, T., Vitale, G. *et al.* (2003). Lethal systemic capillary leak syndrome associated with severe ventilator-induced lung injury: an experimental study, *Crit Care Med*, **31**, 885–892.

[63] Dos Santos, C.C. and Slutsky, A.S. (2000). Mechanotransduction, ventilator-induced lung injury and multiple organ dysfunction syndrome, *Intens Care Med*, **26**, 638–642.

[64] D'Angelo, E., Pecchiari, M. and Gentile, G. (2007). Dependence of lung injury on surface tension during low-volume ventilation in normal open-chest rabbits, *J Appl Physiol*, **102**, 174–182.

[65] Haagsman, H.P. and Diemel, R.V. (2001). Surfactant-associated proteins: functions and structural variation, *Comp Biochem Physiol A Mol Integr Physiol*, **129**, 91–108.

[66] Hamm, H., Fabel, H. and Bartsch, W. (1992). The surfactant system of the adult lung: physiology and clinical perspectives, *Clin Investig*, **70**, 637–657.

[67] Sim, R.B., Clark, H., Hajela, K. *et al.* (2006). Collectins and host defence, *Novartis Found Symp*, **279**, 170–181. Discussion 181–186, 216–219.

[68] Wright, J.R. (2005). Immunoregulatory functions of surfactant proteins, *Nat Rev Immunol*, **5**, 58–68.

[69] Taskar, V., John, J., Evander, E. *et al.* (1995). Healthy lungs tolerate repetitive collapse and reopening during short periods of mechanical ventilation, *Acta Anaesthesiol Scand*, **39**, 370–376.

[70] Bruckner, L., Gigliotti, F., Wright, T. *et al.* (2006). *Pneumocystis carinii* infection sensitizes lung to radiation-induced injury after syngeneic marrow transplantation: role of $CD4^+$ T cells, *Am J Physiol Lung Cell Mol Physiol*, **290**, L1087–L1096.

[71] Panda, A.K., Nag, K., Harbottle, R.R. *et al.* (2004). Effect of acute lung injury on structure and function of pulmonary surfactant films, *Am J Respir Cell Mol Biol*, **30**, 641–650.

[72] Gan, X., Jarstrand, C., Herting, E. *et al.* (2001). Effect of surfactant and specific antibody on bacterial proliferation and lung function in experimental pneumococcal pneumonia, *Int J Infect Dis*, **5**, 9–18.

[73] Gehr, P., Im Hof, V., Geiser, M. *et al.* (2000). [The mucociliary system of the lung–role of surfactants], *Schweiz Med Wochenschr*, **130**, 691–698.

[74] Miranda, D.R., Klompe, L., Meke, l J. *et al.* (2006). Open lung ventilation does not increase right ventricular outflow impedance: an echo-Doppler study, *Crit Care Med*, **34**, 2555–2560.

[75] van den Berg, P.C., Grimbergen, C.A., Spaan, J.A. *et al.* (1997). Positive pressure inspiration differentially affects right and left ventricular outputs in postoperative cardiac surgery patients, *J Crit Care*, **12**, 56–65.

[76] Pinsky, M.R. (2005). Cardiovascular issues in respiratory care, *Chest*, **128** (5, Suppl. 2), 592S–597S.

[77] Shibayama, Y. (1987). The role of hepatic venous congestion and endotoxaemia in the production of fulminant hepatic failure secondary to congestive heart failure, *J Pathol*, **151**, 133–138.

[78] Priebe, H.J., Heimann, J.C. and Hedley-Whyte, J. (1980). Effects of renal and hepatic venous congestion on renal function in the presence of low and normal cardiac output in dogs, *Circ Res*, **47**, 883–890.

[79] Cui ,Y., Urschel, J.D. and Petrelli, N.J. (2001). The effect of cardiopulmonary lymphatic obstruction on heart and lung function, *Thorac Cardiovasc Surg*, **49**, 35–40.

[80] Mortimer, P.S. (2000). Implications of the lymphatic system in CVI-associated edema, *Angiology*, **51**, 3–7.

[81] Rohn, D.A., Stewart, R.H., Elk, J.R. *et al.* (1996). Renal lymphatic function following venous pressure elevation, *Lymphology*, **29**, 67–75.

[82] Pearse, D.B., Searcy, R.M., Mitzner, W. *et al.* (2005). Effects of tidal volume and respiratory frequency on lung lymph flow, *J Appl Physiol*, **99**, 556–563.

[83] Szabo, G. and Magyar, Z. (1967). Effect of increased systemic venous pressure on lymph pressure and flow, *Am J Physiol*, **212**, 1469–1474.

[84] Browse, N.L., Lord, R.S. and Taylor, A. (1971). Pressure waves and gradients in the canine thoracic duct, *J Physiol*, **213**, 507–524.

[85] Laine, G.A., Allen, S.J., Katz, J. *et al.* (1986). Effect of systemic venous pressure elevation on lymph flow and lung edema formation, *J Appl Physiol*, **61**, 1634–1638.

[86] Moore-Olufemi, S.D., Xue H., Allen, S.J. *et al.* (2005). Effects of primary and secondary intra-abdominal hypertension on mesenteric lymph flow: implications for the abdominal compartment syndrome, *Shock*, **23**, 571–575.

[87] Maybauer, D.M., Talke, P.O., Westphal, M. *et al.* (2006). Positive end-expiratory pressure ventilation increases extravascular lung water due to a decrease in lung lymph flow, *Anaesth Intensive Care*, **34**, 329–333.

[88] Blomqvist, H., Frostell, C., Pieper, R. *et al.* (1990). Measurement of dynamic lung fluid balance in the mechanically ventilated dog. Theory and results, *Acta Anaesthesiol Scand*, **34**, 370–376.

[89] Haider, M., Schad, H. and Mendler, N. (1987). Thoracic duct lymph and PEEP studies in anaesthetized dogs. I. Lymph formation and the effect of a thoracic duct fistula on lymph flow, *Intens Care Med*, **13**, 183–191.

[90] van der Zee, H., Cooper, J.A., Hakim, T.S. *et al.* (1986). Alterations in pulmonary fluid balance induced by positive end-expiratory pressure, *Respir Physiol*, **64**, 125–133.

[91] Last, M., Kurtz, L., Stein, T.A. *et al.* (1983). Effect of PEEP on the rate of thoracic duct lymph flow and clearance of bacteria from the peritoneal cavity, *Am J Surg*, **145**, 126–130.

[92] Allen, S.J., Drake, R.E., Laine, G.A. *et al.* (1991). Effect of thoracic duct drainage on hydrostatic pulmonary edema and pleural effusion in sheep, *J Appl Physiol*, **71**, 314–316.

[93] Hersch, M., Bersten, A., Robertson, S. *et al.* (1989). PEEP increases non-pulmonary microvascular fluid flux in healthy and septic sheep, *Chest*, **96**, 1142–1149.

[94] Frostell, C., Blomqvist, H., Pieper, R. *et al.* (1986). Separate thoracic and abdominal lymph flow in the dog, *Acta Chir Scand Suppl*, **530**, 5–7.

[95] Rossaint, R., Krebs, M., Forther, J. *et al.* (1993). Inferior vena caval pressure increase contributes to sodium and water retention during PEEP in awake dogs, *J Appl Physiol*, **75**, 2484–2492.

4

Cellular Physiology in Critical Care

David Brealey and David Howell

4.1 Oxygen Delivery and Cellular Utilisation

Adequate organ function in health and disease is critically dependent on an adequate supply of oxygen for aerobic production of adenosine triphosphate (ATP) generation, i.e. a continuous supply of oxygen from the air to the mitochondria is required in order to sustain aerobic metabolism. This process occurs as a series of steps involving flow from the heart and lungs, efficient transport across the extravascular matrix and extraction at the tissue level. Ultimately, the circulatory transport of O_2 from the lungs, oxygen delivery (DO_2), must meet the metabolic demands of the tissues, oxygen consumption (VO_2), or circulatory shock occurs. The extraction ratio (ERO_2), the ratio of VO_2 to DO_2, describes the amount of oxygen consumed as a fraction of delivery, and in the normal person is about 25%.

In normal subjects the basal tissue DO_2 is sufficient to supply the tissues with oxygen and substrate to allow aerobic respiration at rest. Increasing DO_2 only increases tissue VO_2 slightly, due to increased cardiac work. However, in the face of an increased demand, such as in critical illness, tissue oxygen delivery is increased by both an elevation in cardiac output, and by more oxygen being extracted from haemoglobin. The ERO_2, can increase from a basal level of approximately 0.25 to a maximum of 0.80 at the point of maximum exertion. The increase in ERO_2 is mainly through nutrient capillary recruitment. However, there comes a point where delivery can no longer match consumption, and an oxygen debt is created. This point, the anaerobic threshold (DO_{2crit}), occurs at an ERO_2 of approximately 0.60. At this point VO_2 becomes dependent on DO_2 and is termed physiological supply dependency. Below the DO_{2crit} anaerobic respiration attempts to make up the shortfall in ATP production. This applies to severe exercise in healthy patients and to patients suffering from cardiogenic or hypovolaemic shock.

Patients who maintain high levels of DO_2 fare significantly better than those unable to do so. This has been demonstrated in those undergoing high-risk surgery, trauma patients [1] and those with ARDS [2] and sepsis [3]. A mismatch between DO_2 and VO_2 introduces a concept of oxygen debt. In surgical patients the size of peri-operative oxygen debt was related to outcome [4]. Non-surviving patients had the largest oxygen debt in the early post-operative period (33.5 l/m^2), while those patients who made an uncomplicated recovery had an oxygen debt of only 8.0 l/m^2.

By reducing peri-operative oxygen debt in high-risk surgical patients through targeted oxygen delivery goals using fluid and inotropes, investigators have demonstrated significant improvement in mortality rates.

These results may translate into the treatment of the critically ill in the initial stages of their illness. Rivers and colleagues studied 263 patients admitted to an emergency room (ER) with severe sepsis [5]. Those randomly assigned to an 'early goal-directed group' received a fluid, vasoactive and blood transfusion regimen to a specific protocol to achieve pre-specified haemodynamic targets while in the ER. They had a significantly lower hospital mortality rate compared with those receiving standard care who otherwise received identical treatment (30% versus 46.5%). Multicentre trials in the UK, USA and Australia are currently underway to verify this finding.

In intensive care unit (ICU) patients with already established organ dysfunction, the situation is far more complex. Attempts to enhance DO_2:VO_2 have been generally disappointing with only a slight benefit [6], no difference [7] or harm [8] being reported. These studies suggest that the way patients utilise oxygen is fundamentally different in the early stages of critical illness compared with when organ dysfunction is established.

Sepsis is usually characterised by an increased cardiac output but a decreased arteriovenous oxygen difference and reduced oxygen extraction. This high output state does not appear to be 'luxury flow' in excess of metabolic needs as there is usually a concurrent lactic acidosis (which may or may not be due to tissue hypoxia) and organ dysfunction/failure. This could be explained by a loss of control within the microvasculature where it is unable to locally match oxygen supply and demand resulting in some capillary beds becoming ischaemic, whilst others are over-perfused. However in both septic animal models and patients the tissue oxygen tension (PtO_2) is found to be raised. This is in contrast to low-flow states such as hypovolaemia or cardiogenic shock where PtO_2 falls. This rise is correlated with the severity of sepsis, and in those who go on to survive, the PtO_2 returns to normal but it remains elevated in non-survivors. The decrease in oxygen extraction and raised PtO_2 can be explained as an impairment of oxygen utilisation rather than a problem of oxygen delivery. As mitochondria are responsible for the vast majority (>90%) of a cell's oxygen utilisation, mainly for the process of oxidative phosphorylation and ATP generation, it is now widely believed that mitochondrial dysfunction may play a central role in the organ dysfunction associated with sepsis. To understand this further it is necessary to have a more in-depth look at mitochondria and some of their processes.

4.1.1 *Mitochondria*

Mitochondria are intracellular organelles present in almost all eukaryotic cells and perform the following roles:

- Control of metabolic processes, including ATP generation (by the process of oxidative phosphorylation), fatty acid oxidation and urea formation.
- Control of cell death by the initiation of apoptotic or necrotic processes.
- Ca^{2+} and ion homeostasis.
- Intracellular signalling.
- Heat production.

Mitochondria consist of a central matrix surrounded by an inner and an outer mitochondrial membrane. The outer membrane is permeable whilst the inner membrane, owing to its high cardiolipin content, is highly impermeable. It is this impermeability which allows the mitochondria to carry out many of their functions. The inner membrane is thrown into folds, known as cristae, giving the mitochondrion its classical appearance and massively expanding its surface area (total area estimated to be the equivalent of two football pitches). Mitochondria contain their own circular genome, which in humans encodes 37 different genes. This genome bears some similarity to that of *Rickettsia*, prompting some to suggest that mitochondria were originally prokaryotes that were endocytosed and have formed a symbiotic relationship with their host.

Mitochondrial involvement in certain disease states has been recognised for many years. Spontaneous or inherited defects in mitochondrial or nuclear DNA may affect oxidative phosphorylation and give rise to a large and heterogeneous group of disorders with a prevalence of 1 in 4,000 births. Examples include Leigh Syndrome, mitochondrial encephalomyopathy with lactic acidosis and stroke-like episodes (MELAS) and Kearns–Sayre syndrome. Only more recently have acquired defects in mitochondrial oxidative phosphorylation been postulated as being important in the pathogenesis of disease states, such as Parkinson's and Alzheimer's diseases, heart failure and, of particular relevance to critical care, sepsis and inflammation, which are discussed later in this chapter.

4.1.1.1 *Energy transduction*

All cells require energy to survive. The majority of this energy is used in maintaining ionic gradients, the manufacture and repair of proteins and DNA. Energy is obtained from the cell's environment and through a number of steps transduced into a form that can be readily used; in humans this is ATP. Mitochondria are key to its efficient generation through the process of oxidative phosphorylation fuelled by the process of glycolysis and the oxidation of fatty acids.

Glycolysis is the catabolic process where a six-carbon glucose molecule is metabolised by a series of enzymatic reactions to two pyruvate (three-carbon) molecules. This process results in the net production of two molecules of ATP and, crucially, does not require oxygen. The process occurs in the cytoplasm and is the cell's source of ATP in conditions of low/absent O_2, anaerobic respiration. Pyruvate can undergo oxidative decarboxylation, by pyruvate dehydrogenase, to generate acetyl-CoA and enter the tricarboxylic acid (Krebs) cycle.

Fatty acids are oxidised within mitochondria by most cells (except those of the brain and intestine). The process of fatty acid oxidation is termed β-oxidation since it occurs through the sequential removal of two-carbon units by oxidation at the β-carbon position of the fatty acyl-coenzyme A (CoA) molecule. Each round of β-oxidation produces one molecule of reduced nicotinamide-adenine dinucleotide (NADH), reduced flavin adenine dinucleotide ($FADH_2$) and acetyl-CoA.

The acetyl-CoA molecule, produced by these processes, condenses with oxaloacetate (a four-carbon compound) to generate citrate. Through a series of reactions (comprising the tricaboxylic acid cycle) the two carbons from the acetyl group are then released as carbon dioxide, and the oxaloacetate is regenerated. During this process oxidised nicotinamide-adenine dinucleotide (NAD^+) and fumarate are reduced to NADH and succinate respectively. These two compounds then provide electrons to the mitochondrial respiratory chain. A pyrophosphate bond is also generated in the form of guanosine triphosphate. This is readily transferred to adenosine diphosphate (ADP) to form ATP.

4.1.1.2 *The mitochondrial respiratory chain*

The respiratory chain is the terminal portion of the oxidative phosphorylation pathway and is responsible for the majority of the body's oxygen consumption and ATP generation. Located in the inner membrane, the respiratory chain is composed of four individual complexes (complexes I to IV) and two electron carriers (ubiquinone and cytochrome C (Cyt C)) (see Fig. 4.1). These complexes operate a series of electron transfers with the subsequent oxidation and reduction of the donor and acceptor ultimately transferring electrons down a redox gradient from NADH or succinate to finally oxidise O_2 to water. Electrons cannot be transferred randomly from one complex to another but must follow a sequence

The transfer of electrons through the series of redox centres allows for the extrusion of protons from the matrix to the intermembrane space. This generates a proton motive force (Δp) across the membrane, composed of an electrical potential ($\Delta\psi$) and a pH gradient (ΔpH). It is

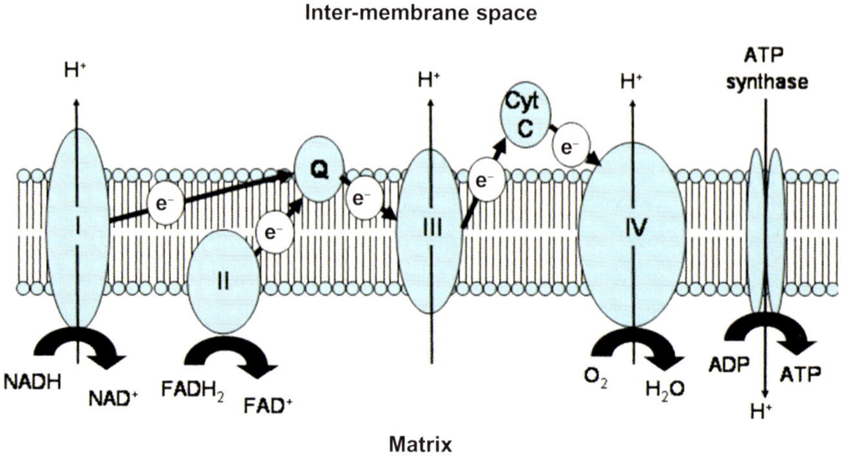

Figure 4.1. The mitochondrial respiratory chain.

estimated that for every molecule of NADH oxidised by the respiratory chain, ten hydrogen ions are extruded (four by complex I, two by complex III and four by complex IV). However, only six hydrogen ions are extruded with the oxidation of succinate (two by complex III and four by complex IV) due to the lower redox potential of the fumarate–succinate couple. The physical movement of protons across the inner mitochondrial membrane is not fully understood.

The Δp generated can then be utilised by the mitochondria in a number of ways;

(i) ATP synthesis, using the ATP synthase enzyme (q.v.).
(ii) Ion and metabolite transport, such as translocation of ATP/ADP and Na^+/H^+ exchange.
(iii) Thermogenesis. Brown adipocytes, common in newborn mammals, contain large numbers of mitochondria. These contain a transmembrane protein known as uncoupling protein-1 (UCP1). Triglyceride stores are hydrolysed to free fatty acids which, in turn, bind to UCP1. This protein now undergoes a conformational change, allowing it to conduct protons, thus lowering Δp and releasing heat. A further four UCPs have been described, two in the brain and two distributed through numerous tissues. UCPs are also thought to be involved in controlling metabolic rate and free radical production [9].

(iv) Proton leak. The inner mitochondrial membrane is not completely impermeable to protons and a proportion will 'leak' back into the matrix lowering Δp. The reason for this is not fully understood. The extent of the leak varies between species; anoxia-tolerant animals have less permeable mitochondrial membranes than mammals. This may allow them to redirect a greater proportion of Δp toward ATP generation when oxygen tensions (and the rate of respiration) fall [10].

4.1.2 *Control of cellular respiration*

In essence respiration is controlled by the thermodynamic disequilibrium between the redox potential across the respiratory chain and Δp. If the inner mitochondrial membrane was impermeable to protons, respiration would generate a proton gradient of approximately −200 mV. At this point equilibrium would be achieved and respiration would stop. However, if the proton gradient is dissipated (e.g. by ATP synthesis, proton leak, etc.) this equilibrium is lost and respiration accelerates.

In health, as metabolic activity increases there is a transient fall in the ATP:ADP ratio, to redress this there is an increase in the activity of ATP synthase and a partial dissipation of Δp. The equilibrium between the redox potential across the respiratory chain and Δp becomes disturbed and so respiration increases to restore the balance.

In disease this equilibrium can be rapidly disrupted. This is most dramatic during episodes of ischaemia; without oxygen, electron transfer ceases, as does proton extrusion, with consequent collapse of Δp, without which ATP synthase ceases to function. The collapse of Δp and dramatic decrease in the ATP:ADP ratio are both triggers for cell apoptosis. Accelerated (anaerobic) glycolysis can partially compensate for this loss of ATP, whilst ATP synthase can potentially work in reverse, hydrolysing ATP to maintain Δp. These mechanisms can only maintain homeostasis for a short period and, unless the supply of oxygen is restored, cell death results.

Inhibitors of mitochondrial respiration may also potentiate a collapse of Δp. A well-recognised example is cyanide, a non-competitive inhibitor of complex IV which rapidly inhibits cellular respiration. Less dramatic examples include carbon monoxide (CO), which will be discussed later (see Section 4.1.4.1), and nitric oxide (NO). Both CO and NO are produced endogenously, particularly during periods of inflammation. NO can be produced in large quantities and has been particularly well studied.

4.1.2.1 *Nitric oxide*

NO is a free radical gas important in numerous other physiological processes such as control of vascular tone, inhibition of platelet aggregation, signalling, memory formation and enhancing neutrophil cytotoxicity. It is produced by numerous cell types, either by the action of nitric oxide synthase (NOS) on L-arginine, or derived from endogenous NO donors, such as nitrosothiols. There are three NOS isoforms, two constitutive (endothelial NOS (eNOS) and neuronal NOS (nNOS)) and one inducible (iNOS), there is also potentially a mitochondrial isoform (mtNOS). The constitutive isoforms maintain a background level of NO to carry out normal physiological functions. The inducible isoform has very little activity in health; however, its production can be markedly and rapidly upregulated in response to stress.

All three NOS isoforms generate NO by the oxidation of L-arginine to citrulline. Each NOS molecule is a homodimer with each monomer comprised of an oxygenase and a reductase domain. These domains are separated by a central region that binds calmodulin (a calcium-binding protein). Calmodulin (and therefore calcium) can control NO production as binding permits the transfer of electrons from the reductase to the oxidase domain. iNOS has a much higher affinity for calmodulin than either eNOS or nNOS, making binding essentially irreversible and therefore persistently active.

NO is rapidly deactivated by binding to haemoglobin [11] (for which it has a high affinity), reaction with thiol residues to form nitrosothiols, (these may then act as a NO reservoir) [12], auto-oxidation to nitrite or by reacting with reactive oxygen species (ROS) to form peroxynitrite ($ONOO^-$) and other derivatives [13].

4.1.3 *Sepsis and mitochondria activity*

Mitochondrial function during a septic illness almost certainly varies as the illness progresses.

The first few hours of a septic insult are difficult to investigate in patients as they rarely present until they are unwell. However it can be reproduced in healthy volunteers given intravenous endotoxin or in animal models. These first few hours tend to be associated with an increased DO_2 but also increased VO_2, and, in the small amount of human data available, enhanced mitochondrial activity. However as time progresses and sepsis becomes established, VO_2 starts to fall and the magnitude of this relates to disease severity. At this point there is often evidence of mitochondrial impairment which is a consequence of the inflammatory response.

As discussed above, an inflammatory response results in a marked increase in iNOS activity and NO production in both animal models and septic patients. Clinically, NO is heavily implicated in the vasodilatation and the refractory hypotension seen in septic shock, which can be restored or prevented by using NOS inhibitors. What is less clinically appreciable is the effect NO may be having on mitochondrial function. That mitochondria are affected by sepsis and NO is beyond doubt; however, it is difficult to quantify the clinical significance of findings to date. Mitochondria isolated from patients and animals with septic shock demonstrate:

- Swelling.
- Alterations in shape and size.
- Disruption to cristae.
- Presence of electron lucent areas (significance unknown).

Cell and animal models have consistently demonstrated that NO, derived either endogenously during a septic insult or exogenously, rapidly inhibits respiration. This is believed to be due to an inhibition of complex IV at either the oxidised copper atom B (Cu_B) or the reduced Fe^{2+} of the cytochrome a_3 [14,15] thus raising the apparent Michaelis constant (Km) (for oxygen) of the complex. Both these inhibitory mechanisms are competitive with oxygen and are rapidly reversible; thus changes in NO concentrations will have rapid effects on the rate of cellular respiration. These inhibitory changes can also be prevented in iNOS knockout models, or by the use of iNOS inhibitors or NO scavengers.

In health a small proportion (~ 1%) of electrons passing through the chain react directly with oxygen to form superoxide (O_2^-), however if electron transfer is inhibited, the 'upstream' complexes become reduced and O_2^- production increases markedly. O_2^- can be dismutated to hydrogen peroxide (H_2O_2) and water by either cytosolic CuZn-superoxide dismutase or mitochondrial Mn-superoxide dismutase. O_2^- is in itself pro-inflammatory, has a potential signalling role but also reacts directly with NO to produce a number of highly reactive molecules such as $ONOO^-$. $ONOO^-$ is capable of denaturing proteins, cleaving DNA [16] and causing prolonged/irreversible inhibition of the respiratory chain, in particular complex I. Thus with more prolonged exposure to NO (hours), the initial rapidly reversible inhibition becomes irreversible. Studies in septic patients have predominantly demonstrated a loss of complex I activity which, in part, may also be due to destruction of the complex. This loss of activity is particularly pronounced in the non-survivors and is directly related to NO levels. Work has also demonstrated an inhibition of the associated ATP synthase, suggesting that oxidative phosphorylation is inhibited at numerous points. The direct effect of these inhibitions on the cell's capability to generate ATP and maintain function is unknown. Muscle biopsies from septic patients have shown significantly depressed ATP levels, though this tells little about rates of ATP production and utilisation. Animal models are often contradictory, but generally short-term models demonstrate enhanced ATP utilisation whilst models extending beyond 24 hours start to show evidence of impaired production

Very little is known about mitochondrial activity and the recovery from critical illness. The work that does exist suggests that complex I activity is restored and that this is associated with evidence of enhanced mitochondrial biogenesis.

The potential of mitochondrial inhibition by reactive nitrogen or oxygen species raises the possibility of therapeutic intervention. iNOS inhibition, mitochondria-targeted antioxidants and substrate supplementation for alternative bioenergetic pathways are all candidates, but none of these have been assessed formally in a clinical trial.

4.1.4 *Mitochondrial inhibitors*

Beyond NO, there are a number of well-known environmental mitochondrial inhibitors such as CO, cyanide and alcohols. Perhaps less well known is that a number of drugs used in routine clinical care have also been implicated in pathologically inhibiting mitochondrial respiration.

4.1.4.1 *Carbon monoxide*

A colourless, odourless gas, usually produced through the incomplete combustion of fossil fuels. Poisoning may be deliberate but is often the unintentional consequence of house fires or poorly maintained/ventilated heating systems. CO accounts for approximately 500 deaths a year in the USA. Acute poisoning is confirmed from the presence of significant carboxyhaemoglobin (COHb). COHb is unable to bind oxygen and thus impairs DO_2 but CO also binds and inhibits mitochondrial complex IV (plus myoglobin and cytochrome P450), thus inhibiting VO_2. This may explain why COHb levels are poorly predictive of outcome. The management of acute CO poisoning is performed through oxygen therapy (normobaric or hyperbaric) as it significantly reduces the time for COHb to revert to Hb, and thus for restoration of DO_2. Oxygen therapy also significantly increases the rate of CO dissociation from complex IV [17], though at a slower rate than that of COHb.

4.1.4.2 *Alcohols*

Ethanol is metabolised via alcohol dehydrogenase to the toxic acetaldehyde and then via aldehydyde dehydrogenase to acetate. Acetaldehyde is capable of inhibiting respiratory chain complexes II/III and IV, generating increased levels of reactive oxygen species and a loss of ATP. Chronic alcoholism is also associated with induction of iNOS and raised levels of NO with the capability of further respiratory chain inhibition [18]. Similarly, the metabolism of methanol results in the generation of formate, which is directly toxic to complex IV. These inhibitions will result in the generation of a lactate acidosis, frequently seen in acute poisonings.

4.1.4.3 *Cyanide*

Like CO, most victims of cyanide poisoning have been involved in a fire, often domestic or vehicular. Other routes include industrial exposure, ingestion of apple, cherry or peach seeds, illicit synthesis of phencyclidine and prolonged exposure to sodium nitroprusside. Cyanide is rapidly absorbed though the gastrointestinal or respiratory tract and mucous membranes. Cyanide is an extremely effective inhibitor of complex IV and various antioxidant pathways such as catalase and glutathione reductase. A 50 mg dose of hydrogen cyanide is usually lethal. The profound respiratory chain inhibition markedly reduces VO_2 and raises venous oxygen saturations. Thus despite profound cardio/respiratory collapse the patient rarely looks cyanotic. Treatment involves chelators of cyanide such as dicobalt edetate or hydroxocobalamin. Sodium thiosulphate can be used a thiol donor to maximise the activity of rhodanese, an enzyme capable of detoxifying cyanide. Sodium nitrite can be used to induce methaemaglobin which can act as an alternative cyanide binding site as opposed to complex IV.

4.1.4.4 *Propofol*

Propofol has been demonstrated to inhibit complex I and to reduce Δp in cell culture. These findings are thought to be the pathological basis for the rare but dangerous propofol infusion syndrome (metabolic acidosis, cardiac failure and rhabdomyolysis), that occurs during prolonged, high-dose infusions.

4.1.4.5 *Metformin*

Metformin is also known to impair complex I activity. This potentially explains its hypoglycaemic action but is also thought to be the mechanism which results in the severe lactic acidosis that occurs when excretion is impaired

4.1.4.6 *Statins*

Statins are all inhibitors of 3-hydroxy-3-methyl-glutaryl-CoA reductase, which catalyses the rate-limiting step in cholesterol, dolichol and ubiquinone synthesis. The inhibition of the dolichol pathway is thought to confer some of the 'pleiotropic', immunomodulatory effects attributed to statins.

These effects have resulted in statins being adopted for conditions as diverse as sepsis, breast cancer and sub-arachnoid haemorrhage. However the inhibition of ubiquinone (an integral component of the respiratory chain) synthesis is believed to be the mechanism behind the statin-associated myopathy. Low levels of ubiquinone, impaired mitochondrial function and structure have been seen in patients suffering from statin-induced rhabdomyolysis.

4.1.4.7 *Nucleos(t)ide*

Nucleos(t)ide reverse transcriptase inhibitors are integral to the management of human immunodeficiency virus (HIV). These drugs act by inhibiting HIV reverse transcriptase enzyme but also inhibit human DNA polymerase gamma, the enzyme responsible for replication of mitochondrial DNA. The resultant defects in mitochondrial DNA have been blamed for the severe lactic acidosis and many other side effects associated with this class of drug.

4.2 Cell Death in Critical Care

Cell death is clearly central to a number of pathologies in critical care. These pathologies are often associated with a very abrupt and severe loss of local oxygen delivery (e.g. stroke or myocardial infarction) or due to physical disruption (e.g. trauma, burns). The management of these conditions aims at reducing any further cell loss by restoring DO_2 and preventing secondary injury. Cells die broadly as a result of two processes; apoptosis and necrosis. Apoptosis is often seen as a physiological response to remove unwanted or defective cells whilst necrosis is often seen as the pathological process of uncontrolled cell death. Such a distinction is artificial and it is becoming apparent that necrotic cell death now has some control elements and that both forms may be important in the critically ill. The role of cell death in other conditions such as sepsis and the multiple organ dysfunction syndrome (MODS) is far less clear. Many of the mediators released during the inflammatory process are pro-apoptotic and numerous cell and animal models have demonstrated that these act through the different apoptotic pathways [19,20]. Enhanced lymphocyte apoptosis has been associated with increased mortality in sepsis [21] and increased morbidity in high-risk surgery. Though lymphocyte apoptosis is part of the normal resolution of inflammation, excessive cell death potentially renders the patient relatively immune-compromised. Post-mortem samples obtained from patients who died of sepsis-induced MODS also demonstrated evidence of ileal and colonic columnar epithelial cell apoptosis [22]. Patients with acute lung injury (ALI) have evidence of alveolar epithelial apoptosis associated with upregulation of pro-apoptotic genes (B cell leukaemia/lymphoma 2 (*Bcl-2*), BCL2-associated X protein (*Bax*)) [23]; there is also some evidence of endothelial cell damage in human sepsis [24]. However, post-mortem studies have demonstrated minimal cell death in other vital organs, including brain, liver, kidney, heart, lung and muscle, despite evidence of biochemical and physiological organ dysfunction in both septic patients and animals [25,26].

The study of apoptosis or necrosis is a rapidly evolving and complex field, the following is a brief overview of the currently understood mechanisms.

4.2.1 *Apoptosis*

Apoptosis is the mechanism by which the body is able to calmly and quietly remove unwanted cells in a controlled manner. It has a minimal effect on surrounding cells and structures and does not generate a marked inflammatory response. An apoptotic cell is recognised by its retraction from neighbouring cells, blebbing of the cell membrane with condensation and fragmentation of its nucleus. The cell is then engulfed by phagocytes. Apoptosis may be initiated by three different routes (though others may exist); however these routes lead to a final common pathway resulting in the activation of a series of cysteine proteases known as caspases. Initiation may be through:

(i) The extrinsic route. Specific agonist ligands (familial autoimmune lymphoproliferative syndrome (Fas)-ligand, apoptosis protein 3(APO-3) ligand or tumour necrosis factor-α (TNF-α) can bind transmembrane death receptors triggering an internal conformational change and exposure of a 'death domain'. This recruits adaptor proteins such as the Fas associated death domain protein (FADD) which in turn recruits and activates pro-caspase 8 to caspase 8. This then cleaves and activates further downstream effector caspases 3 and 7. Caspase 8 also results in the proteolysis and activation of Bcl-2 homology domain 3-interacting domain death agonist (BID), a pro-apoptotic Bcl-2 protein. Bcl-2 is a family of regulator proteins which may be pro-apoptotic (e.g. BCL2-antagonist/killer (BAK), BAX, BID) or anti-apoptotic (Bcl-xL, Bcl-w). In-turn, BID results in a conformational change in BAX (Bcl-2-associated X protein) that forms an oligomeric pore with Bak in the outer mitochondrial membrane. This pore enables the release of mitochondrial cytochrome C. Free cytosolic cytochrome C combines with apoptotic protease activating factor-1 (APAF-1), ATP and procaspase 9 to form an apoptosome that then results in activation of the effector caspases 3 and 7.

(ii) The intrinsic route. Apoptosis may be effected by a number of internal cellular signals or stresses such as the withdrawal of growth factors, heat, radiation or hypoxia. This diverse range of stimuli can activate a number of Bcl-2 homology domain 3 (BH3)-only proteins (e.g. BID, Bcl2-associated agonist of cell death (BAD), Noxa, p53 upregulated modulator of apoptosis (PUMA)), which, in turn inhibit anti-apoptotic members of the Bcl-2 family. This inhibition promotes the assembly of the BAX/BAK mitochondrial pore with the subsequent release of cytochrome C and the formation of the apoptosome.

(iii) Granzyme-B-dependent route. Natural killer and cytotoxic T cells can induce apoptosis in virally infected or tumour cells by delivering a serine protease, granzyme B (in conjunction with perforin and granulysin) into the cell via the mannose 6-phosphate receptor. Granzyme B has the ability to cleave BID (described above) thus recruiting BAX and BAK with the resultant pore formation. Granzyme B can also directly activate caspase 3.

Caspase activation, by any of these routes, results in a controlled destruction of numerous vital cell processes:

(i) Direct cleavage of cellular actin and myosin, thus destroying the cytoskeleton.

(ii) Destruction of the nuclear lamina. This, in conjunction with the loss of cytoskeleton, destroys the nuclear envelope and generates the characteristic nuclear fragmentation. Caspases also activate DNases that fragment nuclear DNA, preventing cell division/repair but also preventing the release of pro-inflammatory unfragmented DNA.
(iii) Fragmentation of the endoplasmic reticulum and Golgi apparatus.
(iv) Destruction of extracellular adhesion molecules, with the consequent withdrawing of the cell from its neighbours and extracellular matrix. Potentially also making the cell more accessible to phagocytosis.

Despite all this, the plasma membrane remains intact and the cell is then removed by phagocytes. Interestingly, the apoptotic cell probably releases chemo-attractants (e.g. lysophosphatidylcholine) signalling to the phagocytic cells the need for disposal; however unlike the removal of bacteria or 'foreign' substances there is very little subsequent inflammatory response.

4.2.2 *Necrosis*

On the other hand, necrotic cell death is less controlled and almost invariably results in an inflammatory response and potential disturbance to surrounding architecture. Necrosis is often the result of overwhelming cell damage from insults such as hypoxia, radiation, direct trauma or infection. These insults may mediate cell death through a collapse of ionic gradients, ATP depletion, DNA damage and production of reactive oxygen species.

Necrosis is characterised by a disruption of the cell membrane and is often seen as uncontrolled and of no benefit to the organism. However the release of cell contents is recognised by the immune system through pattern recognition receptors (e.g. formyl receptor-1 or Toll-like receptors) found on neutrophils, macrophages, dendritic and natural killer cells. Activation of these receptors initiates an inflammatory response. The full range of molecules recognised by these receptors are yet to be fully described but include ATP, uric acid, DNA, high mobility group box-1 (HMGB-1) and heat shock proteins. Collectively they are known as damage-associated molecular patterns (DAMPS) and can be found at high levels following blunt trauma and surgery. This approach may allow the body to contain and eliminate any introduced infection and act as a warning system of distant damage. However in the presence of sterile necrosis this inflammatory response may well bc deleterious, extending the area of damage and impairing organ function.

4.3 Conclusion

The importance of oxygen delivery and its manipulation in the perioperative setting has been recognised for many years. However the inability to translate these interventions to the critically ill has frustrated many. The last decade has seen a marked improvement in the understanding of the pathophysiology behind the organ dysfunction associated with generalised inflammation. Reduced oxygen utilisation, impaired mitochondrial function and cell death have all been implicated. Pre-clinical models manipulating these processes demonstrate encouraging results but, at the time of writing, no clinical study has successfully intervened in any of these processes. Ongoing efforts to address this issue and alter the outcomes of critically ill patients are eagerly awaited.

4.4 Clinical Scenario

4.4.1 *History*

A 31-year-old Somali male presented with a two-day history of left-sided chest pain, shortness of breath and dizziness. His relevant past medical history included schizophrenia (on olanzapine), he was a Qat chewer and he drank five to six cans of strong lager a day.

On examination he was awake, oriented, with a respiratory rate of 40 and had left-sided basal crackles on auscultation.

4.4.2 *Investigations*

Initial chest radiograph showed left basal shadowing.

Electrocardiogram (ECG) showed dynamic lateral T-wave depression.

Arterial blood gas analysis (on air)

pH 7.37, PaO_2 13.2, $PaCO_2$ 1.94, base excess (BE) 10.6.

Haemoglobin (Hb) 12.4, white blood cells (WBC) 19.4, C-reactive protein (CRP) 49, Na 122, Cl^- 93, Urea 1.9, Creatinine 97, Osmol 269.

Troponin 0.06, creatine kinase 143, liver function tests clotting, B12 and folate, thyroid function tests — normal.

(i) What are the differential diagnosis and the initial treatment?

(Answers to questions (i)–(iv) are given in Section 4.4.5.)

4.4.3 *Progress*

Patient deteriorated and was reviewed by medical team.

On examination he was afebrile, Glasgow Coma Scale 15, calm, euvolaemic (2 l intravenous fluid given since admission).

His respiratory rate was 35 breaths per minute and he had a few left-sided basal crackles.

Oxygen saturations were 98% on 4 l/min O_2.

Heart rate was 120 beats per minute, blood pressure 110/50, central venous pressure elevated at 29 cm H_20, central venous oxygen saturation ($ScvO_2$) 84%.

His abdomen was soft and slightly distended.

Limbs had palpable pulses but very cold peripheries.

He was oliguric and urine dipstix showed ketones ++, capillary blood sugar was 13.8 mmol/l.

ECG showed 1mm ST depression and T-wave inversion V3–4, right heart strain.

Repeat arterial blood gas analysis (on air)

pH 7.37 → 7.14

PaO_2 13.2 → 12

$PaCO_2$ 1.94 → 1.9

BE −10.6 → −23

Lactate → 16

(ii) What is the differential diagnosis now?

4.4.4 *Further progress*

A sliding scale of insulin was commenced with potassium supplementation.

Antibiotics and low-molecular-weight heparin were continued.

The severe acidosis did not resolve and a trial of 1.26% sodium bicarbonate at 50 ml/h was commenced.

In view of the ECG changes, intravenous glyceryl trinitrate was commenced and a trial of facial CPAP, which was poorly tolerated.

A repeat chest X-ray was reported as possible atypical pneumonia or left ventricular failure. Urgent echocardiogram showed 'normal' contractility, mild MR/TR with a degree of pulmonary hypertension.

The following morning the patient was progressively oliguric, had increased shortness of breath and was very anxious.

He complained of painful hands and feet which were cold but had good pulses and colour.

He developed crackles in the right side of his chest and oxygen saturation (SaO_2) was 97% (0.4 fraction of inspired oxygen (FiO_2)), ScvO2 79%.

The following graph (Fig. 4.2) shows progress of haemodynamic parameters and acid–base status.

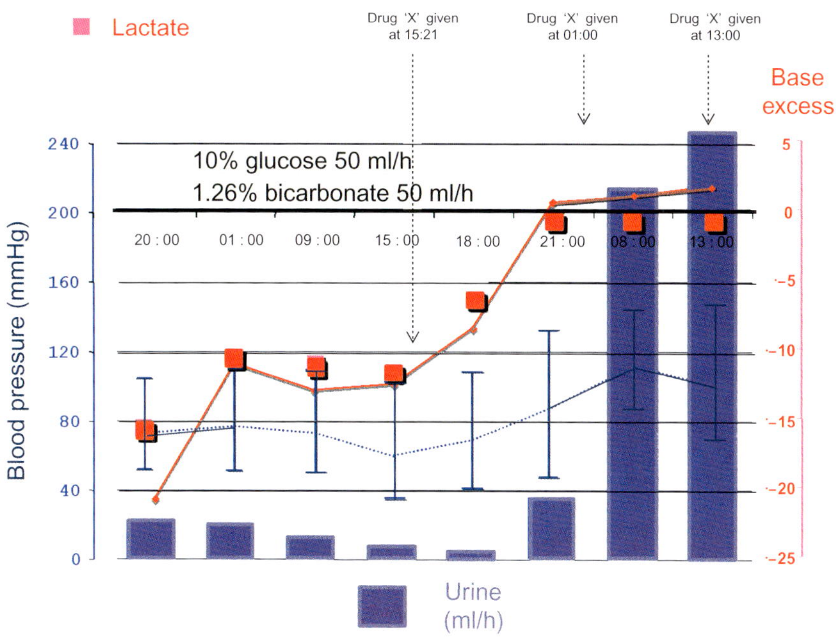

Figure 4.2. Progress of haemodynamic parameters and acid–base status.

(iii) What was Drug 'X'?
(iv) What was the diagnosis?

4.4.5 *Answers*

(i) Differential diagnosis includes community-acquired pneumonia and possible acute coronary syndrome.
Initial treatment was intravenous cefuroxime and oral clarithromycin. The patient was also given treatment dose low-molecular-weight heparin, aspirin and clopidogrel.
(ii) It is still possible this presentation is all related to pneumonia and sepsis. However, the metabolic acidosis raises the possibility of olanzapine-related toxicity, the urinary ketones raise the possibility of diabetic ketoacidosis and the elevated jugular venous pressure, hypoxia and evidence of poor tissue perfusion bring pulmonary embolism or cardiogenic shock into the differential.
(iii) Drug 'X' was intravenous pabrinex (thiamine).
(iv) The diagnosis was confirmed as 'beri beri' with a degree of cardiomyopathy. Blood thiamine level was confirmed as 50 nmol/l (NR 66–200). The patient made a good recovery after treatment.

References

[1] Moore, F.A., Haenel, J.B., Moore, E.E. *et al.* (1992). Incommensurate oxygen consumption in response to maximal oxygen availability predicts postinjury multiple organ failure, *J Trauma*, **33**, 58–65.
[2] Russell, J.A., Ronco, J.J., Lockhat, D. *et al.* (1990). Oxygen delivery and consumption and ventricular preload are greater in survivors than in nonsurvivors of the adult respiratory distress syndrome, *Am Rev Respir Dis*, **141**, 659–665.
[3] Pollack, M.M., Fields, A.I. and Ruttimann, U.E. (1985). Distributions of cardiopulmonary variables in pediatric survivors and nonsurvivors of septic shock, *Crit Care Med*, **13**, 454–459.
[4] Shoemaker, W.C., Appel, P.L. and Kram, H.B. (1988). Tissue oxygen debt as a determinant of lethal and nonlethal postoperative organ failure, *Crit Care Med*, **16**, 1117–1120.

[5] Rivers, E., Nguyen, B., Havstad, S. *et al.* (2001). Early goal–directed therapy in the treatment of severe sepsis and septic shock, *N Engl J Med*, **345**, 1368–1377.
[6] Tuchschmidt, J., Fried, J., Astiz, M. *et al.* (1992). Elevation of cardiac output and oxygen delivery improves outcome in septic shock, *Chest*, **102**, 216–220.
[7] Gattinoni, L., Brazzi, L., Pelosi, P. *et al.* (1995). A trial of goal-oriented hemodynamic therapy in critically ill patients, *N Engl J Med*, **333**, 1025–1032.
[8] Hayes, M.A., Timmins, A.C., Yau, E.H. *et al.* (1994). Elevation of systemic oxygen delivery in the treatment of critically ill patients, *N Engl J Med*, **330**, 1717–1722.
[9] Adams, S.H., Pan, G. and Yu, X.X. (2001). Perspectives on the biology of uncoupling protein (UCP) homologues, *Biochem Soc Trans*, **29**, 798–802.
[10] St Pierre, J., Brand, M.D. and Boutilier, R.G. (2000). Mitochondria as ATP consumers: cellular treason in anoxia, *Proc Natl Acad Sci USA*, **97**, 8670–8674.
[11] Gow, A.J. and Stamler, J.S. (1998). Reactions between nitric oxide and haemoglobin under physiological conditions, *Nature*, **391**, 169–173.
[12] Stamler, J.S., Simon, D.I., Osborne, J.A. *et al.* (1992). S-Nitrosylation of proteins with nitric oxide: Synthesis and characterization of biologically active compounds, *Proc Natl Acad Sci USA*, **89**, 444–448.
[13] Eiserich, J.P., Hristova, M., Cross, C.E. *et al.* (1998). Formation of nitric oxide-derived inflammatory oxidants by myeloperoxidase in neutrophils, *Nature*, **391**, 393–397.
[14] Cooper, C.E. and Davies, N.A. (2000). Effects of nitric oxide and peroxynitrite on the cytochrome oxidase K_m for oxygen: implications for mitochondrial pathology, *Biochim Biophys Acta*, **1459**, 390–396.
[15] Torres, J., Darley-Usmar, V. and Wilson, M.T. (1995). Inhibition of cytochrome *c* oxidase in turnover by nitric oxide: mechanism and implications for control of respiration, *Biochem J*, **312**, 169–173.
[16] Szabo, C., Zingarelli, B. and Salzman, A.L. (1996). Role of poly-ADP ribosyltransferase activation in the vascular contractile and energetic failure elicited by exogenous and endogenous nitric oxide and peroxynitrite, *Circ Res*, **78**, 1051–1063.
[17] Garrabou, G., Inoriza, J.M., Moren, C. *et al.* (2011). Mitochondrial injury in human acute carbon monoxide poisoning: the effect of oxygen treatment, *J Environ Sci Health C Environ Carcinog Ecotoxico Rev*, **29**, 32–51.
[18] Manzo-Avalos, S. and Saavedra-Molina, A. (2010). Cellular and mitochondrial effects of alcohol consumption, *Int J Environ Res Public Health*, **7**, 4281–4304.
[19] Chang, K.C., Unsinger, J., Davis, C.G. *et al.* (2007). Multiple triggers of cell death in sepsis: death receptor and mitochondrial-mediated apoptosis, *FASEB J*, **21**, 708–719.

[20] Hotchkiss, R.S., Osmon, S.B., Chang, K.C. *et al.* (2005). Accelerated lymphocyte death in sepsis occurs by both the death receptor and mitochondrial pathways, *J Immunol*, **174**, 5110–5118.
[21] Hotchkiss, R.S. and Nicholson, D.W. (2006). Apoptosis and caspases regulate death and inflammation in sepsis, *Nat Rev Immunol*, **6**, 813–822.
[22] Hotchkiss, R.S., Swanson, P.E., Freeman, B.D. *et al.* (1999). Apoptotic cell death in patients with sepsis, shock, and multiple organ dysfunction, *Crit Care Med*, **27**, 1230–1251.
[23] Matute-Bello, G. and Martin, T.R. (2003). Science review: apoptosis in acute lung injury, *Crit Care*, **7**, 355–358.
[24] Mutunga, M., Fulton, B., Bullock, R. *et al.* (2001). Circulating endothelial cells in patients with septic shock, *Am J Respir Crit Care Med*, **163**, 195–200.
[25] Hotchkiss, R.S., Swanson, P.E., Freeman, B.D. *et al.* (1999). Apoptotic cell death in patients with sepsis, shock, and multiple organ dysfunction, *Crit Care Med*, **27**, 1230–1251.
[26] Brealey, D., Karyampudi, S., Jacques, T.S. *et al.* (2004). Mitochondrial dysfunction in a long-term rodent model of sepsis and organ failure, *Am J Physiol Regul Integr Comp Physiol*, **286**, R491–R497.

5
Cardiovascular Monitoring

Parind Patel

5.1 Purpose of Monitoring

In the management of critically ill patients, haemodynamic assessment remains an important component in guiding therapy to improve patient outcome. Cardiovascular failure contributes to a large proportion of morbidity and mortality in intensive care units. Therefore gathering as much relevant data and adjusting therapy is assumed to have a positive effect on patient outcome.

There has been significant change in the last 40 years in the development of haemodynamic monitoring. Initial dependence on clinical examination was complemented with direct and invasive central venous pressure and arterial pressure monitoring. In the early 1970s the pulmonary artery flotation catheter was developed and became common practice. With technological advances and more pathophysiological insights, newer, less invasive tools have been developed, providing an ever-increasing choice of monitoring and resulting data for the clinician to reflect upon. Much effort has been made to demonstrate the validity and proposed benefits of the data, when merged with a sensible protocol or care pathway. However the evidence has been conflicting with some studies showing benefit when treatment protocols have been implemented whilst others have shown harm. There are several varying factors that affect the results of these studies, such as whether monitoring and a protocol are instituted early or late in the patient's disease progression.

The data collected from the monitor and the subsequent therapy, whether following evidence-based guidelines or the clinician's experience and judgement are very variable, even within the same hospital and certainly across continents.

Ultimately, it is not in dispute that optimising cardiac function and oxygen delivery is useful and sometimes essential in the critically ill. Current consensus [1] certainly recommends the use of advanced haemodynamic and cardiac output monitoring, although the benefits of the various monitors and devices remain uncertain.

5.2 Clinical Examination and Non-Invasive Monitoring

In the current climate of rapidly advancing technology, clinical history and examination are still the most important monitoring method in assessing the patient's haemodynamic condition. Although it cannot be substantiated by evidence, clinical examination is certainly the most convenient, safe and universally accepted method of monitoring in intensive care units.

Further haemodynamic variables are measured at the bedside, most notably arterial blood pressure, heart rate, central venous pressure (CVP), arterial and central venous saturations along with acid–base balance and lactate as global markers of perfusion.

Some of these parameters have specific thresholds that should be targeted. Blood pressure is regulated through baroreceptor reflex arcs such that it remains constant despite changes in CO, whereas cardiac output varies with changing tissue metabolic demands. Thus, a normal blood pressure does not necessarily reflect hemodynamic stability, but it does reflect normal organ perfusion pressure [2]. For this reason maintaining a normal or a minimum mean arterial blood pressure of 65 mmHg is often used to prevent organ hypoperfusion [3].

CVP is the back pressure to central venous return. It is limited as a target for resuscitation as there is no value that will identify fluid overload or a lack of response to fluid challenges [4]. However a value less than 10 mmHg in ventilated patients correlates with a collapsing vena cava or a relatively empty circulation [5]. Combining these pressure variables with global markers of perfusion such as lactate or base deficit forms a large part of the initial monitoring which can then be followed by measuring changes in trend after therapeutic interventions. Other surrogates for cardiovascular well-being such as capillary refill time and peripheral skin temperature provide reassurance whilst a reduction in urine output, although not useful diagnostically, suggests renal hypoperfusion or dysfunction.

The most useful and proven features of the above measurements are incorporated into dynamic haemodynamic monitoring [6]. Thus preload responsiveness is assessed by rapidly administering a small bolus of fluid and monitoring the changes in clinical signs, heart rate, blood pressure and CVP. However, it is essential to monitor for detrimental effects, particularly in respiratory and gas exchange measurements. Fluid challenges can be replaced by passive leg raising to increase venous return transiently, which in responders causes a rise in cardiac output and blood pressure. This same principle can be extended to information available from more invasive means.

5.3 Pulse Oximetry

The pulse oximeter has become the most frequently used non-invasive patient monitor in intensive care and throughout the hospital. A conventional pulse oximeter monitors the perfusion of blood to the dermis and subcutaneous tissue of the skin. In terms of macrocirculatory monitoring, it has reasonable correlation with systolic blood pressure [7], although limited in the setting of low cardiac output and high systemic vascular resistance. The plethysmographic waveform signal displayed resembles the arterial waveform resulting from beat-to-beat changes in the stroke volume transmitted to the peripheral circulation. The interaction between the heart and lung in mechanical variation allows pulse-pressure variation to be utilised in assessing fluid responsiveness [8]. In hypovolaemic patients it has been demonstrated that the cyclical changes in inspiration result in a rise in intrathoracic and intrapulmonary pressures, which causes a decreased preload leading to a reduction in stroke volume (Frank–Starling's principle). Several indices derived from the plethysmographic waveform signal have proven useful in demonstrating this relative hypovolaemia and fluid responsiveness in mechanically ventilated patients [6,9]. Its benefits have also been demonstrated in spontaneously breathing patients undergoing a passive leg raise, inducing an increase in preload and a corresponding decrease in the variation in plethysmographic waveform amplitude [10]. In daily clinical practice it has limitations in low-perfusion states, such as low cardiac output, vasoconstriction, hypothermia and in conditions such as tricuspid regurgitation, resulting in a pulsatile venous waveform, which may make it difficult for the sensor to distinguish a true signal from background noise and hence its reproducibility is limited.

5.4 Venous Saturations

There are two potentially useful measurements that can be made in critically unwell patients: mixed venous saturation (SvO_2) and central venous saturation ($ScvO_2$).

SvO_2 is the oxygen saturation of the mixed venous blood which is received from all parts of the body, and is sampled from the pulmonary artery before it is oxygenated by the lungs. It therefore reflects the proportion of oxygen that has been extracted by the body which is the oxygen delivery (DO_2) minus the oxygen consumption (VO_2).

Oxygen delivery is the product of the cardiac output and the oxygen content and is normally around 800–1200 ml/min. Cardiac output may be compromised by hypovolaemia and/or cardiac pump failure. Oxygen content is largely dependent on arterial oxygen saturations and haemoglobin concentration.

$$DO_2 = \text{CO} \times \text{Oxygen content}$$
$$\text{Oxygen content} = (10 \times \text{Hb} \times SaO_2 \times 1.34) + (10 \times PO_2 \times 0.0225)$$
$$1.34 = \text{Hufner constant}$$
$$0.0225 = \text{ml of } O_2 \text{ dissolved per 100 ml plasma per kPa}$$
$$PO_2 = \text{Partial pressure of oxygen}$$

Normal oxygen extraction (VO_2) is 20–25% of that delivered and therefore the normal mixed venous saturations (SvO_2) are 75%. A greater proportion is extracted if the delivery is poor, thus resulting in low SvO_2. This, of course, occurs during exercise, but can also be an indicator of cardiogenic or hypovolaemic shock and low haemoglobin.

However, a high SvO_2 may also be pathological as it indicates that the tissues are not able to extract the oxygen delivered, for instance in sepsis. Oxygen extraction is also reduced in sedated or anaesthetised patients, which can lead to false reassurance from a normal SvO_2. Often various causes of shock and anaemia coexist, making the interpretation of SvO_2 difficult; trends, nevertheless, may be useful. The main practical limitation is that a pulmonary artery flotation catheter is required to sample SvO_2.

This has led to the use of central venous saturations ($ScvO_2$) sampled from the superior vena cava via a central venous catheter which is sited in critically unwell patients more routinely.

Mixed venous blood is a mixture of blood from the superior vena cava, inferior vena cava and coronary sinus. Under physiologically normal conditions, the $ScvO_2$ is lower than the SvO_2 mainly because of the higher proportional extraction of oxygen by the brain compared with the kidney. However this is altered in critically unwell patients, where the splanchnic circulation is often compromised, often with increased demands leading to a high extraction ratio and very low oxygen saturations in the inferior vena cava. Hence the SvO_2 is lower than the $ScvO_2$. Studies have shown reasonable correlation between the two [11], but not necessarily consistently and the two values certainly cannot be interchanged.

The use of SvO_2 has declined with the use of the pulmonary artery flotation catheter. In contrast $ScvO_2$ has become increasingly popular particularly as a guide to goal-directed early resuscitation in patients with septic shock [12]. Its use in other areas of critical care has not been proven [13] and it is important to realise its limitations. Despite this, trends in $ScvO_2$ can be useful in guiding therapy along with other markers of perfusion and adequate cardiac output.

5.5 Pulmonary Artery Flotation Catheter

The balloon-tipped, flow-directed, pulmonary artery catheter (PAC), first introduced in 1970 [14] became the gold standard of bedside haemodynamic monitoring in the 1980s.

The device directly measures pressures within the superior vena cava, right heart, pulmonary circulation and, by means of balloon occlusion of the pulmonary artery, the left atrial pressure. As well as pressures, flow can be measured. Intermittent thermodilution with the proximal injection of saline induces a temperature change which is measured by a thermistor at the distal end of the catheter, based on the Stewart–Hamilton principle and allows cardiac output to be derived. Mixed venous oxygen saturations can be measured directly, providing a guide for adequacy of tissue oxygenation. Modern catheters have a thermal filament coil and spectrophotometer allowing the continuous display of cardiac output and mixed venous saturations.

The monitor was used widely during this early phase. Less invasive alternatives were not available, and the additional information it provided was thought to be crucial to managing the complicated severely ill critical care patient. During the late 1990s questions were being raised regarding its negative effect on mortality [15].

Initial concerns were raised regarding the clinicians' ability to extract the data accurately. Considerable skill is required to place the catheter and there are additional risks to central venous catheter placement and, even when experienced staff extract the data, there appears an error of up to 25% [16].

Once the data has been extracted, the additional information often confirms the underlying clinical observations and adds reassurance. However there is little evidence to suggest an improvement in outcome. Of course this is exceptionally difficult to demonstrate. The device is reserved for the most critically ill and complex cases and there is not only variation in the extraction of data but also the treatment that may follow. Not surprisingly an observational case-matched study showed an increase in mortality when a pulmonary catheter had been used [15].

Several studies have failed to demonstrate benefit from using a PAC [17] even in specific conditions such as acute lung injury [18]. Moreover when combined with aggressive goal-directed targets, its use, or more likely the resulting treatment, has been shown to cause harm in mixed intensive care patients [19].

Finally a prospective, randomised controlled trial has demonstrated that not only is there no benefit of using a PAC compared with no PAC, but when compared with alternative cardiac output monitoring devices there is also no difference [20].

Current trend suggests that PACs are not being routinely used to guide hemodynamic management in the intensive care unit [21]. It remains possible that their use may benefit highly selective patient groups [22], but clinicians must carefully consider if the additional data the PAC provides will truly result in a beneficial therapeutic manoeuvre that outweighs the small, but non-zero, risk of harm to the patient.

It is also important to note that the safety and, more importantly, proven efficacy of alternative haemodynamic monitoring tools to be discussed in the remainder of this chapter have also not been demonstrated.

5.6 Pulse Contour Analysis

These monitors encompass a mixture of techniques that allow determination directly from the arterial pressure waveform of either cardiac output or stroke volume. Assuming that the patient requires or has in place an arterial catheter, the main advantages of this technique are that it is minimally invasive and continuous.

There are three devices that use this technology in current general use:

- LiDCOplus/PulseCO system (LiDCO Ltd, UK).
- PiCCO system (Pulsion Medical Systems, Germany).
- Vigileo/FloTrac system (Edwards Lifesciences, USA).

The first two involve calibration while the latter is uncalibrated.

With the LiDCO, initial calibration involves the measurement of cardiac output from lithium transpulmonary thermodilution. A small amount injected via a central venous catheter is detected at the arterial catheter (whichever type is *in situ*). The arterial line is connected to a pump withdrawing the blood at a predetermined rate into a lithium sensor. This generates a lithium concentration–time curve. The cardiac output is hence derived from the area under the curve based on the Stewart–Hamilton equation. Once calibrated the device contains an algorithm relating the pulse power to continuous stroke volume and cardiac output monitoring. There is continuous beat-to-beat monitoring allowing other useful data such as stroke volume and pulse pressure variations to be displayed to help guide fluid therapy. There is an assumption that the compliance of the vascular system remains unchanged once calibrated since it is converting net power data to net flow data. Therefore recalibration is recommended every eight hours and caution encouraged in interpreting the data where there are huge haemodynamic and compliance changes, for example massive haemorrhage [23]. Calibration is affected by lithium therapy, severe hyponatraemia and quaternary ammonium neuromuscular blocking drugs. More relevant in haemodynamically unstable patients, the data is not interpretable in patients requiring intra-aortic balloon counter pulsation therapy.

Significant advantages of this technique include the fact that a regular arterial line is used. The system can also be used without a central line, with calibration from a large intravenous peripheral cannula being just as accurate [24] (although the need for cardiac output monitoring in such a patient must be questionable). Its accuracy has been demonstrated in a wide variety of patients including medical and surgical intensive care patients [25]. Benefits have also been described, with reduced morbidity and hospital stay when lithium-derived cardiac output monitoring is coupled with a sensible goal-directed therapy in the peri-operative setting [26].

The PiCCO system measures cardiac output via transpulmonary thermodilution which is subsequently calibrated against a pulse contour analysis algorithm. A specific proximal (either femoral or brachial) arterial catheter with a thermistor-tip is used to detect blood temperature change following the injection of a set volume of cold saline into a central venous catheter. As with a PAC, three calibrations are performed initially. This cardiac output along with subsequent values derived from the continuous pulse contour analysis have been validated against the PAC in several settings. The temperature differential detected by the arterial thermistor is composed of a series of exponential decay curves as the cold injectate passes through the various compartments of the circulation from the central venous catheter. Most of the temperature change occurs as a result of redistribution within the intrathoracic compartment. Hence other volumetric variables such as intrathoracic blood volume and extravascular lung water as markers of pulmonary oedema can be estimated.

The limitations of the PiCCO system, are similar to those of the LiDCO, relating to conditions that interfere with the calibration process such as intracardiac shunts, or the pulse contour waveform analysis, such as severe aortic valve disease and the use of intra-aortic balloon pump devices. There appears to be inconsistency with the timing intervals between calibrations, the manufacturer recommending every eight hours to observational studies supporting hourly recalibration [27].

Studies have shown a reasonable correlation between pulse contour cardiac output compared with PAC-derived methods [28]. An observational study comparing either PAC- or PiCCO-guided therapy has found no difference in outcome [29]. The lung water indices along with ease of use and ability to have the data presented on the main monitor have accounted for the increased popularity of the latter, but there are no prospective randomised controlled studies with or without a goal-directed therapy suggesting an outcome benefit.

The most uncertain aspect of the above two systems concerns the necessity and timing of recalibration. This most recent addition to the pulse analysers is the Vigileo, and because it requires no calibration it has gained considerable interest. It is based on the principle that the pulse pressure is proportional to the stroke volume. A specific arterial pressure transducer (Edward Lifesciences, Irvine, California, USA, Edward FloTrac sensor) samples at a frequency of 100 Hz to characterise the pulse waveform. This is amalgamated with the patient's demographics to estimate stroke volume and cardiac output. At present there are conflicting reports as to how accurately this device tracks cardiac output when compared with PAC. Certainly initial studies have raised doubts about its accuracy with both underestimation [30,31] and overestimation [32] in separate study populations. However there has been a series of positive studies showing reasonable accuracy and reproducibility when compared with calibrated pulse contour analysis and PAC [33–35]. Also of note, the algorithm used to calculate the stroke volume has been modified further and this may lead to a more consistent performance with future use.

5.7 Oesophageal Doppler

The oesophageal Doppler is a commonly used device to monitor cardiac output. The flexible probe is inserted orally into sedated and ventilated patients and advanced until the tip is at the level of the descending aorta. The tip has a Doppler transducer which measures the blood flow velocity in the descending aorta. The probe is rotated to face the aorta to achieve maximum signal and velocity waveform.

The following assumptions are made: the aorta sits parallel to the oesophagus so that the angle between the Doppler beam and blood flow is the same as that of the transducer and the probe; when measuring the velocity it is assumed that all the red cells are moving at approximately the same speed; once blood leaves the left ventricular outflow tract, a constant 70% of the blood flows into the descending aorta, with the remaining 30% to the brachiocephalic, coronary and carotid circulation; the cross-sectional area of the aorta which is estimated from a nomogram based on the patient's age, weight and height does not change significantly during the cardiac cycle. These assumptions have the potential to cause error in pathophysiological conditions.

The characteristics of the waveform of the blood flow are displayed on the monitor. The flow time is the time of ejection, which is corrected for heart rate. A short ejection time indicates a hypovolaemic circulation. The stroke volume is derived from the stroke distance (or time–velocity integral) multiplied by the estimated cross-sectional area of the descending aorta. The mean acceleration time is the time from the opening of the aortic valve to the time point when the flow rate reaches its maximum velocity, and when combined with the peak velocity, useful information regarding contractility can be derived.

In practice the oesophageal Doppler is a simple technique, with most users able to achieve adequate probe positioning and to obtain reproducible results. There appears to be a steep learning curve with the technique with satisfactory skills achieved within 12 placements. Despite its critics, both the inter-observer variability (10%) and the intra-observer variability (8%) are low compared with the gold standard thermodilution (12%) [36]. Probe displacement can occur during prolonged monitoring as a result of various factors (nursing procedures, deglutition and gravity, amongst others). Therefore the manufacturers recommend rechecking the signal quality regularly and if necessary repositioning on a regular basis, before acquiring and interpreting Doppler-derived data [37].

Correlation with thermodilution has been reported as good with a slight tendency to underestimate, albeit consistently, allowing the clinician to monitor haemodynamic changes in a relatively non-invasive manner in mechanically ventilated patients [38]. Early nurse-led interventions have shown benefits [39]. When combined with a reasonable goal-directed therapy within specific settings there are studies supporting the benefits of the Doppler, particularly in the peri-operative setting [40,41].

5.8 Echocardiography

Echocardiography has been available for 50 years [42]. Enhanced images and information from the transoesophageal approach have been available for more than 30 years [43], and in the last decade this information has become available for the monitoring of haemodynamically unstable critical care patients. Portable battery-operated systems, lower cost and more echocardiography-trained clinicians has permitted greater development and understanding of this tool. Harmonic imaging and the use of contrast has enhanced picture quality.

Advantages over the PAC include:

- Ability to visualise cardiac chamber volumes rather than pressure.
- Ability to monitor ventricular systolic and diastolic function.
- Ability to detect wall motion abnormalities and cardiomyopathies.
- Allows assessment of the pericardial space for inflammation, effusions or haemorrhage.
- Can be used for diagnosis of valvular dysfunction.
- Non-invasive with minimal complications, although this is arguable with the transoesophageal approach.

The initial assessment is based on the two-dimensional short-axis view of each ventricle providing information on global function, wall motion abnormalities, preload and afterload volume indices. Pulsed-wave and continuous-wave Doppler allows the estimation of low- and high-velocity flow across the valves, further enhanced by the superimposition of colour Doppler information. Cardiac output can be accurately measured along with myocardial tissue movement [44].

Adequate views from a transthoracic approach may be compromised in the intensive care patient by hyperinflated ventilated lungs, surgical emphysema, drains, wounds, dressings and general lack of mobility. Multiplane transoesophageal imaging may be indicated in some patients for these reasons. The oesophageal approach is also indicated in the diagnosis and evaluation of endocarditis, thrombus and dissection.

The effect of using echocardiography to influence decision making in critical care patients has been reported as high by its enthusiasts [45]. Although the ability to visualise volume rather than pressures appears attractive, it is still not as helpful as monitoring dynamic changes when evaluating fluid responsiveness [6].

The usefulness of echocardiography is not disputed, but the availability of the equipment, training of clinicians and the time taken to gather the appropriate information limit its use. Although gaining popularity, until it is used regularly by frontline staff i.e. nurses and residents, its use will be reserved for the more complicated patients and therefore require experienced clinicians to interpret the images.

5.9 Current Approach to Monitoring the Critically Ill Patient

The ideal monitor must be easy and quick to use, widely available and of no danger to the patient. The information it provides must be accurate, reproducible and not available from basic clinical assessment.

Evidence indicates that the use of dynamic parameters, such as respiratory changes in right atrial pressure (RAP), arterial pressure and aortic blood velocity is superior to using static parameters in predicting fluid responsiveness in intensive care patients. Thus the raw data provided by the various monitors are limited, but changes and trends may be useful information.

What is done about this useful information in a particular patient is far more important. Using a liberal fluid strategy to improve stroke volume and cardiac output guided by an oesophageal Doppler in peri-operative anaesthetised hip operations improves outcome [41], as does a fluid restrictive strategy guided by PAC in patients with acute respiratory distress syndrome (ARDS) in intensive care units [18]. The difference between the two studies is not the monitor but the patient at that particular moment.

Timing of the therapy is relevant. Acting on abnormal data early with goal-directed therapy has been shown to significantly improve outcome in septic shock patients on admission to the hospital [12]. Similar goal-directed therapy later in the patient's care has been shown to cause harm [19]. Once again the type of monitor or the particular observation or information becomes irrelevant and it is the speed of initiating a therapeutic manoeuvre that is more productive. If implementing the monitor takes time, as it may with transoesophageal echo or PAC, then this limits its usefulness.

The haemodynamic or cardiovascular status is only one aspect of the patient's condition. One also has to consider the renal and respiratory status and the impact haemodynamic manipulation may have on these. If the monitor in question suggests that further fluid challenges are required to improve stroke volume, flow and oxygen delivery, but the patient is currently requiring a high fraction of inspired oxygen (FiO_2) high positive end-expiratory pressure (PEEP) ventilation with considerable lung oedema, then most clinicians may avoid liberal fluid use, whatever the monitor suggests.

One final aspect to consider is the availability of the monitor and the skills and resources required to use it. If the monitor can be used and acted upon by the bedside nurse or resident, then this will result in a speedier therapeutic reaction. A monitor that requires considerable training may result in considerable delay or even avoidance when it is most needed: at the onset of the patient's deterioration.

Considering all of the above factors, it is of no surprise that a consensus has not been reached. Basic monitoring and clinical skills are essential in managing all critical care patients. As the patient becomes more haemodynamically unstable, one has to consider the possible underlying cause, whether further monitoring will help confirm the diagnosis and guide treatment. For this reason in most patients, either oesophageal Doppler or pulse contour analysis could provide additional valuable information with minimal potential for harm. When used regularly, both are relatively easy to use, allowing most members of the critical care team to become involved in goal-directed patient care at an early stage. At this stage it may become necessary to define cardiac abnormalities further by echocardiography, either as a single investigation or repeated to monitor progress of disease and treatment. The latter may be difficult due to limitations in skills, resources and time, and availability will vary between institutions. There will be times where diagnostically echocardiography is essential, particularly with complex cardiac disease, but its use as a routine haemodynamic monitor for critical care patients is unproven. Finally the pulmonary artery flotation catheter, the most controversial of monitoring devices, still has a role for the complicated unstable patient. Trends in pressures provide useful information in a rapidly changing patient, for instance in high-risk cardiac surgery, where treatment may involve numerous vasoactive drugs and an intra-aortic balloon pump.

Current practice appears to follow a ladder, based on skills required, cost and invasiveness in keeping with a common sense approach in the monitoring of critically unwell patients.

Whatever combination of monitoring is used, the most vital component is a rapid and appropriate response to the information provided.

5.10 Clinical Case

A 47-year-old man presents to hospital with a three-day history of shortness of breath, left-sided pleuritic chest pain and a fever. On arrival he is hypoxic and in respiratory failure. He is started on antibiotics to cover severe community-acquired pneumonia. A central line is inserted. He is hypotensive with a CVP of 6 mmHg and receives in total 2 litres of fluid resuscitation. Over the next few hours his respiratory status deteriorates, requiring intubation and mechanical ventilation. Further haemodynamic deterioration occurs on induction, culminating in a peri-arrest situation. Adrenaline is given by bolus followed by an infusion and he is ventilated with high inspiratory pressures. Four hours following arrival he is transferred to the intensive care unit with a FiO_2 of 0.8 and adrenaline infusion of 0.5 μg/kg/min. The electrocardiogram (ECG) shows a left bundle branch block and there is clinical suggestion of both a cardiac and septic pathology. Serial chest radiographs show worsening bilateral infiltrates as well as the original left-sided consolidation. For this reason a pulmonary artery flotation catheter is requested. The insertion is technically difficult and complicated by worsening gas exchange and cardiac arrhythmias. The information from the PAC suggests vasodilatation and sepsis with a normal cardiac output. Mixed venous saturations are low (60%), with arterial saturations at 88% at this stage. Pulmonary artery occlusion pressure (PAOP) is 14 mmHg, excluding a cardiogenic element to the lung oedema.

The diagnosis at present is pneumonia with septic shock and acute respiratory distress syndrome. Further haemodynamic management consists of noradrenaline with weaning of adrenaline and fluid restricted balance.

Over the next three days haemodynamic and respiratory parameters improve. Atrial fibrillation complicates the recovery process and is treated with amiodarone. The PAC is removed since the overall clinical condition is improving. Raised troponin increases suspicion of an ischaemic cardiac component. A transthoracic echocardiogram is performed, showing left anterior descending regional wall hypokinesia with preservation of stroke volume and ejection fraction. In view of the ongoing ischaemia the patient is transferred to the cardiac catheter laboratory for angioplasty and stent insertion of the occluded coronary artery. Rhythm disturbances and haemodynamic parameters continue to improve and the patient eventually recovers fully.

5.10.1 *Comment*

The case highlights the difficulty in interpreting blood pressure and CVP and the strengths of PAC in guiding therapy in a deteriorating patient. Although there was a successful outcome there are several areas of criticisms and improvement.

The initial management could have been vastly improved by better use of monitoring in the first few hours to prevent further deterioration. Numerous haemodynamic variables can be used in conjunction to differentiate the type of shock from which the patient is suffering (Table 5.1). Central venous saturations can correlate with mixed venous saturations and provide an indication of the adequacy of oxygen delivery. This can be combined with global markers of perfusion, such as lactate, acidosis and capillary refill time. Trends in CVP and arterial blood pressure in response to careful fluid challenges and passive straight leg raise whilst monitoring for respiratory side effects are far more informative than isolated values. The above information can be gathered and acted upon within the first few hours with proven benefits. Once intubated or on the intensive care unit there are several other alternatives that allow the information to be

Table 5.1. Haemodynamic profiles characteristic for differentiating shock.

	Hypvolaemic	Cardiogenic	Obstructive	Distributive
Mean Arterial Pressure	↓	↓	↓	↓
Central Venous Pressure	↓	↑	↑	↓
$ScvO_2/SvO_2$	↓	↓	↓	↑
Lactate/ Base Deficit	↑	↑	↑	↑
Cardiac Output	↓	↓	↓	↑
Flow Time	↓	↑	↔	↓
Pulmonary Artery Occlusion Pressure	↓	↑	↕	↓
Systemic Vascular Resistance	↑	↑	↑	↓
Pulse Pressure Variability	↑	↔	↔	↑

gathered faster and require less training for rotating residents. These include the oesophageal Doppler and pulse contour analysis. Finally, although the PAC differentiates the states of shock, it is not a diagnostic tool, and for this reason there are occasions where an echocardiogram performed at an earlier opportunity would be more helpful.

References

[1] Antonelli, M., Levy, M., Andrews, P.J. *et al.* (2007). Hemodynamic monitoring in shock and implications for management, International Consensus Conference, Paris, France, 27–28 April 2006, *Intens Care Med*, **33**, 575–590.

[2] Partrick, D.A, Bensard, D.D, Janik, J.S. *et al.* (2002). Is hypotension a reliable indicator of blood loss from traumatic injury in children? *Am J Surg*, **184**, 555–559.

[3] Lim, S.M., Huang, C.D., Lin, H.C. *et al.* (2006). A modified goal directed protocol improves clinical outcomes in intensive care unit patients with septic shock: a randomised controlled trial, *Shock*, **26**, 551–557.

[4] Kumar, A., Anel, R., Bunnell, E. *et al.* (2004). Pulmonary artery occlusion pressure and central venous pressure fail to predict ventricular filling volume,

cardiac performance, or the response to volume infusion in normal subjects, *Crit Care Med*, **32**, 691–699.

[5] Vieillard-Baron, A., Chergui, K., Rabiller, A. *et al.* (2004). Superior vena caval collapsibility as a gauge of volume status in ventilated septic patients, *Intens Care Med*, **30**, 1734–1739.

[6] Michard, F. and Teboul, J.L. (2002). Predicting fluid responsiveness in ICU patients: a critical analysis of the evidence, *Chest*, **121**, 2000–2008.

[7] Lawson, D., Norley, I., Korbon, G. *et al.* (1987). Blood flow limits and pulse oximeter signal detection, *Anesthesiology*, **67**, 599–603.

[8] Solus-Biguenet, H., Fleyfel, M., Tavernier, B. *et al.* (2006). Non-invasive prediction of fluid responsiveness during major hepatic surgery, *Br J Anaesth*, **97**, 808–816.

[9] Natalini, G., Rosano, A., Taranto, M. *et al.* (2006). Arterial versus plethysmographic dynamic indices to test responsiveness for testing fluid administration in hypotensive patients: a clinical trial, *Anesth Analg*, **103**, 1478–1484.

[10] Delerme, S., Renault, R., Le Manach, Y. *et al.* (2007). Variations in pulse oximetry plethysmographic waveform amplitude induced by passive leg raising in spontaneously breathing volunteers, *Am J Emerg Med*, **25**, 637–642.

[11] Reinhart, K., Kuhn, H.J., Hartog, C. *et al.* (2004). Continuous central venous and pulmonary artery oxygen saturation monitoring in the critically ill, *Intens Care Med*, **30**, 1572–1578.

[12] Rivers, E., Nguyen, B., Havstad, S. *et al.* (2001). Early goal directed therapy in the treatment of severe sepsis and septic shock, *N Engl J Med*, **345**, 1368–1377.

[13] Vincent, J.L. (2008). '$ScvO_2$ as a marker for resuscitation in intensive care', in Kuhlen, R., Moreno, R., Raineri, M. *et al.* (eds), *Controversies in Intensive Care Medicine,* European Society of Intensive Care Medicine, Brussells, pp. 77–82.

[14] Swan, H.J., Ganz, W., Forrester, J. *et al.* (1970). Catheterization of the heart in man with use of a flow-directed balloon-tipped catheter, *N Engl J Med*, **283**, 447–451.

[15] Connors Jr, A.F., Speroff, T., Dawson, N.V. *et al.* (1996). The effectiveness of right heart catheterization in the initial care of critically ill patients, SUPPORT Investigators, *JAMA*, **276**, 889–897.

[16] Gnaegi, A., Feihl, F. and Perret, C. (1997). Intensive care physicians' insufficient knowledge of right-heart catheterisation at the bedside: time to act? *Crit Care Med*, **25**, 213–220.

[17] Rhodes, A., Cusack, R.J., Newman, P.J. *et al.* (2002). A randomised, controlled trial of the pulmonary artery catheter in critically ill patients, *Intens Care Med*, **28**, 256–264.

[18] Richard, C., Warszawski, J., Anguel, N. *et al.* (2003). Early use of the pulmonary artery catheter and outcomes in patients with shock and acute respiratory distress syndrome: a randomized controlled trial, *JAMA*, **290**, 2713–2720.

[19] Hayes, M.A., Timmins, A.C., Yau, E.H. *et al.* (1994). Elevation of systemic oxygen delivery in the treatment of critically ill patients, *N Engl J Med*, **330**, 1717–1722.

[20] Harvey, S., Harrison, D.A., Singer, M. *et al.* (2005). Assessment of the clinical effectiveness of pulmonary artery catheters in management of patients in intensive care (PAC-Man): a randomized controlled trial, *Lancet*, **366**, 472–477.

[21] Wiener, R.S. and Welch, H.G. (2007). Trends in the use of the pulmonary artery catheter in the United States, 1993–2004, *JAMA*, **298**, 423–429.

[22] Rubenfeld, G.D., McNamara-Aslin, E., Rubinson, L. (2007). The pulmonary artery catheter, 1967–2007: rest in peace? *JAMA*, **298**, 458–461.

[23] Cooper, E.S. and Muir, W.W. (2007). Continuous cardiac output monitoring via arterial pressure waveform analysis following severe hemorrhagic shock in dogs, *Crit Care Med*, **35**, 1724–1729.

[24] Jonas, M.M., Kelly, F.E., Linton, R.A. *et al.* (1999). A comparison of lithium dilution cardiac output measurements made using central and antecubital venous injection of lithium chloride, *J Clin Monit Comput*, **15**, 525–528.

[25] Cecconi, M., Fawcett, J., Grounds, R.M. *et al.* (2008). A prospective study to evaluate the accuracy of pulse power analysis to monitor cardiac output in critically ill patients, *BMC Anesthesiol*, **8**, 3.

[26] Pearse, R., Dawson, D., Fawcett, J *et al.* (2005). Early goal-directed therapy after major surgery reduces complications and duration of hospital stay. A randomised, controlled trial, *Crit Care*, **9**, R687–R693.

[27] Hamzaoui, O., Monnet, X., Richard, C. *et al.* (2008). Effects of changes in vascular tone on the agreement between pulse contour and transpulmonary thermodilution cardiac output measurements within an up to 6-hour calibration-free period, *Crit Care Med*, **36**, 434–440.

[28] Della Rocca, G., Costa, M.G., Coccia, C. *et al.* (2003). Cardiac output monitoring: aortic transpulmonary thermodilution and pulse contour analysis agree with standard thermodilution methods in patients undergoing lung transplantation, *Can J Anaesth*, **50**, 707–711.

[29] Della Rocca, G., Costa, M.G., Pompei, L. *et al.* (2002). Continuous and intermittent cardiac output measurement: pulmonary artery catheter versus aortic transpulmonary technique, *Br J Anaesth*, **88**, 350–356.

[30] Lorsomradee, S., Lorsomradee, S.R., Cromheecke, S. *et al.* (2007). Continuous cardiac output measurement: arterial pressure analysis versus thermodilution

technique during cardiac surgery with cardiopulmonary bypass, *Anaesthesia*, **62**, 979–983.
[31] Lorsomradee, S., Lorsomradee, S., Cromheecke, S. *et al.* (2007). Uncalibrated arterial pulse contour analysis versus continuous thermodilution technique: effects of alterations in arterial waveform, *J Cardiothorac Vasc Anesth*, **21**, 636–643.
[32] Sander, M., Spies, C.D., Grubitzsch, H. *et al.* (2006). Comparison of uncalibrated arterial waveform analysis in cardiac surgery patients with thermodilution cardiac output measurements, *Crit Care*, **10**, R164.
[33] McGee, W.T., Horswell, J.L., Calderon, J. *et al.* (2007). Validation of a continuous, arterial pressure-based cardiac output measurement: a multicenter, prospective clinical trial, *Crit Care*, **11**, R105.
[34] Button, D., Weibel, L., Reuthebuch, O. *et al.* (2007). Clinical evaluation of the FloTrac/Vigileo system and two established continuous cardiac output monitoring devices in patients undergoing cardiac surgery, *Br J Anaesth*, **99**, 329–336.
[35] de Waal, E.E., Kalkman, C.J., Rex, S. *et al.* (2007). Validation of a new arterial pulse contour-based cardiac output device, *Crit Care Med*, **35**, 1904–1909.
[36] Freund, P.R. (1987). Transesophageal Doppler scanning versus thermodilution during general anesthesia. An initial comparison of cardiac output techniques, *Am J Surg*, **153**, 490–494.
[37] Lefrant, J.Y., Bruelle, P., Aya, A.G. *et al.* (1998).Training is required to improve the reliability of esophageal Doppler to measure cardiac output in critically ill patients, *Intens Care Med*, **24**, 347–352.
[38] Valtier, B., Cholley, B.P., Belot, J *et al.* (1998). Noninvasive monitoring of cardiac output in critically ill patients using transesophageal Doppler, *Am J Respir Crit Care Med*, **158**, 77–83.
[39] McKendry, M., McGloin, H., Saberi, D. *et al.* (2004). Randomised controlled trial assessing the impact of a nurse delivered, flow monitored protocol for optimisation of circulatory status after cardiac surgery, *BMJ*, **329**, 258.
[40] Wakeling, H.G., McFall, M.R., Jenkins, C.S. *et al.* (2005). Intraoperative oesophageal Doppler guided fluid management shortens postoperative hospital stay after major bowel surgery, *Br J Anaesth*, **95**, 634–642.
[41] Sinclair, S., James, S. and Singer, M. (1997). Intraoperative intravascular volume optimisation and length of hospital stay after repair of proximal femoral fracture: randomised control trial, *BMJ*, **315**, 909–912.
[42] Edler, I. and Hertz, C.H. (2004). The use of ultrasonic reflectoscope for the continuous recording of the movements of heart walls. 1954., *Clin Physiol Funct Imaging*, **24**, 118–136.

[43] Frazin, L., Talano, J.V., Stephanides, L. *et al.* (1976). Esophageal echocardiography, *Circulation*, **54**, 102–108.

[44] Poelart, J. (2004). *Transoesophageal Echocardiography in Anaesthesia and Intensive Care Medicine*, second edition, BMJ Books, London.

[45] Joseph, M.X, Disney, P.J, Da Costa, R. *et al.* (2004). Transthoracic echocardiography to identify or exclude cardiac cause of shock, *Chest*, **126**, 1592–1597.

6
Vasoactive Agents

Gayathri Satkurunath, Raha Rahman West
and Andrew Rhodes

6.1 Definitions

Vasoactive agents are groups of bioactive chemicals that exert effects on the calibre of blood vessels, causing vasoconstriction or vasodilatation. This is achieved by their action on various peripheral receptors or targets. Many of these agents also have inotropic (increasing cardiac contractility) or chronotropic effects (increasing heart rate) as a result of action on the myocardium.

6.2 The Pressure versus Flow Dilemma

Acute circulatory failure causes an inadequate oxygen or nutrient supply to the tissues or inadequate use by the tissues, which can lead to cellular hypoxia and lactic acidosis. This is usually associated with hypotension. It has been shown in shock that the severity and duration of hypotension and reduction of cardiac output worsens patient outcome [1–3]. These factors lead to a decrease in oxygen delivery and development of organ failure. Hence early fluid resuscitation and the control of vascular tone and cardiac contractility with pharmacological agents in indicated critically ill patients are crucial.

Mean arterial pressure (MAP) represents the mean pressure available for tissue perfusion. Flow to tissues is crucially dependent on MAP. In shock, in addition to hypotension, there may also be changes in regional blood flow distribution, the microvasculature and cellular metabolism, which also affect oxygen delivery and usage. However, when arterial pressure is raised by the use of vasoconstrictor agents the microvascular flow may be impaired [4].

It is crucial to find a balance between maintaining arterial pressure to provide the flow to vital organs while at the same time maintaining flow to the microcirculation as a whole where oxygen exchange takes place. The dilemma is in determining the value of the target MAP that is adequate for maintaining the pressure as well as flow to the tissues.

In a 224-patient randomised control study of a goal-directed protocol to improve clinical outcomes in intensive care patients with septic shock, a MAP of 65 mmHg was used as a target in the protocol group. Hospital mortality decreased by 54% in the protocol group compared with 74% in the control group who did not have a goal-directed protocol [5].

In another study of 111 patients with septic shock, four different MAP values were used to define hypotension: 60, 65, 70 and 75 mmHg [6]. It was found that MAP of 65 mmHg during the first 6 and 48 hours of admission separated survivors and non-survivors better than the other MAP values. It seems that a MAP of above 65 mmHg is a reasonable target for the majority of patients and improved outcomes following septic shock.

Two studies showed similar results when MAP was increased from 65 to 85 mmHg. There was no change in tissue perfusion as measured by lactate levels, urine output and gastric tonometry [7,8]. However, these studies are small and so their findings cannot be generalised.

After the initial resuscitation, if there is evidence of ongoing tissue hypoperfusion (e.g. lactic acidosis) despite adequate global haemodynamic targets such as MAP and cardiac output, assessment and optimisation of the microvascular flow may be beneficial. It has been shown that microcirculation impairment was more severe in non-survivors of sepsis and that ongoing impairment was associated with organ failure and death [9,10]. Microvascular resuscitation may include the use of vasodilators, the titration of inotropes and the judicious use of vasopressors [11].

6.3 Tissue Oxygen Consumption and Supply

Oxygen is inspired from the atmosphere and transported through the oxygen cascade to mitochondria in the tissues [12]. This is essential for the maintenance of normal aerobic metabolism and viable cell function. Imbalance in supply versus demand for oxygen may results in cell injury and organ dysfunction. Therefore the understanding of factors determining oxygen delivery to tissues and oxygen consumption is crucial in the management of critically ill patients [13].

6.3.1 *Oxygen supply*

Oxygen (O_2) supply to tissues can be defined as the amount of oxygen delivered to the tissues per unit of time, usually expressed in ml/min. It is the product of cardiac output and arterial oxygen content (CaO_2):

$$\text{Oxygen delivery} = \text{cardiac output} \times CaO_2 \tag{6.1}$$

Cardiac output represents the product of heart rate (HR) and stroke volume (SV). Arterial oxygen content is the sum of the two forms in which oxygen is carried in the blood. These are the oxygen that is bound to haemoglobin (Hb) and the oxygen that is dissolved in the plasma.

In healthy individuals over 98% of the oxygen content is bound to Hb. The amount of oxygen bound to Hb is determined by the Hb concentration in g/dl, arterial oxygen saturation of Hb (SaO_2) as a percentage and oxygen carrying capacity of Hb or Hufner's constant [14]. The value of the constant differs between authors but *in vivo* each gram of Hb binds with 1.34 ml of O_2. The presence of different forms of Hb, e.g. carboxyhaemoglobin and methaemoglobin, gives different values and reduces the oxygen carrying capacity.

The amount of oxygen that is dissolved in plasma depends on the arterial partial pressure of oxygen (PaO_2) in kPa and the solubility coefficient of O_2 at body temperature which is 0.0225 ml of O_2 dissolved per 100 ml of plasma per kPa.

Therefore factors affecting adequacy of oxygen delivery to the tissue can be summarised into an equation:

$$\begin{aligned} O_2\ \text{delivery} = \text{cardiac output} \times ((\text{Hb} \times SaO_2 \times 1.34) \\ + (PaO_2 \times 0.0225)) \end{aligned} \tag{6.2}$$

Therefore in an average healthy adult, ignoring the small amount of dissolved oxygen:

$$1000 \text{ ml } O_2/\text{min} = 5000 \text{ ml/min} \times (0.15 \text{ g Hb/ml} \times 0.99 \times 1.34 \text{ ml } O_2/\text{g Hb}) \quad (6.3)$$

Agents with an inotropic effect therefore can be used in suitable patients to enhance cardiac output and hence oxygen delivery to tissues.

6.3.2 *Oxygen consumption*

Tissue oxygen consumption can be defined as the amount of oxygen uptake by the tissues per unit time, usually expressed in ml/min. A conscious resting person consumes approximately 250 ml of oxygen every minute, hence only approximately 25% of arterial oxygen is used every minute in healthy individuals [13].

Oxygen is consumed to generate energy under aerobic metabolism and this corresponds to the metabolic rate and tissue demand. When the oxygen demand is increased (e.g. in exercise), the raised oxygen consumption is usually provided by an increase in cardiac output [15]. However if oxygen delivery fails to meet the demand initially, more oxygen will be extracted from haemoglobin by the tissues resulting in a fall of mixed venous blood oxygen saturation.

Global oxygen consumption can be measured by analysis of respiratory gases or derived from cardiac output, arterial oxygen content (CaO_2) and venous oxygen contents (CvO_2). The inverse Fick's principle can be used to derive oxygen consumption where:

$$O_2 \text{ consumption} = \text{cardiac output} \times (CaO_2 - CvO_2) \quad (6.4)$$

The relationship between oxygen delivery and oxygen consumption is crucial during critical illness. The ratio of oxygen consumption to oxygen delivery gives the oxygen extraction ratio. The ratio signifies the amount of oxygen delivered to the microcirculation that is taken up by the tissues. When the oxygen delivery continues to fall to a critical point where the oxygen extraction ratio cannot increase further to maintain adequate oxygen supply, the energy production in cells becomes limited. Any reduction beyond this critical point results in tissue hypoxia, anaerobic metabolism and lactic acidosis. The critical oxygen delivery varies dependent on the metabolic activity of the tissue. In humans it has been estimated to be approximately 4 ml/kg/min [14].

It has been suggested that most critically ill patients have inadequate oxygen delivery because when oxygen delivery is optimised in these patients, the oxygen consumption also increased [16]. It has also been observed that patients with a higher oxygen delivery index (DO_2I) are more likely to survive than patients with a lower index suggesting a pathological oxygen supply dependency. Hence goal-directed therapy to optimise oxygen delivery in critically ill patients has been evaluated and will be discussed in Section 6.7.

6.4 Vasodilators: Rationale and Current Treatments

The aim of vasodilators is to reduce pathologically high systemic vascular resistance in situations where it is causing excessive cardiac afterload or poor perfusion (Table 6.1). They are commonly used in acute heart failure without symptomatic hypotension, coronary ischaemia or acute severe hypertension. They should be avoided in patients with a systolic blood pressure of less than 90 mmHg and may cause severe hypotension in patients with aortic stenosis [17].

6.4.1 *Nitrates*

Nitrates are a group of drugs used in acute cardiac failure, acute coronary ischaemia or hypertension control in aortic dissection. They decrease left and right heart pressures, relieve the pulmonary congestion and dyspnoea of acute cardiac failure and can improve cardiac output in appropriate patients without increasing myocardial oxygen demand. They can also cause relaxation of myocardial smooth muscle and improve diastolic dysfunction. High levels of nitrates can also cause oxidation of the iron in haemoglobin, producing methaemoglobinaemia with a reduction in oxygen delivery.

Nitrates produce the free radical nitric oxide (NO) by denitration [18]. The mechanism for this is controversial; theories include denitration

Table 6.1. Vasodilators.

	Mode of action	Dosages (intravenous)	Side effects
Glyceryl trinitrate (GTN)	Nitric oxide release, which activates guanylyl cyclase to increase cyclic guanosine monophosphate (GMP) in smooth muscle	10–200 μg/min	Headache, flushing, hypotension, tachycardia
Nitroprusside	Nitric oxide release	0.3–2 μg/kg/min	Rebound hypertension with abrupt withdrawal, raised intracranial pressure, cyanide toxicity
Nifedipine	Calcium channel antagonist on coronary and vascular smooth muscle	100–200 μg	Headache, flushing, dizziness, peripheral oedema
Esmolol	Cardioselective beta-1-adrenergic antagonist	0.5–1.0 mg/kg loading dose, 50-300 μg/kg/min infusion	Bradycardia, hypotension, sweating, nausea, pain on injection, bronchospasm
Labetolol	Combined alpha-1-, beta- and beta-2-adrenergic antagonist	5–20 mg boluses, 2–8 mg/min infusion, max 300 mg/day	Bradycardia, hypotension, bronchospasm
Hydralazine	Direct acting smooth muscle relaxant	200–300 μg/min infusion initially then 50-150 μg/min	Hypotension, tachycardia, fluid retention, nausea
Phentolamine	Alpha-adrenergic antagonist, mainly alpha-1	0.1–2 mg/min infusion	Postural hypotension, tachycardia, abdominal pain, diarrhoea

by sulfhydryl groups or by enzymatic reaction by cytochrome P450, glutathione S-transferase, xanthine oxidoreductase or mitochondrial aldehyde dehydrogenase. Nitric oxide activates guanylyl cyclase to increase cyclic guanosine monophosphate (GMP) in smooth muscle, which leads to systemic and coronary vasodilatation (with increased coronary flow as long as diastolic blood pressure is maintained).

6.4.1.1 *Glyceryl trinitrate*

Glyceryl trinitrate (GTN) is the most commonly used intravenous nitrate vasodilator. It has predominantly venodilator effects, but at high doses causes arterial dilatation. Cerebral vasodilatation may lead to severe headache and tachyphylaxis occurs after 24 to 48 hours of use. GTN is a short-acting agent with a half-life of three minutes. It is used in a dose of 10–200 μg/min.

6.4.1.2 *Nitroprusside*

Nitroprusside is a more potent nitrate, which causes both arterial and venous dilatation. It is sensitive to light, which causes its breakdown with the release of cyanide. Cyanide is usually broken down in the liver by thiocyanate, but it can interfere with cellular respiration and may also bind with methaemoglobin to produce cyanomethaemoglobin. Due to its toxicity it should not be used for more than 72 hours and cyanide levels should be monitored. It is a potent vasodilator, but due to its toxicity it should only be used in situations where other treatments are unsuccessful or unavailable. It is used in a dose of 0.3–2 μg/kg/min.

6.4.2 *Nesiritide*

Nesiritide is a recombinant form of B-type natriuretic peptide which causes venous, systemic and coronary arterial vasodilatation. It also increases glomerular filtration, inhibits the renin–angiotensin system and causes natriuresis [19]. It has been shown to be more effective in improving haemodynamic status and some symptoms in decompensated congestive cardiac failure than intravenous GTN. In a single-centre randomised controlled trial [20], however, there was only a small difference in overall clinical status at 24 hours. It is not available in many European countries.

6.4.3 *Nifedipine*

Nifedipine is a dihydropyridine calcium channel blocker used in the chronic treatment of angina and hypertension. It has been used sublingually or orally for hypertensive crises. This may cause sudden, uncontrolled, prolonged hypotensive episodes which could increase mortality and morbidity and so the practice has been abandoned [21,22]. It is not recommended in the treatment of acute cardiac failure as it may decrease cardiac contractility [17].

6.4.4 *Nicardipine*

Nicardipine is a second-generation dihydropyridine calcium channel blocker that can be given intravenously and is more titratable. It may be used for the treatment of hypertensive emergencies and can reduce cerebral and coronary ischaemia. The dose used is 5–30 mg/hour.

6.4.5 *Esmolol*

Esmolol is not a vasoactive agent, but is a rapidly acting cardioselective beta-1 blocker that is used for similar clinical purposes. It is quickly hydrolysed by red cell esterases and so levels are not affected by liver or renal failure. It has a negative inotropic and chronotropic action and is also used for control of hypertensive crises. The loading dose is 0.5–1.0 mg/kg followed by an infusion of 50–300 μg/kg/min.

6.4.6 *Labetolol*

Labetolol acts on alpha-1, beta-1 and beta-2 receptors and is another useful titratable agent in controlling hypertensive emergencies. This mixed agent reduces systemic vascular resistance, but has less detrimental effect on cardiac output and total peripheral blood flow than pure β-blockers.

It has a negative chronotropic effect. Minimal amounts cross the placenta and so it is used for severe pregnancy-induced hypertension. It can be given as 20 mg boluses or a maintenance infusion of 2–8 mg/min with a maximum of 300 mg/day.

6.4.7 *Hydralazine*

Hydralazine is a directly acting smooth muscle relaxant that is thought to work by either decreasing release of calcium from intracellular stores or by decreasing calcium entry into the vascular smooth muscle cells. It may cause an unpredictable and prolonged hypotensive effect and so it is currently not recommended in management of hypertensive crises [22].

6.4.8 *Phentolamine*

Phentolamine is an α-blocker, mainly working on the alpha-1 receptor to decrease systemic vascular tone. It is now used only rarely, particularly in the management of phaeochromocytoma or cocaine-induced hypertension where β-blockade alone could cause unopposed alpha agonist action with vasoconstriction.

6.5 Vasoconstrictors: Rationale and Current Agents

The aim of vasopressors is to provide systemic vasoconstriction and an adequate perfusion pressure to organs and tissues (Table 6.2). This should be done after appropriate fluid loading to prevent inadequate tissue flow. They are mainly used in situations of shock with low systemic vascular resistance (SVR), whether spontaneous such as sepsis or secondary to other treatments such as sedation or the use of an inodilator. They may also be used to decrease bleeding when administered locally, for example around the site of a procedure.

The catecholamine vasopressor group includes dopamine, noradrenaline (norepinephrine) and adrenaline (epinephrine). They are endogenously occurring agents which have a common precursor, tyrosine. They are hormones secreted into the bloodstream from the adrenal medulla, and noradrenaline and dopamine are also neurotransmitters.

Table 6.2. Vasoconstrictors.

	Main action	Dosages (intravenous)	Side effects
Noradrenaline	Mainly alpha-1-adrenergic agonist, also alpha-2 and beta agonist	0.02–0.15 μg/kg/min	Bradycardia
Dopamine	Alpha, beta, dopamine receptor agonist	0.05–3.0 μg/kg/min (renal dose), 3–10 μg/kg/min (intermediate dose), 10–20 μg/kg/min (higher dose)	Arrhythmias, nausea
Adrenaline	Non-specific alpha and beta-adrenergic agonist	0.01–0.1 μg/kg/min	Central nervous system excitation, tachycardia, dysrhythmia, lactic acidosis
Vasopressin	V1 and V2 receptors agonist	0.01–0.04 units/min	Pallor, nausea, abdominal cramps, myocardial infarction
Phenylephrine	Alpha-1-adrenergic agonist	100–500 μg boluses, 30–180 μg/min infusion	Palpitation, vomiting
Metaraminol	Mainly alpha-1-adrenergic agonist, some beta agonist action	0.5–5 mg boluses	Headache, dizziness, tremor, nausea, vomiting

Phenylephrine, ephedrine and metaraminol are principally used for hypotension due to regional anaesthesia, general anaesthesia or sedation.

6.5.1 *Noradrenaline*

One of the most commonly used vasoconstrictors in the critical care setting is noradrenaline. It acts via adrenergic receptors, predominantly alpha-1, but also alpha-2 and beta receptors to a lesser effect. Alpha-1 receptors are coupled to Gq proteins, which stimulate the phospholipase enzyme to increase intracellular calcium. This leads to vascular smooth muscle contraction. Its main effect is systemic vasoconstriction; it causes coronary vasodilatation and inotropy to a lesser degree via beta receptors. The dose is 0.02–1.5 μg/kg/min.

Noradrenaline can cause bradycardia via the baroreceptor reflex. At high doses it can cause tissue ischaemia due to intense vasoconstriction, particularly in conjunction with other vasopressors.

6.5.2 *Dopamine*

Dopamine acts via alpha, beta and dopamine (D) receptors. At "renal dose" (0.05–3.0 μg/kg/min) it stimulates postsynaptic D1 receptors in coronary, renal and mesenteric blood vessels and presynaptic D2 receptors in renal tubules. D1 receptors are coupled to Gs proteins, which stimulate adenylyl cyclase to produce cyclic adenosine monophosphate (cAMP). This, via protein kinase, increases calcium uptake into the sarcoplasmic reticulum, leading to vasodilatation and increased blood flow in these organs. D2 are coupled to Gi proteins, which inhibit adenylyl cyclase and lead to natriuresis.

At intermediate doses (3–10 μg/kg/min), it weakly binds to beta-1 receptors, leading to inotropy and chronotropy. At higher doses (10–20 μg/kg/min) it causes vasoconstriction via alpha-1 receptors. It is less potent than noradrenaline at alpha receptors.

"Renal dose" dopamine does not increase the glomerular filtration rate and has not been found to protect from renal failure [23]. Dopamine can cause arrhythmias and nausea. It has also been found to inhibit cytokines, chemokines, cell adhesion molecules and chemotaxis and may have immunomodulatory effects [24].

Noradrenaline and dopamine have both been recommended as the first-line vasopressors in septic shock [25]. Noradrenaline use in shock was associated with a lower 30-day mortality than dopamine and adrenaline in the Sepsis Occurrence in Acutely Ill Patients (SOAP) study [26]. However a randomised controlled trial comparing the use of noradrenaline and dopamine by the same investigators showed no difference in mortality or length of stay in the intensive care unit. There was a higher incidence of arrhythmia with dopamine, which caused an increase in early termination of this drug. In subgroup analysis, noradrenaline did show an improved outcome in cardiogenic shock, it was proposed that this was due to the tachycardia from dopamine.

6.5.3 *Adrenaline*

Adrenaline is a potent non-specific agent which acts on all adrenoceptors. It causes inotropy and chronotropy and increases coronary blood flow via beta receptors. It increases systemic and pulmonary vascular resistance and causes splanchnic vasoconstriction via alpha-1 receptors. The standard dose for infusion is 0.01–0.1 μg/kg/min.

This stress hormone increases the supply of oxygen and glucose to the brain and skeletal muscles (for the "fight and flight" reaction) whilst suppressing other non-emergency functions such as gastrointestinal function. It acts on alpha-1 receptors in the liver and beta receptors in liver and muscle to promote glycogenolysis. The increase in metabolism can cause hyperlactaemia. Like dopamine it is known to have immunosuppressive effects [27].

Adrenaline is recommended as a second-line vasopressor in septic shock resistant to dopamine or noradrenaline [25]. Although there is no good evidence of worse outcome with adrenaline, it causes tachycardia with increased myocardial demand, raised lactate and splachnic vasoconstriction.

Due to its potency it remains the first choice vasopressor in anaphylactic shock, with an initial dose of 500 μg intramuscularly or 50 μg intravenously [28]. The activation of the beta-2 receptors on mast cells by adrenaline inhibits activation [29,30] and attenuates the immunoglobulin-E-mediated reaction. Adrenaline when used with subcutaneous lignocaine causes vasoconstriction and less absorption of lignocaine systemically and hence a larger dose of local anaesthetic can be used.

6.5.4 *Vasopressin*

Vasopressin (antidiuretic hormone, 1-deamino-8-d-arginine vasopressin (DDAVP)) is an endogenous peptide hormone synthesised in the hypothalamus and released into the bloodstream from the posterior pituitary. It is released in response to hypovolaemia, hypotension, increased extracellular osmolality, angiotensin II stimulation or sympathetic activation. It acts on V1 receptors on vascular smooth muscle, via the inositol triphosphate transduction pathway, to cause vasoconstriction. It also acts on V2 receptors in the renal collecting duct and distal convoluted tubule to increase water permeability, allowing water reabsorption and increased blood volume, which can aid in increasing blood pressure.

Some studies have shown that low-dose infusion vasopressin also causes cerebral, pulmonary and renal dilatation (mediated by endothelial release of NO) while constricting other vascular beds [31].

Endogenous vasopressin levels have been shown to be initially high and then inappropriately low in later stages of vasodilatory shock.

There have been two small randomised controlled trials which showed an improvement in haemodynamic variables in vasodilatory catecholamine-resistant shock. These were not however designed to look at mortality outcome. The first trial had 13 patients in the vasopressin arm and showed a significant decrease in noradrenaline requirements and increased urine output [32]. The second trial involved 24 patients in the vasopressin arm and patients were enrolled when they had a MAP less than 70 mmHg on 0.5 μg/kg/min noradrenaline [33]. The vasopressin group had a high-dose infusion of 4 U/hour (0.067 U/min) and was found to have a higher MAP and cardiac index, lower noradrenaline requirements, a lower frequency of arrhythmias and higher gastrointestinal perfusion.

The Vasopressin and Septic Shock Trial (VASST) study [34] was a multicentred randomised study on patients receiving a minimum of 5 μg of noradrenaline/min with 396 patients in the vasopressin arm receiving 0.01–0.03 U/min, this showed no overall improvement in mortality with low-dose vasopressin. In the patient sub-group with less severe septic shock there was a significant decrease in 28-day mortality. It remains unclear how to fully interpret this data.

6.5.5 *Phenylephrine*

Phenylephrine is an alpha-1 agonist. It is currently the recommended vasoconstrictor in obstetric anaesthesia as it causes less foetal acidosis than the previously recommended agent ephedrine [35]. It has no beta effects and so can cause an unopposed reflex bradycardia. It is very short acting and is often used as an infusion to prevent hypotension.

6.5.6 *Ephedrine*

Ephedrine is an alpha and beta agonist. It also has indirect effects as it causes the release of noradrenaline from sympathetic terminals. Its effects are less potent but longer lasting than those of adrenaline as it is not metabolised by monoamine oxidase or catechol O-methyl transferase (COMT). Due to its beta stimulation it may cause tachycardia.

6.5.7 *Metaraminol*

Metaraminol acts mainly on alpha-1 receptors, but also has some beta and indirect actions. Despite its beta adrenoceptor activity, cardiac output may drop due to the raised systemic vascular resistance and reflex bradycardia.

6.6 Cardiac Output: Advantages and Disadvantages of Pharmacological Augmentation

Inotropes are used to increase cardiac contractility and stroke volume. Chronotropes are used to increase heart rate. Both these mechanisms increase cardiac output and hence oxygen delivery to the tissues. Most agents used to increase cardiac output have both inotropic and chronotropic effects. These may be required in cardiogenic shock.

The increase in cardiac contractility causes an increase in myocardial oxygen requirements that, if not offset by an adequate increase in coronary artery oxygen delivery, will cause myocardial ischaemia. The increase in heart rate causes less time for coronary flow in diastole. Most inotropes also cause an increased incidence of atrial and ventricular arrhythmias.

Although inotropes may produce an immediate haemodynamic and clinical improvement, they may cause further myocardial damage and increase patient mortality. Inotropes should therefore be started early, the minimal amount of inotrope to produce a cardiac output with adequate perfusion or decreased congestion should be used and patients should be weaned off as early as possible.

In cardiogenic shock, it is recommended that vasopressors should only be used if a combination of fluid challenge and inotrope with an increase in cardiac output has been insufficient to correct hypotension and hypoperfusion.

6.6.1 *Adrenaline*

Adrenaline is the most potent inotrope and so remains the first choice agent in cardiac arrest, where it is used at dose of 1 mg every three to five minutes. In the current European Society of Cardiology guidelines for heart failure [17], it is recommended that adrenaline is not used as an inotrope or vasopressor in cardiogenic shock.

6.6.2 *Dobutamine*

Dobutamine is a beta-1 agonist with weak beta-2 properties. It is used in a dose of 2–20 μg/kg/min. Beta adrenoceptors in cardiac myocytes are coupled to Gs proteins, which stimulate adenylyl cyclase to produce cAMP. This raises intracellular calcium which increases actin–myosin myofilament interaction leading to an increase in the force and frequency of contraction.

The racemic mixture of dobutamine used has both alpha-1 agonist and antagonist properties. In addition to its inotropic and chronotropic effects (beta-1 activation), the systemic vascular resistance may either fall, causing hypotension due to the peripheral beta-2 activation, or it may be maintained by the opposing alpha-1 agonist effect. Its use therefore may require the addition of a vasopressor. It is rapidly metabolised by COMT to inactive metabolites and has a half-life of two minutes.

Dobutamine is the recommended first line inotrope in septic shock with measured or suspected low cardiac output in the presence of adequate fluid resuscitation [25].

6.6.3 *Dopexamine*

Dopexamine is a beta-2 and D1 receptor antagonist that produces an increase in cardiac output from positive inotropy due to cardiac beta-2 receptors and a decreased afterload from peripheral beta-2 stimulation. Beta-2 receptors on vascular smooth muscle are coupled to Gs proteins, which stimulate protein kinase. This increases calcium uptake by the sarcoplasmic reticulum leading to vasodilatation. It improves mesenteric and renal blood flow by reducing vascular resistance and so, like dopamine, has a diuretic effect. It is used in a dose of 0.5–6.0 μg/kg/min and has a half-life of seven minutes.

6.6.4 *Dopamine*

Dopamine at low doses will stimulate D1 and beta receptors, producing inotropy, chronotropy and some diuresis. If used at higher doses it will stimulate alpha receptors and maintain or increase blood pressure with increased SVR, but there will be an increase in arrhythmias.

6.6.5 *Phosphodiesterase inhibitors*

Phosphodiesterase inhibitors include milrinone and enoximone. They inhibit the type III phosphodiesterase enzyme that breaks down cAMP, therefore increasing cAMP, intracellular calcium and myocardial contractility. The increase in cAMP peripherally increases uptake of calcium into the sarcoplasmic reticulum and causes vasodilatation. This effect is preserved in patients who have been on chronic β-blocker therapy as the mechanism of action is distal to the beta receptor [36].

The inodilator effect is particularly useful in acute cardiac failure as there is an increase in cardiac output and decrease in SVR and pulmonary vascular resistance (PVR), thereby decreasing ventricular filling pressures. A bolus is given prior to the infusion if there is no hypotension.

6.6.6 *Levosimendan*

Levosimendan is a class II calcium channel sensitiser. It binds and stabilises troponin C in a calcium-dependent manner and increases the actin–myosin crossbridge formation. It increases the sensitivity of the myofilaments to calcium without increasing the actual level of intracellular calcium. It also has a vasodilatory effect on venous, systemic and coronary arterial systems. This is via the increased opening of adenosinetriphosphate (ATP)-sensitive potassium channels in vascular smooth muscle [37], this causes hyperpolarisation, a decrease in intracellular calcium and vasodilatation.

It has been shown to improve contractility in patients with left ventricle dysfunction and post coronary artery bypass graft surgery [38,39]. It is unique in comparison to other inotropic agents as it does not significantly increase myocardial energy demand [40]. Unlike the other inotropes it is non-arrhythmogenic as it does not increase intracellular calcium levels. In patients without hypotension a bolus is given prior to infusion.

There have been a number of randomised controlled trials comparing dobutamine and levosimendan. The Levosimendan Infusion versus Dobutamine (LIDO) study [41], with 103 patients with acute heart failure, showed that levosimendan produced a significant improvement in haemodynamics and also survival at 180 days. Subsequent trials in patients with heart failure and symptoms at rest, showed an early greater symptom response but no improvement in mortality. The largest trial, Survival of Patients with Acute Heart Failure in Need of Intravenous Inotropic Support (SURVIVE), with 1,327 patients in acute heart failure requiring inotropes, showed a trend to decreased mortality at day 5 and 31, but no benefit was seen at 180 days [42].

6.6.7 *Isoprenaline*

Isoprenaline is a sympathomimetic drug which is structurally similar to adrenaline but acts only on beta-1 and beta-2 receptors. It has positive chronotropic, inotropic and dromotropic (increases conduction through atrioventricular node) actions, but is used mainly for its chronotropic actions in bradycardia. It has significant systemic and mild pulmonary vasodilatory actions. It mainly increases cardiac output via its chronotropic actions, as the inotropic effect is offset by the decrease in systemic vascular resistance. It is used at a dose of 2–10 μg/min.

6.7 A Rational Evidence-Based Approach to Inotropes

In hypotensive states, inotropes and vasopressors may be a necessary part of management. During the resuscitation process, it is necessary to consider the cause of the hypotension and what the pre-morbid blood pressure is in order to understand the pressure required to maintain adequate tissue perfusion. Cardiac output monitoring helps titrate the agents used appropriately to obtain targets which may be supra-normal for peri-operative patients, but adequate and appropriate for the majority of critically ill patients.

In septic shock, the current evidence [25] suggests early goal-directed therapy with dopamine or noradrenaline if the targets are not being reached. These are mixed vasoconstrictor–inotrope agents and so are also useful before cardiac output monitoring can be established. The target MAP suggested is 65 mmHg. Adrenaline is the recommended first alternative if the patient is inadequately responsive to dopamine or noradrenaline. If the patient has low cardiac output, despite adequate left ventricular filling pressures or adequate fluid optimisation, dobutamine is recommended for its inotropic effect.

In acute cardiac failure, the European Society of Cardiology guidelines [17] recommend vasodilators and levosimendan (if available). In cardiogenic shock with a systolic blood pressure 90–100 mmHg and adequate filling pressures, inodilators such as dobutamine, phosphodiesterase inhibitors or levosimendan are recommended. With significant systolic hypotension (less than 90 mmHg) dopamine is recommended, as this inotrope has no vasodilating effect and noradrenaline should be added if a vasopressor is required.

6.8 Clinical Case

A 63-year-old gentleman was admitted to the intensive care unit with community-acquired pneumonia and septic shock. Four years previously he had a myocardial infarction and coronary artery bypass grafting, but he had been able to walk up two flights of stairs.

Initial management of septic shock was commenced and he was intubated for type 1 respiratory failure. Being unresponsive to fluid resuscitation, noradrenaline was started to maintain a MAP above 65 mmHg. Cardiac output monitoring showed an initial cardiac index (CI) of 4.2 $l/min/m^2$ and SVR of 600 $dyn.s/cm^5$.

A period of 24 hours later he became hypotensive despite an increasing dose of noradrenaline. His CI decreased to 1.8 $l/min/m^2$, his electrocardiogram showed a new right bundle branch block and he had a raised troponin level. Echocardiography showed an ejection fraction of 20% (previously 45% one year ago).

He had developed cardiogenic shock from a further non-ST-elevation myocardial infarction and at this point a dobutamine infusion was also commenced. His MAP was sustained at between 65 and 75 mmHg. Once the required dosage of dobutamine was established the CI rose to 4.1 l/min^2 gradually and the SVR increased from 400 to 700 $dyn.s/cm^5$ with manipulation of the noradrenaline infusion. The patient had episodes of supraventricular tachycardia (SVT). Subsequently, levosimendan was introduced and he was weaned off dobutamine. His cardiac function was sustained at an adequate level and, after prolonged weaning from inotropes and the ventilator, he was discharged from the intensive care unit after four weeks.

In conclusion, noradrenaline was used to treat fluid-resistant hypotension in this patient with septic shock. When he subsequently developed cardiogenic shock and persistent hypotension despite increasing doses of noradrenaline, dobutamine was commenced, which caused the cardiac output to rise to baseline values. However, as the patient developed SVT, dobutamine was replaced with levosimendan because of its non-arrhythmogenic properties. This case study demonstrates how different vasoactive agents can be used in the clinical setting.

References

[1] Shoemaker, W.C., Appel, P.L., Kram, H.B. *et al.* (1993). Sequence of physiologic patterns in surgical septic shock, *Crit Care Med*, **21**, 1876–1889.

[2] Shoemaker, W.C., Appel, P.L., Kram, H.B. *et al.* (1993). Temporal hemodynamic and oxygen transport patterns in medical patients: septic shock, *Chest*, **104**, 1529–1536.

[3] Tuchschmidt, J., Fried, J., Astiz, M. *et al.* (1992). Elevation of cardiac output and oxygen delivery improves outcome in septic shock, *Chest*, **102**, 216–220.

[4] Krejci, V., Hiltebrand, L.B. and Sigurdson, G.H. (2006). Effects of epinephrine, norepinephrine, and phenylephrine on microcirculatory blood flow in the gastrointestinal tract in sepsis, *Crit Care Med*, **34**, 1456–1463.

[5] Lin, S.M., Huang, C.D., Lin, H.C. *et al.* (2006). A modified goal-directed protocol improves clinical outcomes in intensive care units patients with septic shock: a randomized controlled trial, *Shock*, **26**, 551–557.
[6] Varpula, M., Tallgren, M., Saukkonen, K. *et al.* (2005). Hemodynamic variables related to outcome in septic shock, *Intens Care Med*, **31**, 1066–1071.
[7] LeDoux, D., Astiz, M.E., Carpati, C.M. *et al.* (2000). Effects of perfusion pressure on tissue perfusion in septic shock, *Crit Care Med*, **28**, 2729–2732.
[8] Bourgoin, A., Leone, M., Delmas, A. *et al.* (2005). Increasing mean arterial pressure in patients with septic shocks: effects on oxygen variables and renal function, *Crit Care Med*, **33**, 780–786.
[9] Trzeciak, S., Dellinger, R.P., Parrilo, J.E. *et al.* (2007). Early microcirculatory perfusion derangements in patients with severe sepsis and septic shock: relationship to hemodynamics, oxygen transport and survival, *Ann Emerg Med*, **49**, 88–98.
[10] Sakr, Y., Dubois, M.J., De Backer, D. *et al.* (2004). Persistant microvasculatory alterations are associated with organ failure and death in patients with septic shock, *Crit Care Med*, **32**, 1825–1831.
[11] Bateman, R.M. and Walley, K.R. (2005). Microvascular resuscitation as a therapeutic goal in severe sepsis. *Crit Care*, **9** (Suppl. 4), S27–S32.
[12] Taneja, R. and Vaughan, R.S. (2001). Oxygen, *Brit J Anaesth. CEPD reviews*, **1**, 104–107.
[13] Nunn, J.F. (1993). *Nunn's Applied Respiratory Physiology*, fourth edition, Butterworth-Heinemann, Oxford.
[14] Mclellan, S.A. and Walsh, T.S. (2004). Oxygen delivery and haemoglobin, *Continuing Education in Anaesthesia, Critical Care & Pain*, **4**, 123–126.
[15] Sibbald, W.J., Mesmer, K. and Fink, M.P. (eds) (1998). 'Tissue oxygenation in acute medicine', in Vincent, J-.L. (ed.), *Update in Intensive Care and Emergency Medicine*, **33**, Springer, Berlin.
[16] Herbert, P.C., Wells, G., Blajchman, M.A. *et al.* (1999). A multicenter, randomized, controlled clinical trial of transfusion requirements in critical care, *N Engl J Med*, **340**, 409–417.
[17] Dickstein, K., Cohen–Solal, A., Filippatos, G. *et al.* (2008). ESC Guidelines for the diagnosis and treatment of acute and chronic heart failure 2008, *Eur Heart J*, **29**, 2388–2442.
[18] Hashimoto, S. and Kobayashi, A. (2003). Clinical pharmacokinetics and pharmacodynamics of glyceryl trinitrate and its metabolites, *Clin Pharmacokinet*, **42**, 205–221.
[19] Hobbs, R.E. and Mills, R.M. (1999). Therapeutic potential of neseritide (recombinant b-type natriuretic peptide) in the treatment of heart failure, *Exp Opinion Invest Drugs*, **8**, 1063–1072.

[20] Publication Committee for the VMAC investigators (2002). Intravenous neseritide vs nitroglycerin for treatment of decompensated congested cardiac failure, *JAMA*, **287**, 1531–1540.
[21] Grossman, E., Messerli, F.H., Grodzicki, T. *et al.* (1996). Should a moratorium be placed on sublingual nifedipine capsules given for hypertensive emergencies and pseudoemergencies? *JAMA*, **276**, 1328–1331.
[22] Varon, J. and Marik, P.E. (2003). Clinical review: The management of hypertensive crises, *Crit Care*, **7**, 374–384.
[23] Bellomo, R., Chapman, M., Finfer, S. *et al.* (2000). Low-dose dopamine in patients with early renal dysfunction: a placebo-controlled randomized trial, *Lancet*, **356**, 2139–2143.
[24] Beck, G.C., Brinkkoetter, P., Hanusch, C. *et al.* (2004). Clinical review: immunomodulatory effects of dopamine in general inflammation, *Crit Care*, **8**, 485–491.
[25] Dellinger, R.P., Levy, M.M., Carlet, J.M. *et al.* (2008). Surviving Sepsis Campaign: International Guidelines for management of severe sepsis and septic shock: 2008, *Intens Care Med*, **34**, 17–60.
[26] Sakr, Y., Reinhart, K., Vincent, J.L. *et al.* (2006). Does dopamine administration in shock influence outcome? Results of the Sepsis Occurrence in Acutely ill Patients (SOAP) study, *Crit Care Med*, **34**, 589–597.
[27] Pederson, B.K. and Toft, A.D. (2000). Effects of exercise on lymphocytes and cytokines, *Br J Sports Med*, **34**, 246–251.
[28] Nolan, J.P., Deakin, C.D., Soar, J. *et al.* (2005). European Resuscitation Council Guidelines for Resuscitation 2005. Section 4: Advanced Life Support, *Resuscitation*, **6**, 7S1, S39–S86.
[29] Chong, L.K., Morice, A.H., Yeo, W.W. *et al.* (1995). Functional desensitization of beta agonist responses in human lung mast cells, *Am J Respir Cell Mol Biol*, **13**, 540–546.
[30] Kay, L.J. and Peachell, P.T. (2005). Mast cell β_2-adrenoceptors, *Chem Immunol Allergy*, **87**, 145–153.
[31] Den Ouden, D.T. and Meinders, A.E. (2005). Vasopressin: physiology and clinical use in patients with vasodilatory shock: a review, *Neth J Med*, **63**, 4–13.
[32] Holmes, C., Walley, K., Chittock, R. *et al.* (2001). The effects of vasopressin on hemodynamics and renal function in severe septic shock: a case series, *Intens Care Med*, **27**, 1416–1421.
[33] Dunser, M.W., Mayr, A.J., Ulmer, H. *et al.* (2003). Arginine vasopressin in advanced vasodilatory shock. A prospective randomized controlled study, *Circulation*, **107**, 2313–2319.

[34] Russell, JA., Walley K.R., Singer J. *et al.* (2008). Vasopressin versus norepinephrine infusion in patients with septic shock, *N Engl J Med*, **358**, 877–887.
[35] Macarthur, A. and Riley, E. (2007). Obstetric anesthesia controversies: Vasopressor choice for postspinal hypotension during cesarean delivery, *Int Anesthesiol Clin*, **45**, 115–132.
[36] Metra, M., Nodari S., D'Aloia, A. *et al.* (2002). Beta blocker therapy influences the haemodynamic response to inotropic agents in patients with heart failure: a randomized comparison of dobutamine and enoximone before and after chronic treatment with metoprolol or carvedolol, *J Am Coll Cardiol*, **40**, 1248–1258.
[37] Yokoshiki, H. and Sperelakis, N. (2003). Vasodilating mechanisms of levosimendan, *Cadiovasc Drugs Ther*, **17**, 111–113.
[38] Lilleburg, J., Sundberg, S., Nieminen, M.A. (1995). Dose-range study of a new calcium sensitizer, levosimendan, in patients with left ventricular dysfunction, *J Cardiovasc Pharmacol*, **26** (Suppl. 1), S63–S69.
[39] Lilleburg, J., Sundberg, S., Akkila, J. *et al.* (1998). Effects of a new calcium sensitizer, levosimendan, on haemodynamics, coronary blood flow and myocardial substrate utilization early after coronary artery bypass grafting, *Eur Heart J*, **19**, 660–668.
[40] Figgitt, D.P., Gillies, P.S. and Goa, K.L. (2001). Levosimendan, *Drugs*, **61**, 613–627.
[41] Follath, F., Cleland, J.G., Just, H. *et al.* (2002). Efficacy and safety of intravenous levosimendan compared with dobutamine in severe low-output heart failure (the LIDO study): a randomized double-blind trial, *Lancet*, **360**, 196–202.
[42] Mebazaa, A., Nieminen, M.S., Packer, M. *et al.* (2007). Levosimendan vs dobutamine for patients with acute decompensated heart failure: the SURVIVE Randomized Trial, *JAMA*, **297**, 1883–1891.
[43] Bland, R.D., Shoemaker, W.C., Abraham E. *et al.* (1985). Haemodynamic and oxygen transport patterns in surviving and non-surviving patients, *Crit Care Med*, **13**, 85–90.
[44] Shoemaker, W.C., Appel, P.L., Kram, H.B. *et al.* (1988). Prospective trial of supranormal values of survivors as therapeutic goals in high-risk patients, *Chest*, **94**, 1176–1186.
[45] Boyd, O., Grounds, R.M. and Bennett, E.D. (1993). A randomized clinical trial of the effect of deliberate perioperative increase of oxygen delivery on mortality in high-risk surgical patients, *JAMA*, **270**, 2699–2707.
[46] Hayes, M.A., Timmins, A.C., Yau, E. *et al.* (1994). Elevation of systemic oxygen delivery in the treatment of critically ill patients, *N Engl J Med*, **330**, 1717–1722.

[47] Gattinoni, L., Brazzi, L., Pelosi, P. *et al.* (1995). A trial of goal-oriented hemodynamic therapy in critically ill patients, *N Engl J Med*, **333**, 1025–1032.

[48] Weil, M.H. and Henning, R.J. (1979). New concepts in the diagnosis and fluid treatment of circulatory shock. Thirteenth annual Becton, Dickinson and Company Oscar Schwidetsky Memorial Lecture, *Anesth Analg*, **58**, 124–132.

[49] Michard, F., Boussat, S., Chemla, D. *et al.* (2000). Relation between respiratory changes in arterial pulse pressure and fluid responsiveness in septic patients with acute circulatory failure, *Am J Respir Crit Care Med*, **162**, 134–138.

[50] Coriat, P., Vrillon, M., Perel, A. *et al.* (1994). A comparison of systolic blood pressure variations and echocardiographic estimates of end-diastolic left ventricular size in patients after aortic surgery, *Anesth Analg*, **78**, 46–53.

[51] Bekenstadt, H., Margalit, N., Hadani, M. *et al.* (2001). Stroke volume variation as a predictor of fluid responsiveness in patients undergoing brain surgery, *Neurosurg Anaesth*, **92**, 984–989.

[52] Rivers, E., Nguyen, B., Havsted, S. *et al.* (2001). Early goal-directed therapy in the treatment of severe sepsis and septic shock, *N Engl J Med*, **345**, 1368–1377.

[53] Dellinger, R.P., Carlet, J.M., Masur, H. *et al.* (2004). Surviving Sepsis Campaign guidelines for management of severe sepsis and septic shock, *Intens Care Med*, **30**, 536–555.

7

Mechanical Ventilation

Amisha V. Barochia, Charles Natanson and Peter Q. Eichacker

7.1 Overview

While acute lung injury (ALI) and the acute respiratory distress syndrome (ARDS), severe asthma and decompensated chronic obstructive pulmonary disease are all common causes of acute respiratory failure, the methods and adjunctive measures used for their ventilatory support vary. Despite these differences, all patients requiring such support are at risk of ventilator-acquired pneumonia. This chapter examines issues regarding the ventilatory management of these conditions.

7.2 Acute Lung Injury (ALI)/Acute Respiratory Distress Syndrome (ARDS)

7.2.1 *Introduction*

ALI and the more severe ARDS result from diffuse inflammatory injury of the alveolar–capillary interface. This injury is typically related to precipitating conditions such as sepsis, pneumonia, aspiration, massive blood product transfusion and trauma, which stimulate host cellular and humoral responses [1–4]. The American–European Consensus (AECC) on ARDS definition for these conditions includes the acute onset of bilateral pulmonary infiltrates on a chest X-ray (CXR) with a partial pressure of oxygen in arterial blood:fraction of inspired oxygen (PaO_2:FiO_2) ratio ≤ 200 for ARDS and ≤ 300 for ALI, in a patient without evidence of left atrial hypertension [1]. Patients with ALI/ARDS typically require early mechanical ventilatory support and mortality remains high [5,6]. Research has increasingly highlighted the complex and heterogeneous nature of this syndrome and, repeatedly, new therapies introduced to augment conventional ones have not shown clear benefit in randomised trials [7,8]. Initiation of ventilatory support followed by control of the underlying cause of ALI/ARDS, prevention of secondary infection and further lung injury and judicious use of other supportive measures remain mainstays of treatment.

7.2.2 *Histopathological and pathophysiological changes*

The histological and pathophysiological changes during ALI/ARDS evolve in three stages [9,10]. An early exudative stage (days 1–7) is characterised by widespread disruption of type I and II alveolar cell function along with endothelial cell swelling and widening of intracellular junctions [9–12]. Alveoli fill with neutrophils, oedema, platelet and fibrin aggregates and cellular debris that organise into hyaline membranes. A variety of host inflammatory mediators contribute to this stage [13]. Computerised chest tomography shows that alveolar injury and filling is heterogeneous [14–16]. Some alveoli are spared or partially filled and some show no aeration. Independent lung regions show greater sparing than dependent ones. Arterial hypoxemia results from perfusion of non-ventilated alveolar units (i.e. shunt) and can be resistant to increased oxygen concentrations [17,18]. Application of positive end expiratory pressure (PEEP) may recruit or stabilise reversibly collapsed alveoli and improve oxygenation. Reduced pulmonary compliance during this stage relates to the presence of fluid and impaired surfactant function as well as to the loss of inflatable lung volume.

The proliferative stage follows (days 7–14). Type II cell numbers increase and there is myofibrocyte infiltration and collagen deposition [9,10]. While the proliferative phase is necessary for repair, it may also progress into a final fibroproliferative phase characterised by excessive myofibroblast proliferation and collagen deposition [19,20]. This fibrotic response can obliterate normal alveolar and vascular structures. Regeneration of normal lung architecture during ALI/ARDS appears to be dependent upon the net balance between lung recruitment of endothelial precursor cells necessary for normal repair versus myofibroblast infiltration and proliferation [21]. Pathophysiologic changes during these later stages reflect organisation of the protein-rich alveolar exudate and fibrosis of alveolar and vascular tissue. Hypoxemia with intrapulmonary shunt and reductions in compliance persist and become resistant to PEEP [22,23]. Pulmonary vasculature is lost and dead space ventilation results in hypercarbia [24].

7.2.3 *Ventilator-induced lung injury (VILI)*

While mechanical ventilation is essential for the management of ALI/ARDS, it may also aggravate injury. Excessive distending pressures, over-inflation of spared lung and repetitive opening and closing of partially collapsed alveoli can cause injury referred to as barotrauma, volutrauma and atelectrauma [25,26]. This trauma may itself stimulate release of host mediators that propagate injury [27,28]. A major direction of ALI/ARDS research has been to define methods capable of limiting the potential adverse effects of mechanical ventilation.

7.2.4 *Conventional mechanical ventilation*

7.2.4.1 *Modes of ventilation*

Two basic modes of conventional mechanical ventilation are applied during ALI/ARDS; either volume- or pressure-limited [29,30]. The former is set to deliver a prescribed tidal volume independent of airway pressures while the latter is set based on airway pressure independent of the administered volume. Pressure-regulated volume control ventilation is a combination mode in which set volumes may or may not be achieved based on pressures generated during a series of respiratory cycles [31]. No large controlled trials support one of these modes over the other although clinical surveys suggest that volume mode is used most frequently [32,33].

7.2.4.2 *Arterial oxygen and carbon dioxide goals*

Oxygen goals for ALI/ARDS have decreased related to the findings that (i) hypoxemia is not a direct cause of death in most cases of ALI/ARDS and (ii) adjunctive treatments that improve oxygenation do not alter outcome [7,34]. To what degree oxygen toxicity is a factor in patients with ALI/ARDS is unclear [35]. At this time it is recommended that FiO_2 be maintained at levels of less than 70% while ensuring that arterial oxygen pressure produces haemoglobin oxygen saturation (SaO_2) levels of 90% or greater.

Accepted carbon dioxide levels (partial pressure of arterial CO_2 ($PaCO_2$)) have increased to avoid ventilatory injury [5,7]. Recent studies in ALI/ARDS report $PaCO_2$ levels well above 40 mmHg with mean values approaching 50 mmHg in some subgroups. The safety of this approach is based largely on the ARDS Network low-tidal-volume trial (Respiratory Management in Acute Lung Injury/Acute Respiratory Distress Syndrome (ARMA)), although questions regarding this trial have been raised [36,37]. The use of bicarbonate to counter the pH changes occurring with increased $PaCO_2$ may not be advantageous since it may itself increase $PaCO_2$ and can cause volume overload and lower potassium levels. Increased $PaCO_2$ is contraindicated in some subgroups, such as those with increased intracranial pressure or cardiac ischemia [7].

7.2.4.3 *Tidal volume and airway pressure goals*

Maintaining airway pressures less than 30–35 cm H_20 to reduce VILI has been advocated for ALI/ARDS for the past 20 years [35]. Based on the widespread use of volume-control ventilation, reduction in tidal volume was often used to accomplish this goal. To help define optimal tidal volumes for ALI/ARDS patients, randomised trials were conducted comparing higher and lower tidal volumes [36,38–41]. The results of five such trials were inconsistent and overall did not support the use of any single tidal volume [37]. An updated analysis of these trials, including one additional trial, concluded that 'clinical heterogeneity, such as different lengths of follow up and higher plateau pressures in control arms in two trials, make interpretation of the combined results difficult' [42,43]. However, the largest of these trials (the ARMA trial) reported that a low tidal volume of 6ml/kg predicted body weight (PBW) improved survival compared with a 'traditional' control tidal volume of 12 ml/kg PBW [36]. The high airway pressures in the 'traditional' control arm raised questions about whether 6ml/kg was beneficial or 12ml/kg was disadvantageous, compared with the usual practice of titrating tidal volume to maintain airway pressures below 30–35 cm H_2O. Regardless, some experts in the field came to recommend a tidal volume of 6 ml/kg PBW for all ALI/ARDS patients [2,44]. Despite such recommendations, physicians have been slow to incorporate such a discrete low tidal volume for all patients [45]. In recent trials testing different PEEP levels in ALI/ARDS, patients were assigned to 6ml/kg PBW tidal volumes following randomisation, but before randomisation, tidal volumes (mean ± standard deviation) varied between 7.4 ± 1.4 and 8.4 ± 2.2 ml/kg PBW [46–48]. Consistent with this pre-randomisation clinical trial data, surveys show physicians vary tidal volumes based in part on lung compliance to achieve airway pressures generally less than 30 cm H_20 [49–52]. All patients require a lung-protective strategy to minimise VILI. However, inappropriately low tidal volumes may increase sedation needs, aggravate hemodynamic function and increase atelectasis [53–55]. Thus caution must be used when decreasing tidal volume. Even proponents of 6 ml/kg tidal volumes agree, because 'mechanical ventilation with low tidal volume (V_t) and plateau pressure (P_{plat}) may cause more atelectasis and increase requirements for higher FiO_2 and positive end-expiratory pressure' [56]. The population of patients with ALI/ARDS is heterogeneous in terms of cause and severity of lung injury as well as other comorbidities. Although some experts recommend strict adherence to a fixed low-tidal-volume regimen, others recognise that patient heterogeneity requires each ALI/ARDS patient be considered individually [45,57,58]. Tidal volume and other settings should be titrated to avoid injurious airway pressures while maintaining patient comfort and avoiding the risk of atelectasis and other sequelae of under-ventilation.

7.2.4.4 *Use of positive end expiratory pressure*

PEEP improves oxygenation and compliance during ALI/ARDS by recruiting or stabilising partially collapsed alveoli in areas of lung continuing to receive blood flow [59]. PEEP may be less effective during ALI/ARDS related to pulmonary causes (e.g. bacterial pneumonia) as opposed to non-pulmonary ones (e.g. intra-abdominal sepsis) [10]. The beneficial effects of PEEP on oxygenation decrease as fibrosis progresses [23,60]. PEEP can also have adverse cardiovascular effects and may itself worsen ventilation and perfusion matching [61,62].

There has been recent interest in determining whether the use of higher PEEP levels during ALI/ARDS to maintain maximal lung inflation (i.e. open lung) and prevent injury related to repetitive opening and closing of partially filled alveoli (i.e. atelectrauma) would improve outcome [8]. This interest relates in part to recognition that low-tidal-volume ventilation may increase atelectasis. None of three large randomised controlled trials however has shown a beneficial effect of higher compared with lower PEEP (Table 7.1) [46–48]. Lack of benefit has been attributed to patient heterogeneity [8]. Increased PEEP may only be effective for the subgroup of patients with ALI/ARDS with a large component of lung oedema and alveolar collapse and more severe hypoxemia. Prior work with CTT has shown that recruitment manoeuvers (e.g., high and briefly sustained PEEP levels) result in substantial improvement in aeration in some ALI/ARDS patients but not others [63]. At this time physicians must titrate PEEP, balancing oxygen goals with the potential detrimental effects of PEEP on haemodynamics and airway pressures.

7.2.5 *Alternate modes of mechanical ventilation and adjunctive treatments*

7.2.5.1 *High-frequency oscillatory ventilation*

High-frequency oscillatory ventilation (HFOV) employs rapid pressure oscillations of 3 to 10 Hz in the setting of continuous high distending

Table 7.1. Summary of randomised controlled trials comparing low and high PEEP levels in ALI/ARDS.

Study/Author (year) [ref]	PEEP group	PEEP level (mean ± standard deviation)	Percentage of patients surviving (total studied)
ARDS Network (2004) [36]	Low	8.9 ± 3.5	75.1 (273)
	High	14.7 ± 3.5	72.5 (276)
Meade *et al.* (2008) [47]	Low	10.1 ± 3.0	59.6 (508)
	High	15.6 ± 63.6	63.6 (475)
Mercat *et al.* (2008) [48]	Low	7.1 ± 1.8	61.0 (382)
	High	14.6 ± 3.2	64.6 (385)

airway pressure [64]. This produces very small tidal volumes resulting in gas exchange via interregional gas mixing between alveoli and convective and axial transport. The potential attributes of HFOV for ALI/ARDS are that the small tidal volumes minimise barotrauma and volutrauma while the high distending airway pressures promote improved oxygenation and reduced atelectrauma [65]. Case series suggested that HFOV could be applied safely in adult ALI/ARDS although hypotension and pneumothorax were reported [64–66]. In one randomised trial in 48 patients, HFOV was associated with a lower but not significantly different mortality rate than conventional mechanical ventilation (CMV) (37 versus 52%, $p = 0.102$) while complication rates did not differ [67]. In a second randomised trial in 61 patients, HFOV was associated with a higher but not statistically different mortality rate compared with CMV (43% versus 33%, $p = 0.59$) [68]. A third randomised trial enrolling 39 patients reported mortality rates in patients receiving HFOV in the supine position (38%), CMV in the prone position (31%) and HFOV in the prone position (23%) but small group sizes contradict this study [69]. The OSCILLATE trial investigators reported the results of a multicentre, multinational, randomised, controlled trial comparing HFOV with conventional ventilation in moderate to severe ARDS [215]. The trial was stopped early after 548 of 1200 planned patients due to increased mortality in the HFOV compared with the conventional group (47% ve 35%, respectively).

7.2.5.2 *Airway pressure release ventilation*

Airway pressure release ventilation (APRV) has also been referred to as an open-lung approach to the ventilation of patients with ALI/ARDS [70,71]. Airway pressure is maintained at a constant high level (P_{High}) with intermittent brief releases in pressure to a low level (P_{Low}) permitting ventilation. Patients continue to breathe spontaneously during APRV. Clinical trials of APRV have been limited however. One trial of 50 patients who were crossed over between APRV and CMV for 30 minute periods noted reductions in airway pressure and no clear adverse effects with the former [72]. In three small randomised controlled trials, APRV was associated with lower but not significantly different mortality rates (20% versus 26%, $n = 30$; 8% versus 14%, $n = 33$; and 17% versus 18%, $n = 58$) [73–75]. Although spontaneous breathing with APRV may promote recruitment of dependent lung regions, whether the net effects of this on VILI outweigh the potential risks of prolonged exposure to P_{High} is unclear. Further study is necessary to define the place of APRV in ALI/ARDS.

7.2.5.3 *Prone ventilation*

Rationales for ventilating patients in the prone position include reduction of lung compression by the heart, improved matching of ventilation and perfusion to the dorsal lung regions and increased alveolar recruitment [76–78]. A recent systematic literature search identified five randomised controlled trials (RCTs) testing prone-positioning in patients with ALI/ARDS and one testing it in coma patients without lung injury [79–85]. Across the five trials in patients with lung injury ($n = 1372$), although prone positioning resulted in significant increases in oxygenation, it did not alter survival ($p = 0.79$). However, many aspects of these trials, including the types of patients studied, the methods and duration of prone positioning and the severity of lung injury, differed. Overall, the complication rate with prone positioning was not significantly increased although the incidence of pressure sores showed a trend. At present prone positioning cannot be widely recommended for ALI/ARDS.

7.2.5.4 *Partial liquid ventilation*

The rationale for partial liquid ventilation (PLV) was that perfluorocarbons would support oxygen transport, open-lung units and increase gas exchange [86]. However, neither a phase II/III trial ($n = 90$) nor a larger phase III trial ($n = 311$) showed any benefit with PLV compared with CMV [87,88]. In fact mortality rate was higher in the low- and high-dose PLV groups in the phase III trial. Thus, PLV cannot be recommended for ALI/ARDS.

7.2.5.5 *Nitric oxide*

Nitric oxide (NO) is a selective pulmonary artery vasodilator which if inhaled directs blood flow to better ventilated lung regions [89]. Based on early studies in ALI/ARDS showing that inhaled NO improved oxygenation, it was rapidly introduced into clinical use without controlled trials [90].

Subsequently, controlled trials were undertaken. Following an earlier smaller meta-analysis, a recent one analysing 12 such trials was published [89,91–103]. Although NO reduced pulmonary artery pressure and improved oxygenation in a highly consistent pattern, it had an unfavourable effect on survival and overall increased the risk ratio of death (risk ratio 1.10, 95% confidence interval 0.94–1.30) [93–96,98,101,103]. Furthermore, in four trials including almost three quarters of the patients studied, NO consistently increased the relative risk of renal dysfunction (1.5, 95% confidence interval 1.11–2.02) [94,97,99,102]. Use of inhaled NO cannot be widely recommended for ALI/ARDS.

7.2.5.6 *Surfactant*

Surfactant is important not only for normal gas-exchange and lung compliance but also for pulmonary host defence [104] Abnormalities of surfactant protein appear to correlate with severity of ALI/ARDS. Despite these associations, attempts to replace surfactant in adults with ALI/ARDS, while improving oxygen exchange, have not altered overall outcome [105–108]. Although surfactant replacement continues to be studied for ALI/ARDS, at present it cannot be recommended as treatment.

7.2.5.7 *Extracorporeal membrane oxygenation*

Extracorporeal membrane oxygenation (ECMO), sometimes referred to as extracorporeal life support (ECLS), removes venous blood from a patient, pumps it through a membrane oxygenator, warms and returns it either to the venous (VV ECMO) or arterial (VA ECMO) circulations [109–111]. Thus VV ECMO provides oxygenated blood in series with the lung while VA ECMO does so in parallel. While on ECMO, patients continue to receive mechanical ventilation, although tidal volume and respiratory rate settings can be minimised to limit the potential for ventilator-associated lung injury. Treatment with VV ECMO is employed to provide oxygenation or ventilatory support while VA ECMO can also provide cardiac support.

Use of ECMO for respiratory failure was originally shown to be effective in the neonatal and then the paediatric population [111]. The role of ECMO for the treatment of adult patients with ARDS is unclear. An early randomised trial did not show any benefit of VA ECMO, although many criticisms of this trial have been raised [112]. A subsequent randomised trial employing VV ECMO for carbon dioxide removal in adults with ARDS also gave negative results [113]. Despite these negative trials, experience with ECMO for patients with ARDS has grown at several specialised centres. Accumulating results from such patients has suggested that for some adult patients with ARDS unresponsive to conventional or salvage (e.g. nitric oxide or prone positioning) ventilatory therapy, ECMO may provide effective support until lung repair can occur [111–114]. Based in part on this type of experience, a third randomised intention-to-treat trial was conducted (Conventional Ventilation or ECMO for Severe Adult Respiratory Failure (CESAR) trial) in the United Kingdom [115]. Mortality or disability in the ECMO group was 37% at six months whether patients did (n = 68) or did not (n = 22) receive ECMO compared with 53% in the control group (n = 90) (p = 0.03). At this time, use of ECMO for adult ARDS may be indicated in those patients with severe but potentially reversible ARDS. However, such support should only be conducted at centres with the experience and resources that this treatment demands.

7.3 Asthma

7.3.1 *Introduction*

The National Asthma Education and Prevention Program 2007 Expert Panel Report-3 (NAEPP EPR-3) [116] defines asthma as a common chronic disorder of the airways characterised by airflow obstruction, bronchial hyper-responsiveness, and underlying inflammation. In 2004, there were nearly 1.8 million emergency room visits and 0.5 million hospitalisations for asthma in the USA [117]. An estimated 32.6 million people in the USA (4% of the population) have been diagnosed with asthma at some time in their lives based on data from the year 2005. The incidence of asthma appears to be increasing and the mortality rate is substantial. There were 4,055 deaths from asthma reported in the USA in 2003; adults were more likely to die than children and women more so than men. Racial disparities were also noted, with higher mortality rates in African–Americans and Puerto Ricans compared with non-Hispanic whites [117]. More asthma deaths have also been noted in the UK in those over 45 years of age with other comorbidities such as respiratory infections, heart disease and diabetes [118].

Two clinical phenotypes of severe or fatal asthma have been described [119]. One presents acutely, with a sudden onset of bronchospasm occurring over minutes to hours, associated with a neutrophilic bronchitis. This presentation has been linked to massive exposure to allergen or psychological stress, and appears to respond rapidly to therapy. The other pattern has a slower onset of worsening symptoms occurring over days to weeks. It is associated with extensive mucous plugging, mucus gland hypertrophy and airway wall oedema. Moderate to severe airflow obstruction and increasing respiratory symptoms that respond slowly to treatment are typical of this phenotype [120–123].

Risk factors associated with near fatal asthma include previous life-threatening asthmatic episodes, prior mechanical ventilation, steroid dependence, non-adherence to inhaled corticosteroids, poorly controlled asthma and hospital admission within the past year due to asthma. A lower forced expiratory volume in one second (FEV_1), current cigarette smoke exposure, lack of access to health care and psychosocial or psychological problems are other risk factors that have been identified [121,124].

The classic symptoms of an asthma attack are dyspnoea, wheezing and cough, but it may be difficult to appreciate the severity of an exacerbation clinically. The NAEPP 2007 guidelines recommend admission to the intensive care unit (ICU) if the peak expiratory flow (PEF) or FEV_1 values are below 25% predicted and improve by less than 10% after initial treatment [116].

7.3.2 *Pathophysiology*

Asthma is characterised by airway inflammation, probably resulting from an interaction between genetic susceptibility and environmental factors such as viruses, allergens or other stressors. This inflammation is mediated by numerous cell types and cytokines [116,125–127]. Variable airway obstruction results from inflammation of the airway wall, oedema, increased mucus secretion, bronchial hyper-reactivity and constriction and, eventually, airway remodelling, which may be irreversible [128]. During an acute exacerbation of asthma, airflow obstruction results in incomplete exhalation and an elevated end-expiratory pressure in the lungs, often termed intrinsic positive end-expiratory pressure (iPEEP, occult PEEP or auto PEEP) that in turn produces dynamic hyperinflation. With this, the inspiratory muscles have to generate a transpulmonary pressure to first overcome iPEEP before inspiration can occur, thus leading to increased work since breathing is occurring at a higher, less compliant part of the pressure–volume curve. If this is excessive, respiratory muscle fatigue and respiratory failure occurs.

7.3.3 *Non-invasive mechanical ventilation*

Non-invasive ventilation (NIV) remains controversial in the management of asthmatics with respiratory failure [129]. A trial of NIV, administered as continuous positive airway pressure (CPAP) or as non-invasive positive pressure ventilation (NIPPV), may be considered in addition to aggressive medical therapy in carefully chosen patients. It reduces the work of breathing by offsetting iPEEP and may decrease the hemodynamic effects secondary to large swings in transpulmonary pressures. It also improves lung function parameters and decreases airway obstruction [130]. Potential advantages of NIPPV include improved comfort and lower sedative needs with fewer associated complications [124]. NIV has also been found to improve gas exchange and reduce dyspnoea in severe acute asthma with hypercarbia [131]. Details regarding titration of NIPPV can be found elsewhere [131].

A Cochrane review of NIV for asthma [129] identified 11 studies of NIPPV use in asthmatics, but excluded 10 of those studies due to lack of randomisation or inclusion of non-asthmatic patients. The remaining trial analysed 30 patients [130], half of whom were assigned to conventional therapy and the other half to NIPPV. NIPPV improved FEV_1, forced vital capacity (FVC) and respiratory rate, and decreased the frequency of hospitalisation without increasing complications.

7.3.4 *Conventional (invasive) mechanical ventilation*

7.3.4.1 *Indications*

The decision to intubate the asthmatic patient with respiratory failure is based on clinical assessment. Necessary intubation should not be delayed.

Hypercapnia is often a sign of impending respiratory failure, but in an otherwise alert and co-operative patient, may not mandate intubation [132,133]. Intubation is indicated if the patient develops an altered mental status, hemodynamic instability, fatigue, persistent hypoxia or progressive hypercapnia and respiratory acidosis despite adequate support. Intubating an asthmatic in extremis can be challenging, as it may be difficult to ventilate the patient with a bag–valve device. Rapid sequence intubation by the most experienced operator, with the largest diameter endotracheal tube possible, is recommended to minimise complications. Laryngospasm and reflex bronchoconstriction may occur [124,134].

7.3.4.2 *Drugs for intubation and sedation*

Propofol and ketamine are intravenous agents with bronchodilator properties, and are useful during intubation and as sedatives thereafter for the mechanically ventilated patient [124]. However, both can cause significant hemodynamic instability, especially in those who are volume contracted. Prolonged use of propofol has been associated with pancreatitis and increased risk of infection [135,136]. Ketamine can heighten laryngeal reflexes and increase tracheobronchial secretion; it also has sympathomimetic effects which can be deleterious in those with hypertension and increased intracranial pressure. It should therefore be avoided in those with suspected anoxic brain injury [137]. Etomidate is a rapidly acting hypnotic agent with a short duration of action with minimal hemodynamic effects that may be useful in the unstable patient [138].

Benzodiazepines are often used during intubation, but may produce inadequate relaxation/sedation; they are valuable thereafter for reducing over-breathing and patient–ventilator dyssynchrony and for their amnesic properties. Opioids are used for controlling pain and suppressing the respiratory drive, but they can cause histamine release and potentially worsen bronchospasm [139]. Synthetic opioids such as fentanyl may be preferable to morphine for this reason.

A neuromuscular blocking agent is helpful during the intubation process, and succinylcholine is regarded by some as the drug of choice [124]. Rocuronium, a short acting, non-depolarising agent is an alternative.

7.3.4.3 *Methods*

Increased airway resistance in asthma leads to incomplete exhalation and air-trapping [140]. The aim of mechanical ventilation is to improve alveolar ventilation while minimising dynamic hyperinflation. Oxygenation is usually not a significant problem. Attempts to achieve normal $PaCO_2$ levels are likely to lead to hyperinflation, barotrauma and hemodynamic instability. Therefore, to avoid lung injury, permissive hypercapnia is recommended as a ventilatory strategy [141].

Mechanical ventilation may be achieved with either pressure control (PC) or volume control (VC) modes. The former may be helpful in averting barotrauma but, if not closely monitored, can lead to severe hypoventilation or hyperventilation (depending on how fast the obstruction resolves) due to fluctuating levels of airway resistance and air-trapping. Although VC may be an easier mode with which to control minute ventilation, it requires close, continuous monitoring of airway pressures to prevent barotrauma. No randomised trials exist to show superiority of one mode over the other.

Suggested initial settings for the ventilator include V_t of 6–10 ml/kg predicted body weight, respiratory rate 10–14/min, PEEP 0 cm H_2O, minute ventilation < 10 l/min, inspiratory flow 60–80 l/min, expiratory time 4–5 seconds keeping end-expiratory plateau pressures < 30 cm H_2O, and titrating the oxygen to keep SaO_2 > 90% [142]. Since these settings can be uncomfortable for those in respiratory extremis and cause dyssynchronous ventilation, patients often require deep sedation and occasionally paralysis, although use of both should be kept to a minimum due to potential complications [143].

To counteract alveolar hypoventilation while attempting to minimise hyperinflation, V_t may be cautiously adjusted by monitoring both plateau pressures (end-inspiratory occlusion pressure; goal <30 cm H_2O) and iPEEP [144–146]. The most effective method of decreasing air-trapping is to reduce minute ventilation by decreasing V_t and respiratory rate. Adjunctive measures include increasing the inspiratory flow rate to about 60–80 l/sec in a volume cycled setting to maximise expiratory time. Higher flow rates generally add only marginal benefit and increasing expiratory time to over 4 seconds has little further effect on decreasing hyperinflation [142,145,147].

7.3.4.4 *Intrinsic and extrinsic PEEP*

Intrinsic PEEP can be identified and measured by studying the ventilator graphics, and by performing an end-expiratory occlusion manoeuvre [144]. If inspiratory flow begins before expiratory flow ends (i.e. returns to zero) on the flow versus time graphics on the ventilator screen, air-trapping is occurring. Dynamic iPEEP is measured at the moment when flow equals zero, while static iPEEP is measured by occluding the airway at the end of expiration and allowing the airway pressures to equilibrate [148]. Increasing iPEEP leads to decreasing lung compliance, worsening gas exchange, reduced venous return to the heart and increased work of breathing. Application of extrinsic PEEP (ePEEP) can overcome the increased workload on the respiratory muscles and improve the ventilator–patient interaction in a spontaneously breathing patient [149]. If ePEEP is used, close monitoring of airway pressures is mandatory. If ePEEP exceeds iPEEP, it can increase hyperinflation and end-expiratory lung volumes [150,151]. Passive exhalation from the smaller airways may not be flow-limited in this situation, and applied ePEEP may extend all the way to the alveoli, resulting in increased end-inspiratory volumes. It is therefore important to be able to accurately determine the true value of iPEEP.

7.3.4.5 *Adjunctive therapies*

In addition to supporting ventilation, pharmacological treatment of acute asthma includes use of bronchodilators, steroids and oxygen. Adjunctive therapies considered in refractory cases, but which lack clinical evidence to support their use, include heliox, buffers, general anaesthetics and extracorporeal membrane oxygenation. Inhaled steroids, methylxanthines, mucolytics, aggressive hydration, chest physical therapy and routine antibiotics for the management of acute asthma exacerbations are not recommended [116]. Cysteinyl leukotriene inhibitors may be considered, though their use in severe exacerbations has not been studied. Epinephrine administered subcutaneously is recommended if other bronchodilators cannot be administered by emergency medical services personnel, and no benefit is noted from administering intravenous preparations over inhaled medication [116]. Nebulised epinephrine may be as safe as inhaled Salbutamol, based on several small studies, and could be considered for refractory patients [152].

Oxygen should be used to counteract hypoxia from alveolar hypoventilation, and it should be titrated using pulse oximetry to keep $SaO_2 > 90\%$ ($> 95\%$ in pregnant women and those with cardiovascular disease [116]). Excessive use of oxygen should be avoided, as it can mask hypoventilation and worsen CO_2 retention.

Short-acting beta agonists and steroids reduce expiratory resistance and hyperinflation during asthma. It may be difficult to deliver adequate amounts of inhaled drug to the mechanically ventilated patient, since not all ventilators include nebulisers. An in-line nebuliser attached to the ventilator circuit may interfere with airway pressure measurement, and should be turned off before such manoeuvers are carried out. It may also necessitate adjustment of volume delivered during nebuliser treatments, since the treatment itself will add to the amount of air going to the lungs [153].

Heliox is a mixture of oxygen and helium gas, usually in a 20:80 or 30:70 ratio, which has a density lower than air. Its use reduces turbulent flow, thereby decreasing resistance to flow and air-trapping. Clinical studies done with heliox are small and not all consistent; a Cochrane review involving 544 patients with acute asthma recommends against routine use of heliox, but found that heliox may be useful for those with the most severe obstruction [154]. Heliox has been shown to deliver aerosolised bronchodilators more effectively than an oxygen–air mixture [155], though it is less effective than air–oxygen mixtures for nebulising albuterol into small particles [156]. Though its use has not been associated with any complications, it should be noted that it may be difficult to use with mechanical ventilation, since accurate titration of flow and volumes delivered may be problematic. Correction factors have been calculated that can be used to calibrate ventilators when using heliox [157].

Inhaled anaesthetic agents have not been rigorously studied in the treatment of asthma, though they have been noted anecdotally to be potent bronchodilators, useful for decreasing air-trapping and relieving airflow obstruction. Use of these agents is complicated, as the ventilators used to supply them are often not suited to ventilating patients with increased airway resistance [158].

7.3.5 *Outcome*

Mechanical ventilation plays a supportive role in the treatment of severe asthma. In general, most patients requiring such support survive. Of 2,152 asthmatic patients admitted to ICUs in the United Kingdom between 1995 and 2001, 57% required mechanical ventilation, 7.1% of whom died in the ICU [159]. When death does occur in asthmatics requiring mechanical ventilation it is usually associated with pre-hospital cardiac arrests or cerebral anoxia, or with complications from mechanical ventilation such as barotrauma, hypotension, nosocomial infections or premature extubation [153,159]. Long-term mortality and morbidity is significantly higher in asthmatics requiring mechanical ventilation, and aggressive measures to prevent further exacerbations should be instituted prior to discharge.

7.4 Chronic Obstructive Pulmonary Disease

7.4.1 *Introduction*

Chronic obstructive pulmonary disease (COPD) is characterised by airflow limitation that is not fully reversible [160]. COPD is the fourth leading cause of death in the USA and is expected to increase in incidence over the coming decades. Nearly 24 million people in the USA are believed to have this condition, about half of whom remain undiagnosed [161].

The airflow limitation characteristic of COPD is thought to be secondary to inflammation in the small airways (obstructive bronchiolitis) and parenchymal destruction (emphysema) caused by noxious particles or gases. Acute respiratory failure from COPD exacerbations occurs when an increase in minute ventilation leads to air-trapping from airflow limitation, hyperinflation, worsening ventilation and finally respiratory muscle fatigue [162]. Many stimuli may result in increased minute ventilation in these patients but a common one is an upper or lower respiratory tract infection. Inadequate emptying of the lungs in COPD also leads to worsening ventilation–perfusion (VQ) matching (by compressing the healthier areas of the lungs), decreased venous return to the heart and barotrauma.

The primary goals of mechanical ventilation in the COPD patient with respiratory failure are to provide ventilatory support, to improve gas exchange while minimising lung injury and to allow the respiratory muscles to rest and recover. Mechanical ventilation in the form of NIPPV or conventional ventilation via an endotracheal tube should be considered when medical treatment fails to improve respiratory function.

7.4.2 *Non-invasive positive pressure ventilation*

Short-term respiratory support with NIPPV may be used in patients during an exacerbation of COPD to allow time for medical therapies to reverse airflow limitation and airway inflammation. Many randomised clinical trials have tested the role of NIPPV in the management of respiratory failure due to COPD, and several meta-analyses have been performed based on these [163–166]. Unless contraindicated, NIPPV is now considered first-line therapy for COPD patients with respiratory failure needing ventilatory support, as it has reduced the need for intubation and conferred a mortality benefit in several studies. More severely ill patients appeared to have a greater mortality benefit. Criteria for benefit from NIPPV include a $PaCO_2 > 55$ or $pH < 7.37$ [165]. NIPPV should not be used if there is hemodynamic instability, impaired consciousness, high aspiration risk, copious secretions or other contraindication to a tight-fitting facial mask [167]. Patients who are placed on NIPPV should be closely monitored, and if they fail to improve in the first few hours, NIPPV should be discontinued in favour of invasive mechanical ventilation. NIPPV is most effectively administered as CPAP with some pressure support (PS). Initial settings that may be tried are CPAP 4–8 cm H_2O with PS 10–15 cm H_2O [160].

COPD patients who received NIPPV rather than optimal medical therapy alone or medical therapy with invasive ventilation had a lower one-year mortality [168,169]. NIPPV is also cost effective [170]. NIPPV has been used to wean intubated COPD patients off mechanical ventilation [171,172].

7.4.3 *Invasive mechanical ventilation*

7.4.3.1 *Methods*

Patients with an acute exacerbation of COPD and hyperinflation may be at increased risk of alveolar over-distension and volutrauma during mechanical ventilation. Based on this, controlled hypoventilation with permissive hypercapnia using tidal volumes in the range of 5–7 ml/kg may decrease dynamic hyperinflation and VILI [173]. The aim is not to correct the pH or the $PaCO_2$ to a normal physiological value but to achieve levels that the patient had tolerated prior to the episode of acute respiratory failure. Many patients with advanced COPD have $PaCO_2$ levels that exceed normal physiological ranges and are compensated for by higher serum bicarbonate levels. If the $PaCO_2$ level is corrected to a 'normal' value, it may lead to renal bicarbonate losses. During spontaneous breathing, these losses can lead to metabolic acidosis, increased minute ventilation and failure to wean from mechanical ventilation [174].

Hyperinflation during a COPD exacerbation may be eased by decreasing the minute ventilation, increasing the time available for expiration and decreasing airflow resistance. Increasing inspiratory flow to achieve longer expiratory time can help with air-trapping, but may result in high peak airway pressures. These pressures are dissipated in the larger airways, and may be less likely to result in barotrauma to the alveoli. However, it is possible that due to the heterogeneous distribution of airway disease in COPD, some normal areas of the lungs will be exposed to transient high pressures at the alveolar level, leading to stretch injury [173]. As in asthmatics with acute respiratory failure, decreasing both the respiratory rate and tidal volume may be quite distressing for the dyspnoeic COPD patient, and adequate sedation during mechanically ventilation is necessary for patient comfort and for patient–ventilator synchrony.

Prone ventilation in a small trial of severely hypoxic COPD patients improved oxygenation, but also increased aspiration of secretions without any significant change in outcomes [175]. Negative-pressure ventilation may be useful but lacks sufficient evidence to support its use in respiratory failure from COPD [160].

7.4.3.2 *Intrinsic and extrinsic PEEP*

Respiratory failure in COPD results from respiratory muscle fatigue due to the increased work from breathing at a higher part of the pressure–volume curve. This occurs because of the presence of iPEEP, which has to be overcome before airflow into the lungs can occur. As in asthma, ePEEP applied through the ventilator may help in spontaneously breathing ventilated COPD patients by decreasing the gradient of the transpulmonary pressure necessary to generate flow and improving pressure-triggered ventilation. However, not all patients respond well to ePEEP, and in some, it may even worsen hyperinflation, especially when ePEEP is more than 85–90% of iPEEP [176]. A trial of ePEEP set at about 80% of iPEEP is recommended if other measures are ineffective in reducing air-trapping [177]. An alternative in spontaneously breathing COPD patients is to set the ventilator to deliver flow-triggered breaths [178], which may improve tidal volume and minute ventilation.

7.4.3.3 *Adjunctive therapies*

Medical therapy of COPD exacerbations entails the use of bronchodilators, systemic steroids and antibiotics, along with judicious amounts of supplemental oxygen. Concerns with regard to the use of inhaled medications during mechanical ventilation are similar to those discussed in the section on asthma. Bronchodilators may be delivered either via in-line circuit nebulisers or metered-dose inhalers with inspiratory circuit holding chambers. Drugs may be given as continuous aerosols or at three-fold to four-fold higher intermittent doses to ensure adequate delivery, since endotracheal tubes significantly interfere with aerosol delivery [173].

Overuse of oxygen can worsen hypercapnia by various mechanisms, including dead space ventilation, worsened VQ mismatch, Haldane effect and decreased ventilatory drive. Therefore, oxygen should be titrated to a minimal amount that will achieve adequate SpO_2 levels (~ 90%) [173].

A 2002 Cochrane review concluded that there was insufficient evidence to recommend heliox for treating either ventilated or non-ventilated COPD patients with respiratory failure [179]. However, heliox has been shown to reduce iPEEP, the work of breathing, intrathoracic pressure and airway resistance, as well as duration and cost of hospitalisation. It has also been used with NIPPV, and has been used for weaning patients from MV [176]. NO has not been demonstrated to be beneficial in cases of respiratory failure from COPD [180].

7.4.3.4 *Outcomes*

Acute COPD exacerbations accelerate decline in FEV_1, increase mortality and worsen quality of life in patients. In-hospital mortality rates range around 10%, but are higher in those admitted to the ICU. In-hospital mortality for mechanically ventilated patients in one study was approximately

25%; one-year mortality was close to 40% and five-year mortality was greater than 70% [173]. Respiratory failure requiring mechanical ventilation increases the risk of rehospitalisation and reintubation markedly in COPD patients, especially if mechanical ventilation was necessary for more than 72 hours [167]. However, surviving a prior episode of mechanical ventilation actually predicted better survival.

7.5 Weaning

Weaning encompasses the assessment of a mechanically ventilated patient's readiness for and liberation from mechanical ventilation. It is often delayed [181]. While mechanical ventilation is essential for patients in respiratory failure, increased duration of mechanical ventilation is associated with increased morbidity and mortality [182]. Weaning should begin as early as possible. A systematic daily evaluation for weaning readiness shortens the weaning process and duration of mechanical ventilation, and is an independent predictor of survival.

Depending on the local ICU practices and the patient population, a protocol-driven weaning process, implemented by physicians, respiratory therapists or ICU nurses may hasten the weaning process and shorten the duration of mechanical ventilation [183–188]. A protocol may help in systematically decreasing sedative use and therefore improve patient readiness for weaning and extubation. Computer-based automated protocols have also been developed using closed-loop feedback systems which gradually decrease the level of support provided by the ventilator and alert the clinician when the patient passes certain criteria.

About two-thirds of mechanically ventilated patients are extubated successfully following the initial spontaneous breathing trial. These patients have been classified as the simple-weaning group. The remaining one-third, the difficult-weaning group, follow a prolonged weaning process, partly due to underlying illness and partly from complications of prolonged mechanical ventilation itself. This latter population has a much higher ICU mortality of about 25% compared with the former, which has a good prognosis with an ICU mortality of approximately 5% [181].

Weaning should be initiated based on clinical criteria such as hemodynamic stability, adequate oxygenation/ventilation and ability to clear secretions and protect the airway. Many parameters to assess for readiness for weaning and extubation have been proposed [189,190]. These include maximal inspiratory pressure (MIP), or negative inspiratory force (NIF), minute ventilation, respiratory frequency, tidal volume and respiratory frequency:tidal volume ratio. However, the capacity of these parameters to predict successful weaning is modest [191]. Routine use of weaning predictors is not recommended as this may actually delay extubation [181]. On the other hand, these parameters may be helpful in certain situations, and could be used to identify causes of weaning failure.

When a patient is ready for weaning, a spontaneous breathing trial (SBT) is the best assessment for readiness for extubation. This may be done without any assistance from the ventilator (T-piece trial) or low levels of pressure support (≤ 7mmHg) or CPAP; all three have been shown to be equivalent [192–195]. Many ventilators allow the use of automatic tube compensation (ATC) whereby the increased work of breathing associated with resistance within the endotracheal tube is compensated for by applying continuously adjusted pressure support [261]. Low levels of pressure support have been used to the same purpose. The ideal duration of a SBT may depend on the underlying cause of respiratory failure and the duration of mechanical ventilation. A 30-minute SBT has been shown to be equivalent to a 2-hour SBT with either pressure support or T-piece [196,197]. Patients who have passed a SBT, determined by the patient's comfort, gas exchange, hemodynamic stability and respiratory pattern, should be extubated if they have a patent airway and can clear secretions. Less than 15% of patients who have passed a SBT and are extubated require reintubation [181].

Weaning failure is defined as failure of a SBT or reintubation within 48 hours of extubation [181]. It can be associated with increased mortality, either as a marker of disease severity, or because of associated complications from reintubation. However, the risks of complications from delay in weaning are greater, and therefore weaning attempts should continue. When weaning fails, the underlying cause should be determined and corrected, if possible. Weaning success or failure depends on several factors. Respiratory and cardiovascular load, neuromuscular and neuropsychological, as well as nutritional and metabolic factors play a role in successful liberation from mechanical ventilation. Cardiac dysfunction is becoming an increasingly recognised cause of weaning failure [198–201]. Spontaneous breathing is associated with increased venous return to the heart and increased workload to the heart, which can induce myocardial ischemia, and decreased left ventricular compliance, resulting in pulmonary oedema. A positive fluid balance can also predispose a patient to weaning failure [202].

Further weaning efforts may be either in the form of daily SBTs with full ventilator support in between, or gradually decreasing pressure support from the ventilator. Synchronised intermittent mandatory ventilation mode should not be used during the weaning process as it does not allow adequate rest to the respiratory muscles in between weaning trials [192]. In a select group of patients with acute respiratory failure with a history of chronic lung disease, non-invasive mechanical ventilation has been used to facilitate weaning. Extubation to NIV was associated with a decreased duration of mechanical ventilation, ICU and hospital stay in this population of patients who had failed SBTs. It also resulted in better survival, with fewer occurrences of nosocomial pneumonia and septic shock [203,204].

Once a SBT has been successful, an evaluation for extubation is performed. Depending on the population studied, up to 5–20% of patients fail extubation, i.e. require reintubation within 24 to 72 hours [205]. Reintubation is associated with higher hospital mortality, longer hospital and ICU stays and increased morbidity [206]. Excessive secretions, upper airway disorders as well as mechanical ventilation of longer than 72 hours and a prior failed weaning attempt have been associated with unsuccessful extubations [181]. Arterial blood gases following a SBT do not help predict extubation failure [207,208]. Patients with medical and neurologic illness are also considered to be at higher risk [209]. A positive fluid balance and a pathogen cultured from tracheobronchial secretions within 72 hours of extubation of COPD patients are other predictors of failure. An approach combining three parameters: peak cough flow rates (< 60 l/min), secretions (>2.5 ml/h) and abnormal mental status, has also been used to predict extubation failure. The absence of all three was associated with a reintubation risk of only 3%, while the presence of all three was almost certain to result in extubation failure [184]. Other parameters have been proposed to predict extubation failure, and include the time to return to baseline minute ventilation after resumption of full ventilatory support, and the degree of expiratory flow limitation with measurement of airway occlusion pressure at 0.1s [210].

While NIV has been advocated as an alternative weaning technique or as a prophylactic measure after extubation for patients at high risk for reintubation, it should generally not be used as a treatment for extubation failure [181,211]. One cause of extubation failure is upper airway oedema. Assessment for upper airway oedema may be performed using an air- or cuff-leak test. If no leak is present, methylprednisolone injection during the 24 hours prior to extubation can decrease post-extubation stridor and the need for reintubation [212–214].

7.6 Clinical Case

A middle-aged, obese male was found lying on the ground outside of a bar in the early morning hours. When paramedics arrived he was found to be arousable but lethargic. He was haemodynamically stable and his oxygen saturation was 92%. There was no evidence of trauma, but there was fresh emesis on his clothing and on the ground next to him. With face mask oxygen his saturation increased to 98%. He was transported to an emergency room for further evaluation at which time he was noted to vomit, aspirate and desaturate. He was rapidly endotracheally intubated with cervical neck precautions, and a nasogastric (NG) tube and central venous lines were placed. On an assist control mode, respiratory rate 16,V_t 600 ml, PEEP 5 cm H_2O, and FiO_2 100% the patient's transcutaneous oxygen saturation was 98%. Transient hypotension following intubation responded to a 1000 ml normal saline bolus. Physical examination showed poor dentition, bilateral rhonchi on chest ausculation and persistent lethargy, but was otherwise unremarkable. His height was 178 cm and weight 90 kg. Post-intubation chest radiograph showed good endotracheal and NG tube position and possible early bilateral lower lobe infiltrates. Contacted family members indicated that the patient was 45 years old, and besides a history of heavy alcohol use, did not have other known past medical history. Laboratory data was unremarkable with the exception of an arterial blood gas of pH 7.38, $PaCO_2$ 42 mmHg and PaO_2 240 mmHg while still on 100% FiO_2. Plateau airway pressure was 28 cm H_2O. A radial arterial catheter was placed. Full body computed tomography (CT) scan an hour later was negative except for patchy bilateral lower and upper lobe infiltrates. The patient was transported to an ICU where increasing agitation necessitated initiation of both fentanyl and midazolam infusions. Fluid support was continued, and stress ulcer and deep venous thrombosis prophylaxis were started along with full vitamin supplementation. Over the next 24 hours, the patient's oxygenation worsened and airway pressures increased. CXR showed worsening bilateral infiltrates. Tidal volumes were reduced and PEEP increased to maintain airway pressures $\leq$ 30 cm H_2O and $FiO_2 \leq 70\%$. Increasing temperature prompted blood, sputum and urine cultures and the patient was empirically treated with piperacillin/tazobactam and levofloxacin. The patient remained febrile however, and bronchoalveolar lavage (BAL) was performed. Gram-staining of both endotracheal aspirate and BAL showed inflammatory cell infiltrate and occasional Gram-positive cocci, but all cultures were negative. Enteral feedings were initiated. Despite antibiotic coverage, fever persisted, white blood cell (WBC) count increased to 35×10^3 cells/mm^2, and oxygenation did not show improvement despite escalation of PEEP to 16 cm H_2O. With tidal volumes of 450 ml/kg, airway pressures were maintained at 32–35 cm H_2O. One attempt to change the patient to pressure-control ventilation was associated with desaturation, and volume-control mode was continued. CXR on the fifth hospital day showed a possible air fluid level in the right lower lobe (RLL). After discussion with the family, the patient was transported for further imaging and possible intervention. Chest CT showed a RLL abscess and an associated loculated pleural effusion. Bilateral upper and lower lobe infiltrates persisted, but these were densest in the dependent lung regions. Percutaneous drainage of the abscess and pleural collection were attempted by interventional radiology, and pig-tail catheters were left in place. A small amount of pleural fluid that was drained had a pH of 7.15, a glucose level of 35 g/dl (serum, glucose 100 g/dl) and a lactate dehydrogenase level of 2000 units/l. Cultures were negative. Over the next 72 hours, FiO_2 requirement decreased to 65% and PEEP was decreased to 12 cm H_2O. However, fever and an elevated WBC count persisted despite a change of all indwelling catheters. There was limited drainage from the pig-tail catheters and no change in radiological appearance of the RLL air fluid level, loculated effusion or chest infiltrates. After further discussions with the family, on the ninth day of hospitalisation, the patient was taken to the operating room, where a partial right lower lobe resection and decortication were performed, with placement of a wide-bore chest tube as well as a tracheostomy. By the 14th day of hospitalisation, there had been a gradual reduction in the patient's febrile course and WBC count and improvement in both oxygenation and infiltrates on CXR. Midazolam and fentanyl infusions were weaned.

Spontaneous breathing trials with tracheal collar were initiated once the patient's FiO_2 and PEEP had been reduced to 40% and 5 cm H_2O respectively. After the patient could be supported with tracheal collar alone, he was transferred to a step-down unit for further rehabilitation.

References

[1] Bernard, G.R., Artigas, A., Brigham, K.L. *et al.* (1994). The American-European Consensus Conference on ARDS. Definitions, mechanisms, relevant outcomes, and clinical trial coordination, *Am J Respir Crit Care Med*, **149**, 818–824.

[2] Ware, L.B. and Matthay, M.A. (2000). The acute respiratory distress syndrome, *N Engl J Med*, **342**, 1334–1349.

[3] Hudson, L.D., Milberg, J.A., Anardi, D. *et al.* (1995). Clinical risks for development of the acute respiratory distress syndrome, *Am J Respir Crit Care Med*, **151**, 293–301.

[4] Ashbaugh, D.G., Bigelow, D.B., Petty, T.L. *et al.* (1967). Acute respiratory distress in adults, *Lancet*, **2**, 319–323.

[5] Piantadosi, C.A. and Schwartz, D.A. (2004). The acute respiratory distress syndrome, *Ann Intern Med*, **141**, 460–470.

[6] Rubenfeld, G.D., Caldwell, E., Peabody, E. *et al.* (2005). Incidence and outcomes of acute lung injury, *N Engl J Med*, **353**, 1685–1693.

[7] Girard, T.D. and Bernard, G.R. (2007). Mechanical ventilation in ARDS: a state-of-the-art review, *Chest*, **131**, 921–929.

[8] Gattinoni, L. and Caironi, P. (2008). Refining ventilatory treatment for acute lung injury and acute respiratory distress syndrome, *JAMA*, **299**, 691–693.

[9] Katzenstein, A.L., Bloor, C.M. and Leibow, A.A. (1976). Diffuse alveolar damage: the role of oxygen, shock, and related factors. A review, *Am J Pathol*, **85**, 209–228.

[10] Penuelas, O., Aramburu, J.A., Frutos-Vivar, F. *et al.* (2006). Pathology of acute lung injury and acute respiratory distress syndrome: a clinical-pathological correlation, *Clin Chest Med*, **27**, 571–578. Abstract vii–viii.

[11] Ware, L.B. and Matthay, M.A. (2001). Alveolar fluid clearance is impaired in the majority of patients with acute lung injury and the acute respiratory distress syndrome, *Am J Respir Crit Care Med*, **163**, 1376–1383.

[12] Gregory, T.J., Longmore, W.J., Moxley, M.A. *et al.* (1991). Surfactant chemical composition and biophysical activity in acute respiratory distress syndrome, *J Clin Invest*, **88**, 1976–1981.

[13] Suratt, B.T. and Parsons, P.E. (2006). Mechanisms of acute lung injury/acute respiratory distress syndrome, *Clin Chest Med*, **27**, 579–589. Abstract viii.

[14] Gattinoni, L., Caironi, P., Cressoni, M. *et al.* (2006). Lung recruitment in patients with the acute respiratory distress syndrome, *N Engl J Med*, **354**, 1775–1786.
[15] Gattinoni, L., Mascheroni, D., Torresin, A. *et al.* (1986). Morphological response to positive end expiratory pressure in acute respiratory failure. Computerized tomography study, *Intens Care Med*, **12**, 137–142.
[16] Maunder, R.J,, Shuman, W.P., McHugh, J.W. *et al.* (1986). Preservation of normal lung regions in the adult respiratory distress syndrome. Analysis by computed tomography, *JAMA*, **255**, 2463–2465.
[17] Dantzker, D.R. (1986). Gas exchange in acute lung injury, *Crit Care Clin*, **2**, 527–536.
[18] Petty, T.L. Reiss, O.K., Paul, G.W. *et al.* (1977). Characteristics of pulmonary surfactant in adult respiratory distress syndrome associated with trauma and shock, *Am Rev Respir Dis*, **115**, 531–536.
[19] Bachofen, M. and Weibel, E.R. (1982). Structural alterations of lung parenchyma in the adult respiratory distress syndrome, *Clin Chest Med*, **3**, 35–56.
[20] Bitterman, P.B. (1992). Pathogenesis of fibrosis in acute lung injury, *Am J Med*, **92**(6A), 39S–43S.
[21] Hashimoto, N., Jin, H., Liu, T. *et al.* (2004). Bone marrow-derived progenitor cells in pulmonary fibrosis, *J Clin Invest*, **113**, 243–252.
[22] Matamis, D., Lemaire, F., Harf, A. *et al.* (1984). Total respiratory pressure-volume curves in the adult respiratory distress syndrome, *Chest*, **86**, 58–66.
[23] Lamy, M., Fallat, R.J., Koeniger, E. *et al.* (1976). Pathologic features and mechanisms of hypoxemia in adult respiratory distress syndrome, *Am Rev Respir Dis*, **114**, 267–284.
[24] Nuckton, T.J., Alonso, J.A., Kallet, R.H. *et al.* (2002). Pulmonary dead-space fraction as a risk factor for death in the acute respiratory distress syndrome, *N Engl J Med*, **346**, 1281–1286.
[25] Webb, H.H. and Tierney, D.F. (1974). Experimental pulmonary edema due to intermittent positive pressure ventilation with high inflation pressures. Protection by positive end-expiratory pressure, *Am Rev Respir Dis*, **110**, 556–565.
[26] Frank, J.A. and Matthay, M.A. (2003). Science review: mechanisms of ventilator-induced injury, *Crit Care*, **7**, 233–241.
[27] Pugin, J., Dunn, I., Jolliet, P. *et al.* (1998). Activation of human macrophages by mechanical ventilation in vitro, *Am J Physiol*, **275**, L1040–1050.
[28] Ranieri, V.M., Suter, P.M., Tortorella, C. *et al.* (1999). Effect of mechanical ventilation on inflammatory mediators in patients with acute respiratory distress syndrome: a randomized controlled trial, *JAMA*, **282**, 54–61.
[29] Gali, B. and Goyal, D.G. (2003). Positive pressure mechanical ventilation, *Emerg Med Clin North Am*, **21**, 453–473.

[30] Brower, R.G., Ware, L.B., Berthiaume, Y. *et al.* (2001). Treatment of ARDS, *Chest*, **120**, 1347–1367.

[31] Kallet, R.H., Campbell, A.R., Dicker, R.A. *et al.* (2005). Work of breathing during lung-protective ventilation in patients with acute lung injury and acute respiratory distress syndrome: a comparison between volume and pressure-regulated breathing modes, *Respir Care*, **50**, 1623–1631.

[32] Thompson, B.T., Hayden, D., Matthay, M.A. *et al.* (2001). Clinicians' approaches to mechanical ventilation in acute lung injury and ARDS, *Chest*, **120**, 1622–1627.

[33] Esteban, A., Ferguson, N.D., Meade, M.O. *et al.* (2008). Evolution of mechanical ventilation in response to clinical research, *Am J Respir Crit Care Med* 15, **177**, 170–177.

[34] Vincent, J.L. and Zambon, M. (2006). Why do patients who have acute lung injury/acute respiratory distress syndrome die from multiple organ dysfunction syndrome? Implications for management, *Clin Chest Med*, **27**, 725–731. Abstract x–xi.

[35] Slutsky, A.S. (1993). Mechanical ventilation, American College of Chest Physicians' Consensus Conference, *Chest*, **104**, 1833–1859.

[36] The Acute Respiratory Distress Syndrome Network (2000). Ventilation with lower tidal volumes as compared with traditional tidal volumes for acute lung injury and the acute respiratory distress syndrome, *N Engl J Med*, **342**, 1301–1308.

[37] Eichacker, P.Q., Gerstenberger, E.P., Banks, S.M. *et al.* (2002). Meta-analysis of acute lung injury and acute respiratory distress syndrome trials testing low tidal volumes, *Am J Respir Crit Care Med*, **166**, 1510–1514.

[38] Amato, M.B., Barbas, C.S., Medeiros, D.M. *et al.* (1998). Effect of a protective-ventilation strategy on mortality in the acute respiratory distress syndrome, *N Engl J Med*, **338**, 347–354.

[39] Brochard, L., Roudot-Thoraval, F. Roupie, E. *et al.* (1998). Tidal volume reduction for prevention of ventilator-induced lung injury in acute respiratory distress syndrome, *Am J Respir Crit Care Med*, **158**, 1831–1838.

[40] Brower, R.G., Shanholtz, C.B., Fessler, H.E. *et al.* (1999). Prospective, randomized, controlled clinical trial comparing traditional versus reduced tidal volume ventilation in acute respiratory distress syndrome patients, *Crit Care Med*, **27**, 1492–1498.

[41] Stewart, T.E., Meade, M.O., Cook, D.J. *et al.* (1998). Evaluation of a ventilation strategy to prevent barotrauma in patients at high risk for acute respiratory distress syndrome, *N Engl J Med*, **338**, 355–361.

[42] Petrucci, N. and Iacovelli, W. (2007). Lung protective ventilation strategy for the acute respiratory distress syndrome, *Cochrane Database Syst Rev* CD003844.

[43] Villar, J., Kacmarek, R.M., Perez-Mendez, L., *et al.* (2006). A high positive end-expiratory pressure, low tidal volume ventilatory strategy improves outcome in persistent acute respiratory distress syndrome: a randomized, controlled trial, *Crit Care Med*, **34**, 1311–1318.

[44] Dellinger, R.P., Carlet, J.M., Masur, H. *et al.* (2004). Surviving Sepsis Campaign guidelines for management of severe sepsis and septic shock, *Crit Care Med*, **32**, 858–873.

[45] Umoh, N.J., Fan, E., Mendez-Tellez, P.A. *et al.* (2008). Patient and intensive care unit organizational factors associated with low tidal volume ventilation in acute lung injury, *Crit Care Med*, **36**, 1463–1468.

[46] Brower, R.G., Lanken, P.N., MacIntyre, N. *et al.* (2004). Higher versus lower positive end-expiratory pressures in patients with the acute respiratory distress syndrome, *N Engl J Med*, **351**, 327–336.

[47] Meade, M.O., Cook, D.J., Guyatt, G.H. *et al.* (2008). Ventilation strategy using low tidal volumes, recruitment maneuvers, and high positive end-expiratory pressure for acute lung injury and acute respiratory distress syndrome: a randomized controlled trial, *JAMA*, **299**, 637–645.

[48] Mercat, A., Richard, J.C., Vielle, B. *et al.* (2008). Positive end-expiratory pressure setting in adults with acute lung injury and acute respiratory distress syndrome: a randomized controlled trial, *JAMA*, **299**, 646–655.

[49] Carmichael, L.C., Dorinsky, P.M., Higgins, S.B. *et al.* (1996). Diagnosis and therapy of acute respiratory distress syndrome in adults: an international survey, *J Crit Care*, **11**, 9–18.

[50] Deans, K.J., Minneci, P.C., Cui, X. *et al.* (2005). Mechanical ventilation in ARDS: One size does not fit all, *Crit Care Med*, **33**, 1141–1143.

[51] Ferguson, N.D., Frutos-Vivar, F., Esteban, A. *et al.* (2005). Airway pressures, tidal volumes, and mortality in patients with acute respiratory distress syndrome, *Crit Care Med*, **33**, 21–30.

[52] Weinert, C.R., Gross, C.R. and Marinelli, W.A. (2003). Impact of randomized trial results on acute lung injury ventilator therapy in teaching hospitals, *Am J Respir Crit Care Med*, **167**, 1304–1309.

[53] Kallet, R.H., Alonso, J.A., Luce, J.M. *et al.* (1999). Exacerbation of acute pulmonary edema during assisted mechanical ventilation using a low-tidal volume, lung-protective ventilator strategy, *Chest*, **116**, 1826–1832.

[54] Muscedere, J.G., Mullen, J.B., Gan, K. *et al.* (1994). Tidal ventilation at low airway pressures can augment lung injury, *Am J Respir Crit Care Med*, **149**, 1327–1334.

[55] Pohlman, M.C., McCallister, K.E., Schweickert, W.D. *et al.* (2008). Excessive tidal volume from breath stacking during lung-protective ventilation for acute lung injury, *Crit Care Med*, **36**, 3019–3023.

[56] Hager, D.N., Krishnan, J.A., Hayden, D.L. *et al.* (2005). Tidal volume reduction in patients with acute lung injury when plateau pressures are not high, *Am J Respir Crit Care Med*, **172**, 1241–1245.
[57] Marini, J.J. and Gattinoni, L. (2004). Ventilatory management of acute respiratory distress syndrome: a consensus of two, *Crit Care Med*, **32**, 250–255.
[58] Ricard, J.D. (2003). Are we really reducing tidal volume–and should we? *Am J Respir Crit Care Med*, **167**, 1297–1298.
[59] MacIntyre, N. (2006).Ventilatory management of ALI/ARDS, *Semin Respir Crit Care Med*, **27**, 396–403.
[60] Holzapfel, L., Robert, D., Perrin, F. *et al.* (1983). Static pressure–volume curves and effect of positive end-expiratory pressure on gas exchange in adult respiratory distress syndrome, *Crit Care Med*, **11**, 591–597.
[61] Maisch, S., Reissmann, H., Fuellekrug, B. *et al.* (2008). Compliance and dead space fraction indicate an optimal level of positive end-expiratory pressure after recruitment in anesthetized patients, *Anesth Analg*, **106**, 175–181.
[62] Pinsky, M.R. (2007). Heart–lung interactions, *Curr Opin Crit Care*, **13**, 528–531.
[63] Pelosi, P., D'Onofrio, D., Chiumello, D. *et al.* (2003). Pulmonary and extrapulmonary acute respiratory distress syndrome are different, *Eur Respir J Suppl*, **42**, 48s–56s.
[64] Chan, K.P., Stewart, T.E., Mehta, S. (2007). High-frequency oscillatory ventilation for adult patients with ARDS, *Chest*, **131**, 1907–1916.
[65] Mehta, S., Lapinsky, S.E., Hallett, D.C. *et al.* (2001). Prospective trial of high-frequency oscillation in adults with acute respiratory distress syndrome, *Crit Care Med*, **29**, 1360–1369.
[66] Mehta, S., Granton, J., MacDonald, R.J. *et al.* (2004). High-frequency oscillatory ventilation in adults: The, Toronto experience, *Chest*, **126**, 518–527.
[67] Derdak, S., Mehta, S., Stewart, T.E. *et al.* (2002). High-frequency oscillatory ventilation for acute respiratory distress syndrome in adults: a randomized, controlled trial, *Am J Respir Crit Care Med*, **166**, 801–808.
[68] Bollen, C.W. van, Well, G.T., Sherry, T. *et al.* (2005). High frequency oscillatory ventilation compared with conventional mechanical ventilation in adult respiratory distress syndrome: a randomized controlled trial [ISRCTN24242669], *Crit Care*, **9**, R430–439.
[69] Papazian, L., Gainnier, M., Marin, V. *et al.* (2005). Comparison of prone positioning and high-frequency oscillatory ventilation in patients with acute respiratory distress syndrome, *Crit Care Med*, **33**, 2162–2171.
[70] Fan, E. and Stewart, T.E. (2006). New modalities of mechanical ventilation: high-frequency oscillatory ventilation and airway pressure release ventilation, *Clin Chest Med*, **27**, 615–625. Abstract viii–ix.

[71] Downs, J.B. and Stock, M.C. (1987). Airway pressure release ventilation: a new concept in ventilatory support, *Crit Care Med*, **15**, 459–461.
[72] Rasanen, J., Cane, R.D., Downs, J.B. *et al.* (1991). Airway pressure release ventilation during acute lung injury: a prospective multicenter trial, *Crit Care Med*, **19**, 1234–1241.
[73] Putensen, C., Zech, S., Wrigge, H. *et al.* (2001). Long-term effects of spontaneous breathing during ventilatory support in patients with acute lung injury, *Am J Respir Crit Care Med*, **164**, 43–49.
[74] Varpula, T., Jousela, I., Niemi, R. *et al.* (2003). Combined effects of prone positioning and airway pressure release ventilation on gas exchange in patients with acute lung injury, *Acta Anaesthesiol Scand*, **47**, 516–524.
[75] Varpula, T., Valta, P., Niemi, R. *et al.* (2004). Airway pressure release ventilation as a primary ventilatory mode in acute respiratory distress syndrome, *Acta Anaesthesiol Scand*, **48**, 722–731.
[76] Mutoh, T., Guest, R.J., Lamm, W.J. *et al.* (1992). Prone position alters the effect of volume overload on regional pleural pressures and improves hypoxemia in pigs *in vivo*, *Am Rev Respir Dis*, **146**, 300–306.
[77] Lamm, W.J., Graham, M.M. and Albert, R.K. (1994). Mechanism by which the prone position improves oxygenation in acute lung injury, *Am J Respir Crit Care Med*, **150**, 184–193.
[78] Broccard, A., Shapiro, R.S., Schmitz, L.L. *et al.* (2000). Prone positioning attenuates and redistributes ventilator-induced lung injury in dogs, *Crit Care Med*, **28**, 295–303.
[79] Abroug, F., Ouanes-Besbes, L., Elatrous, S. *et al.* (2008). The effect of prone positioning in acute respiratory distress syndrome or acute lung injury: a meta-analysis. Areas of uncertainty and recommendations for research, *Intens Care Med*, **34**, 1002–1011.
[80] Beuret, P., Carton, M.J., Nourdine, K. *et al.* (2002). Prone position as prevention of lung injury in comatose patients: a prospective, randomized, controlled study, *Intens Care Med*, **28**, 564–569.
[81] Curley, M.A., Hibberd, P.L., Fineman, L.D. *et al.* (2005). Effect of prone positioning on clinical outcomes in children with acute lung injury: a randomized controlled trial, *JAMA*, **294**, 229–237.
[82] Gattinoni, L., Tognoni, G., Pesenti, A. *et al.* (2001). Effect of prone positioning on the survival of patients with acute respiratory failure, *N Engl J Med*, **345**, 568–573.
[83] Guerin, C., Gaillard, S., Lemasson, S. *et al.* (2004). Effects of systematic prone positioning in hypoxemic acute respiratory failure: a randomized controlled trial, *JAMA*, **292**, 2379–2387.

[84] Mancebo, J., Fernandez, R., Blanch, L. *et al.* (2006). A. multicenter trial of prolonged prone ventilation in severe acute respiratory distress syndrome, *Am J Respir Crit Care Med*, **173**, 1233–1239.

[85] Voggenreiter, G., Aufmkolk, M., Stiletto, R.J. *et al.* (2005). Prone positioning improves oxygenation in post-traumatic lung injury–a prospective randomized trial, *J Trauma*, **59**, 333–341. Discussion 341–343.

[86] Hirschl, R.B., Pranikoff, T., Wise, C. *et al.* (1996). Initial experience with partial liquid ventilation in adult patients with the acute respiratory distress syndrome, *JAMA*, **275**, 383–389.

[87] Hirschl, R.B., Croce, M., Gore, D. *et al.* (2002). Prospective, randomized, controlled pilot study of partial liquid ventilation in adult acute respiratory distress syndrome, *Am J Respir Crit Care Med*, **165**, 781–787.

[88] Kacmarek, R.M., Wiedemann, H.P., Lavin, P.T. *et al.* (2006). Partial liquid ventilation in adult patients with acute respiratory distress syndrome, *Am J Respir Crit Care Med*, **173**, 882–889.

[89] Adhikari, N.K., Burns, K.E., Friedrich, J.O. *et al.* (2007). Effect of nitric oxide on oxygenation and mortality in acute lung injury: systematic review and meta-analysis, *BMJ*, **334**, 779.

[90] Rossaint, R., Falke, K.J., Lopez, F. *et al.* (1993). Inhaled nitric oxide for the adult respiratory distress syndrome, *N Engl J Med*, **328**, 399–405.

[91] Sokol, J., Jacobs, S.E. and Bohn, D. (2003). Inhaled nitric oxide for acute hypoxic respiratory failure in children and adults: a meta-analysis, *Anesth Analg*, **97**, 989–998.

[92] Day, R.W., Allen, E.M. and Witte, M.K. (1997). A randomized, controlled study of the 1–hour and 24–hour effects of inhaled nitric oxide therapy in children with acute hypoxemic respiratory failure, *Chest*, **112**, 1324–1331.

[93] Schwebel, C., Beuret, P., Perdrix, J.P. *et al.* (1997). Early inhaled nitric oxide inhalation in acute lung injury: results of a double-blind randomized study [abstract]. *Intens Care Medicine*, **23** (Suppl. 1), S2.

[94] Dellinger, R.P., Zimmerman, J.L., Taylor, R.W. *et al.* (1998). Effects of inhaled nitric oxide in patients with acute respiratory distress syndrome: results of a randomized phase II trial. Inhaled Nitric Oxide in ARDS Study Group, *Crit Care Med*, **26**, 15–23.

[95] Michael, J.R., Barton, R.G., Saffle, J.R. *et al.* (1998). Inhaled nitric oxide versus conventional therapy: effect on oxygenation in ARDS, *Am J Respir Crit Care Med*, **157**, 1372–1380.

[96] Troncy, E., Collet, J.P., Shapiro, S. *et al.* (1998). Inhaled nitric oxide in acute respiratory distress syndrome: a pilot randomized controlled study, *Am J Respir Crit Care Med*, **157**, 1483–1488.

[97] Dobyns, E.L., Cornfield, D.N., Anas, N.G. *et al.* (1999). Multicenter randomized controlled trial of the effects of inhaled nitric oxide therapy on gas exchange in children with acute hypoxemic respiratory failure, *J Pediatr*, **134**, 406–412.

[98] Lundin, S., Mang, H., Smithies, M. *et al.* (1999). Inhalation of nitric oxide in acute lung injury: results of a European multicentre study. The European Study Group of Inhaled Nitric Oxide, *Intens Care Med*, **25**, 911–919.

[99] Payen, D., Vallet, B., Group d'étude du NO dans l'ARDS, (1999). Results of the French prospective multicentric randomized double-blind placebo-controlled trial on inhaled nitric oxide (NO) in ARDS [abstract], *Intens Care Med*, **25**(Suppl. 1), S166.

[100] Gerlach, H., Keh, D., Semmerow, A. *et al.* (2003). Dose-response characteristics during long-term inhalation of nitric oxide in patients with severe acute respiratory distress syndrome: a prospective, randomized, controlled study, *Am J Respir Crit Care Med*, **167**, 1008–1015.

[101] Park, K.J., Lee, Y.J., Oh, Y.J. *et al.* (2003). Combined effects of inhaled nitric oxide and a recruitment maneuver in patients with acute respiratory distress syndrome, *Yonsei Med J*, **44**, 219–226.

[102] Taylor, R.W., Zimmerman, J.L., Dellinger, R.P. *et al.* (2004). Low-dose inhaled nitric oxide in patients with acute lung injury: a randomized controlled trial, *JAMA*, **291**, 1603–1609.

[103] Mehta, S., Simms, H., Levy, M.M., *et al.* (2001). Inhaled nitric oxide improves oxygenation acutely but not chronically in acute respiratory distress syndrome: a randomized, controlled trial, *J Appl Res*, **1**, 73–84.

[104] Anzueto, A. and Guntapalli, K. (2006). Adjunctive therapy to mechanical ventilation: surfactant therapy, liquid ventilation, and prone position, *Clin Chest Med*, **27**, 637–654. Abstract ix.

[105] Anzueto, A., Baughman, R.P., Guntupalli, K.K. *et al.* (1996). Aerosolized surfactant in adults with sepsis-induced acute respiratory distress syndrome. Exosurf Acute Respiratory Distress Syndrome Sepsis Study Group, *N Engl J Med*, **334**, 1417–1421.

[106] Spragg, R.G., Lewis, J.F., Walmrath, H.D. *et al.* (2004). Effect of recombinant surfactant protein C-based surfactant on the acute respiratory distress syndrome, *N Engl J Med*, **351**, 884–892.

[107] Cochrane, C.G., Revak, S.D., Merritt, T.A. *et al.* (1996). The efficacy and safety of KL4-surfactant in preterm infants with respiratory distress syndrome, *Am J Respir Crit Care Med*, **153**, 404–410.

[108] Wiswell, T.E., Smith, R.M., Katz, L.B. *et al.* (1999). Bronchopulmonary segmental lavage with Surfaxin (KL-surfactant) for acute respiratory distress syndrome, *Am J Respir Crit Care Med*, **160**, 1188–1195.

[109] Brown, J.K., Haft, J.W., Bartlett, R.H. *et al.* (2006). Acute lung injury and acute respiratory distress: extracorporeal life support and liquid ventilation for severe acute respiratory distress syndrome, *Semin Respir Crit Care Med*, **27**, 416 – 425.

[110] Kopp, R., Dembinski, R. and Kuhlen, R. (2006). Role of extracorporeal lung assist in the treatment of acute respiratory failure, *Minerva Anestesiologica*, **72**, 587–595.

[111] Schuerer, D.J., Kolovos, N.S., Boyd, K.V. *et al.* (2008). Extracorporeal membrane oxygenation: Current clinical practice, coding and reimbursement, *Chest*, **134**, 179–184.

[112] Zapol, W.M., Snider, M.T., Hill, J.D. *et al.* (1979). Extracorporeal membrane oxygenation in severe acute respiratory failure: a randomized prospective study, *JAMA*, **242**, 2193–2196.

[113] Morris, A.H., Wallace, C.J., Menlove, R.L. *et al.* (1994). Randomized clinical trial of pressure-controlled inverse ratio ventilation and extracorporeal CO_2 removal for adult respiratory distress syndrome, *Am J Respir Crit Care Med*, **149**, 295–305.

[114] Hemmila, M.R., Rowe, S.A., Boules, T.N. *et al.* (2004). Extracorporeal life support for severe acute respiratory distress syndrome in adults, *Ann Surg*, **240**, 595–605.

[115] Peek, G.J., Mugford, M., Tiruvoipati, R. *et al.* (2009). Efficacy and economic assessment of conventional ventilator support versus extracorporeal membrane oxygenation for severe adult respiratory failure (CESAR): A multicentre randomised controlled trial, *Lancet*, **374**, 1351–1363.

[116] The National Asthma Education and Prevention Program. (2007). *Expert, Panel, Report - 3. Guidelines for the Diagnosis and Management of Asthma*, [Online]. Available at: http://www.nhlbi.nih.gov/guidelines/asthma/asthgdln.htm [Accessed 17 January 2013].

[117] Akinbami, L. (2006). *Asthma Prevalence, Health Care Use and, Mortality: United States, 2003–05*, [Online]. Available at: http://www.cdc.gov/nchs/products/pubs/pubd/hestats/ashtma03–05/asthma03–05.htm [Accessed 17 Jan 2013].

[118] Watson, L., Turk, F., James, P. *et al.* (2007). Factors associated with mortality after an asthma admission: a national United Kingdom database analysis, *Respir Med*, **101**, 1659–1664.

[119] Picado, C. (1996). Classification of severe asthma exacerbations: a proposal, *Eur Respir J*, **9**, 1775–1778.

[120] Barr, R.G., Woodruff, P.G., Clark, S. *et al.* (2000). Sudden-onset asthma exacerbations: clinical features, response to therapy, and 2–week follow-up,

Multicenter Airway Research Collaboration (MARC) investigators, *Eur Respir J*, **15**, 266–273.

[121] Lugogo, N.L. and MacIntyre, N.R. (2008). Life-threatening asthma: pathophysiology and management, *Respir Care*, **53**, 726–735. Discussion 735–729.

[122] Ramnath, V.R., Clark, S. and Camargo, C.A. Jr. (2007). Multicenter study of clinical features of sudden-onset versus slower-onset asthma exacerbations requiring hospitalization, *Respir Care*, **52**, 1013–1020.

[123] Wasserfallen, J.B., Schaller, M.D., Feihl, F. *et al.* (1990). Sudden asphyxic asthma: a distinct entity? *Am Rev Respir Dis*, **142**, 108–111.

[124] Marik, P.E., Varon, J. and Fromm, R. Jr. (2002). The management of acute severe asthma, *J Emerg Med*, **23**, 257–268.

[125] Busse, W.W. and Lemanske, R.F. Jr. (2001). Asthma, *N Engl J Med*, **344**, 350–362.

[126] Holgate, S.T. and Polosa, R. (2006). The mechanisms, diagnosis, and management of severe asthma in adults, *Lancet*, **368**, 780–793.

[127] Stevenson, D.D. and Szczeklik, A., (2006). Clinical and pathologic perspectives on aspirin sensitivity and asthma, *J Allergy Clin Immunol*, **118**, 773–786. Quiz 787–778.

[128] Martin, J.G., Shore, S.A. and Engel, L.A. (1983). Mechanical load and inspiratory muscle action during induced asthma, *Am Rev Respir Dis*, **128**, 455–460.

[129] Ram, F.S., Wellington, S., Rowe, B. *et al.* (2005). Non-invasive positive pressure ventilation for treatment of respiratory failure due to severe acute exacerbations of asthma, *Cochrane Database Syst Rev*, CD004360.

[130] Soroksky, A., Stav, D. and Shpirer, I. (2003). A pilot prospective, randomized, placebo-controlled trial of bilevel positive airway pressure in acute asthmatic attack, *Chest*, **123**, 1018–1025.

[131] Meduri, G.U., Cook, T.R., Turner, R.E. *et al.* (1996). Noninvasive positive pressure ventilation in status asthmaticus, *Chest*, **110**, 767–774.

[132] Bondi, E. and Williams Jr, M.H. (1977). Severe asthma. Course and treatment in hospital, *N Y State J Med*, **77**, 350–353.

[133] Mountain, R.D. and Sahn, S.A. (1988). Clinical features and outcome in patients with acute asthma presenting with hypercapnia, *Am Rev Respir Dis*, **138**, 535–539.

[134] Mansel, J.K., Stogner, S.W., Petrini, M.F. *et al.* (1990). Mechanical ventilation in patients with acute severe asthma, *Am J Med*, **89**, 42–48.

[135] Fudickar, A., Bein, B. and Tonner, P.H. (2006). Propofol infusion syndrome in anaesthesia and intensive care medicine, *Curr Opin Anaesthesiol*, **19**, 404–410.

[136] Bennett, S.N., McNeil, M.M., Bland, L.A. *et al.* (1995). Postoperative infections traced to contamination of an intravenous anesthetic, propofol, *N Engl J Med*, **333**, 147–154.

[137] L'Hommedieu, C.S. and Arens, J.J. (1987). The use of ketamine for the emergency intubation of patients with status asthmaticus, *Ann Emerg Med*, **16**, 568–571.

[138] Bergen, J.M. and Smith, D.C. (1997). A review of etomidate for rapid sequence intubation in the emergency department, *J Emerg Med*, **15**, 221–230.

[139] Lakshminarayan, S., Sahn, S.A. and Hudson, L.D. (1973). Treatment of status asthmaticus, *BMJ*, **1**, 611–612.

[140] Tuxen, D.V. (1994). Permissive hypercapnic ventilation, *Am J Respir Crit Care Med*, **150**, 870–874.

[141] Darioli, R. and Perret, C. (1984). Mechanical controlled hypoventilation in status asthmaticus, *Am Rev Respir Dis*, **129**, 385–387.

[142] Oddo, M., Feihl, F., Schaller, M.D. *et al.* (2006). Management of mechanical ventilation in acute severe asthma: practical aspects, *Intens Care Med*, **32**, 501–510.

[143] Shapiro, J.M. (2002). Management of respiratory failure in status asthmaticus, *Am J Respir Med*, **1**, 409–416.

[144] Blanch, L., Bernabe, F. and Lucangelo, U. (2005). Measurement of air trapping, intrinsic positive end-expiratory pressure, and dynamic hyperinflation in mechanically ventilated patients, *Respir Care*, **50**, 110–123. Discussion 123–114.

[145] Leatherman, J.W., McArthur, C. and Shapiro, R.S. (2004). Effect of prolongation of expiratory time on dynamic hyperinflation in mechanically ventilated patients with severe asthma, *Crit Care Med*, **32**, 1542–1545.

[146] Slutsky, A.S. (1994). Consensus conference on mechanical ventilation–January 28–30 1993 at Northbrook Illinois USA. Part 2. *Intens Care Med*, **20**, 150–162.

[147] McFadden, E.R. Jr., Kiser, R. and DeGroot, W.J. (1973). Acute bronchial asthma. Relations between clinical and physiologic manifestations, *N Engl J Med*, **288**, 221–225.

[148] Stather, D.R. and Stewart, T.E. (2005). Clinical review: mechanical ventilation in severe asthma, *Crit Care*, **9**, 581–587.

[149] Smith, T.C. and Marini, J.J. (1988). Impact of PEEP on lung mechanics and work of breathing in severe airflow obstruction, *J Appl Physiol*, **65**, 1488–1499.

[150] Marini, J.J. (1989). Should PEEP be used in airflow obstruction? *Am Rev Respir Dis*, **140**, 1–3.

[151] Pepe, P.E. and Marini, J.J. (1982). Occult positive end-expiratory pressure in mechanically ventilated patients with airflow obstruction: the auto-PEEP effect, *Am Rev Respir Dis*, **126**, 166–170.

[152] Wiebe, K. and Rowe, B.H. (2007). Nebulized racemic epinephrine used in the treatment of severe asthmatic exacerbation: a case report and literature review, *CJEM*, **9**, 304–308.

[153] Leatherman, J.W. (1996). Mechanical ventilation in obstructive lung disease, *Clin Chest Med*, **17**, 577–590.

[154] Rodrigo, G., Pollack, C., Rodrigo, C. *et al.* (2006). Heliox for nonintubated acute asthma patients, *Cochrane Database Syst Rev*, CD002884.

[155] Anderson, M., Svartengren, M., Bylin, G. *et al.* (1993). Deposition in asthmatics of particles inhaled in air or in helium-oxygen, *Am Rev Respir Dis*, **147**, 524–528.

[156] Hess, D.R., Acosta, F.L., Ritz, R.H. *et al.* (1999). The effect of heliox on nebulizer function using a beta-agonist bronchodilator, *Chest*, **115**, 184–189.

[157] Tassaux, D., Jolliet, P., Thouret, J.M. *et al.* (1999). Calibration of seven ICU ventilators for mechanical ventilation with helium-oxygen mixtures, *Am J Respir Crit Care Med*, **160**, 22–32.

[158] Maltais, F., Sovilj, M., Goldberg, P. *et al.* (1994). Respiratory mechanics in status asthmaticus,, Effects of inhalational anesthesia, *Chest*, **106**, 1401–1406.

[159] Gupta, D., Keogh, B., Chung, K.F. *et al.* (2004). Characteristics and outcome for admissions to adult, general critical care units with acute severe asthma: a secondary analysis of the ICNARC Case Mix Programme Database, *Crit Care*, **8**, R112–121.

[160] American Thoracic Society / European Respiratory Society Task Force (2004). *Standards for the Diagnosis and Management of Patients with COPD*, [Online]. Available at: http://www.thoracic.org/go/copd [Accessed 17 January 2013].

[161] National Heart Lung and Blood Institute (2007). *COPD: Learn More. Breathe Better*, [Online]. Available at: http://www.nhlbi.nih.gov/health/public/lung/copd/health-care-professionals/index.htm [Accessed 17 January 2013].

[162] O'Donnell, D.E. and Parker, C.M. (2006). COPD exacerbations. 3: Pathophysiology, *Thorax*, **61**, 354–361.

[163] Ram, F.S., Picot, J., Lightowler, J. *et al.* (2004). Non-invasive positive pressure ventilation for treatment of respiratory failure due to exacerbations of chronic obstructive pulmonary disease, *Cochrane Database Syst Rev*, CD004104.

[164] Keenan, S.P., Sinuff, T., Cook, D.J. *et al.* (2003). Which patients with acute exacerbation of chronic obstructive pulmonary disease benefit from non-invasive positive-pressure ventilation? A systematic review of the literature, *Ann Intern Med*, **138**, 861–870.

[165] Peter, J.V. and Moran, J.L. (2004). Noninvasive ventilation in exacerbations of chronic obstructive pulmonary disease: implications of different meta-analytic strategies, *Ann Intern Med*, **141**, W78–W79.

[166] Peter, J.V., Moran, J.L., Phillips-Hughes, J. *et al.* (2002). Noninvasive ventilation in acute respiratory failure — a meta-analysis update, *Crit Care Med*, **30**, 555–562.

[167] Schumaker, G.L. and Epstein, S.K. (2004). Managing acute respiratory failure during exacerbation of chronic obstructive pulmonary disease, *Respir Care*, **49**, 766–782.

[168] Plant, P.K., Owen, J.L. and Elliott, M.W. (2001). Non-invasive ventilation in acute exacerbations of chronic obstructive pulmonary disease: long term survival and predictors of in-hospital outcome, *Thorax*, **56**, 708–712.

[169] Conti, G., Antonelli, M., Navalesi, P. *et al.* (2002). Noninvasive vs, conventional mechanical ventilation in patients with chronic obstructive pulmonary disease after failure of medical treatment in the ward: a randomized trial, *Intens Care Med*, **28**, 1701–1707.

[170] Plant, P.K., Owen, J.L., Parrott, S. *et al.* (2003). Cost effectiveness of ward based non-invasive ventilation for acute exacerbations of chronic obstructive pulmonary disease: economic analysis of randomised controlled trial, *BMJ*, **326**, 956.

[171] Nava, S., Ambrosino, N., Clini, E. *et al.* (1998). Noninvasive mechanical ventilation in the weaning of patients with respiratory failure due to chronic obstructive pulmonary disease. A randomized, controlled trial, *Ann Intern Med*, **128**, 721–728.

[172] Ferrer, M., Esquinas, A., Arancibia, F. *et al.* (2003). Noninvasive ventilation during persistent weaning failure: a randomized controlled trial, *Am J Respir Crit Care Med*, **168**, 70–76.

[173] MacIntyre, N. and Huang, Y.C. (2008). Acute exacerbations and respiratory failure in chronic obstructive pulmonary disease, *Proc Am Thorac Soc*, **5**, 530–535.

[174] Gladwin, M.T. and Pierson, D.J. (1998). Mechanical ventilation of the patient with severe chronic obstructive pulmonary disease, *Intens Care Med*, **24**, 898–910.

[175] Reignier, J., Lejeune, O., Renard, B. *et al.* (2005). Short-term effects of prone position in chronic obstructive pulmonary disease patients with severe acute hypoxemic and hypercapnic respiratory failure, *Intens Care Med*, **31**, 1128–1131.

[176] Ward, N.S. and Dushay, K.M. (2008). Clinical concise review: mechanical ventilation of patients with chronic obstructive pulmonary disease, *Crit Care Med*, **36**, 1614–1619.

[177] Caramez, M.P., Borges, J.B., Tucci, M.R. *et al.* (2005). Paradoxical responses to positive end-expiratory pressure in patients with airway obstruction during controlled ventilation, *Crit Care Med*, **33**, 1519–1528.

[178] Ranieri, V.M., Mascia, L., Petruzzelli, V. *et al.* (1995). Inspiratory effort and measurement of dynamic intrinsic PEEP in COPD patients: effects of ventilator triggering systems, *Intens Care Med*, **21**, 896–903.

[179] Rodrigo, G., Pollack, C., Rodrigo, C. *et al.* (2002). Heliox for treatment of exacerbations of chronic obstructive pulmonary disease, *Cochrane Database Syst Rev*, CD003571.

[180] Baigorri, F., Joseph, D., Artigas, A. *et al.* (1999). Inhaled nitric oxide does not improve cardiac or pulmonary function in patients with an exacerbation of chronic obstructive pulmonary disease, *Crit Care Med*, **27**, 2153–2158.

[181] Boles, J.M., Bion, J., Connors, A. *et al.* (2007). Weaning from mechanical ventilation, *Eur Respir J*, **29**, 1033–1056.

[182] Esteban, A., Anzueto, A., Frutos, F. *et al.* (2002). Characteristics and outcomes in adult patients receiving mechanical ventilation: a 28–day international study, *JAMA*, **287**, 345–355.

[183] Ely, E.W., Baker, A.M., Dunagan, D.P. *et al.* (1996). Effect on the duration of mechanical ventilation of identifying patients capable of breathing spontaneously, *N Engl J Med*, **335**, 1864–1869.

[184] Kollef, M.H., Shapiro, S.D., Silver, P. *et al.* (1997). A randomized, controlled trial of protocol-directed versus physician-directed weaning from mechanical ventilation, *Crit Care Med*, **25**, 567–574.

[185] Marelich, G.P., Murin, S., Battistella, F. *et al.* (2000). Protocol weaning of mechanical ventilation in medical and surgical patients by respiratory care practitioners and nurses: effect on weaning time and incidence of ventilator-associated pneumonia, *Chest*, **118**, 459–467.

[186] Krishnan, J.A., Moore, D., Robeson, C. *et al.* (2004). A prospective, controlled trial of a protocol-based strategy to discontinue mechanical ventilation, *Am J Respir Crit Care Med*, **169**, 673–678.

[187] Rose, L., Presneill, J.J., Johnston, L. *et al.* (2008). A randomised, controlled trial of conventional versus automated weaning from mechanical ventilation using SmartCare/PS, *Intens Care Med*, **34**, 1788–1795.

[188] Meade, M., Guyatt, G., Cook, D. *et al.* (2001). Predicting success in weaning from mechanical ventilation, *Chest*, **120**(Suppl. 6), 400S–424S.

[189] Epstein, S.K. (2000). Weaning parameters, *Respir Care Clin N Am*, **6**, 253–301, v–vi.

[190] Epstein, S.K. (2009). Weaning from ventilatory support, *Curr Opin Crit Care*, **15**, 36–43.

[191] Esteban, A., Frutos, F., Tobin, M.J. *et al.* (1995). A comparison of four methods of weaning patients from mechanical ventilation. Spanish Lung Failure Collaborative Group, *N Engl J Med*, **332**, 345–350.

[192] Esteban, A., Alia, I., Gordo, F. *et al.* (1997). Extubation outcome after spontaneous breathing trials with T-tube or pressure support ventilation. The Spanish Lung Failure Collaborative Group, *Am J Respir Crit Care Med*, **156**, 459–465.

[193] Farias, J.A., Retta, A., Alia, I. *et al.* (2001). A comparison of two methods to perform a breathing trial before extubation in pediatric intensive care patients, *Intens Care Med*, **27**, 1649–1654.

[194] Jones, D.P., Byrne, P., Morgan, C. *et al.* (1991). Positive end-expiratory pressure vs T-piece. Extubation after mechanical ventilation, *Chest*, **100**, 1655–1659.

[195] Haberthur, C., Mols, G., Elsasser, S. *et al.* (2002). Extubation after breathing trials with automatic tube compensation. T-tube, or pressure support ventilation, *Acta Anaesthesiol Scand*, **46**, 973–979.

[196] Esteban, A., Alia, I., Tobin, M.J. *et al.* (1999). Effect of spontaneous breathing trial duration on outcome of attempts to discontinue mechanical ventilation. Spanish Lung Failure Collaborative Group, *Am J Respir Crit Care Med*, **159**, 512–518.

[197] Perren, A., Domenighetti, G., Mauri, S. *et al.* (2002). Protocol-directed weaning from mechanical ventilation: clinical outcome in patients randomized for a 30-min or 120-min trial with pressure support ventilation, *Intens Care Med*, **28**, 1058–1063.

[198] Richard, C. and Teboul, J.L. (2005). Weaning failure from cardiovascular origin, *Intens Care Med*, **31**, 1605–1607.

[199] Chatila, W., Ani, S., Guaglianone, D., Jacob, B. *et al.* (1996). Cardiac ischemia during weaning from mechanical ventilation, *Chest*, **109**, 1577–1583.

[200] Frazier, S.K., Stone, K.S., Moser, D. *et al.* (2006). Hemodynamic changes during discontinuation of mechanical ventilation in medical intensive care unit patients, *Am J Crit Care*, **15**, 580–593. Quiz 594.

[201] Frazier, S.K., Brom, H., Widener, J. *et al.* (2006). Prevalence of myocardial ischemia during mechanical ventilation and weaning and its effects on weaning success, *Heart Lung*, **35**, 363–373.

[202] Upadya, A., Tilluckdharry, L., Muralidharan, V. *et al.* (2005). Fluid balance and weaning outcomes, *Intens Care Med*, **31**, 1643–1647.

[203] Ferrer, M., Esquinas, A., Arancibia, F. *et al.* (2003). Noninvasive ventilation during persistent weaning failure: a randomized controlled trial, *Am J Respir Crit Care Med*, **168**, 70–76.

[204] Girault, C., Daudenthun, I., Chevron, V. *et al.* (1999). Noninvasive ventilation as a systematic extubation and weaning technique in acute-on-chronic respiratory failure: a prospective, randomized controlled study, *Am J Respir Crit Care Med*, **160**, 86–92.

[205] Epstein, S.K. (2002). Decision to extubate, *Intens Care Med*, **28**, 535–546.

[206] Coplin, W.M., Pierson, D.J., Cooley, K.D. *et al.* (2000). Implications of extubation delay in brain-injured patients meeting standard weaning criteria, *Am J Respir Crit Care Med*, **161**, 1530–1536.

[207] Pawson, S.R. and DePriest, J.L. (2004). Are blood gases necessary in mechanically ventilated patients who have successfully completed a spontaneous breathing trial? *Respir Care*, **49**, 1316–1319.

[208] Salam, A., Smina, M., Gada, P. *et al.* (2003). The effect of arterial blood gas values on extubation decisions, *Respir Care*, **48**, 1033–1037.

[209] Salam, A., Tilluckdharry, L., Amoateng-Adjepong, Y. *et al.* (2004). Neurologic status, cough, secretions and extubation outcomes, *Intens Care Med*, **30**, 1334–1339.

[210] Martinez, A., Seymour, C. and Nam, M. (2003). Minute ventilation recovery time: a predictor of extubation outcome, *Chest*, **123**, 1214–1221.

[211] Esteban, A., Frutos-Vivar, F., Ferguson, N.D. *et al.* (2004). Noninvasive positive-pressure ventilation for respiratory failure after extubation, *N Engl J Med*, **350**, 2452–2460.

[212] Cheng, K.C., Hou, C.C., Huang, H.C. *et al.* (2006). Intravenous injection of methylprednisolone reduces the incidence of postextubation stridor in intensive care unit patients, *Crit Care Med*, **34**, 1345–1350.

[213] Francois, B., Bellissant, E., Gissot, V. *et al.* (2007). 12-h pretreatment with methyl-prednisolone versus placebo for prevention of postextubation laryngeal oedema: a randomised double-blind trial, *Lancet*, **369**, 1083–1089.

[214] Lee, C.-H., Peng, M.-J. and Wu, C.-L. (2007). Dexamethasone to prevent postextubation airway obstruction in adults: a prospective, randomized, double-blind controlled study, *Crit Care*, **11**, R72.

[215] Ferguson, N.D., Cook, D.J., Guyatt, G.H. *et al.* (2013) High-frequency oscillation in early acute respiratory distress syndrome, *N Engl J Med*, **368**, 795–805.

8
Non-Invasive Ventilation

Borja G. Cosío and José M. Echave Sustaeta

8.1 Principles of Non-Invasive Ventilation

8.1.1 *Non-invasive ventilation at a glance*

Mechanical ventilation (MV) provides respiratory support using a mechanical ventilator. This can be done through the endotracheal route (oro- or nasotracheal intubation or tracheotomy) in invasive mechanical ventilation (IMV), or with a nasal or facial interface respecting the natural airway of the patient, known in this case as non-invasive mechanical ventilation (NIMV). In the acute setting, NIMV is usually provided with devices that deliver positive pressure, and this is also known as non-invasive positive pressure ventilation (NIPPV).

8.1.1.1 *Indications of NIMV*

NIMV is currently considered the initial treatment of choice in acute ventilatory failure, regardless of its cause [1–3]. Conditions known to respond to NIPPV include:

- Exacerbations of chronic obstructive pulmonary disease (COPD) complicated by hypercapnic acidosis (partial pressure of arterial carbon dioxide ($PaCO_2$) > 45 mmHg and pH < 7.30).
- Cardiogenic pulmonary oedema.

- Hypoxemic respiratory failure including immunocompromised patients.
- Post-extubation respiratory failure.

8.1.1.2 *Contraindications of NIMV*

In general, there are no absolute contraindications [4] other than the need for urgent intubation. There are however relative contraindications to the administration of NIMV:

- Cardiac or respiratory arrest.
- Inability to cooperate, protect the airway or clear secretions.
- Severely impaired consciousness.
- Non-respiratory organ failure.
- Facial surgery, trauma or deformity.
- High aspiration risk.
- Prolonged duration of mechanical ventilation anticipated.
- Recent oesophageal anastomosis.

8.1.1.3 *Advantages of NIMV*

NIMV has several advantages over IMV [4]:

- It does not require sedation.
- It can be intermittent and can therefore be adjusted to the individual needs of each patient.
- It does not interfere with phonation, deglution and spontaneous expectoration.
- It reduces the incidence of complications associated with endotracheal intubation: respiratory infections, etc.
- It facilitates disconnection ('weaning').
- It can be applied out of the intensive care unit (ICU).
- It does not alter the possibilities for endotracheal intubation.

8.1.1.4 *Consequences of NIMV*

The respiratory consequences of NIMV are shown in Table 8.1. The adverse hemodynamic side effects are less significant than in IMV, and in most patients these are not a limiting factor.

Table 8.1. Outcomes of NIMV: immediate and long-term consequences.

Primary outcome	Secondary outcome
Increased ventilation	Muscle function improvement
Alveolar recruitment	Lung volume improvement
Increased functional residual capacity	Sleep quality improvement
Mucle rest	Re-setting of respiratory centre
Decreased $PaCO_2$	Arterial blood gas improvement
Increased partial pressure of oxygen in arterial blood (PaO_2)	

8.2 Procedures in Non-Invasive Ventilation

8.2.1 *Accessing the airway*

This is a key aspect of success of the technique. It is necessary to make every possible effort to choose an appropriate mask which fits correctly without air leaks or pain.

Desirable characteristics of the ideal mask are [4]:

- Tight fitting in order to avoid air leaks and ensure adequate ventilation.
- Comfortable such that prolonged use is tolerated and does not cause side effects (such as pressure areas).
- As small as possible in order to minimise dead space and optimise ventilation.
- Easy to place and remove so that the patient can do so without assistance.
- Easy to clean.
- Light and transparent in order to avoid claustrophobia.
- Non-allergenic.
- Of various sizes and compatible with different ventilators.
- Low in cost.

8.2.1.1 *Interface*

Different systems are available: nasal masks, oro-nasal masks, full-face masks and nasal pillows. In a randomised, prospective study performed in patients with chronic respiratory failure comparing oro-nasal masks, nasal masks and nasal plugs, the first provided greatest physiological benefits, but the nasal mask was best tolerated [5]. The choice of mask should be determined on an individual basis. Sometimes it is appropriate to commence NIV treatment with an oro-nasal mask, and later change to a nasal mask when consciousness and/or dyspnoea improve. In severe situations, oro-nasal masks are most widely used, while full-face masks are another good alternative.

More recently, the ventilation helmet [6] has gained popularity. Although it may be better tolerated than conventional masks, it seems more appropriate for hypoxemic than for hypercapnic failure due to problems with elimination of CO_2 caused by the increased dead space. This problem can, however, be solved by increasing air flows.

8.2.2 *Ventilation technique*

Timing of initiation of NIMV determines its success, especially if it is the patient's first experience with mechanical ventilation. Before initiating NIMV, the following aspects must be considered (Table 8.2) [7]:

(i) Patient collaboration is necessary.
(ii) Although it is important not to delay administration of NIMV, it is worth taking measures to increase acceptance of therapy by the patient

Table 8.2. Procedure prior to initiating NIMV.

(i)	Inform the patient and monitor patient's vital signs.
(ii)	Program initial ventilator settings, including fraction of inspired oxygen (FiO_2), prepare the bed at 45° and check the mask size before starting ventilation.
(iii)	Place the mask without harness and start the ventilator with the initial settings.
(iv)	Place the mask with harness, without ventilator in order to get the patient used to the mask on their face.
(v)	Start the ventilator and fit the mask to avoid air leaks.
(vi)	Increase ventilator settings gradually according to patient's tolerance and ventilation efficacy.

In addition, it must not be forgotten that NIMV is a part of the patient's overall treatment, and other necessary measures must also be maintained, such as treatments for COPD exacerbation, cardiac failure, pneumonia, etc. Parameter setting varies in patients with hypercapnic and non-hypercapnic respiratory failure (Tables 8.3 and 8.4).

Table 8.3. Ventilator adjustment for hypercapnic respiratory failure.

Initial settings	**Adjustment**
• Bilevel positive airway pressure (BPAP) type ventilator.	Increase IPAP gradually to achieve:
• Expiratory positive airway pressure (EPAP)/ continuous positive airway pressure (CPAP): 4.	• Respiratory frequency < 25 per minute and/or
• Inspiratory positive airway pressure (IPAP): 8–12.	• Tidal volume (Vt) > 7 ml/kg and/or
• Mode: spontaneous/timed.	• IPAP 20 cm H_2O and/or
• Respiratory frequency > 15 per minute.	• Tolerance problems.
• Trigger: sensitive.	
• Inspiration:expiration (I:E) ratio: ± 20–40%.	
• Rise time: short.	
• FiO_2: increase as needed to get oxygen saturation (SaO_2) > 90%.	

Table 8.4. Ventilator adjustment for non-hypercapnic respiratory failure.

- BPAP or CPAP ventilator.
- EPAP/CPAP: between 5 and 10 to get $SaO_2 > 90\%$ with $FiO_2 < 60\%$.
- IPAP: start on 8–12, but increase gradually to get $V_t \geq 7$ ml/kg.
- Respiratory frequency > 15 rpm.
- Trigger: sensitive.
- I/E ratio: ± 20–40%.
- Rise time: short.
- FiO_2: increase as needed to get SaO2 > 90%.

8.2.3 *Monitoring non-invasive mechanical ventilation (NIMV)*

Once NIMV has been initiated, it is necessary to monitor its effects (Fig. 8.1) [4,8,9]. It is essential to monitor the following factors:

- Clinical evaluation:
  - Coordination between the patient and respirator: comfort.
  - Accessory muscle use.
  - Respiratory frequency and cardiac rate (probably the earliest change).
  - Presence of air leaks.
  - Level of consciousness.
- Continuous pulse oximetry.
- Arterial blood gas analyses before commencement of NIMV and at regular intervals thereafter (1–2 hours, 4–6 hours and every 24 hours).

8.2.4 *NIMV failure*

NIMV failure should be defined on an individual basis depending upon the objectives determined prior to initiating NIMV. Some of the criteria used are:

- Intolerance or failure of coordination between patient and ventilator.
- Deterioration in the overall clinical condition.

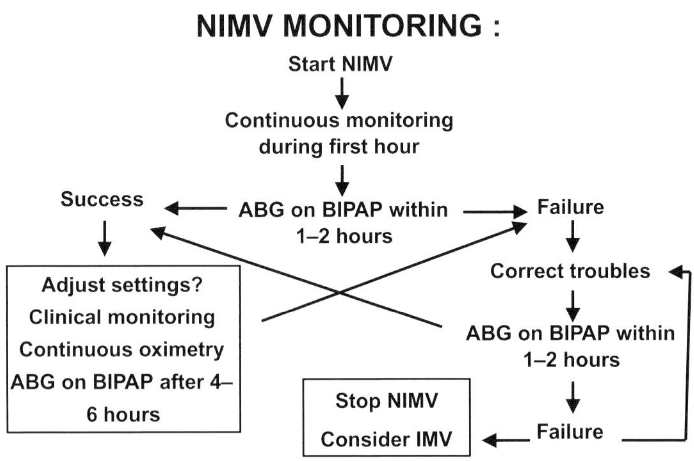

Figure 8.1. Suggested flowchart for monitoring and adjustment of non-invasive ventilation.

- Deterioration or lack of improvement in arterial blood gasses.
- Development of complications: pneumothorax, retention of secretions, etc.

8.2.5 *Discontinuation*

The duration of NIMV is quite variable. In a study by Brochard *et al.* [10] it ranged from 1 to 21 days. In patients with hypercapnic failure, the treatment is no longer necessary when the patient is able to withstand pauses in the treatment without:

- An increase in dyspnoea.
- An increase in respiratory rate (>24 per minute or an increase of 5 per minute above the NIMV rate).
- $pH < 7.35$.
- $SaO_2 < 90\%$ with $FiO_2 < 40\%$.
- A decrease in level of consciousness.

On occasions, it is the patient who discontinues treatment ('self-weaning'). These patients must be observed very carefully in the days immediately following, as there may be a later deterioration with a high incidence of mortality.

In patients in whom NIMV has been applied for hypoxemic failure, once the FiO_2 has been reduced to below 50% an attempt should be made at spontaneous ventilation with a venturi mask and $FiO_2 \leq 50$.

8.2.6 *Nursing time*

In a non-controlled study with a small patient population and in an ICU setting with little NIMV experience, Chevrolet *et al.* [7] reported that NIMV was a procedure that required great amounts of time on the part of the nurses, even more so than IMV. This brought into question the clinical usefulness of NIMV. Later studies have not confirmed these data [11,12]. In general, the first hour of NIMV requires intensive supervision for mask and ventilator adjustments. After this, however, constant presence is not usually necessary.

8.3 Modes and Equipment

8.3.1 *Ventilators*

One of the most important characteristics of NIMV is that it is a ventilation method in which there are air leaks. It is not a closed system like invasive ventilation [4]. These leaks can compromise the efficacy of ventilation. NIMV ventilators should therefore be designed to compensate for this air loss. NIMV ventilators automatically detect the amount of air leakage and alter the airflow supplied accordingly, thereby maintaining the pressure delivered relatively constant.

The most important characteristics of NIMV ventilators are:

(i) A variable flow circuit with turbine generator.
(ii) Pressure stabilisation.
(iii) Compensation for air leaks.
(iv) Air-flow-activated trigger.
(v) Breath-to-breath sensitivity.
(vi) Open circuit without expiratory valve.

There are other NIMV respirators that have double circuits and expiratory valves, which allow for many other parameters to be monitored and which provide better control of MV.

The most commonly used respirators can be divided into two groups depending on their size and capabilities, although their function is similar: ICU-type respirators and portable respirators. The former are those usually used for IMV and can be used in patients with higher MV requirements. The latter have certain advantages in that they do not need compressed air intake, usually weigh between 3 and 7 kg and therefore can be transported more easily.

8.3.2 *Concepts*

There are a series of concepts and terms widely used in NIMV and it is necessary to be familiar with them:

- Trigger: Sensor by which the respirator detects changes in either air pressure or flow created by the patient's inspiratory efforts, at which time the respirator delivers the inspiratory support as dialled.

Insufficiently sensitive triggers can be difficult to activate. Conversely, overly sensitive triggers can discharge too easily and interfere with spontaneous ventilation. In most NIMV ventilators, these triggers are automatic, with flows between 0.5 and 2 l/min.

- Cycle: This determines the change from inspiration to expiration, i.e. when the ventilators should cease applying IPAP and initiate expiration. This trigger can be activated by either flow or time elapsed. In NIMV, cycle changes are usually determined by flow, meaning that the fall in inspiratory flow is detected (which is decelerating; as the programmed pressure is being reached, the flow decreases), and the trigger to initiate expiration can be either a percentage of the maximum peak flow (12–25%) or a previously established absolute value.
- IPAP (inspiratory positive airway pressure): This is the programmed level of positive pressure which is reached during the inspiratory phase of respiration. This pressure is what actually provides ventilatory support.
- EPAP (expiratory positive airway pressure): This is the positive pressure level programmed for the expiratory phase of respiration. It is especially useful in single-tube systems in order to avoid the rebreathing of CO_2. In patients with hyperinflation, it allows for compensation of autoPEEP. In addition, it increases the functional residual capacity, favouring gas exchange and therefore improving hypoxemia.
- PEEP (positive end-expiratory pressure). This is the level of positive pressure programmed for the end of expiration. In NIMV devices, this concept is usually comparable to EPAP.
- I:E ratio: This refers to the percentage of inspiration time relative to the entire respiratory cycle. It is not applicable in the spontaneous mode as this ratio is then determined by the patient.
- Rise time: This is the slope of the pressure curve on inspiration. The greater the slope, the sooner the IPAP level is reached. This may be deemed advisable for patients with acute respiratory insufficiency, who are usually more tachypnoeic and need high flows, but in other patients this may cause discomfort and increase air leaks.
- PSV (pressure support ventilation): The difference in pressure between IPAP and EPAP is considered to be the pressure support administered. There are devices in which PSV and PEEP are specifically programmed as inspiratory and expiratory support, respectively, much the same way as IPAP/EPAP.

8.3.3 *Modes*

NIMV can be delivered using the same modes that are used for invasive mechanical ventilation, although certain modes are used more frequently:

- Assist control (AC) is normally chosen when a guaranteed minimal minute ventilation is desired.
- PSV is chosen when the priority is to maximise patient comfort and synchronisation.
- Continuous positive airway pressure (CPAP) is often used for patients with acute respiratory failure due to cardiogenic pulmonary oedema, for reasons discussed below.

Controlled mechanical ventilation (CMV), intermittent mandatory ventilation, synchronised intermittent mandatory ventilation (SIMV) and pressure-controlled ventilation (PCV) are seldom used during NIPPV. In addition to the modes that can be delivered by either NIPPV or invasive positive pressure ventilation, there are modes that are only applicable to NIPPV. They include bilevel positive airway pressure (BPAP) and proportional assist ventilation (PAV). Like PSV, these tend to be comfortable modes that are triggered by patient effort:

- BPAP delivers both IPAP and EPAP. It is similar to PSV plus PEEP during invasive positive pressure ventilation. The term "BiPAP" is often used incorrectly to refer to NIPPV in the BPAP mode. BiPAP® is a brand name of a portable ventilator, one of many that can deliver BPAP.
- PAV delivers an inspiratory pressure that is proportional to patient effort. Specifically, it is determined by patient-generated volume and flow. PAV provides automatic synchrony between the patient and the ventilatory cycle.

8.4 Special Indications

8.4.1 *Avoidance of intubation: post-extubation*

Weaning from mechanical ventilation can be difficult, especially in patients with chronic respiratory insufficiency, cardiac failure or neurological diseases [13]. Difficult weaning affects up to 42% of intensive care patients, and this proportion rises to 67% of patients with COPD. Clearly this has a major effect on resource utilisation. In addition, survival decreases with each day that a patient continues to be intubated [14]. Chronically ventilated patients represent 6% of all mechanically ventilated patients but consume 37% of intensive care unit resources [15].

Currently, the two most widely used weaning techniques are the clinical tolerance to a two-hour spontaneous breathing trial using a T-tube, and the use of pressure support [16].

Over the last few years, some authors have proposed using NIMV as an alternative to more conventional weaning in three different situations [17]: (i) patients in whom weaning fails; (ii) patients who develop symptoms of ventilatory failure shortly after extubation; and (iii) patients at high risk of re-intubation, as a prophylactic measure after extubation.

8.4.1.1 *NIMV as an alternative technique in patients with weaning failure*

The early experiences reported in the literature come from non-controlled studies, some of which included tracheotomised patients, which facilitated the change back to invasive ventilation again if the NIMV failed. These studies observed improvements in gas exchange parameters, respiratory rate and decrease in respiratory effort and a high percentage of patients reached spontaneous breathing successfully without requiring reintubation.

Nava *et al.* [18] were, to our knowledge, the first to carry out a prospective, controlled, randomised study in 50 patients with COPD exacerbation who required orotracheal intubation due to acute respiratory failure. All the patients selected had failed at a disconnection attempt 48 hours after receiving IMV, by means of a two-hour spontaneous breathing trial with a T-tube. They were randomly chosen to either receive conventional treatment before being extubated, following the usual protocol for ventilator removal (control group) or to receive support pressure through a facial mask (experimental group). The patients treated with NIMV presented a greater number of successful extubations (88% versus 68%), shorter invasive mechanical ventilation treatments (10.2 versus 16.6 days), shorter ICU stays (15.1 versus 24 days) and a greater 60-day survival rate (92% versus 72%). In addition, no patient treated with NIMV presented nosocomial pneumonia, while in the control group this occurred in seven patients.

Girault *et al.* [19] performed a study of similar design in 33 patients with chronic exacerbated respiratory insufficiency, most of whom had COPD. The group of patients treated with NIMV remained intubated for fewer days (4.6 versus 7.7 days). Although there were no differences in mortality, ICU stay or total hospital stay, there was a tendency towards fewer complications in the group of patients treated with NIMV.

Ferrer *et al.* [20], in a study with patients with respiratory failure of different aetiology, reported a significant reduction in the duration of invasive mechanical ventilation, shorter ICU and hospital stays, fewer incidences of complications and higher ICU and 90-day survival rates in the group treated with NIMV.

In a systematic review including 171 patients [21] mainly with hypercapnic respiratory failure caused by COPD, it was concluded that NIMV reduces mortality (relative risk, (RR): 0.41, 95% confidence interval (CI): 0.22–0.76), the incidence of pneumonia associated with ventilator use (RR: 0.28, 95% CI: 0.09–0.85), ICU stay, hospital stay and total duration of mechanical ventilation (−7.33 days, 95% CI: −11.45 to −3.22 days). The analysis of subgroups showed a greater effect in COPD patients when compared with the mixed population, although the differences were not significant.

Therefore, in intubated patients with ventilatory failure due to COPD exacerbation and a failed spontaneous breathing test who would be good candidates for NIMV, the use of NIMV should be considered [22,23].

The appearance of NIMV as an alternative in the process of weaning while continuing MV has led to the coining of the phrase 'weaning in process' for such situations [17]. These results come mainly from patients with COPD and ventilatory failure and are therefore difficult to extrapolate to patients with hypoxemic failure.

The former studies refer to patients without tracheostomy, but experiences with the use of NIMV in the weaning of patients with COPD, prolonged MV and tracheotomy have also been published [24]. In this group of patients, 66% were able to be weaned with the use of NIMV.

8.4.1.2 *NIMV as a prophylactic measure in patients with high risk for reintubation after extubation*

Prophylactic NIMV was studied initially in post-operative patients after abdominal and vascular surgery. In such studies, the use of CPAP (mean 7.5 cm H_2O) demonstrated an improvement in oxygenation, a reduction in infections and in one study reintubations were decreased.

Later, three randomised studies were published. In the Ferrer *et al.* [25] study, the use of NIMV as a prophylactic measure in patients with high risk for reintubation after extubation (at least one of the following factors: age > 65, cardiac failure causing the intubation and Acute Physiology and Chronic Health Evaluation (APACHE) > 12 the day of the extubation) reduced post-extubation respiratory failure and ICU mortality, but there were no differences in the 90-day mortality rate. In an analysis by subgroups, those with $PaCO_2$ > 45 mmHg during the spontaneous breathing test, 90-day mortality rate also decreased. Nava *et al.* [26] reported that the use of NIMV (more than 8 hours/day for 48 hours) in a high-risk population (hypercapnia, cardiac insufficiency, unproductive cough, excessive respiratory secretions, comorbility, failure of more than one attempt at weaning) was associated with a reduction in the need for intubation and mortality.

A recently published, randomised study [27] did not find differences in mortality and mean ICU stay, but did so in the incidence of infections and need for tracheotomy. A work on obese patients [28] (body mass index (BMI) > 35 kg/m^2) found that NIMV (compared with a historical cohort), reduced mortality in the group of hypercapnic patients.

8.4.1.3 *NIMV as a treatment for post-extubation ventilatory failure*

According to various studies, post-extubation ventilatory failure has a prevalence ranging from 6% to 18% and is associated with high mortality. Two initial studies performed with few patients and in solid-organ transplant recipients [29,30] found that NIMV (compared with oxygen) reduced respiratory rate and improved oxygenation. None of the studies found advantages in mortality, even though in one of them [30] the need for reintubation and ICU stays were lower.

Two later large, randomised studies [31,32] did not find any advantages in using NIMV. However, in a post-hoc analysis by Esteban *et al.* [32], the COPD patients presented a decrease in reintubation rate. Therefore, the information currently available does not support the utilisation of NIMV for post-extubation failure [17,33].

8.4.2 *In chronic obstructive pulmonary disease (COPD)*

8.4.2.1 *Demonstrated benefits:*

COPD is a disease that has frequent exacerbations. The mortality rate of a COPD exacerbation requiring hospital admission ranges between 11% and 14%, reaching 25% if MV is required. Respiratory acidosis in COPD exacerbation is associated with an increase in the need for intubation and mortality [34]. In addition, an acute exacerbation is associated with poor prognosis, and some studies report one-year mortality rates over 40% [35].

In most cases, acute respiratory insufficiency secondary to a COPD exacerbation can be managed conservatively, although MV is sometimes necessary [36].

IMV exposes the patient to a variety of complications derived from the necessity of an endotracheal access. NIMV is undoubtedly useful in treating severe COPD exacerbation with respiratory acidosis. This has been reflected in numerous randomised clinical trials and systematic reviews [37–39].

Observed benefits:

- Decrease in mortality: RR 0.41 (95% CI: 0.26–0.64), with a number needed to treat (NNT) of 8 (95% CI: 6–13).
- Decrease in need for intubation: RR 0.42 (95% CI: 0.31–0.59) with an NNT of 5 (95% CI: 4–7).
- Decrease in mean hospital stay of −3.24 days (−4.42 to −2.06 days).

Other benefits observed are faster improvement of pH, $PaCO_2$, PaO_2, dyspnoea and respiratory rate, and reductions in complications, duration of MV, mean ICU stay, and a considerable reduction in cost [40].

Another aspect of great relevance is that of long-term prognosis. This group of patients with severe COPD, chronic respiratory insufficiency and episodes of either acute or chronic exacerbations of ventilatory failure has poor mid-term prognosis. In a study [41] completed one year after having required NIMV for acute exacerbation, 79.9% of patients had been rehospitalised for COPD exacerbation, 63.3% had presented another life-threatening event, 49% had died, and the survivors had required an average of 12 days of hospitalisation.

The development of strategies aimed at decreasing mortality is very important, given the poor prognosis of these patients. In this regard, various authors consider this group to be candidates for home NIMV [42].

8.4.2.2 *Where should NIMV be administered?*

NIMV can be applied in different settings: the emergency room, hospital wards and in recovery, high-dependency and intensive care units. Each offers advantages, which can vary depending on many factors (Table 8.4.). Most authors agree that what is more important than the setting is the experience and knowledge of the doctors and nurses involved in NIMV application. 75% of patients included in studies considered for a systematic review [37] had received treatment in conventional hospital wards and the remaining 25% in ICUs.

8.4.2.3 *Patient selection*

A crucial factor in the different NIMV studies in acute respiratory insufficiency is patient selection. The most widely used published criteria are: (i) patients hospitalised with a diagnosis of COPD exacerbation; (ii) respiratory rate > 25 per min.; (iii) pH < 7.35 with $PaCO_2$ > 45 mmHg; and (iv) lack of response to standard medical treatment.

Some authors set the pH limit under 7.30 [43], although the work by Plant *et al.* [11] demonstrated a benefit in the pH group from 7.30–7.35. Even in especially severely affected patients (pH < 7.20), NIMV has demonstrated an efficacy similar to IMV [44,45].

8.4.2.4 *NIMV success*

The aim of NIMV is to reduce mortality and the need for intubation and IMV, and it is therefore considered successful if these objectives are reached. However, other intermediate objectives can be established as predictors of the aforementioned goals. The following could be considered to be intermediate objectives:

- Comfort and good tolerance.
- More than one of the following:
  - Reduce respiratory rate ≥ 5 per min.
  - Reduce $PaCO_2 \geq 5$ mmHg.
  - Increase pH ≥ 0.03.
  - Improvement in level of consciousness.
  - Increase $PaO_2 > 10$ mmHg with no deterioration in $PaCO_2$ or pH.

Although in most patients much more important improvements are obtained than those described, the former were chosen based on the average changes reported in a systemic review [37]: mean decrease in respiratory rate of −3.08 (95% CI: −4.26 to −1.89), mean increase in pH of 0.03 (95% CI: 0.02 to 0.04), mean decrease in $PaCO_2$ of −3.03 mmHg (95% CI: −5.91 to −0.22).

8.4.2.5 *Predictive factors of response*

Even with NIMV, between 15–30% of COPD patients with severe exacerbation require intubation and 10% die [37–39]. It is very important to identify those in whom NIMV is not going to be effective, as prolonging NIMV can delay IMV, which has been associated with an increase in mortality [46].

Studies specifically designed to predict NIMV success indicate that information available just prior to initiating NIMV as well as shortly after initiation (30 min to 3 hours) can only predict the possibilities for success rather than measure them precisely [47–48].

Among the data available at the start of treatment are predictors of patient evolution: low level of consciousness; initial agitation; severity determined by more acidosis, more hypercapnia and/or a higher Simplified Acute Physiology Score (SAPS) or APACHE II; lack of teeth; cause of the acute respiratory insufficiency; presence of excessive respiratory secretions; breathing with pursed lips; important comorbidity; orofacial deformities; low weight; previous lung function; etc.

Among the information obtained after a short period of time with NIMV, the most important is an improvement in pH and $PaCO_2$ in the first hour of treatment, decrease in respiratory rate, and improvement in encephalopathy. The tolerance and maintenance of the treatment [47,48] have been cited as prognostic factors of treatment efficacy, while the presence of air leaks is an unfavourable prognostic factor [39].

Nevertheless, despite initial improvement in blood gases and symptoms, and even after a few days of successful NIMV, some 15–28% of patients require intubation or die [37–39,49]. The overall mortality in this group of patients with late ventilatory failure was 68%; this can be subdivided into 53% for those who received IMV treatment and 92% for those who were maintained on NIMV. In the study by Brochard *et al.* [10] of patients necessitating orotracheal intubation, 45% did so in the first four hours, 82% in the first 12 hours and 15% after 48 hours.

8.4.2.6 *Timetable and duration of NIMV*

On the first day, NIMV should be applied the maximum number of hours possible. While initially the treatment is constant, after four to six hours there should be an attempt at a rest of 30–60 min in order to ingest food and liquids, etc. NIMV should be reinitiated if during this resting period one of the following signs or symptoms develops: increase in respiratory rate>5 per minute, increase in dyspnoea or a decrease in SaO_2. Similar resting periods should be programmed every four to six hours depending on the response to the first period.

On the second day, ideally 14–16 hours of NIMV should be applied, normally as night-time rest with an additional two hours in the morning and in the afternoon. On the following days, the number of hours and/or level of support should be reduced. It is important to remember that once NIMV has been established, priority should be shifted more or less immediately towards weaning of the same.

It is not always possible to achieve these objectives. In one study, Plant *et al.* [11] set initial objectives of NIMV duration for the first three days, and the actual number of hours was quantified (Table 8.5).

Table 8.5. Initial objective and number of hours of NIMV in the study of Plant *et al.* [11].

	Objective	**Actual**
First day:	As much as possible	8 hours
Second day:	16 hours	7 hours
Third day:	12 hours	5 hours

8.4.3 *In pulmonary oedema*

8.4.3.1 *Introduction*

An aging population together with improvement in survival after acute myocardial infarction has produced a rapid increase in the number of patients with chronic heart failure, with an increase in the number of hospitalisations for decompensated cardiac failure [50]. 75% of medical expenses linked to cardiac insufficiency are hospital expenses. Hospital mortality from acute pulmonary oedema (APO) ranges from 10% to 20%, and reaches 30% when associated with acute myocardial infarction. 40% of patients hospitalised for APO require at least one rehospitalisation in the subsequent 12 months, in which mortality reaches 40%.

Patients that do not respond to medical treatment frequently need intubation and invasive mechanical ventilation. In the last ten years, numerous studies trying to explore the role of NIMV in APO of cardiogenic origin have been published. The first article published on NIMV in acute respiratory failure was a series of cases including patients with APO [51].

Two NIMV methods have been assayed: CPAP and support pressure. Compared with CPAP, support pressure produces greater improvement in respiratory work, $PaCO_2$ and oxygenation [52].

8.4.3.2 *Available information*

Two initial randomised, controlled studies of CPAP (10–15 cm H_2O) administered by face mask showed faster improvement in oxygenation and a reduced need for endotracheal intubation. Later, a study [53] that compared PSV + CPAP versus CPAP found an increase in myocardial infarction in the PSV group; however these patients had higher incidence of chest pain prior to recruitment.

In the following years, various studies were published using CPAP and/or BPAP versus standard treatment. Most reported favourable results in the NIMV group although, as in COPD studies, recruitment was low and in one study [54] only 30% of the eligible patients were included.

In 2006, a meta-analysis was published [55] that included 23 articles: 12 comparing CPAP versus standard treatment (295 patients), seven comparing BPAP versus standard treatment (171 patients) and ten comparing CPAP versus BPAP (178 patients). Treatment with CPAP was associated with lower mortality (RR: 0.59, 95% CI: 0.38–0.90, $p = 0.015$), and the group treated with BPAP showed a tendency towards lower mortality (RR: 0.63, 95% CI: 0.37–1.1, $p = 0.11$) compared with the standard treatment group. There were no differences in mortality between the CPAP and the BPAP groups ($p = 0.38$). In both the CPAP (0.44, 0.29–0.66, $p = 0.0003$) and BPAP groups (0.50, 0.27–0.90, $p = 0.02$) the incidence of orotracheal intubation and IMV decreased, again with no differences between either ($p = 0.86$). When compared with CPAP there was a trend towards more acute myocardial infarctions in the BPAP group (RR: 1.49, 95% CI: 0.92–2.42, $p = 0.11$) which did not reach statistical significance.

Recently, a randomised multicentre study was published with three treatment types: standard treatment with oxygen, CPAP (5–15 cm H_2O) and BPAP (inspiratory pressure 8–20 cm H_2O and expiratory 4–10 cm H_2O). The main outcome was death seven days after treatment was started, but other variables were measured: orotracheal intubation, dyspnoea, physiological variables, hospital stay, ICU admittance and death after 30 days. The inclusion criteria were: age > 16, clinical symptoms compatible with cardiac insufficiency, APO on imaging, respiratory rate higher than 20 per minute and pH < 7.35. A population of severely affected patients was included: pH 7.22, $PaCO_2$ 7.6 kiloPascales (kp), respiration rate 33 per minute and dyspnoea at rest. There were no differences between the NIMV group versus the standard treatment group in seven-day mortality (9.5% versus 9.8%, $p = 0.87$), 30-day mortality (15.2% versus 16.4%, $p = 0.64$), intubation at seven days (2.9% versus 2.8%, $p = 0.90$), need for ICU admittance (45.2% versus 40.5%, $p = 0.15$), myocardial infarction and mean hospital stay. The NIMV group presented faster improvement in pH, $PaCO_2$, dyspnoea and heart rate. Once again, there were no differences between the NIMV and CPAP groups. There was a greater percentage of patients who withdrew from the study due to discomfort in the NIMV group (8.4%) and in the CPAP group (5.2%) than in the standard treatment group (0.3%), $p < 0.001$.

In conclusion, it seems clear that in acute cardiogenic pulmonary oedema, treatment with BPAP is no better than treatment with CPAP. Although a CPAP trial is used frequently, available evidence regarding whether CPAP offers advantages over standard oxygen treatment is contradictory in the setting of pulmonary oedema (meta-analysis versus randomised study), but the current clinical perception is that it probably does not.

8.4.4 *In other diseases*

8.4.4.1 *Immunocompromised*

Among immunocompromised patients who have acute respiratory failure, NIPPV is associated with a decreased ICU mortality, intubation rate and ICU length of stay compared with invasive mechanical ventilation [57]. This is probably a consequence of fewer nosocomial infections.

8.4.4.2 *Pneumonia*

Difficulty managing secretions is an accepted contraindication to NIPPV. However, NIPPV may be beneficial in patients with pneumonia if they are able to manage their secretions. In one trial, 105 patients with acute hypoxemic respiratory failure of varying aetiologies were randomly assigned to receive standard medical therapy alone or NIPPV plus standard medical therapy [58]. NIPPV decreased ICU mortality (18% versus 39%) and the intubation rate (25% versus 5%). These effects were particularly strong in the subgroup of patients with hypoxemic respiratory failure due to pneumonia.

8.4.4.3 *Asthma*

Most patients with asthma do not present with acute respiratory failure; as a result, the number of studies investigating the use of NIPPV in acute asthma exacerbations is limited. In one trial, 30 patients with an acute asthma exacerbation were randomly assigned to receive NIPPV (in the BPAP mode) or sham (subtherapeutic BPAP) in the emergency room [59]. NIPPV reduced the rate of hospitalisation (18% versus 63%) and increased the likelihood of a significant improvement in forced expiratory volume in one second (FEV_1) (80% versus 20%). Although these findings are encouraging, more rigorous controlled trials are needed before NIPPV becomes a routine part of managing asthma exacerbations.

8.5 Summary

NIPPV refers to positive pressure ventilation delivered through a non-invasive interface (nasal mask, face mask, nasal plugs, or helmet).

A trial of NIPPV is worthwhile for a variety of patients. The following recommendations pertain to patients who do not require emergency intubation and for whom there are no contraindications to NIPPV.

- For patients with an exacerbation of COPD complicated by hypercapnic acidosis ($PaCO_2$ >45 mmHg or pH <7.30), we recommend a trial of NIPPV rather than proceeding directly to IMV (Grade 1A).
- For patients with cardiogenic pulmonary oedema, we recommend a trial of NIPPV rather than proceeding directly to IMV (Grade 1A). CPAP is an appropriate choice for normocarbic patients, while other modes of NIPPV are preferable for hypercarbic patients.
- For patients with hypoxemic respiratory failure due to causes other than cardiogenic pulmonary oedema, we suggest a trial of NIPPV rather than proceeding directly to IMV (Grade 2B).
- NIPPV may be beneficial to some patients who develop respiratory failure after extubation.

Once a patient has been selected to receive a trial of NIPPV, it should be initiated as soon as possible. Patients who fail to improve or stabilise within one and a half to two hours should be promptly intubated. NIPPV is generally safe. Most complications are local and related to the tightly fitting mask.

References

[1] Brochard, L., Mancebo, J. and Elliott, M.W. (2002). Non-invasive ventilation for acute respiratory failure, *Eur Respir J*, **19**, 712–721.

[2] Brochard, L. (2003). Mechanical ventilation: invasive versus noninvasive, *Eur Respir J Suppl*, **47**, 31s–37s.

[3] Antro, C., Merico, F., Urbino, R. *et al.* (2005). Non-invasive ventilation as a first-line treatment for acute respiratory failure: "real life" experience in the emergency department, *Emerg Med J*, **22**, 772–777.

[4] American Thoracic Society, the European Respiratory Society, the European Society of Intensive Care Medicine, and the Société de Réanimation de Langue Française (2001). International Consensus Conferences in Intensive Care Medicine: noninvasive positive pressure ventilation in acute respiratory failure, *Am J Respir Crit Care Med*, **163**, 283–291.

[5] Navalesi, P., Fanfulla, F., Frigerio, P. *et al.* (2000). Physiologic evaluation of noninvasive mechanical ventilation delivered with three types of masks in patients with chronic hypercapnic respiratory failure, *Crit Care Med*, **28**, 1785–1790.

[6] Antonelli, M., Pennisi, M.A., Pelosi, P. *et al.* (2004). Noninvasive positive pressure ventilation using a helmet in patients with acute exacerbation of chronic obstructive pulmonary disease: a feasibility study, *Anesthesiology*, **100**, 16–24.

[7] Chevrolet, J.C., Jolliet, P., Abajo, B. *et al.* (1991). Nasal positive pressure ventilation in patients with acute respiratory failure. Difficult and time-consuming procedure for nurses, *Chest*, **100**, 775–782.

[8] Meduri, G.U. and Spencer, S.E. (2001). Noninvasive mechanical ventilation in the acute setting. Technical aspects, monitoring and choice of the interface, *Eur Respir Mon*, **6**, 106–124.

[9] British Thoracic Society Standards of Care Committee (2002). Non-invasive ventilation in acute respiratory failure, *Thorax*, **57**, 192–211.

[10] Brochard, L., Mancebo, J., Wysocki, M. *et al.* (1995). Noninvasive ventilation for acute exacerbations of chronic obstructive pulmonary disease, *N Engl J Med*, **333**, 817–822.

[11] Plant, P.K., Owen, J.L. and Elliott, M.W. (2000). Early use of non-invasive ventilation for acute exacerbations of chronic obstructive pulmonary disease on general respiratory wards: a multicentre randomised controlled trial, *Lancet*, **355**, 1931–1935.

[12] Nava, S., Evangelisti, I., Rampulla, C. *et al.* (1997). Human and financial costs of noninvasive mechanical ventilation in patients affected by COPD and acute respiratory failure, *Chest*, **111**, 1631–1638.

[13] Alia, I. and Esteban, A. (2000). Weaning from mechanical ventilation, *Crit Care*, **4**, 72–80.
[14] Ferrer, M. (2005). Non-invasive ventilation as a weaning tool, *Minerva Anestesiol*, **71**, 243–247.
[15] Wagner, D.P. (1989). Economics of prolonged mechanical ventilation, *Am Rev Respir Dis*, **140**, S14–S18.
[16] Esteban, A., Frutos, F., Tobin, M.J. *et al.* (1995). A comparison of four methods of weaning patients from mechanical ventilation, *N Engl J Med*, **332**, 345–350.
[17] Boles, J.M., Bion, J., Connors, A. *et al.* (2007). Weaning from mechanical ventilation, *Eur Respir J*, **29**, 1033–1056.
[18] Nava, S., Ambrosino, N., Clini, E. *et al.* (1998). Noninvasive mechanical ventilation in the weaning of patients with respiratory failure due to chronic obstructive pulmonary disease. A randomized, controlled trial, *Ann Intern Med*, **128**, 721–728.
[19] Girault, C., Daudenthun, I., Chevron, V. *et al.* (1999). Noninvasive ventilation as a systematic extubation and weaning technique in acute-on-chronic respiratory failure. A prospective, randomized controlled study, *Am J Respir Crit Care Med*, **160**, 86–92.
[20] Ferrer, M., Esqinas, A., Arancibia, F. *et al.* (2003). Noninvasive ventilation during persistent weaning failure, *Am J Respir Crit Care Med*, **168**, 70–76.
[21] Burns, K.E., Adhikari, N.K. and Meade, M.O. (2006). A meta-analysis of noninvasive weaning to facilitate liberation from mechanical ventilation, *Can J Anaesth*, **53**, 222–225.
[22] Ambrosino, N. and Vagheggini, G. (2008). Noninvasive positive pressure ventilation in the acute care setting: where are we? *Eur Respir J*, **31**, 874–886.
[23] Garpestad, E., Brennan, J. and Hill, N.S. (2007). Noninvasive ventilation for critical care, *Chest*, **132**, 711–720.
[24] Quinnell, T.G., Pilsworth, S., Shneerson, J.M. *et al.* (2006). Prolonged invasive ventilation following acute ventilatory failure in COPD: weaning results, survival, and the role of noninvasive ventilation, *Chest*, **129**, 133–139.
[25] Ferrer, M., Valencia, M., Nicolas, J.M. *et al.* (2006). Early noninvasive ventilation averts extubation failure in patients at risk. A randomized trial, *Am J Respir Crit Care Med*, **173**, 164–170.
[26] Nava, S., Gregoretti, C., Fanfulla, F. *et al.* (2005). Noninvasive ventilation to prevent respiratory failure after extubation in high-risk patients, *Crit Care Med*, **33**, 2465–2470.
[27] Trevisan, C.E, Vieira, S.R and Research Group in Mechanical Ventilation Weaning (2008). Noninvasive mechanical ventilation may be useful in treating patients who fail weaning from invasive mechanical ventilation: a randomized clinical trial, *Crit Care*, **12**, R51.

[28] El-Solh, A.A., Aquilina, A., Pineda, L. *et al.* (2006). Noninvasive ventilation for prevention of post-extubation respiratory failure in obese patients, *Eur Respir J*, **28**, 588–595.

[29] Kilger, E., Briegel, J., Haller, M. *et al.* (1999). Effects of non-invasive positive pressure ventilatory support in non-COPD patients with acute respiratory insufficiency after early extubation, *Intens Care Med*, **25**, 1374–1380.

[30] Antonelli, M., Conti, G., Bufi, M. *et al.* (2000). Noninvasive ventilation for treatment of acute respiratory failure in patients undergoing solid organ transplantation: a randomized trial, *JAMA*, **283**, 235–241.

[31] Keenan, S.P., Powers, C., McCormack, D.G. *et al.* (2002). Noninvasive positive-pressure ventilation for postextubation respiratory distress: a randomized controlled trial, *JAMA*, **287**, 3238–3244.

[32] Esteban, A., Frutos-Vivar, F., Ferguson, N.D. *et al.* (2004). Noninvasive positive-pressure ventilation for respiratory failure after extubation, *N Engl J Med*, **350**, 2452–2460.

[33] Agarwal, R., Aggarwal, A.N., Gupta, D. *et al.* (2007). Role of noninvasive positive-pressure ventilation in postextubation respiratory failure: a meta-analysis, *Respir Care*, **52**, 1472–1479.

[34] Soo Hoo, G.W., Hakimian, N. and Santiago, S.M. (2000). Hypercapnic respiratory failure in COPD patients. Response to therapy, *Chest*, **117**, 169–177.

[35] Connors, A.F., Dawson, N.V., Thomas, C. *et al.* (1996). Outcomes following acute exacerbations of severe chronic obstructive lung disease, *Am J Respir Crit Care Med*, **154**, 959–967.

[36] Wedzicha, J.A. (2003). 'Exacerbations', in Calverley, P.M.A., MacNee, W., Pride, N.B., Rennard, S.I. (eds), *Chronic Obstructive Pulmonary Disease*, Arnold, London, pp. 390–401.

[37] Lightowler, J.V., Wedzicha, J.A., Elliott, M.W. *et al.* (2003). Non-invasive positive pressure ventilation to treat respiratory failure resulting from exacerbations of chronic obstructive pulmonary disease: Cochrane systematic review and meta-analysis, *BMJ*, **326**,185.

[38] Keenan, S.P., Sinuff, T., Cook, D.J. *et al.* (2003). Which patients with acute exacerbation of chronic obstructive pulmonary disease benefit from non-invasive positive-pressure ventilation? A systematic review of the literature, *Ann Intern Med*, **138**, 861–870.

[39] Wark, P. (2005). 'Non-invasive ventilation in acute respiratory failure', in Gibson, P.G., Abramson, M., Wood-Baker, R. *et al.* (eds), *Evidence-Based Respiratory Medicine*, Blackwell Publishing, Oxford, pp. 429–436.

[40] Plant, P.K., Owen, J.L., Parrott, S. *et al.* (2003). Cost effectiveness of ward based non-invasive ventilation for acute exacerbations of chronic obstructive

pulmonary disease: economic analysis of randomised controlled trial, *BMJ*, **326**, 956.

[41] Chu, C.M., Chan, V.L., Lin, A.W. *et al.* (2004). Readmission rates and life threatening events in COPD survivors treated with non-invasive ventilation for acute hypercapnic respiratory failure, *Thorax*, **59**,1020–1025.

[42] Elliott, M.W. (2004). Non-invasive ventilation in acute exacerbations of COPD: what happens after hospital discharge? *Thorax*, **59**, 1006–1008.

[43] Antón, A., Güell, R., Gómez, J. *et al.* (2000). Predicting the result of noninvasive ventilation in severe acute exacerbation of patients with chronic airflow limitation, *Chest*, **117**, 828–833.

[44] Diaz, G.G., Alcaraz, A.C., Talavera, J.C. *et al.* (2005). Noninvasive positive-pressure ventilation to treat hypercapnic coma secondary to respiratory failure, *Chest*, **127**, 952–960.

[45] Gay, P.C., Hess, D.R. and Hill, N.S. (2001). Noninvasive proportional assist ventilation for acute respiratory insufficiency. Comparison with pressure support ventilation, *Am J Respir Crit Care Med*, **164**, 1606–1611.

[46] Wood, K.A., Lewis, L., Von Harz, B. *et al.* (1998). The use of noninvasive positive pressure ventilation in the emergency department, *Chest*, **113**, 1339–1346.

[47] Soo Hoo, G.W., Santiago, S. and Williams, A.J. (1994). Nasal mechanical ventilation for hypercapnic respiratory failure in chronic obstructive pulmonary disease, determinants of success and failure, *Crit Care Med*, **22**, 1253–1261.

[48] Ambrosino, N., Foglio, K., Rubino, F. *et al.* (1995). Noninvasive mechanical ventilation in acute respiratory failure due to chronic obstructive pulmonary disease, correlates for success, *Thorax*, **50**, 755–757.

[49] Moretti, M., Cilione, C., Tampieri, A. *et al.* (2000). Incidence and causes of non-invasive mechanical ventilation failure after initial success, *Thorax*, **55**, 819–825.

[50] Dickstein, K., Cohen-Solal, A., Filippatos, G. *et al.* (2008). ESC Guidelines for the diagnosis and treatment of acute and chronic heart failure. 2008: The Task Force for the Diagnosis and Treatment of Acute and Chronic Heart Failure 2008 of the European Society of Cardiology. Developed in collaboration with the Heart Failure Association of the ESC (HFA) and endorsed by the European Society of Intensive Care Medicine (ESICM), *Eur J Heart Fail*, **10**, 933–989.

[51] Meduri, G.U., Conoscenti, C.C., Menashe, P. *et al.* (1989). Noninvasive face mask ventilation in patients with acute respiratory failure, *Chest*, **95**, 865–870.

[52] Chadda, K., Annane, D., Hart, N. *et al.* (2002). Cardiac and respiratory effects of continuous positive airway pressure and noninvasive ventilation in acute cardiac pulmonary edema, *Crit Care Med*, **30**, 2457–2461.

[53] Metha, S., Jay, G.D., Woolard, R.H. *et al.* (1997). Randomized prospective trial of bilevel versus continuous positive airway pressure in acute pulmonary edema, *Crit Care Med*, **25**, 620–628.

[54] Masip, J., Betbesé, A.J., Páez, J. *et al.* (2000). Non-invasive pressure support ventilation versus conventional oxygen therapy in acute cardiogenic pulmonary oedema: a randomised trial, *Lancet*, **356**, 2126–2132.

[55] Peter, J.V., Moran, J.L, Phillips-Hughes, J.K. *et al.* (2006). Effect of noninvasive positive pressure ventilation (NIPPV) on mortality in patients with acute cardiogenic pulmonary oedema: a meta-analysis, *Lancet*, **367**, 1155–1163.

[56] Gray, A., Goodacre, S., Newby, D.E. *et al.* (2008). Noninvasive ventilation in acute cardiogenic pulmonary edema, *N Engl J Med*, **359**, 142–151.

[57] Girou, E., Schortgen, F., Delclaux, C. *et al.* (2000). Association of noninvasive ventilation with nosocomial infections and survival in critically ill patients, *JAMA*, **284**, 2361–2367.

[58] Ferrer, M., Esquinas, A., Leon, M. *et al.* (2003). Noninvasive ventilation in severe hypoxemic respiratory failure: a randomized clinical trial, *Am J Respir Crit Care Med*, **168**, 1438–1444.

[59] Soroksky, A., Stav, D. and Shpirer, I. (2003). A pilot prospective, randomized, placebo-controlled trial of bilevel positive airway pressure in acute asthmatic attack, *Chest*, **123**, 1018–1025.

9 Nutrition

Richard Leonard

9.1 Introduction

The vast majority of patients receiving intensive care for more than a short period of time also receive nutritional support. Yet despite this nearly universal practice, there remains considerable uncertainty about crucial aspects of its delivery. Much of the evidence is conflicting, and of lamentably poor quality [1]. The resulting debates often have similar failings, and tendentious positions are defended with absurd vigour [2]. With tedious inevitability, those in search of enlightenment have been drawn like moths to the illusory flame of meta-analysis. Since this technique appears to get the answer wrong more often than not [3], it should come as no surprise that the two most recent meta-analyses addressing the critical question of the optimal route of feeding reach opposite conclusions [4,5]. It seems that the major legacy of evidence-based medicine is to leave clinicians with a choice of meta-analyses to believe, instead of original papers. As clinicians are generally better trained to evaluate scientific methods than statistical ones, it is hard to see this as the advance into lucid scientific medical practice claimed by the cultists of evidence-based medicine.

The situation is hardly improved by a plethora of clinical practice guidelines, which differ in important respects [6–11]. Nonetheless, one at least has some degree of clinical validation. The Algorithms for Critical-Care Enteral and Parenteral Therapy (ACCEPT) study was a cluster-randomised trial of a nutrition guideline and supporting education programme [6]. The investigators found a 10% reduction in mortality in those units using the guideline, which just failed to reach statistical significance. Naturally, this does not necessarily mean that every element of the ACCEPT guidelines is optimal.

The pragmatic intensivist attempting to make sense of this mess in order to manage patients faces six questions:

(i) Why do we feed patients in intensive care?
(ii) Which patients need to be fed?
(iii) When should feeding start?
(iv) How much feed should critically ill patients receive?
(v) Which route should be used to feed intensive care unit (ICU) patients?
(vi) What should the feed contain?

This chapter will seek to provide answers that are supported by the presently available evidence, and to make clear the shortcomings of that evidence when necessary. Practical considerations concerning nutritional management will be addressed as they arise.

9.2 Why do we Feed Patients in Intensive Care?

This apparently trivial question conceals some important uncertainties. It is obvious that patients who are unable by virtue of their illness to meet their own nutritional needs will ultimately starve if not artificially supported. In healthy humans, starvation takes weeks before it is fatal. Critically ill patients however are significantly catabolic, with a high energy expenditure and high rate of nitrogen loss compared with resting healthy individuals. The consensus conference in 1997 between the US National Institutes of Health, the American Society for Parenteral and Enteral Nutrition and the American Society for Clinical Nutrition calculated that dangerous depletion of lean body mass would occur in critically ill patients in around 14 days if nutritional support was not forthcoming [10]. Given that a significant proportion of ICU patients recover in less than this time, the justification for nutritional support is based primarily on the close association between pre-existing malnutrition, negative nitrogen and energy balance and death.

Unsurprisingly, there are few trials comparing the feeding of ICU patients with the withholding of feed. However, one study has approached these conditions. It was carried out in patients who had undergone surgery for severe acute pancreatitis, and compared jejunal feeding with electrolyte and fluid support alone [12] and found a reduction in mortality in patients receiving nutritional support. Even with optimal support, though, it is not possible to completely prevent depletion of lean body mass [13].

The purpose of feeding critically ill patients in intensive care, then, is two-fold: to treat existing malnutrition, and to minimise its development as far as possible.

9.2.1 *Nutritional assessment*

In order to treat existing malnutrition in intensive care patients, it is necessary first to identify it. Objective methods used in the general population are useless in the critically ill. Anthropometric measurements such as skin-fold thickness and mid-arm circumference are confounded by oedema, while voluntary hand-grip strength is of no value in unconscious patients. The same problem exists with laboratory measures like transferrin, pre-albumin and albumin levels, all of which are abnormal in critical illness.

Simple clinical evaluation using the so-called Subjective Global Assessment is better at predicting nutrition-related morbidity [14]. A history of weight loss, poor diet, gastrointestinal symptoms, reduced functional capacity, and a diagnosis associated with poor intake suggests that the patient is likely to be malnourished. Physical findings of muscle wasting, loss of subcutaneous fat, oedema and ascites support the conclusion.

One important exception to the inapplicability of laboratory tests of nutritional status to intensive care patients exists. Intensivists are increasingly involved in the pre-operative evaluation and preparation of candidates for major surgery. In this population, the serum albumin and operative site were closely associated with the risk of post-operative complications [15]. The opportunity may exist to improve outcomes by identifying and treating nutritional deficits before the surgical insult is inflicted.

9.3 Which Patients Need to be Fed?

Some patients admitted to intensive care are likely to recover nutritional independence within a few days. The question then arises of how long they can safely be left without support while awaiting that recovery.

Data addressing this question are few. The 1997 consensus conference cited above opined that in view of the likelihood of dangerous nutritional depletion after 14 days of critical illness without feeding, artificial nutritional support should be provided to all patients thought unlikely to feed themselves within seven to ten days [10]. Others have suggested that the maximum permitted delay in establishing full intake should be seven days [16].

It therefore appears that head-injured patients may tolerate up to five days without feeding. It is not known whether this can be extrapolated to other groups of patients, however, and indeed, in light of studies aiming to answer the next question, it seems likely that more catabolic patients will start to develop complications sooner. Certainly, the ACCEPT trial fed all patients not likely to regain oral intake within 24 hours [6].

9.4 When Should Feeding Start?

If a patient will clearly exceed the maximum permissible period without feed (say five days), is it better to start to feed them before that time elapses? A reasonable body of evidence now suggests that this is indeed the case, inasmuch as two meta-analyses have at least reached similar conclusions. The first compared early enteral feeding starting within the first 48 hours of admission to ICU with later enteral feeding started thereafter, and showed a reduction in infectious complications [17]. The second compared early parenteral feeding with delayed enteral feeding, and found a reduction in mortality with earlier support [18]. Although these findings are tarred with the weaknesses inherent in all meta-analyses, they are at least concordant, logical, and in line with Macbeth's view that 'If it were done when 'tis done, then 'twere well/It were done quickly'.

It is worth noting that the ACCEPT study placed stress both on tolerating only a very limited period of starvation, and on starting to feed early. All patients not expected to regain oral intake within 24 hours were fed, and the aim of the guideline was to reach the prescribed intake within 24 hours of starting [6].

The current trend is therefore to feed all patients not likely to regain oral intake within a very limited period of time (certainly five days, and probably only 48 hours), and to commence feeding as soon as practical once preliminary stabilisation of the patient has occurred, but again within 48 hours.

9.5 How Much Feed Should Critically Ill Patients Receive?

9.5.1 *Energy*

It appears that optimal nutritional support can hope only to minimise rather than completely prevent the muscle depletion associated with critical illness [13]. Moreover, there seems to be an upper limit to the amounts of both energy and protein that critically ill patients can utilise [13,19]. Feed provided above these limits, far from being simply of no benefit, is actually deleterious, producing serious metabolic complications [20]. Over the past 20 years there has been a downward trend in the estimation both of the degree of catabolism seen in most intensive care patients and in their energy requirements, and it is possible that this trend will continue. In 1997, the American College of Chest Physicians (ACCP) recommended a daily energy intake of 25 kCal/kg, and this has remained the standard prescription. However, there is some evidence from observational studies that this may still be too much, with patients whose measured energy intake was between 9 and 18 kCal/kg/day showing lower mortality than those with both higher and lower intakes [21]. As a result, so-called 'hypocaloric' feeding is being investigated, as yet with no prospectively demonstrable benefits to the general ICU population. Despite this present fashion, it is crucially important to remember that enterally fed patients frequently receive far less than their target intake, and that this under-feeding is very clearly linked to worse outcomes [21–23].

Energy requirements vary both between patients (depending on such factors as age, sex, diagnosis and treatment) and in the same patient over time, as their illness progresses and then hopefully recedes, and the patient becomes more active as he or she weans from mechanical ventilation [24]. It is therefore common practice to attempt to tailor the energy provided to the patient, using either indirect calorimetry or predictive equations.

The most precise method is to use indirect calorimetry to measure the resting energy expenditure (REE). In the past, this has been a cumbersome technique, and although more modern devices designed for the intensive care setting are making it easier, it is still far from usual practice. The resulting value excludes the energy consumed in physical activity, and in ICUs using this approach it is usual to provide the patient with approximately 1.3 times the measured REE [25]. Calorimetry certainly reveals wide deviation from energy requirements predicted from equations [26]. However, the only study to test whether it improved outcomes did not show a benefit [27].

Predictive equations estimate an individual's basal metabolic rate (BMR) based on age, weight and sex. The Harris–Benedict equation is the best known, but is nearly a century old, and Schofield's more modern version is now widely used [28]. Correction factors accounting for variables such as diagnosis, presence of pyrexia, and activity are then applied to convert BMR into an estimated energy requirement. The British Association for Parenteral and Enteral Nutrition has produced guidelines for doing this [29].

Despite the popularity of predictive equations, as with calorimetry, there is no direct evidence that their use improves patient outcomes. It remains acceptable simply to provide the ACCP's recommended 25 kCal/kg/day.

9.5.2 *Protein*

Once again, it is difficult to adjust protein or nitrogen provision to an individual patient's needs. In the past, daily nitrogen balance was calculated and intake adjusted accordingly, but this measurement has long been shown to be too variable to be of clinical use [30] and the practice has been largely abandoned. Given the upper limit to the amount of nitrogen that can be used during critical illness of around 0.2 g/kg/day, there is no purpose in providing more. A daily nitrogen intake of 0.15–0.2 g/kg/day is therefore recommended in ICU patients. This is equivalent to a protein intake of 1–1.25 g/kg/day. In certain circumstances of extreme hypercatabolism such as major burn injuries, the nitrogen intake may be increased to 0.3 g/kg/day.

9.5.3 *Vitamins and trace elements*

Intensive care patients have higher requirements than healthy humans for vitamins A, E, K, thiamine (B_1), B_3, B_6, vitamin C and pantothenic and folic acids [31]. Water-soluble vitamins and trace elements may be depleted during renal replacement therapy, while thiamine, folic acid and vitamin K are vulnerable to depletion during total parenteral nutrition (TPN). Deficiency syndromes have been described in critically ill patients for iron, selenium, zinc, copper and manganese. Suggested daily intakes of micronutrients vary depending on the route of administration and on the source of the recommendation. Comprehensive guidelines have recently been published [31]. Supplementation of micronutrients in excess of recommended intakes has been popular, despite a dearth of conclusive evidence to support the practice. Whether such interventions are pharmacological or nutritional is open to question; they are considered below.

9.5.4 *Water and electrolytes*

Needs vary greatly according to the patient's condition. Basal requirements are summarised in Table 9.1.

9.6 Which Route Should be Used to Feed ICU Patients?

Enteral feeding is on present evidence preferable to parenteral on the basis that it is

- cheaper
- easier
- possibly associated with fewer infective complications.

Table 9.1. Basal requirements for water and electrolytes.

Water	25–35 ml/kg/day
Sodium	0.9–1.2 mmol/kg/day
Potassium	1 mmol/kg/day

Despite the debate which this question has aroused, these appear to be the only demonstrable benefits of using the enteral route. The widespread belief that enteral feeding provides clear and unassailable advantages in terms of outcome has little basis in fact. This belief seems to be based upon two hypothetical considerations.

First, it does seem that the lipid contained in parenteral feeding solutions suppresses immune function. It is certainly known to reduce neutrophil and reticulo-endothelial cell activity *in vitro*. The belief is supported by a comparison of TPN with and without lipid in trauma patients, which showed fewer complications in the (nearly) lipid-free group [32]. Of course, this comparison also offers a simple solution to this problem, by giving lipid in TPN only in the minimal quantities required to provide essential fatty acids.

Secondly, it is argued that enteral feeding may itself protect against infectious complications of critical illness. In rats, lack of complex molecules from the gut lumen is associated with villus atrophy and a reduction in the gut-associated lymphoid tissue (GALT). Lymphocytes produced in the GALT move to the respiratory mucosa, and contribute to immunity there, a contribution which is lost in mice fed intravenously. The starvation-related changes in villus architecture and GALT mass are seen to a much lesser extent in humans. Despite this, the findings have been extrapolated to critically ill patients to form the basis of the theory that 'the gut is the motor of multiple organ failure'. According to this theory, the multiple organ dysfunction seen later in critical illness is produced by translocation of bacteria or endotoxin across an impaired intestinal mucosal barrier. The extrapolation then permits its protagonists to argue that enteral feeding protects against this sequence of events.

Unfortunately, this venerable, if not actually archaic, hypothesis has never been proven. Despite the association between TPN and increased intestinal permeability to large molecules [33], there is no corresponding association with translocation of bacteria [34]. While translocation does seem to follow surgery, and may be associated with sepsis [35], it has not been shown to cause multiple organ dysfunction.

Turning from theory to clinical evidence, once again the advantages of the enteral route are much less apparent than is commonly believed. A reduction in infectious complications has only been shown in certain groups, primarily victims of blunt abdominal trauma. In two studies of such patients, enteral feeding reduced the incidence of abdominal abscesses and pneumonia [36,37], although a third study showed no effect [38]. The evidence in patients with head injuries is balanced, with one study supporting either route and one showing no effect [39,40]. The antiquity of these studies is noticeable — the most recent is 16 years old, and practical methods of enteral and parenteral feeding have evolved considerably since then. In particular, the past tendency to overfeed intravenously, with the attendant increase in infectious complications, has been reversed. In patients with pancreatitis, a meta-analysis claims to support the use of the enteral route. Route of feeding appeared to have no effect in septic patients, perhaps the most numerous single group in most British ICUs, although enteral support was commenced late [41]. When he reviewed 31 trials looking at the effect of the route used for nutritional support, Lipman was unable to discern a clear effect [42].

In addition to the general inflation of the disadvantages of intravenous feeding, which have probably decreased over time, there is a tendency to under-recognise the complications of the enteral route. Firstly, because of the practical difficulties in establishing the full target rate of some patients, there is a significant risk that enterally fed patients receive insufficient nutrition. As discussed below, this is associated with worse outcomes, and it may be more of a problem in patients outside clinical trials, where close attention is being paid to establishing and maintaining adequate support. Secondly, use of the enteral route for nutrition is an independent risk factor for the development of ventilator-associated pneumonia [43], although this is rarely viewed as a complication of enteral feeding.

As mentioned in the introduction, the two most recent systematic reviews of this subject have reached opposite conclusions. The first found that enteral feeding reduced infectious complications, but had no effect on mortality [5]. The second, much more robust, analysis had more stringent selection criteria for trials to be included, and limited itself to those using an intention-to-treat principle [4]. It found a clear reduction in mortality in patients fed parenterally. When a sub-group analysis was performed comparing early enteral with parenteral feeding, it showed no difference in mortality. Another recent meta-analysis of this question reached the same conclusion [44].

At present, then, it seems that the timing of nutritional support matters as much as or more than the route used. On this basis, the ACCEPT study recommended early use of enteral feeding, with rapid conversion to TPN if the enteral route proved problematic.

A well-powered, randomised multicentre comparison of early enteral and early parenteral nutritional support has recently been commissioned by the UK National Institute for Health Research's Health Technology Assessment programme in the hope of resolving this vexed question. However, in view of the practical and economic advantages of the enteral route, it is likely to continue to be preferred unless a significant reduction in mortality with parenteral feeding can be demonstrated.

9.6.1 *Enteral feeding in practice*

Nasal tubes are generally preferable to oral, except in patients with a basal skull fracture. At first, a large bore (12–14 French gauge) nasogastric tube is used, as it provides gastric drainage and the ability to check residual volumes. Later, once feeding is well established, it can be replaced with a more comfortable fine-bore tube. Fine-bore tubes should not be aspirated, as they easily become blocked; various methods of unblocking have been tried, including the instillation of Coca-Cola™, fruit juice and pancreatic enzyme supplements. These methods frequently fail, necessitating replacement of the tube.

Confirmation of tube position within the stomach is essential before feeding commences, as intrapulmonary delivery of feed is a serious and sometimes fatal complication. How such confirmation is achieved is a matter of some debate. The UK National Patient Safety Agency (NPSA) mandates the daily use of litmus paper to confirm an acidic aspirate in all tube-fed patients, but there are difficulties in extending this to the intensive care population, whose gastric pH is frequently abnormally high as a result of either continuous feeding or drugs used to protect against mucosal ulceration. Chest radiographs are not immune to misinterpretation, but remain probably the most practical method of confirming correct positioning. They are much easier to interpret if the tube has a radio-opaque line along its length.

Common practice is to start feeding at around 30 ml/h, and to increase to the target intake depending on tolerance, as assessed by four-hourly aspiration of the tube to determine gastric residual volumes. Such a gradual approach does not definitely increase tolerance, and head-injured patients fed with target intake from the start had fewer infective complications [45]. On the other hand, patients with significant pre-existing malnutrition may be at risk of refeeding syndrome (see Section 9.6.2) if feed is started too rapidly.

The gastric residual volume that indicates intolerance is uncertain — one study has shown that volumes over 150 ml are associated with an increase in the incidence of ventilator-associated pneumonia [46] while others could not identify any link between residual volume and risk of aspiration [47]. Treatment with prokinetic agents such as metoclopramide or erythromycin appears to improve tolerance if gastric residual volumes exceed 200 ml, though without exerting any effect on morbidity or mortality [48]. If this does not resolve the problem, a nasojejunal tube often does, because gastric emptying restarts later than small bowel motility. Blind insertion does not reliably result in a position beyond the pylorus, although a single 200 mg dose of erythromycin may increase the success rate [48] and radiological or endoscopic assistance is frequently necessary. Predictably, the two meta-analyses of small and inconclusive studies have reached opposite conclusions on the question of whether nasojejunal feeding reduces the risk of aspiration or ventilator-associated pneumonia [7,49]. If a nasojejunal tube is used, it becomes important to ensure the sterility of the feed, as the stomach is being bypassed, and to continue to keep a nasogastric tube in place to ensure that the stomach does not dilate and produce a serious risk of aspiration.

Numerous enteral feeding solutions are available, with different compositions. Polymeric feeds contain intact proteins (derived from whey, meat, soy isolates and caseinates) and carbohydrates in the form of oligosaccharides and polysaccharides. These substances must be broken down by pancreatic enzymes in order to be absorbed. So-called elemental feeds provide nitrogen from either amino-acids or peptides. Although their routine use is not indicated, they can be better absorbed than polymeric feeds in certain circumstances, such as pancreatic insufficiency, or when the small bowel mucosa is atrophic following prolonged starvation.

The lipids contained in enteral feeds usually consist mainly of long-chain triglycerides from vegetable oils. There is some enthusiasm for the inclusion of medium-chain triglycerides, which are more easily absorbed. Normally one-third of the energy requirement is provided as lipid, and two-thirds as carbohydrate.

Sodium- and potassium-restricted formulations are available, as are more concentrated solutions. Vitamins and trace elements are usually added during manufacture so that daily requirements are present in a volume containing a typical day's energy intake of around 2000 kCal.

Complications of enteral feeding tend to be under-recognised. Despite the enthusiastic condemnation by some of intravenous nutrition, it is the use of the enteral route that has been firmly established as an independent risk factor for ventilator-associated pneumonia. This was established in a large trial which demonstrated a reduction in pneumonia resulting from the simple measure of nursing all ventilated patients with a 30° head-up tilt [43]. Nasogastric tubes can cause sinusitis, which can be managed by replacing the tube via the mouth. All tubes, but particularly fine-bore ones, can be misplaced in the bronchial tree, or perforate the oesophagus, stomach or bowel. Percutaneous endoscopic gastrostomy may be useful in neurologically impaired patients who are approaching the chronic stage of their illness, but has little place in the acute phase, when it is associated with a high all-cause mortality at 30 days [50,51]. Other complications of this technique and of surgically placed jejunostomies include serious abdominal wall infection, peritonitis and bowel obstruction.

Diarrhoea is a frequent and very distressing problem in ICU patients, especially those fed enterally. Among the commoner causes are antibiotic therapy, *Clostridium difficile* infection, faecal impaction and a non-specific effect of critical illness upon the gut. Less common causes include malabsorption, lactose intolerance, prokinetic agents, magnesium, aminophylline, quinidine and medications containing sorbitol (for instance, paracetamol syrup). Management requires the exclusion or treatment of faecal impaction, drug causes and *Clostridium difficile* infection. The rate at which feed is delivered may also be relevant; slowing it may help, while diluting the formula does not. If other measures do not help and *Clostridium difficile* has been ruled out, then agents such as loperamide or codeine may alleviate symptoms. Depending on the cause, malabsorption may improve with an elemental feed.

9.6.2 *Parenteral feeding in practice*

Parenteral nutrition is indicated when adequate intake cannot be achieved enterally. In some patients, gastrointestinal failure is obvious, while in others it may only become apparent after considerable time and effort has been spent in trying and failing to use the enteral route. Early recourse to intravenous feeding is increasingly being used if any significant difficulty in establishing enteral feeds is encountered.

Parenteral feeding solutions can be prepared from their constituent parts under sterile conditions. Ready-made solutions are commercially available; any additions to their content must also be made aseptically.

In intensive care, parenteral feeding is performed continuously, with the daily requirements being infused over 24 hours. Close clinical and biochemical monitoring is essential.

Energy is provided either as carbohydrate alone or as a combination of carbohydrate and lipid in an approximately 2:1 ratio. As mentioned above, there may be fewer infective complications in patients in whom carbohydrates alone are given, with lipid intake in the form of soybean oil emulsified with glycerol and egg phosphatides limited to twice weekly provision of essential fatty acids (linoleic and linolenic acids) [32]. Carbohydrate is given as concentrated dextrose solution. There is a limit to the septic patient's capacity to metabolise glucose of around 4 mg/kg/min; exceeding this produces hyperglycaemia and excess carbon dioxide production. Many patients will require exogenous insulin infusions to control blood sugar levels, but if hyperglycaemia persists, it is better to reduce the glucose infusion rate than to escalate the insulin infusion to very high levels. Once insulin requirements are stable, it can be added to the TPN solution. Nitrogen is provided as crystalline solutions of amino acids; the exact composition of the commercially available solutions varies, but it is important to note that glutamine, tyrosine and cysteine may be absent because they are unstable in solution. Micronutrients are added to TPN solutions in appropriate doses.

The list of complications of intravenous feeding is dominated by the risk of catheter-related sepsis. In relation to line insertion, it is important to note that [52]:

- Subclavian lines are less likely to become infected than those placed into the jugular or femoral veins.
- Infection rates fall with increasing experience of the operator.
- 2% chlorhexidine in alcohol is the most effective form of skin preparation. Remarkably, this has only very recently become available in the United Kingdom.
- Use of maximal barrier precautions (mask, cap, gown, gloves and large drape) reduces the risk of catheter-related bacteraemia six-fold. The continued resistance to the use of such procedures still commonly encountered outside intensive care units represents an incomprehensible and unpardonable abdication of responsibility for the most basic standards of care.
- Catheters coated with either antiseptic agents (chlorhexidine and silver sulphadiazine) or antimicrobials (rifampicin and minocycline) are several times less likely to become infected than standard catheters. The effect appears to last for two weeks in the case of antibiotic-treated catheters, rather than one week in those treated with antiseptics.
- Patients receiving TPN in the long term (more than two months) may benefit from specialised catheters with a tunnelled cuff or subcutaneous port.

Once inserted, certain aspects of care of the catheter are also important [52]:

- Permeable transparent polyurethane dressings are superior to impermeable ones.
- Nurse staffing levels in ICUs have a significant effect on the incidence of catheter-related bacteraemia.
- Scheduled exchange of central venous catheters has not been shown to reduce infection rates.
- Guide-wire exchange is associated with a reduction in mechanical complications, but in routine use this is outweighed by an increase in catheter-related bacteraemias.
- If a multi-lumen catheter is used, one lumen should be used exclusively for delivery of TPN, three-way taps should not be used, and the infusion set should be changed daily under sterile conditions.

Other complications of intravenous feeding include:

- Refeeding syndrome, which can follow the restoration of normal intake after a period of starvation. It may also be seen in enterally fed patients, and is associated with profound hypophosphataemia, often with hypokalaemia and hypomagnesaemia as well. Once glucose becomes available as a substrate again, insulin levels rise, causing phosphate, potassium and magnesium ions to be transported into the cells. The subsequent depletion of adenosine triphosphate (ATP) and 2,3-diphosphoglycerate (2,3-DPG) causes a failure of cellular energy metabolism, manifesting as cardiovascular and respiratory failure, and sometimes also in neurological problems, including paraesthesiae and even seizures.
- Rebound hypoglycaemia may follow the sudden cessation of intravenous feeding. If possible, TPN should be weaned over at least 12 hours; if this is not possible, it should be replaced by an infusion of concentrated glucose and blood sugar levels closely monitored.
- The electrolyte abnormalities mentioned above may occur without the other manifestations of the refeeding syndrome.
- Hyperchloraemic metabolic acidosis may be due to amino acid solutions containing chloride as the major anion. Replacing some or all of the chloride with acetate resolves the problem.
- Biochemical liver dysfunction is common in patients fed intravenously, but it can be difficult to tell whether this is due to the TPN itself or to the condition necessitating the use of TPN. Hepatic steatosis and intrahepatic cholestasis are commonly seen.

9.6.3 *Nutrition in specific conditions*

Although it is tempting to believe that the application of nutritional support must necessarily be different in different conditions necessitating intensive care, there is little evidence of this. In general, good nutritional practice seems to be similar in the vast majority of patients. Some specific points follow:

- Acute renal failure no longer necessitates dietary fluid and protein restriction or the use of specialised lipid or amino acid formulations for TPN.

- Chronic liver disease similarly has little effect on nutritional practice [10,53]. Energy requirements are not affected, although lipid should be used with caution to avoid hypertriglyceridaemia in view of the increase in lipolysis. This is likely to pale into insignificance compared with the effect of using propofol for sedation, however. Severely encephalopathic patients may occasionally require a reduction in nitrogen intake, perhaps starting at 0.5 g/kg/day and increasing towards a normal intake. If a normal protein intake is absolutely precluded by refractory encephalopathy, feed enriched with branched-chain amino acids may help. Routine use of such feed is not indicated in critically ill patients [18].
- Fulminant hepatic failure is accompanied by failure of gluconeogenesis; the resulting hypoglycaemia can be profound and often requires infusion of concentrated glucose solutions. There are no other nutritional implications.
- Respiratory failure is of no particular concern other than the crucial importance of avoiding over-feeding in patients in whom hypercarbia is delaying weaning from mechanical ventilation.
- Acute pancreatitis was until recently regarded as an absolute indication for TPN. Recently, jejunal feeding has been shown to be safe and effective, and possibly associated with reductions in infective complications [54]. However, enteral feeding still fails in a significant number of patients, and TPN then remains necessary. Malabsortion due to pancreatic dysfunction can be a problem; the use of elemental feeds and pancreatic enzyme supplements may be of help.
- Obesity has been suggested as a specific circumstance in which hypocaloric feeding may be of benefit. A reduction in the length of ICU stay was shown in obese patients fed less than 20 kCal/kg/day compared with controls fed 25–30 kCal/kg/day, but no other benefit could be shown [55]. There seems no basis at present to alter usual nutritional practice on grounds of obesity.

9.7 What Should the Feed Contain?

It is apparent from what has gone before that there are certain basic necessities which must be provided. These are energy, in the form of carbohydrate and at least some lipid (needed for the essential fatty acids), nitrogen, water, electrolytes and trace elements. The form in which these necessities are delivered depends on whether the feed is enteral or parenteral. Their nature and amount has been discussed in detail above.

However, it is intermittently fashionable to supplement the preparations fed to patients in intensive care with various substances, usually designed to treat postulated deficiencies or modulate the immune response in one way or another. While such fashions are certainly less glamorous than those of Milan or Paris, with one or two exceptions they have a similar relationship to reality. Many studies are marred by a tendency to study multiple compounds at once, at arbitrary doses (or before a dose–effect relationship has been established) and in populations often including large numbers of patients outside ICU. Retrospective sub-group analysis or extrapolation to intensive care patients are then used in order to argue an effect. Until such time as individual compounds with established therapeutic windows are studied in isolation, the situation will remain unclear. These interventions are more pharmacological than nutritional, and should be evaluated accordingly.

The exceptions to these strictures are the use of glutamine and selenium.

9.7.1 *Glutamine*

Glutamine is used by enterocytes and immune cells as an oxidative fuel and nucleotide precursor. It is also involved in regulating signal transduction and cellular defence and repair. It is therefore in high demand during an episode of critical illness, when it is released in large quantities from skeletal muscle. Normally, glutamine is not an essential amino acid, as the body is able to synthesise it. However, during critical illness, demand is such that it may become depleted, and is then often referred to as 'conditionally essential'. It has therefore been postulated that patients depleted of glutamine during a prolonged critical illness may suffer impairment in their ability to survive.

Inevitably, the evidence on glutamine supplementation is somewhat confusing. It appears that in patients fed enterally, there is little benefit in providing additional glutamine. Although reductions in secondary endpoints such as infectious complications and ICU stay were shown in smaller studies in trauma and burns patients, a large Australian study in unselected ICU patients (containing many patients from these groups) found no effect on any outcome measure [56].

The position of patients fed parenterally is perhaps more positive. In the past, parenteral feeding solutions have not contained glutamine owing to its instability and insolubility. Dipeptide solutions are now available, and several studies have investigated their use in patients receiving TPN, both inside and outside ICU. Results have varied, and once again, one group of meta-analysts has felt able to endorse its use in higher doses on the basis of a claimed demonstrable effect on mortality [57], while another declined to make any recommendation on the basis of excessive heterogeneity in the primary studies [18]. However, for those who prefer their evidence unmediated, there is one early trial exclusively in ICU patients requiring prolonged TPN, which showed a reduction in late mortality [58]. This only became apparent after 20 days, but persisted for at least six months. Such results are consistent with the hypothesis that in prolonged critical illness glutamine becomes 'conditionally essential'. For now, it seems that patients most likely to benefit from glutamine supplementation are those requiring TPN for more than ten days [58] and, in this group at least, many clinicians now provide supplementary intravenous glutamine at around 20–30 g/day.

9.7.2 *Selenium*

Selenium is necessary for the regulation of the body's major free radical scavenging system, glutathione peroxidase. Low plasma levels are common during critical illness, and supplementation (or treatment of this deficiency) has been postulated to be beneficial. Once again, larger doses by the intravenous route seem to be necessary to produce any effect, a result shown by a number of smaller studies. A recent larger randomised trial of selenium, given intravenously at a dose of 1 mg for 14 days, showed a reduction in mortality [59]. However, this study was flawed — the effect on mortality did not reach statistical significance when an intention-to-treat analysis was used, and although 11 ICUs were involved, only 249 patients were recruited over a four-year period. While parenteral selenium supplementation may well soon be proven to be beneficial in unselected ICU patients, this has not yet occurred.

References

[1] Doig, G.S., Simpson, F. and Delaney, A. (2005). A review of the true methodological quality of nutritional support trials conducted in the critically ill: time for improvement, *Anesth Analg*, **100**, 527–533.

[2] Marik, P.E. and Pinsky, M. (2003). Death by parenteral nutrition, *Intens Care Med*, **29**, 867–869.

[3] LeLorier, J., Gregoire, G., Benhaddad, A. *et al.* (1997). Discrepancies between meta-analyses and subsequent large randomized, controlled trials, *N Engl J Med*, **337**, 536–542.

[4] Simpson, F. and Doig, G.S. (2005). Parenteral vs. enteral nutrition in the critically ill patient: a meta-analysis of trials using the intention to treat principle, *Intens Care Med*, **31**, 12–23.

[5] Gramlich, L., Kichian, K., Pinilla, J. *et al.* (2004). Does enteral nutrition compared to parenteral nutrition result in better outcomes in critically ill adult patients? A systematic review of the literature, *Nutrition*, **20**, 843–848.

[6] Martin, C.M., Doig, G.S., Heyland, D.K. *et al.* (2004). Multicentre, cluster-randomized clinical trial of algorithms for critical-care enteral and parenteral therapy (ACCEPT), *CMAJ*, **170**, 197–204.

[7] Heyland, D.K., Dhaliwal, R., Drover, J.W. *et al.* (2003). Canadian clinical practice guidelines for nutrition support in mechanically ventilated, critically ill adult patients, *JPEN*, **27**, 355–373.

[8] Jacobs, D.G., Jacobs, D.O., Kudsk, K.A. *et al.* (2004). Practice management guidelines for nutritional support of the trauma patient, *J Trauma*, **57**, 660–678.

[9] Cerra, F.B., Benitez, M.R., Blackburn, G.L. *et al.* (1997). Applied nutrition in ICU patients. A consensus statement of the American College of Chest Physicians, *Chest*, **111**, 769–778.

[10] Klein, S., Kinney, J., Jeejeebhoy, K. *et al.* (1997). Nutrition support in clinical practice: review of published data and recommendations for future research directions. Summary of a conference sponsored by the National Institutes of Health, American Society for Parenteral and Enteral Nutrition, and American Society for Clinical Nutrition, *Am J Clin Nutr*, **66**, 683–706.

[11] Kreymann, K.G., Berger, M.M., Deutz, N.E. *et al.* (2006). ESPEN Guidelines on Enteral Nutrition: intensive care, *Clin Nutr*, **25**, 210–223.

[12] Pupelis, G., Selga, G., Austrums, E. *et al.* (2001). Jejunal feeding, even when instituted late, improves outcomes in patients with severe pancreatitis and peritonitis, *Nutrition*, **17**, 91–94.

[13] Streat, S.J., Beddoe, A.H. and Hill, G.L. (1987). Aggressive nutritional support does not prevent protein loss despite fat gain in septic intensive care patients, *J Trauma*, **27**, 262–266.

[14] Baker, J.P., Detsky, A.S., Wesson, D.E. *et al.* (1982). Nutritional assessment: a comparison of clinical judgement and objective measurements, *N Engl J Med*, **306**, 969–972.

[15] Kudsk, K.A., Tolley, E.A., DeWitt, R.C. *et al.* (2003). Preoperative albumin and surgical site identify surgical risk for major postoperative complications, *JPEN*, **27**, 1–9.

[16] Woodcock, N.P., Zeigler, D., Palmer, M.D. *et al.* (2001). Enteral versus parenteral nutrition: a pragmatic study, *Nutrition*, **17**, 1–12.

[17] Marik, P.E. and Zaloga, G.P. (2001). Early enteral nutrition in acutely ill patients: a systematic review, *Crit Care Med*, **29**, 2264–2270.

[18] Doig, G. and Simpson, F. (2005). *Evidence-based guidelines for nutritional support of the critically ill: results of a bi-national guideline development conference*, [Online]. Available at: www.evidencebased.net/files/EBGforNutSupportofICUpts.pdf [Accessed 19 December 2012].

[19] Larsson, J., Lennmarken, C., Martensson, J. *et al.* (1990). Nitrogen requirements in severely injured patients, *Br J Surg*, **77**, 413–416.

[20] Klein, C.J., Stanek, G.S., Wiles, C.E. 3rd (1998). Overfeeding macronutrients to critically ill adults: metabolic complications, *J Am Diet Assoc*, **98**, 795–806.

[21] Krishnan, J.A., Parce, P.B., Martinez, A. *et al.* (2003). Caloric intake in medical ICU patients: consistency of care with guidelines and relationship to clinical outcomes, *Chest*, **124**, 297–305.

[22] Rubinson, L., Diette, G.B., Song, X. *et al.* (2004). Low caloric intake is associated with nosocomial bloodstream infections in patients in the medical intensive care unit, *Crit Care Med*, **32**, 350–357.

[23] Villet, S., Chiolero, R.L., Bollmann, M.D. *et al.* (2005). Negative impact of hypocaloric feeding and energy balance on clinical outcome in ICU patients, *Clin Nutr*, **24**, 502–509.

[24] Plank, L.D. and Hill, G.L. (2000). Sequential metabolic changes following induction of systemic inflammatory response in patients with severe sepsis or major blunt trauma, *World J Surg*, **24**, 630–638.

[25] Streat, S.J., Plank, L.D. and Hill, G.L. (2000). Overview of modern management of patients with critical injury and severe sepsis, *World J Surg*, **24**, 655–663.
[26] Makk, L.J., McClave, S.A., Creech, P.W. *et al.* (1990). Clinical application of the metabolic cart to the delivery of total parenteral nutrition, *Crit Care Med*, **18**, 1320–1327.
[27] Saffle, J.R., Larson, C.M. and Sullivan, J. (1990). A randomized trial of indirect calorimetry-based feedings in thermal injury, *J Trauma*, **30**, 776–782.
[28] Schofield, W. (1985). Predicting basal metabolic rate; new standards and review of previous work, *Hum Nutr Clin Nutr*, **39** (Suppl 1), 5–41.
[29] Working Party of the British Association for Parenteral and Enteral Nutrition. (1999). *Current perspectives on enteral nutrition in adults*, British Association for Parenteral and Enteral Nutrition (BAPEN), Maidenhead.
[30] Konstantinides, F.N., Konstantinides, N.N., Li, J.C. *et al.* (1991). Urinary urea nitrogen: too insensitive for calculating nitrogen balance studies in surgical clinical nutrition, *JPEN*, 15, 189–193.
[31] Demling, R.H. and DeBiasse, M.A. (1995). Micronutrients in critical illness, *Crit Care Clin*, **11**, 651–673.
[32] Battistella, F.D., Widergren, J.T., Anderson, J.T. *et al.* (1997). A prospective, randomized trial of intravenous fat emulsion administration in trauma victims requiring total parenteral nutrition, *J Trauma*, **43**, 52–58.
[33] Hadfield, R.J., Sinclair, D.G., Houldsworth, P.E. *et al.* (1995). Effects of enteral and parenteral nutrition on gut mucosal permeability in the critically ill, *Am J Respir Crit Care Med*, **152**, 1545–1548.
[34] Sedman, P.C., MacFie, J., Palmer, M.D. *et al.* (1995). Preoperative total parenteral nutrition is not associated with mucosal atrophy or bacterial translocation in humans, *Br J Surg*, **82**, 1663–1667.
[35] MacFie, J., O'Boyle, C., Mitchell, C.J. *et al.* (1999). Gut origin of sepsis: a prospective study investigating associations between bacterial translocation, gastric microflora, and septic morbidity, *Gut*, **45**, 223–228.
[36] Moore, F.A., Moore, E.E., Jones, T.N. *et al.* (1989). TEN versus TPN following major abdominal trauma–reduced septic morbidity, *J Trauma*, **29**, 916–922.
[37] Kudsk, K.A., Croce, M.A., Fabian, T.C. *et al.* (1992). Enteral versus parenteral feeding. Effects on septic morbidity after blunt and penetrating abdominal trauma, *Ann Sur*, **215**, 503–511.
[38] Adams, S., Dellinger, E.P., Wertz, M.J. *et al.* (1986). Enteral versus parenteral nutritional support following laparotomy for trauma: a randomized prospective trial, *J Trauma*, **26**, 882–891.

[39] Grahm, T.W., Zadrozny, D.B. and Harrington, T. (1989). The benefits of early jejunal hyperalimentation in the head-injured patient, *Neurosurgery*, **25**, 729–735.

[40] Young, B., Ott, L., Twyman, D. *et al.* (1987). The effect of nutritional support on outcome from severe head injury, *J Neurosurg*, **67**, 668–676.

[41] Cerra, F.B., McPherson, J.P., Konstantinides, F.N. *et al.* (1988). Enteral nutrition does not prevent multiple organ failure syndrome (MOFS) after sepsis, *Surgery*, **104**, 727–733.

[42] Lipman, T.O. (1998). Grains or veins: is enteral nutrition really better than parenteral nutrition? A look at the evidence, *JPEN*, **22**, 167–182.

[43] Drakulovic, M.B., Torres, A., Bauer, T.T. *et al.* (1999). Supine body position as a risk factor for nosocomial pneumonia in mechanically ventilated patients: a randomised trial, *Lancet*, **354**, 1851–1858.

[44] Peter, J.V., Moran, J.L. and Phillips-Hughes, J. (2005). A metaanalysis of treatment outcomes of early enteral versus early parenteral nutrition in hospitalized patients, *Crit Care Med*, **33**, 213–220.

[45] Taylor, S.J., Fettes, S.B., Jewkes, C. *et al.* (1999). Prospective, randomized, controlled trial to determine the effect of early enhanced enteral nutrition on clinical outcome in mechanically ventilated patients suffering head injury, *Crit Care Med*, **27**, 2525–2531.

[46] Mentec, H., Dupont, H., Bocchetti, M. *et al.* (2001). Upper digestive intolerance during enteral nutrition in critically ill patients: frequency, risk factors, and complications, *Crit Care Med*, **29**, 1955–1961.

[47] McClave, S.A., Lukan, J.K., Stefater, J.A. *et al.* (2005). Poor validity of residual volumes as a marker for risk of aspiration in critically ill patients, *Crit Care Med*, **33**, 324–330.

[48] Booth, C.M., Heyland, D.K. and Paterson, W.G. (2002). Gastrointestinal promotility drugs in the critical care setting: a systematic review of the evidence, *Crit Care Med*, **30**, 1429–1435.

[49] Marik, P.E. and Zaloga, G.P. (2003). Gastric versus post-pyloric feeding: a systematic review, *Crit Care*, **7**, R46–R51.

[50] Abuksis, G., Mor, M., Segal, N. *et al.* (2000). Percutaneous endoscopic gastrostomy: high mortality rates in hospitalized patients, *Am J Gastroenterol*, **95**, 128–132.

[51] Abuksis, G., Mor, M., Plaut, S. *et al.* (2004). Outcome of percutaneous endoscopic gastrostomy (PEG): comparison of two policies in a 4-year experience, *Clin Nutr*, **23**, 341–346.

[52] Fraenkel, D.J., Rickard, C. And Lipman, J. (2000). Can we achieve consensus on central venous catheter-related infections? *Anaesth Intensive Care*, **28**, 475–490.
[53] Mizock, B.A. (1999). Nutritional support in hepatic encephalopathy, *Nutrition*, **15**, 220–228.
[54] Marik, P.E. and Zaloga, G.P. (2004). Meta-analysis of parenteral nutrition versus enteral nutrition in patients with acute pancreatitis, *BMJ*, **328**, 1407.
[55] Dickerson, R.N., Boschert, K.J., Kudsk, K.A. *et al.* (2002). Hypocaloric enteral tube feeding in critically ill obese patients, *Nutrition*, **18**, 241–246.
[56] Hall, J.C., Dobb, G., Hall, J. *et al.* (2003). A prospective randomized trial of enteral glutamine in critical illness, *Intens Care Med*, **29**, 1710–1716.
[57] Nova, F., Heyland, D.K., Avenell, A. *et al.* (2002). Glutamine supplementation in serious illness: a systematic review of the evidence. *Crit Care Med*, **30**, 2022–2029.
[58] Griffiths, R.D., Jones, C. and Palmer, T.E. (1997). Six-month outcome of critically ill patients given glutamine-supplemented parenteral nutrition, *Nutrition*, **13**, 295–302.
[59] Angstwurm, M.W., Engelmann, L., Zimmermann, T. *et al.* (2007). Selenium in Intensive Care (SIC), results of a prospective randomized, placebo-controlled, multiple-center study in patients with severe systemic inflammatory response syndrome, sepsis, and septic shock, *Crit Care Med*, **35**, 118–126.

10
Microbiology and Infection Control

Annette Jepson

10.1 Introduction

Critically ill patients in the intensive care unit (ICU) are at high risk of developing nosocomial infections (defined as an infection occurring more than 48 hours after admission to hospital): a recent UK study reported a prevalence rate of 23% [1].

Such infections are associated with increased morbidity and mortality; it is therefore essential that ICU physicians are provided with timely microbiological data to ensure that only appropriate antimicrobials are used, that empirical regimes are promptly discontinued (or changed based upon culture and sensitivity data) and that patients with resistant organisms are cohorted or isolated appropriately.

10.2 Pathophysiology of ICU-Acquired Infections

ICU patients are at increased risk of infection for the following reasons:

- Impaired host defences, which may be physical, for example:
  - Breached skin with intravascular devices (may increase the risk of developing a hospital-acquired infection up to seven-fold).

  - Presence of an endotracheal tube or urinary catheter that bypasses normal defence mechanisms and permits direct access of microorganisms to lungs or bladder.
- Impaired host defences may also result from modified cytokine responses or treatment-related issues, e.g. following immunosuppressive therapy.
- The underlying disease process itself and/or poor nutritional status may also compromise the ICU patient's ability to respond to stress.

In addition to the above, there is an increased infection risk because highly vulnerable patients are grouped together, antibiotics are likely to be used more frequently than in general wards and the organisms that comprise the hospital flora (and especially the ICU flora) are frequently more resistant than those found in the community [2].

10.3 Implicated Organisms

The infecting organisms may be both exogenous and endogenous. Patients who have had extensive exposure to the healthcare environment, particularly those with chronic or relapsing conditions who may have received multiple rounds of treatment for persistent infections, are more likely to be colonised by resistant organisms [3]. Colonisation places patients at increased risk for subsequent infection [4]. However, understanding how such organisms behave in the ICU environment and the routes of cross-transmission are essential for the planning of successful infection control programmes [5].

The commonest sites of nosocomial infection among ICU patients are not the same as those in non-ICU patients (where urinary tract infections tend to predominate). A European point-prevalence study carried out in 1992 found that pneumonia accounted for 47% of the ICU-acquired infections, with other lower respiratory tract and urinary tract infections each accounting for 18% of infections, laboratory-confirmed septicaemia accounted for 12% and wound infections for 7% [6].

In terms of the nosocomial pathogens most frequently implicated, *Staphylococcus aureus* accounted for 30% of infections, *Pseudomonas aeruginosa* for 29%, *Escherichia coli* for 13%, with the remainder mostly being *Enterococci*, *Acinetobacter* and *Klebsiella* spp. Interestingly, the proportion of yeasts has been increasing in recent years with significant increases in the incidence of non-albicans *Candida* isolates [7].

Other groups of organisms are more rarely implicated in ICU infections, but must be considered in patients with particular risk factors or unexplained prolonged fever. Such infections include:

- Cytomegalovirus (CMV) antigenaemia — in one study (which excluded transplant recipients and patients with human immunodeficiency virus (HIV) infection), 17% of patients with prolonged fever were found to have a positive CMV antigenaemia assay [8]; risk factors included steroid use and renal failure. CMV reactivation has also been documented in critically ill immunocompromised patients [9].
- Respiratory viruses can be transmitted between patients (or between staff and patients) if there are poor infection control procedures in place.

Risks of viral transmission by blood components are low (approximately 1 in 50,000 to 1.6 million for hepatitis B virus (HBV), hepatitis C virus (HCV), and HIV1/2 [10]); however other viruses such as Epstein–Barr virus (EBV), human parvovirus B19 and Hepatitis A and G viruses can be transmitted by blood products and these may be a rare cause of nosocomial infection.

10.4 Specific Nosocomial Infections

10.4.1 *Pneumonia*

Pneumonia is the most common nosocomial infection in ICUs, accounting for almost half of the infections [11]. Moreover, pneumonia is associated with a high crude mortality rate, having an attributable mortality of at least 27% and a risk ratio for death of 2.0 in mechanically ventilated patients [12]. The risk of developing ventilator-associated pneumonia (VAP) is highest during the first five days of ventilation (approximately 3% per day), followed by 2% per day up to day ten of ventilation and 1% per day thereafter [13]. It should be noted, however, that ICU patients may develop pneumonia in the absence of mechanical ventilation, as microaspiration of oropharyngeal secretions and altered mental status are particular risk factors: a recent European study of more than 87,000 patients having an ICU stay of more than two days reported that 7.2% developed pneumonia, 10% of which were non-ventilated patients [14]. The relative frequency of the microorganisms isolated varied between the countries surveyed, but, overall, almost 50% of the infections were caused by Gram-negative bacilli (24.1% Enterobacteriaceae; 18.8% *Pseudomonas aeruginosa*); *Staphylococcus aureus* accounted for almost 20% of infections with approximately 40% of these being methicillin-resistant (MRSA).

Cultures of the lower respiratory tract are essential for the diagnosis and management of ICU-acquired pneumonia. Sputum is not adequate, as it may reflect oro-pharyngeal colonising flora only. Many techniques have been suggested for the collection of lower respiratory tract samples and these are summarised in the recently published guidelines for the management of hospital-acquired pneumonia in the UK [15]. There appears to be no evidence to recommend any one invasive sampling method over any other, and our practice at St Mary's Hospital is to use the non-bronchoscopic ('blind') bronchoalveolar lavage (BAL) technique unless the patient requires a formal bronchoscopy, in which case specific sites of inflammation may be targeted and sampled.

Depending upon the patient's underlying diagnosis and the suspected aetiology of the pneumonia, specimens should be separately submitted for bacteriological (including fungal and mycobacterial) culture, as well as virological and cytological investigations. If suspected, a separate specimen should be sent for investigation of *Pneumocystis jurovecii*. In the majority of cases when a new fever or neutrophilia develops in a ventilated patient on the ICU, however, submission of a non-directed BAL for bacteriological and fungal culture should be adequate.

The role of quantitative or semi-quantitative microbiological culture in the diagnosis of VAP is not clear-cut, given the range of reported sensitivities and specificities [16]; at St Mary's we use quantitative bacterial cultures to distinguish between colonisation and infection, with a cut-off of 10^4–10^5 colony-forming units (c.f.u.)/ml. Whilst recognising the caveats, we have found this technique a valuable tool when assessing the response to therapy and for determining or confirming when to discontinue antibiotic therapy.

The choice of empirical antimicrobial therapy for patients with pneumonia on the ICU should be guided by the local knowledge of organisms that are prevalent on that unit and their susceptibility patterns. In general, however, our practice is to regard those patients who develop pneumonia within 48 hours of admission to hospital, who have not previously received antibiotics and in the absence of other risk factors, as having an infection caused by a community-type organism (e.g. *Haemophilus influenzae, Moraxella catarrhalis, Streptococcus pneumoniae* or *Staphylococcus aureus*) for whom cefuroxime (plus metronidazole if aspiration is suspected) or co-amoxiclav is appropriate.

Patients hospitalised (whether or not on the ICU) for more than 48 hours will be at risk of pneumonia caused by more resistant pathogens and we recommend a combination of piperacillin–tazobactam (Tazocin®) and vancomycin (after collecting cultures). After 24–48 hours, the vancomycin can be discontinued if there is no MRSA present and the Tazocin may be changed to an alternative (less broad-spectrum) antimicrobial, depending upon the culture and susceptibility data.

Our practice is treat patients for 5–7 days, depending upon the clinical and microbiological response to therapy. This practice is supported by the findings of Chastre *et al* [17]. Longer courses of therapy (including antibiotic combinations) may be required for the treatment of pneumonia caused by *Pseudomonas aeruginosa* or *Staphylococcus aureus* (MRSA or methicillin-sensitive *Staphylococcus aureus* (MSSA)) and these are summarised in [18] and [19], respectively.

At St Mary's, we have gained some experience in the use of topical aminoglycoside instilled via the endotrachael tube in the management of ventilated patients with recurrent pseudomonal infections [20]. In selected cases, this approach may be warranted, although supporting evidence is limited (see Section 4.3.10 in reference [15]).

In terms of preventing the development of pneumonia among ICU patients, there are general issues based upon good infection control practices (see Section 10.6.5 in this chapter) and a range of specific recommendations relating to the best use of equipment (ventilation, ventilator circuits, heated humidifiers, etc.); these are summarised in reference [15], Sections 2.2–2.3.

In the UK, the NHS Saving Lives campaign [21] has produced a care bundle (high impact intervention #5, revised June 2007) to prevent the development of VAP. Specifically in this context is the recommendation that the head of the bed should be elevated to 30–45°; the inspired gas should be approximately humidified (to prevent inspissation of secretions); ventilator tubing should be replaced when visibly soiled or malfunctioning and routinely replaced according to the manufacturer's guidance; condensate should be prevented from entering the patients airway. The care bundle also recommends the wearing of examination gloves when suctioning respiratory sections and advises that hands should be decontaminated before and after the suction procedure. The recommendations are based on Tablan *et al* [22].

The role of selective decontamination of the digestive tract (SDD) in the prevention of VAP remains controversial and individual units may need to make local decisions regarding its suitability (a good, up-to-date review is available in reference [23]).

Another option worthy of further study is the use of a silver-coated endotracheal tube; a recent report indicated that patients who were ventilated using such tubes had a statistically significant reduction in VAP incidence and delayed time to VAP occurrence compared with controls using uncoated tubes [24].

10.4.2 *Blood stream infections (BSIs)*

In the European study [14], BSIs occurred in 3.1% of patients staying in the ICU for more than two days, with a higher incidence occurring in those units with a higher proportion of ventilated patients. The majority of BSIs (60%) were catheter-associated (defined as a primary BSI in patients with a central venous catheter (CVC) used in the 48 hours proceeding the infection onset); in 31% of cases, the bacteraemia was associated with an infection at another site (most commonly, the respiratory tract); in 9% of cases the origin was unknown (without a CVC in use in the 48 hours preceding infection).

Almost 30% of the BSIs were caused by coagulase-negative Staphylococci, with Enterobacteriaceae (*Escherichia coli, Enterobacter* spp., *Klebsiella* spp. and *Serratia* spp.) accounting for approximately 18%. *Staphylococcus aureus* was responsible for approximately 14% of episodes (with 32–53% of these being methicillin-resistant; the proportion varying according to the country surveyed). Enterococci were isolated in 10.8% of cases and *Candida* spp. accounted for 6.3%.

Estimating the attributable mortality associated with an episode of a BSI in the ICU accurately is difficult owing to the effect of confounding by the severity of the illness. An American study that attempted to address this issue, taking into account the illness severity using the Acute Physiology and Chronic Health Evaluation (APACHE) III score, found no clear association between primary nosocomial BSIs and increased ICU mortality; nevertheless, such infections were associated with an increased length of ICU stay (a median of five days) and increased direct costs [25]. Earlier studies had estimated the crude mortality for ICU BSIs to be in excess of 50%, with a range between 31.5% and 82.4% [26,27], although underlying illness severity was not taken into account.

Whatever the true figure, every possible attempt must be made to limit the development of nosocomial BSIs. Given that the majority of BSIs occurring in ICU are catheter-related, attention should be focussed upon basic standards of hygiene and the use of full aseptic technique when inserting CVCs. Studies such as those of Sheretz *et al.* [28] have demonstrated that an education programme combined with the use of full-size sterile drapes can produce a significant reduction in the rate of catheter-related BSIs. Such data (and related studies, e.g. [29–31]) underpin the current UK-based guidelines [21]. The guidelines make the following recommendations for catheter insertion:

- Use a single-lumen cannula unless otherwise indicated.
- Consider using an antibacterial-impregnated catheter if the likely duration of insertion is one to three weeks and the risk of catheter-related BSI is high.
- Insert the lines into the subclavian or internal jugular veins (associated with the lowest infection risks).
- Prepare the skin using 2% chlorhexidine gluconate in 70% isopropyl alcohol and allow to dry (if the patient has sensitivity to these agents, use a single-patient-use application of povidone-iodine).
- In terms of personal protective clothing, the guidance notes that gloves are single-use items which should be removed and discarded upon

completion of the care activity and that eye/face protection is indicated if there is a risk of splashing with blood or body fluids.

- Correct hand hygiene technique is emphasised (including the need to decontaminate hands before and after each patient contact).
- Aseptic technique must be used (including use of gown, gloves and drapes).
- Following line insertion, a sterile, transparent, semipermeable dressing is recommended (to allow observation of the insertion site).

In terms of ongoing line care, the guidelines highlight the importance of hand hygiene (decontamination of hands before and after each patient contact) and regular observation of the catheter site (at least daily) for signs of infection. Whenever the line is accessed (e.g. for administration of fluids or injections), it is important that an aseptic technique is first used to swab the ports or hub with 2% chlorhexidine gluconate in 70% isopropyl alcohol.

Whilst there is no routine catheter replacement guideline (clinical judgement should be used, e.g. if the exit site becomes inflamed or in the presence of a rising white cell count or signs of sepsis of unknown origin), administration sets should be replaced as indicated:

- Immediately following administration of blood or blood products.
- Within 24 hours following total parenteral nutrition (TPN) (72 hours if no lipid)
- Within 72 hours for all other fluid sets.

10.4.3 *Other sites of infection*

As mentioned above, other sites of nosocomial infection in ICU patients are less commonly encountered but need to be considered when searching for a focus of sepsis. Urinary tract infections are relatively uncommon in the ICU and are rarely the cause of a secondary BSI unless there is urinary tract obstruction or there has been a recent urological procedure [32,33]. The incidence of nosocomial sinusitis has decreased, as fewer patients are intubated via the orotracheal than the nasotracheal route [34].

Nevertheless, a sinus computed tomography (CT) scan may be required in the investigation of unresolved sepsis in an intubated patient.

Patients may have a fever or inflammatory response in the absence of infection:

- Fever may commonly occur in the first 48 hours after surgery and is usually not infectious in origin [35].
- Haematoma formation.
- Pulmonary embolus.
- Deep vein thrombosis.
- Acute myocardial infarction.
- Pancreatitis.

Other causes are summarised in the excellent review by O'Grady *et al.* [36].

10.5 Investigations

Whenever sepsis is suspected in an ICU patient, it is essential that a septic screen is preformed prior to commencing antimicrobial therapy. A core screen comprises the following:

- Blood cultures (from both a peripheral site and CVC, if present).
- Urine culture.
- Non-directed BAL (if patient is intubated) or sputum culture (if possible) from an unintubated patient.
- Swabs from wound site (if appropriate).
- Stool sample (if diarrhoea).

Other specimens will depend upon the patient's individual circumstances and therefore will be indicated in particular situations (e.g. lumbar puncture, submission of respiratory or other specimens for tuberculosis or viral immunofluorescence; fluid from newly inserted drains (abdominal or pleural) but, in general, culture of fluid from existing drains is often unhelpful as there tends to be a preponderance of colonising skin or overgrowth flora).

Other investigations, such as chest X ray (CXR) or more extensive imaging, will also be dictated by the individual circumstances.

10.6 Antimicrobial Therapy on the ICU

Given the rise in antibiotic resistance and the frequent occurrence of multiple-drug-resistant organisms in the ICU, never has there been a greater need for a multi-disciplinary approach to management of infections in the ICU. Different units will vary in the composition of the team, but a daily review of all patients by the intensivist and a clinical microbiologist (who will have the latest results from the microbiology laboratory) together with the ICU pharmacist should constitute the core members of the team.

Ground rules should be established (e.g. 'no third-generation cephalosporins to be prescribed unless specifically indicated' — ceftriaxone for a patient admitted with suspected bacterial meningitis, for example — or upon recommendation of a consultant microbiologist) and the antibiotic management of ICU patients should be strictly controlled (intensivist and microbiologist/identification physician only).

An antibiotic policy for the ICU should be prepared, outlining the empiric regimes for use in the unit (including antifungal drugs), and describing dose reductions for patients with renal or hepatic impairment or patients receiving continuous veno-venous haemodialysis (CVVHD).

In order to understand why certain classes of antibiotic should be limited, and how resistant sub-populations of an infecting organism may develop during a course of treatment, it is necessary to explain firstly how antibacterial agents work and then explain a little about the mechanisms of acquired antimicrobial resistance — particularly in Gram-negative organisms where the problem is most acute.

10.6.1 *Mechanisms of antibacterial action*

The most important principle of antibacterial therapy is that of selective toxicity i.e. the drug should kill (or impair the metabolism of) the infecting organism without harming the host. Most antimicrobials therefore target prokaryotic structures or pathways that are not present in eukaryotes;

there are therefore four main sites of action: the bacterial cell wall synthetic pathways; inhibition of protein or nucleic acid synthesis or inhibition of a metabolic pathway. Some of the antibiotic classes most frequently used in the ICU are described below:

- β-lactams (penicillins, cephalosporins, carbapenems) interfere with cell-wall synthesis; they are bactericidal and act against rapidly dividing bacteria; they are ineffective against bacteria that lack peptidoglycan cell walls (e.g. *Mycoplasma* or *Chlamydia* spp.). These are relatively non-toxic, have a short half-life (so that multiple dosing or a continuous infusion may be required to ensure that the tissue concentration of the antibiotic is always well above the minimal inhibitory concentration (MIC) needed to kill the organism). β-lactams are renally excreted, so that dose adjustment is required in the presence of renal impairment. It is important to enquire about a history of allergic reactions to β-lactams, as the penicillins are cross-allergenic (and share approximately 10% cross-reactivity with cephalosporins and carbapenems).
- Glycopeptides (e.g. vancomycin, teicoplanin) also interfere with cell wall synthesis, but are very large molecules with activity restricted to Gram-positive organisms. They are not absorbed when administered orally and so must be administered parenterally (except in the treatment of *Clostridium difficile* colitis, which is one of the few uses for an oral glycopeptide). They are slowly bactericidal and nephrotoxic and ototoxic, so that drug levels must be monitored on treatment.
- Aminoglycosides (e.g. gentamicin, tobramycin, amikacin) interfere with protein synthesis by binding to the 30S bacterial ribosomal subunit. They have a rapid, concentration-dependent bactericidal action, which is one of the important principles underlying the use of a once-daily dose of aminoglycoside in the treatment of sepsis. They are active against almost all aerobic Gram-negative bacilli, but they have minimal activity in a low-pH environment (e.g. within an abscess) and are ineffective against anaerobes. Aminoglycosides are ototoxic and nephrotoxic, so serum levels must be monitored during treatment; furthermore, as they are renally excreted, it is important that appropriate dose reductions are made for patients with impaired renal function.

- Macrolides (e.g. clarithromycin, erythromycin, azithromycin) bind to the 50S bacterial ribosome to inhibit RNA-dependent protein synthesis. They are largely bacteriostatic and have a limited role in the ICU except in the management of patients admitted with severe community-acquired pneumonia (they are active against *Legionella* spp. and atypical bacteria such as *Mycoplasma* and *Chlamydia* spp.).
- The fluoroquinolones (e.g. ciprofloxacin, levofloxacin) inhibit the action of the bacterial DNA gyrase, which impairs the DNA supercoiling mechanism. They are active against a broad range of Gram-negative aerobic bacteria (including *Pseudomonas* spp., particularly ciprofloxacin) and also some Gram-positive bacteria (the third- and fourth-generation fluoroquinolones, e.g. levofloxacin and moxifloxacillin are active against penicillin-resistant and penicillin-susceptible strains of *Streptococcus pneumoniae*). The fluoroquinolones are also active against some strains of *Staphylococcus aureus*, but caution is advised as there is evidence that fluoroquinolone use may select for MRSA colonisation [37] as the commonest hospital strains of MRSA in the UK are resistant to this class of antimicrobials. In the ICU, fluoroquinolones have a role in the management of Gram-negative infections (particularly in patients with a significant allergic reaction to β-lactams). They have a concentration-dependent killing mechanism (similar to the aminoglycosides); dose modifications for ciprofloxacin and levofloxacin are required in patients with impaired renal function. Due to the increasing prevalence of fluoroquinolone resistance among the Enterobacteriaceae (23% of UK *Escherichia coli* bacteraemia isolates demonstrated ciprofloxacin resistance in 2007 [38], for example), we recommend that fluoroquinolones are not used alone in the 'blind' treatment of suspected Gram-negative sepsis.
- The nitroimidazoles (e.g. metronidazole) damage microbial DNA under anaerobic conditions and are rapidly bactericidal. Metronidazole is an essential component of any antimicrobial regimen used in the management of suspected anaerobic (or mixed aerobic/anaerobic) infections (usually intra-abdominal, pelvic or deep soft tissue).
- Linezolid is an oxazolidenone antibacterial that inhibits protein synthesis at the 50S ribosomal level. It is active against Gram-positive bacteria, including MRSA and vancomycin-resistant enterococci

(VRE). It has a role to play in the management of significant VRE infections and serious MRSA infections (e.g. pneumonia). There are some significant side effects, however, which may limit its use (particularly haematopoietic disorders) and close monitoring of the full blood count is recommended.

- Tigecycline is a glycylcycline antibacterial (related structurally to the tetracyclines). It has a broad range of antibacterial activity that includes MRSA, VRE and many multi-resistant Gram-negative bacteria. However, it is essentially bacteriostatic and has minimal activity against many strains of *Proteus* spp. or *Pseudomonas aeruginosa*. We do not therefore recommend its use as an empiric antibacterial agent, except in certain cases of complicated abdominal or soft-tissue infections caused by mixed multiple-resistant organisms.

10.6.2 *There are four principal mechanisms of resistance: 'BEAT'*

Bypass: The bacteria may acquire genes for a metabolic pathway that enable them to bypass an existing pathway that is the target of a particular class of antimicrobial agent.

Enzymes: The organism may acquire genes that encode enzymes, such as β-lactamases, that destroy the antibacterial agent before it can affect the bacterium. Some β-lactamases (called extended spectrum β-lactamases (ESBLs)) are able to inactivate a broad range of β-lactam antimicrobials, including third-generation cephalosporins such as ceftazidime. Alternatively, the expression of chromosomal β-lactamase enzymes may be upregulated upon exposure to particular classes of antibacterials (this will be explained in further detail later).

Accumulation/Impairment: The bacteria may acquire efflux pumps that prevent the antibiotic agent from reaching its target or mutations in porins, or downregulation of porin genes may limit the ability of the antibiotic to enter the cell at all.

Target modification: Mutant organisms that possess a modified target or binding site will be selected in the pressure of an antimicrobial that binds to such a target.

Awareness of the types of resistance mechanisms and the rapidity with which resistant subpopulations of bacteria will develop on treatment in the ICU will help to determine appropriate antimicrobial selection and use.

Units will differ in terms of the resistant bacterial organisms that they harbour, and so the treatment regimes that follow may need to be modified for local use. However, there are a few sensible rules:

(i) Antimicrobial therapy should be guided by good laboratory data and knowledge of the known susceptibility patterns of frequently cultured organisms.

(ii) Never commence therapy without collecting specimens for a 'septic screen' (blood cultures, urine if available, respiratory specimens and wound swabs, etc.).

(iii) Use the shortest course of therapy that is safe — in most cases, an 'empirical' course should not exceed five days. Specific infections (e.g. *Pseudomonal* or *Staphylococal* pneumonia, faecal peritonitis or mediastinitis) will require longer courses.

(iv) Discontinue any unnecessary antimicrobial at the earliest opportunity (e.g. empiric vancomycin can be discontinued after 48 hours if there is no evidence of MRSA or an amplicillin-resistant entercoccal infection).

(v) Avoid fluoroquinolones (unless specifically indicated). These are associated with an increased risk of *Clostridium difficile* infection and may rapidly select for fluoroquinolone-resistant strains of *Pseudomonas aeruginosa* and appear to increase the risk of MRSA colonisation [37].

(vi) Avoid third-generation cephalosporins (e.g. ceftazidime). Not only are they associated with an increased risk of *Clostridium difficile* infection, but they are strong inducers of the chromosomal (amp C) β-lactamase enzymes of most strains of *Enterobacter* spp., *Citrobacter* spp., *Morganella morganii*, *Serratia* spp., *Providencia* spp. and indole-positive *Proteus* spp. Infections caused by these organisms should be treated with a carbapenem, fluoroquinolone or aminoglycoside (not a cephalosporin or penicillin).

(vii) Avoid long courses or empirical use of carbapenems unless specifically indicated as there is a risk of selecting for bacteria that are intrinsically resistant to carbapenems (e.g. *Stenotrophomonas maltophilia*). If used in the treatment of *Pseudomonas aeruginosa* infections, there is a risk that carbapenem-resistant mutants (lacking the D2-porin) will be selected.

(viii) No routine 'prophylactic' antibiotics (except for indicated surgical procedures).

(ix) No routine use of antibiotics for line changes.

On the whole we do not recommended routine antibiotic cycling [39] — it is likely that, based on our guidelines (see Section 10.6.3) a variety of anti-infectives will be in use at any one time.

10.6.3 *Simple guide to antimicrobial usage in the ICU*

(i) There is evidence that the use of piperacillin–tazobactam (Tazocin) — rather than a third generation cephalosporin — is associated with a lower risk of promoting colonisation by ESBL-producing Gram-negative infections [40,41] and also a less frequent association with VRE [42] and *Clostridium difficile* infection [43]. We recommend that the initial combination of vancomycin plus Tazocin should be the empirical regimen to be used if an ICU patient (present in hospital for over 48 hours) develops signs of sepsis. Of course, a septic screen should be carried out before commencing the antimicrobial therapy and steps should be taken to modify the regimen (e.g. discontinue vancomycin and/or 'step down' the Tazocin based upon the culture and susceptibility results).

(ii) Discontinue the empirical therapy after a maximum of five days unless there is a compelling reason to continue for longer (see above).

(iii) Should the patient become unwell with a new onset of sepsis whilst on a recommended antimicrobial regimen, we like to leave an 'SOS' in the notes. In general, such an SOS will comprise an empirical antimicrobial upgrade (e.g. moving from single-agent Tazocin to a combination of a glycopeptide and carbapenem) or adding an aminoglycoside and possibly an antifungal if the patient is already on a maximal regimen. In some cases, a more unusual combination may be required to cover two different organisms that are known to be present (e.g. co-trimoxazole and a carbapenem for a patient with, for example, a *Stenotrophomonas maltophilia* respiratory tract infection and an *Enterobacter* spp. abdominal infection). As always, whenever an empirical antimicrobial switch is made, the patient should be fully cultured beforehand. It should also be remembered that an antifungal may be required in a patient who has already been receiving broad-spectrum antimicrobials and particularly in the presence of abdominal sepsis. Antifungal therapy will be discussed in more detail below.

(iv) Different ICUs will have different antimicrobial flora and known local resistance patterns should be taken into account when planning particular antimicrobial regimes or SOS upgrades. There may also be a role for newer antimicrobials (such as linezolid or tigecycline), or a very much older antimicrobial (colistin), under certain circumstances.

10.6.4 *Antifungal therapy*

The prevalence of BSIs caused by *Candida* spp. varies between countries; two recent UK-based surveys have reported a prevalence rate of between 3.0 cases per 10^5 bed days [44] and 5.9 cases per 10^5 bed days [45]. A significant proportion of these cases occurred in ICU patients (45% in [44]). As stated previously, *Candida* spp. infections accounted for approximately 6% of ICU BSIs [14]. Whilst *Candida albicans* (most isolates of which are fluconazole-susceptible) tends to account for the majority of these cases [44], there is evidence that the epidemiology of the candidaemia-causing species is changing, with an increasing proportion of BSIs caused by non-*albicans* species such as *Candida glabrata* and *Candida parapsilosis* (21% and 12% respectively according to the study by Odds *et al.* [45]). A recent Spanish study of 1,765 adult patients admitted to a general ICU for at least seven days reported an incidence rate of 1.5 candidaemia episodes per 1,000 days of ICU stay. Independent risk factors for candidaemia included colonisation by *Candida* spp., TPN, elective surgery and haemofiltration [46].

Risk factors for the development of non-*albicans* candidaemia include the duration of CVC use and length of prior fluconazole exposure [7]. Indeed, fluconazole prophylaxis has previously been suggested as an explanation for the increased prevalence of low-susceptibility *Candida* spp. [47], which is one of the reasons why we do not advocate its routine use in the ICU. A recent randomised trial from the USA has also confirmed that there is no significant improvement in outcome among ICU patients receiving untargeted antifungal prophylaxis [48].

A candida colonisation index has been proposed [49] in an attempt to identify ICU patients most at risk of developing invasive candidiasis. A candida colonisation index was defined as the ratio of the number of distinct body sites (dbs) (other than blood) colonised with identical strains divided by the total number of dbs tested. The initial study was carried out among patients admitted to a surgical and a neonatal ICU and formed the basis for subsequent studies which have attempted to define a threshold ratio which should be the trigger to initiate systemic antifungal therapy.

Given that the mortality of disseminated candidiasis remains high (there is a broad range — between 5 and 71% according to Falgas *et al.*, who carried out a systematic review of matched cohort studies [50]), early initiation of appropriate therapy is important. Certainly antifungals should be commenced when *Candida* spp. have been isolated from blood cultures or from usually sterile body finds, from abscesses or from wounds in burns patients. The difficulty comes in deciding when to commence therapy in an unwell colonised patient on the ICU. Muñoz *et al.* [51] have reviewed the various risk factors and recommended that antifungal therapy may be required when *Candida* spp. colonisation is detected in two or more non-contiguous anatomical sites, or when the colonisation index is >0.5. Our own practice is broadly based upon an awareness of the above criteria: an antifungal is always commenced when a yeast is isolated from blood or a sterile body site. The addition of an antifungal drug is recommended in the management of any ICU patient with new-onset sepsis in whom no other source is found — especially if they have evidence of *Candida* spp. colonisation at two or more sites, if they have had abdominal surgery or if they have already been exposed to a prolonged course of broad spectrum antibiotics.

The choice of which antifungal to use depends upon the species of *Candida* with which the patient is colonised and their clinical status. Susceptibility to antifungals varies between the different *Candida* spp.: broadly, *Candida albicans*, *Candida parapsilosis* and *Candida tropicalis* are susceptible to the azoles (usually including fluconazole) and the polyenes (e.g. amphotericin), while *Candida glabrata* and *Candida krusei* are generally resistant to fluconazole but susceptible to second-generation triazoles (e.g. voriconazole) and the echinocandins (eg caspofungin).

A recent review outlines the current therapeutic options for the treatment of invasive candidosis in critically ill patients [52], but individual ICUs will put policies in place for the use of antifungal agents, based upon clinical efficacy and cost.

In broad terms, we tend to include fluconazole in the empirical management of a patient who is known to be colonised by *Candida albicans* (or a known fluconazole-susceptible *Candida* spp.) if their condition is relatively stable. Fluconazole is largely excreted unchanged in the urine and is therefore particularly effective for the treatment of clinically significant candiduria caused by susceptible organisms. For the empirical management of candidaemia, or developing/worsening sepsis in a patient colonised with a non-albicans yeast (or upon the culture of a non-*albicans* yeast from a sterile site), we would commence therapy with an echinocandin (caspofungin is currently available in our ICU). This is active against most *Candida* spp. (*Candida guilliermondii* and *Candida parapsilosis* appear less susceptible *in vitro* than other *Candida* spp.) and has a low level of toxicity (but dose reduction is required in patients with severe hepatic impairment). It is not renally excreted and is unsuitable for the treatment of *Candida* infection arising in the renal tract.

The second generation azole, voriconazole, also demonstrates a broad spectrum of activity and has a good bioavailability (including significant central nervous system (CNS) penetration), but its use in the ICU is somewhat restricted by the fact that the intravenous formulation contains the excipient sulfobutyl ether β-cyclodextrin, which may accumulate in patients with renal insufficiency. Voriconazole is also hepatically metabolised and should be avoided in patients with severe hepatic insufficiency. There are also several potentially significant drug interactions in patients who may concurrently be receiving medications that are metabolised by the cytochrome P450 enzymes.

In terms of older antifungal agents, there is probably little role for conventional amphotericin B (apart perhaps from use in bladder washouts in patients with significant *Candida* spp. infections of the lower urinary tract) owing to the problems associated with nephrotoxicity, electrolyte disturbances and acute infusion-related side effects. The lipid formulations have significantly fewer side effects and have a role in the treatment of invasive fungal infections that are not susceptible to the azoles or echinocandins.

In summary, the possibility of a fungal infection (particularly invasive candidiasis) should always be considered in an ICU patient with an ongoing inflammatory response that is failing to respond to conventional antimicrobial therapy, particularly if the patient has been on the ICU for more than seven days, or has received prolonged courses of broad-spectrum antimicrobials, or is known to be extensively colonised by *Candida* spp.

10.6.5 *Infection control in the ICU*

The measures to control nosocomial infections are based at three levels: administrative controls (guidelines and policies to be followed by all healthcare workers); engineering controls (such as the provision of negative pressure rooms for the management of patients with airborne infections); and use of personal protective equipment, such as gloves, aprons and face masks.

Best practice recommendations have been published by the Department of Health [21]. Essentially, the actions that have been associated with the most significant reduction in nosocomial infections in the ITU are:

- MRSA screening followed by decolonisation of colonised or infected patients. There should be a clear and agreed policy which is audited and reviewed regularly.
- If facilities exist, MRSA-positive patients should be managed separately from non-infected or colonised patients. However, where side rooms are limited, a risk assessment must be carried out. Preference should be given to patients with open tuberculosis (see separate guidance below) or infectious diarrhoea. MRSA-positive patients may then be cohorted in a separate area of the unit (and preferably away from surgical patients, particularly those who may have had recent implant surgery).

- Use of care bundles/high-impact interventions to ensure best practice with:
  - Central vascular line: insertion and continuing care.
  - Aseptic techniques.
  - Hand hygiene.
  - Treatment of sepsis.
  - VAP.
  - *Clostridium difficile* management.
- Appropriate use and disposal of personal protective equipment (such as gloves, gowns and masks).

In addition to the above, the Department of Health also recommends that there should be planned monitoring of cleaning standards within the ICU and a schedule for regular deep cleaning. An agreed antibiotic prescribing policy for the ICU should be established, based upon local microbiological resistance data.

Patients with open tuberculosis, confirmed or suspected cases of infectious pulmonary tuberculosis in ICUs that are not ventilated via a closed ventilation circuit must be nursed in a single room preferably with negative-pressure ventilation. If the patient is intubated/ventilated via a closed system and secretions are contained, masks do not need to be worn except when exposure to secretions is likely to occur, e.g. whenever the closed system is disconnected.

If the patient is known or suspected to be infected with multidrug resistant tuberculosis (MDR-TB), they must be managed in a single room with negative pressure facilities [53] and staff and visitors managing the patient should wear high filtration filtering face piece class 3 masks.

The full guidance should be available in the hospital's infection control policy.

References

[1] Smyth, E.T., McIlvenny, G., Enstone, J.E. *et al.* (2008). Four country healthcare associated infection prevalence survey 2006: overview of the results, *J Hosp Infect*, **69**, 230–248.

[2] Bryce, E.A. and Smith, J.A. (1995). Focused microbiological surveillance and Gram-negative β-lactamase-mediated resistance in an intensive care unit, *Infect Control Hosp Epidemiol*, **16**, 331–334.

[3] Rodríguez-Baño, J., Navarro, M.D., Romero, L. *et al.* (2004). Epidemiology and clinical features of infections caused by extended-spectrum Beta-lactamase-producing *Escherichia coli* in nonhospitalized patients, *J Clin Microbiol*, **42**, 1089–1094.

[4] Huang, S.S. and Platt, R. (2003). Risk of methicillin-resistant *Staphylococcus aureus* infection after previous infection or colonization, *Clin Infect Dis*, **36**, 281–285.

[5] Pelupessy, I., Bonten, M.J. and Diekmann, O. (2002). How to assess the relative importance of different colonization routes of pathogens within hospital settings, *Proc Natl Acad Sci USA*, **99**, 5601–5605.

[6] Spencer, R.C. (1994). Epidemiology of infection in ICUs, *Intens Care Med*, **20** (Suppl. 4), S2–S6.

[7] Chow, J.K., Golan, Y., Ruthazer, R. *et al.* (2008). Factors associated with candidaemia caused by non-*albicans Candida* species versus *Candida albicans* in the intensive care unit, *Clin Infect Dis*, **46**, 1206–1213.

[8] Jaber, S., Chanques, G., Borry, J. *et al.* (2005). Cytomegalovirus Infection in critically ill patients, *Chest*, **127**, 233–241.

[9] Limaye, A., Kirby, K.A., Rubenfeld, G.D. *et al.* (2008). Cytomegalovirus reactivation in critically ill immunocompetent patients, *JAMA*, **300**, 413–422.

[10] Vrielink, H. and Reesink, H.W. (1998). Transfusion-transmissible infections, *Curr Opin Haem*, **5**, 396–405.

[11] Vincent, J.L., Bihari, D.J., Suter, P.M. *et al.* (1995). The prevalence of nosocomial infection in intensive care units in Europe. Results of the European Prevalence of Infection in Intensive Care (EPIC) Study, *JAMA*, **274**, 639–644.

[12] Fagon, J.-Y, Chastre, J., Hance, A.J. *et al.* (1993). Nosocomial pneumonia in ventilated patients: a cohort study evaluating attributable mortality and hospital stay, *Am J Med*, **94**, 281–288.

[13] Cook, D.J., Walter, S.D., Cook, R.J. *et al.* (1998). Incidence of and risk factors for ventilator-associated pneumonia in critically ill patients, *Ann Int Med*, **129**, 433–440.

[14] Suetens, C., Morales, I., Savey, A. *et al.* (2007). European surveillance of ICU-acquired infections (HELICS-ICU): methods and main results, *J Hosp Inf*, **65** (Suppl. 2), 171–173.

[15] Masterton, R.G., Galloway, A., French, G. *et al.* (2008). Guidelines for the management of hospital-acquired pneumonia in the UK: Report of the working party on hospital-acquired pneumonia of the British society for antimicrobial chemotherapy, *J Antimicrob Chemother*, **62**, 5–34.

[16] Torres, A. and El-Ebiary, M. (2000). Bronchoscopic BAL in the diagnosis of ventilator-associated pneumonia, *Chest*, **117** (4, Suppl. 2), 198–202.

[17] Chastre, J., Wolff, M., Fagon, J.-Y. *et al.* (2003). Comparison of 8 vs 15 days of antibiotic therapy for ventilator-associated pneumonia in adults: a randomized trial, *JAMA*, **290**, 2588–2598.

[18] American Thoracic Society and Infectious Diseases Society of America (2005). Guidelines for the management of adults with hospital-acquired, ventilator-associated, and healthcare-associated pneumonia, *Am J Respir Crit Care Med*, **171**, 388–416.

[19] Bartlett, J.G., Dowell, S.F., Mandell, L.A. *et al.* (2000). Practice guidelines for the management of community-acquired pneumonia in adults, *Clin Infect Dis*, **31**, 347–382.

[20] Brown, R.B., Kruse, J.A., Counts, G.W. *et al.* (1990). Double-blind study of endotracheal tobramycin in the treatment of Gram-negative bacterial pneumonia, *Antimicrob Agents Chemother*, **34**, 269–272.

[21] Department of Health. (2005). *Clean, Safe Care. Reducing MRSA and other healthcare associated infections: Saving lives*, [Online]. Available at: http://webarchive.nationalarchives.gov.uk/20101125133833/http://www.clean-safe-care.nhs.uk/index.php?pid=2 [Accessed 20 January 2013].

[22] Tablan, O.C., Anderson, L.J., Besser, R. *et al.* (2004). Guidelines for preventing healthcare-associated-pneumonia, 2003: recommendations of CDC and the Healthcare Infection Control Practices Advisory Committee, *MMWR Recomm Rep*, **53** (RR-3), 1–36.

[23] de Smet A.M.G.A. and Bonten, M.J.M. (2008). Selective decontamination of the digestive tract, *Curr Opin Infect Dis*, **21**, 179–183.

[24] Kollef, M.H., Afessa, B., Anzueto, A. *et al.* (2008). Silver-coated endotracheal tubes and incidence of ventilator-associated pneumonia: the NASCENT randomized trial, *JAMA*, **300**, 805–813.

[25] Digiovine, B., Chenoweth, C., Watts, C. *et al.* (1999). The attributable mortality and costs of primary nosocomial bloodstream infections in the intensive care unit, *Am J Respir Crit Care Med*, **160**, 976–981.

[26] Smith, R., Meixler, S. and Simberkoff, M. (1991). Excess mortality in critically ill patients with nosocomial bloodstream infections, *Chest*, **100**, 164–167.

[27] Pittet, D., Tarara, D. and Wenzel, R.P. (1994). Nosocomial bloodstream infection in critically ill patients. Excess length of stay, extra costs, and attributable mortality, *JAMA*, **271**, 1598–1601.

[28] Sherertz, R.J., Ely, E.W., Westbrook, D.M. *et al.* (2000). Education of physicians-in-training can decrease the risk for vascular catheter infection, *Ann Int Med*, **132**, 641–648.

[29] Berenholtz, S.M., Pronovost, P.J., Lipsett, P.A. *et al.* (2004). Eliminating catheter-related bloodstream infections in the intensive care unit, *Crit Care Med*, **32**, 2014–2020.

[30] Centers for Disease Control and Prevention (CDC) (2005). Reduction in central line-associated bloodstream infections among patients in intensive care units — Pennsylvania, April 2001–March 2005, *MMWR Morb Mortal Wkly Rep*, **54**, 1013–1016.

[31] Pronovost, P., Needham, D., Berenholtz, S. *et al.* (2006). An intervention to decrease catheter-related bloodstream infections in the ICU, *N Engl J Med*, **355**, 2725–2732.

[32] Bryan, C.S. and Reynolds, K.L. (1984). Hospital-acquired bacteremic urinary tract infection, epidemiology and outcome, *J Urol*, **132**, 494–498.

[33] Quintiliani, R., Klimek, J., Cunha, B.A. *et al.* (1978). Bacteraemia after manipulation of the urinary tract, the importance of pre-existing urinary tract disease and compromised host defences, *Postgrad Med J*, **54**, 668–671.

[34] Rouby, J.J., Laurent, P., Gosnach, M. *et al.* (1994). Risk factors and clinical relevance of nosocomial maxillary sinusitis in the critically ill, *Am J Respir Crit Care Med*, **150**, 776–783.

[35] Garibaldi, R.A., Brodine, S., Matsumiya, S. *et al.* (1985). Evidence for the non-infectious etiology of early post-operative fever, *Infect Control*, **6**, 273–277.

[36] O'Grady, N.P., Barie, P.S., Bartlett, J.G. *et al.* (2008). Guidelines for evaluation of new fever in critically ill adult patients: 2008 update from the American College of Critical Care Medicine and the Infectious Diseases Society of America, *Crit Care Med*, **36**, 1330–1349.

[37] Venezia, R.A., Domaracki, B.E., Evans, A.M. *et al.* (2001). Selection of high-level oxacillin resistance in heteroresistant *Staphylococcus aureus* by fluoroquinolone exposure, *J Antimicrob Chemother*, **48**, 375–381.

[38] Health Protection Agency (2008), Annual Report 2008. London: HPA.

[39] Brown, E.M. and Nathwani, D. (2005). Antibiotic cycling or rotation: a systematic review of the evidence of efficacy, *J Antimicrob Chemother*, **55**, 6–9.

[40] Lan C.K., Hsueh, P.R., Wong, W.W. *et al.* (2003). Association of antibiotic utilization measures and reduced incidence of infections with extended-spectrum β-lactamase-producing organisms, *J Microbiol Immunol Infect*, **36**, 182–186.

[41] Bantar, C., Vesco, E., Heft, C. *et al.* (2003). Replacement of broad-spectrum cephalosporins by piperacillin-tazobactam: impact on sustained high rates of bacterial resistance, *Antimicrob Agents Chemother*, **48**, 392–395.

[42] Quale, J., Landman, D., Saurina, G. *et al.* (1996). Manipulation of a hospital antimicrobial formulary to control an outbreak of vancomycin-resistant enterococci, *Clin Infect Dis*, **23**, 1020–1025.

[43] Wilcox, M.H., Freeman, J., Fawley, W. *et al.* (2004). Long-term surveillance of cefotaxime and piperacillin-tazobactam prescribing and incidence of *Clostridium difficile* diarrhoea, *J Antimicrob Chemother*, **54**, 168–172.

[44] Kibbler, C.C., Seaton, S., Barnes, R.A. *et al.* (2003). Management and outcome of bloodstream infections due to *Candida* species in England and Wales, *J Hosp Inf*, **54**, 18–24.
[45] Odds, F.C., Hanson, M.F., Davidson, A.D. *et al.* (2007). One year prospective survey of *Candida* bloodstream infections in Scotland, *J Med Microbiol*, **56**, 1066–1075.
[46] Jordà-Marcos, R., Álvarez-Lerma, F., Jurado, M. *et al.* (2007). Risk factors for candidaemia in critically ill patients: a prospective surveillance study, *Mycoses*, **50**, 302–310.
[47] Price, M.F., LaRocco, M.T. and Gentry, L.O. (1994). Fluconazole susceptibilities of *Candida* species and distribution of species recovered from blood cultures over a 5-year period, *Antimicrob Agents Chemother*, **38**, 1422–1424.
[48] Schuster, M.G., Edwards, J.E., Sobel, J.D. *et al.* (2008). Empirical fluconazole versus placebo for intensive care unit patients: a randomized trial, *Ann Intern Med*, **149**, 83–90.
[49] Pittet, D., Monod, M., Suter, P.M. *et al.* (1994). *Candida* colonization and subsequent infections in critically ill surgical patients, *Ann Surg*, **220**, 75–78.
[50] Falagas, M.E., Apostolou, K.E. and Pappas, V.D. (2006). Attributable mortality of candidaemia: a systemic review of matched cohort and case-control studies, *Eur J Clin Microbiol Infect Dis*, **25**, 419–425.
[51] Muñoz, P., Burillo, A. and Bouza, E. (2000). Criteria used when initiating antifungal therapy against *Candida* spp. in the intensive care unit, *Int J Antimicrob Agents*, **15**, 83–90.
[52] Ruhnke, M., Hartwig, K. and Kofla, G. (2008). New options for treatment of candidaemia in critically ill patients, *Clin Micrbiol Inf*, **14** (Suppl. 4), 46–54.
[53] Joint Tuberculosis Committee of the British Thoracic Society (2000). Control and prevention of tuberculosis in the United Kingdom: Code of Practice 2000, *Thorax*, **55**, 887–901.

11

Radiological Imaging in Intensive Care

Kanupriya Agrawal and Andrew R. Wright

11.1 Introduction

Radiological imaging is an intrinsic part of the everyday management of the intensive care unit (ICU) patient. Increasingly sophisticated imaging techniques are invaluable in the initial diagnosis of conditions which might lead to an ICU stay, as well as evaluating later complications of the underlying illness and its treatment.

Because of the highly dependent nature of most ICU patients, radiological imaging is generally limited to techniques which can be carried out at the bedside (such as plain radiography and ultrasound scanning), or computed tomography (CT), where transfer is necessary to the radiology department, but where monitoring of the patient is relatively straightforward. Magnetic resonance imaging is generally not employed in the acute care of ICU patients owing to difficulty monitoring patients in the high-magnetic-field-strength environment.

This chapter will describe the indications and typical radiological findings encountered in the ICU setting for the three principal radiological modalities, plain chest radiography, ultrasound scanning and CT.

11.2 The Chest Radiograph

ICU professionals are required to interpret chest radiographs frequently when treating critically ill patients. It is essential to be able to recognise common pathological appearances on portable chest radiographs as well as correct positioning of medical lines and their common complications.

Chest radiographs are frequently taken in surgical or medical ICUs. As these examinations are generally carried out using mobile equipment, the possibility of obtaining optimal films is reduced. The films are often taken supine as patients may be unable to sit up in bed. The post-operative patient also has difficulty with deep inspiration, so that the air content is often reduced in the basal segments of the lungs. Use of digital radiography has, however, considerably improved the quality of these examinations.

As the portable film is taken in the antero–posterior (AP) projection, this will lead to magnification of the cardiac shadow. The upper limit of a cardiothoracic ratio in the AP film has been reported as 57%.

Various life-support and monitoring devices may be used in the care of patients in the ICU. An ICU radiograph of the chest is valuable for identifying the position of and possible complications relating to endotracheal tubes, tracheostomy tubes, nasogastric tubes, intravenous catheters, pulmonary artery catheters, pacemakers, chest tubes, mediastinal tubes and ectopic gas related to mechanical ventilation [1].

11.2.1 *Tubes and lines on chest-radiographs*

11.2.1.1 *Endotracheal tube*

In an adult, the tip of the tube should be situated approximately 5 cm above the tracheal carina, so that excursions of 2 cm upward or downward (with neck extension or flexion) can be safely accommodated [2].

Accidental right main bronchus intubation (Fig. 11.1) is associated with left-sided atelectasis, right-sided tension pneumothorax and decreased survival. Conversely, failure to place the tube several cm beyond the vocal cords may result in inadvertent extubation, aspiration pneumonia or laryngeal spasm.

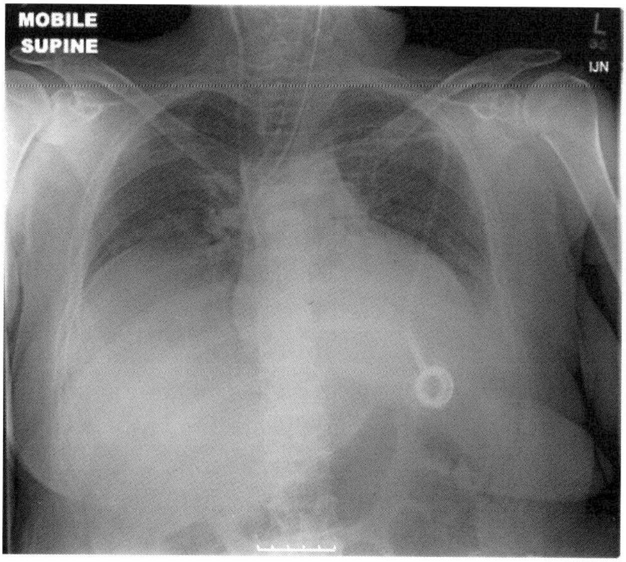

Figure 11.1. Malpositioned endotracheal tube in the right main bronchus.

Besides being placed into the right bronchus, endotracheal tubes can also be inadvertently placed in the oesophagus or in the soft tissues of the neck.

11.2.1.2 *Tracheostomy tube*

Patients with a prolonged post-operative course, who require respirator support, will usually require tracheostomy. A chest radiograph should always be performed after tracheostomy to check the correct position of the tracheal cannula, and to diagnose possible bleeding into the mediastinum, indicated by mediastinal widening.

11.2.1.3 *Nasogastric tube*

Nasogastric tubes and feeding tubes are frequently visualised passing through the mediastinum on their way to the stomach and intestines. Not infrequently, chest radiographs reveal medical devices in abnormal locations and unexpected foreign bodies.

Complications of malpositioned nasogastric tubes [3] include tracheopulmonary intubation, leading to atelectasis and consolidation, bronchial perforation and pleural cavity penetration, leading to pneumothorax. Tube knotting and impaction in the posterior nasopharynx, tube double-backing and kinking, tube obstruction, tube breakage and enteric perforation are other complications (Fig. 11.2).

11.2.1.4 *Central venous catheters*

Central venous catheters are now routinely used for monitoring central venous pressure, for renal replacement and for infusion of medications and parental nutrition. Access is usually obtained by percutaneous puncture of the subclavian, internal jugular or femoral veins.

A catheter tip positioned in the right atrium increases the risk of perforation and cardiac arrhythmia. At the same time, the catheter must be placed centrally in order to avoid damage when parenteral nutrition is infused via a peripheral vein (perforation, thrombosis).

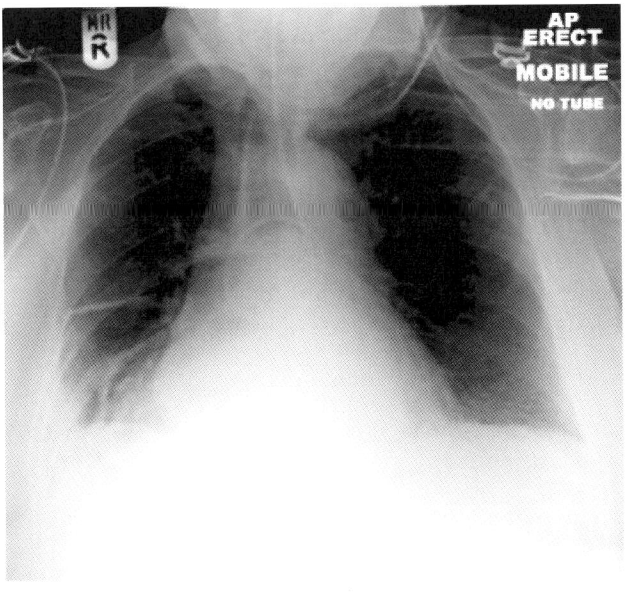

Figure 11.2. Nasogastric tube coiled in oesophagus.

Pneumothorax is a common complication of unsuccessful attempts at subclavian or low-jugular catheter insertion. Looping of catheters may lead to knotting. Pinching of catheters and catheter shearing usually occur at the site of entry and suture fixation. Vessel lacerations and perforations can produce haematomas, haemothorax, and infusion of fluid into the mediastinum, thorax or other inappropriate spaces.

11.2.1.5 *Pulmonary artery catheters*

Accurate measurement of pulmonary arterial wedge pressure in a supine patient requires the catheter tip to be in the lower lobe so that left atrial, not alveolar pressure, is measured.

Over time, pulmonary artery catheters may migrate toward the periphery of the pulmonary bed and become lodged in a small pulmonary artery. Such migration can cause vessel injury by prolonged occlusion or by overdistension of the vessel when the catheter balloon is inflated. Also, pulmonary infarction can result from this situation. A central location of the catheter tip near the lung hilum helps prevent pulmonary artery perforation and is a good 'parking' position for the catheter when it is not being used to measure pulmonary arterial wedge pressure.

Catheter malposition usually involves the catheter passing into a tributary vessel rather than the one sought. The internal jugular vein, azygous arch, and internal mammary vein are frequent sites of catheter malpositioning. Catheters may take an unusual course or position because of a congenital anomaly.

11.2.2 *Post-operative pathological conditions*

11.2.2.1 *Atelectasis and consolidation*

Partial or complete loss of volume of a lung is referred to as collapse or atelectasis. Atelectasis is frequently seen in the post-operative phase, and may be caused either by hypoventilation, retained secretions, or aspiration [4].

The radiological appearances depend on the mechanism of collapse, the degree of collapse and the presence or absence of consolidation. Signs of collapse include displacement of interlobar fissures, loss of aeration and increased density and crowding of vessels and bronchi. Indirect signs include elevation of a hemidiaphragm, mediastinal or hilar displacement and compensatory hyperinflation [5].

Consolidation implies replacement of air in one or more acini by fluid or solid material but does not imply a particular pathology or aetiology. A common cause of consolidation in the post-operative period is acute inflammatory exudate associated with pneumonia. An air bronchogram is often visible when consolidation is associated with a patent conducting airway. Consolidation and atelectasis often co-exist.

Atelectasis/consolidation in different sites have typical appearances on chest radiographs as shown in Figs 11.3–11.6.

11.2.2.2 *Aspiration pneumonia*

The posterior segment of the upper lobes and the superior segment of the lower lobes are the most commonly involved lung sites in aspiration disease [6]. Classic radiographic findings in acute gastric acid aspiration include bilateral perihilar, ill-defined, alveolar consolidation, multifocal

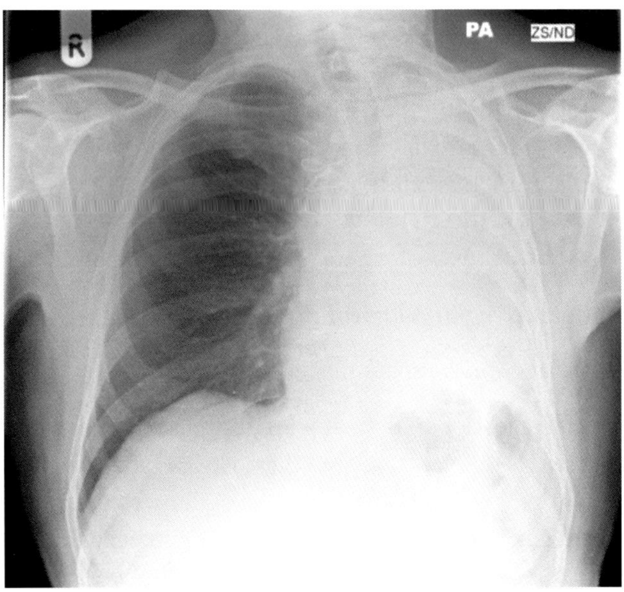

Figure 11.3. Complete collapse of the left lung with mediastinal shift.

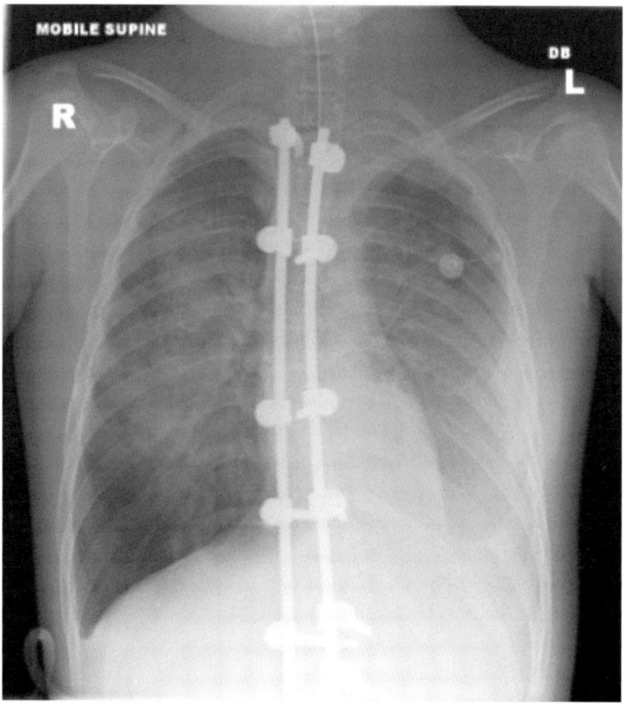

Figure 11.4. Left lower lobe collapse with loss of the left hemidiaphragmatic silhouette and bilateral patchy consolidation in this patient with aspiration pneumonitis. Harrington's rods are also visualised.

patchy infiltrates and segmental or lobar consolidation, which is usually localised to one or both lung bases.

11.2.2.3 *Pulmonary congestion/oedema*

Post-operative pulmonary congestion or oedema can be due either to heart failure or overhydration. Sepsis and shock may also cause pulmonary oedema as a consequence of increased capillary permeability.

Cardiogenic pulmonary oedema is characterised by the transudation of excess fluid into the lungs secondary to an increase in left atrial and subsequently pulmonary venous pressures in the absence of a primary change in the permeability of the pulmonary vasculature. The spectrum

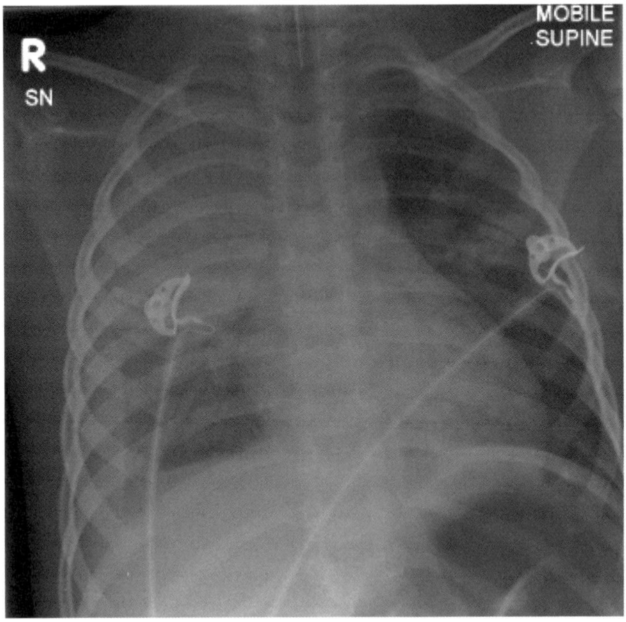

Figure 11.5. Air-space opacification with air-bronchograms (consolidation) in the right upper and mid zones. Associated right pleural fluid is also present.

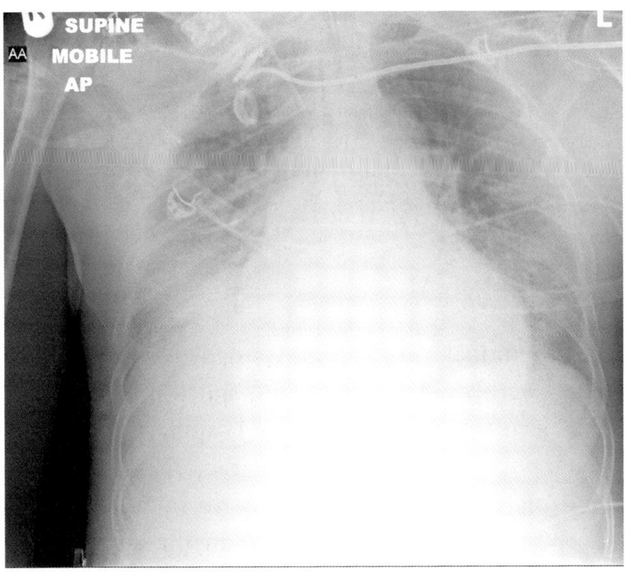

Figure 11.6. Air-space opacification with air-bronchograms in the right lower and mid zones.

and progression of radiographic findings of congestive cardiac failure and pulmonary oedema include cardiomegaly and redistribution of pulmonary vascularity, with attenuation of the lower zone vessels and prominence of the upper zone vessels. As congestive cardiac failure worsens, fluid may be seen in the interlobular septa as septal (Kerley B) lines, horizontal subpleural lines, 1–3 mm in thickness and up to 1 cm in length most frequently identified at the costophrenic angles. With pronounced congestive cardiac failure, fluid accumulates in the alveolar spaces and frank pulmonary oedema becomes apparent. This is seen as effusions and bilateral basilar and perihilar alveolar infiltrates (Fig. 11.7).

11.2.2.4 *Acute respiratory distress syndrome (ARDS)*

ARDS is seen most frequently after major surgery with complications such as infection, aspiration, contusion, fat embolism and disseminated intravascular coagulation (DIC).

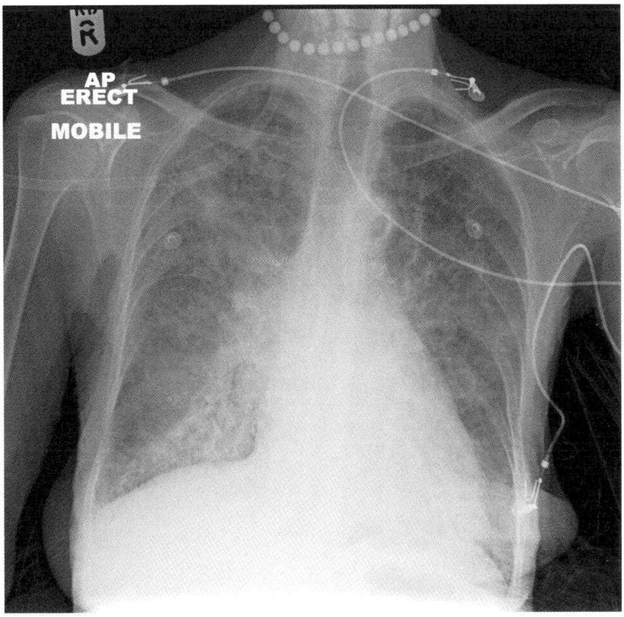

Figure 11.7. Cardiomegaly, pleural fluid, prominence of upper zone vessels, interlobular septal lines and perihilar infiltrates in cardiogenic pulmonary oedema.

There are three stages in the evolution and resolution of ARDS with corresponding radiographic features. In the first stage (0–24 hours) of the syndrome, the chest radiograph is frequently normal despite marked pathological changes. Stage II (24–36 hours) radiographically manifests as opacification in the lungs, nearly always bilateral, usually diffusely scattered, which may be both central and peripheral in the lungs. Air bronchograms and the absence of pleural fluid are other findings (Fig. 11.8). Consolidation of lung tissue is usual in advanced cases of ARDS. Appearances often remain static for two to three days until Stage III (3–14 days) with radiological resolution with interstitial fibrosis and scarring [7].

11.2.2.5 *Pulmonary embolism*

Subjects presenting with symptoms of pulmonary embolism (PE) often have an abnormal chest radiograph. Plain radiographs of the chest are essential in the evaluation of patients with cardiopulmonary symptoms but the chest radiograph findings associated with pulmonary thromboem-

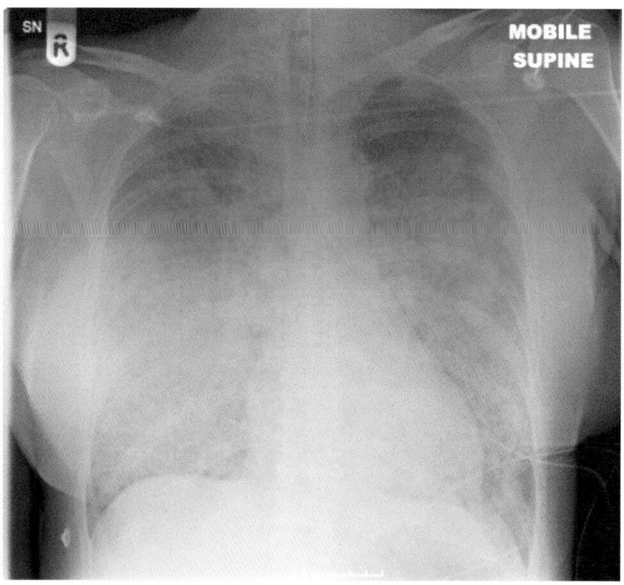

Figure 11.8. Bilateral diffusely scattered opacification with air bronchograms. The absence of pleural fluid is another finding in ARDS.

bolism are usually non-specific. The most common chest radiographic findings are cardiac enlargement (27%), normal (24%), pleural effusion (23%), elevated hemidiaphragm (20%), pulmonary artery enlargement (19%), atelectasis (18%) and parenchymal pulmonary infiltrates (17%). In subjects investigated for PE, an abnormal chest radiograph increases the prevalence of non-diagnostic scintigrams [8]. A normal pre-test chest radiograph is more often associated with a definitive (normal or high probability) scintigram result [9]. In practice most patients in an intensive care setting will require CT pulmonary angiography to exclude PE.

11.2.2.6 *Pleural fluid*

Standard posteroanterior and lateral chest radiography remains the most important technique for the initial diagnosis of pleural effusion. The classical signs of pleural effusion on erect chest X-ray are blunting of the costophrenic angle (Fig. 11.9), homogeneous opacification of the lung fields with no air bronchograms, meniscus sign and accentuation of the right minor fissure [10].

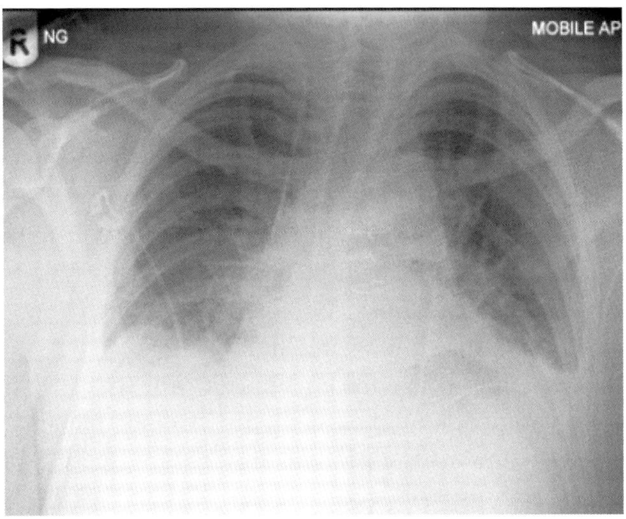

Figure 11.9. Small left-sided pleural effusion with blunting of the costophrenic angle. Median sternotomy, right internal jugular central line and electrocardiogram leads are also present.

On supine chest radiography moderate-to-large pleural effusions may escape detection because the pleural fluid settles posteriorly and no change in the diaphragm or lateral pleural edges may be noted. In these cases, a pleural effusion must be suspected from increased homogeneous density superimposed over the lung fields with preserved vascular markings [11].

In massive effusion there is a complete white-out of the hemithorax with displacement of the mediastinum to the opposite side and flattening or inversion of the ipsilateral hemidiaphragm.

If an effusion is suspected but not clear on plain chest X-ray, ultrasonography should be performed.

11.2.2.7 *Pneumothorax*

On an erect chest radiograph, free air within the pleural space usually collects at the apex. The sharp white line of the displaced visceral pleura separates the retracted lung from the radiolucent pleural space, which is devoid of lung markings (Figs 11.10 and 11.11). A lateral decubitus film with the affected side uppermost is occasionally helpful for a small pneumothorax when an erect radiograph cannot be performed. A horizontal beam shoot through lateral film may be useful in supine patients.

Signs of tension pneumothorax include mediastinal and hilar displacement and depression of the ipsilateral hemidiaphragm (Fig. 11.12).

11.2.2.8 *Pneumonectomy*

Initial chest radiographs after pneumonectomy should demonstrate the trachea close to the midline, slight plethora in the remaining lung, and a postpneumonectomy space that contains gas and fluid (Fig. 11.13). A drainage tube may or may not be present in the space.

Over the next several days, the pneumonectomy space begins to obliterate by accumulation of fluid. The mediastinum either remains stationary or gradually shifts toward the postpneumonectomy space as a result of continuing fluid reabsorption and herniation of the remaining lung across the midline to a position anterior to the heart and aorta.

In the immediate post-operative period, a rapid mediastinal shift toward the non-operated side indicates atelectasis of the lung or an abnormal accumulation of air or fluid in the postpneumonectomy space, most

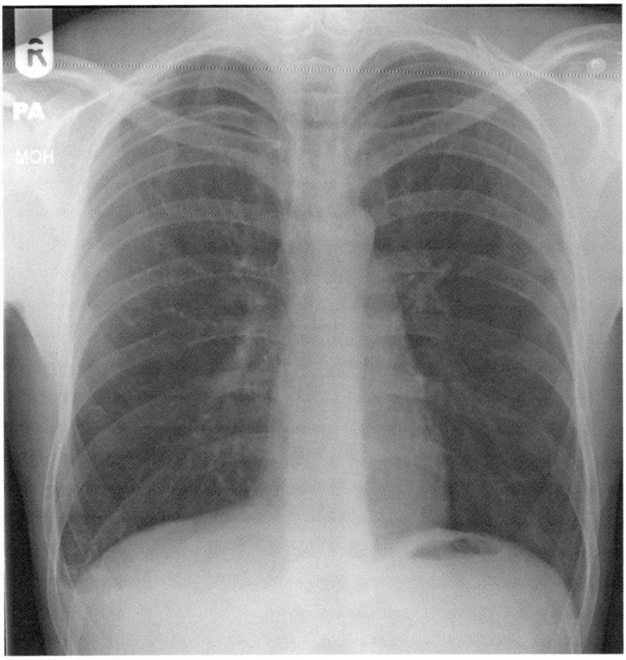

Figure 11.10. Small right apical pneumothorax and a small amount of pleural fluid. The sharp white line of the displaced visceral pleura separates the retracted lung from the radiolucent pleural space, which is devoid of lung markings.

often resulting from a bronchopleural fistula, haemothorax, chylothorax or empyema [12].

11.2.2.9 *Lobectomy*

In the immediate post-operative period after lobectomy, pleural drains are present to prevent pleural fluid accumulation and to maintain negative pressure in the pleural cavity and thus expand the remaining lobes of the lung. A bronchopleural fistula may result in prolonged collection of air in the chest cavity post-operatively.

11.2.2.10 *Cardiac surgery*

Most cardiac surgery is performed through a median sternotomy and wire sutures are often seen on the post-operative radiographs. In the early

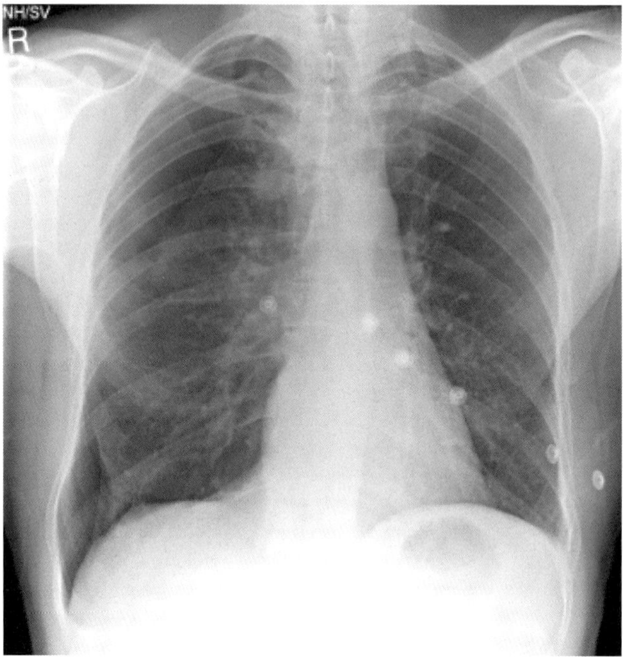

Figure 11.11. Moderate right pneumothorax.

post-operative phase, knowledge of the exact position of the inserted catheters/tubes is important. Small pleural effusions, basal atelectasis and pulmonary congestion indicating either heart failure or overhydration are common. It may be necessary to take lateral decubitus views with a horizontal beam in these patients to evaluate for pleural fluid or pneumothorax.

A widened mediastinum may indicate post-operative bleeding. If the heart shadow increases in size, this may be a sign of a haemopericardium, which may presage cardiac tamponade. Sternal dehiscence and osteomyelitis are diagnosed clinically and alteration in position of the sternal sutures on consecutive films may be suggestive.

11.3 Ultrasound

Many technological developments including increased portability, decreased image acquisition time and improved data resolution have

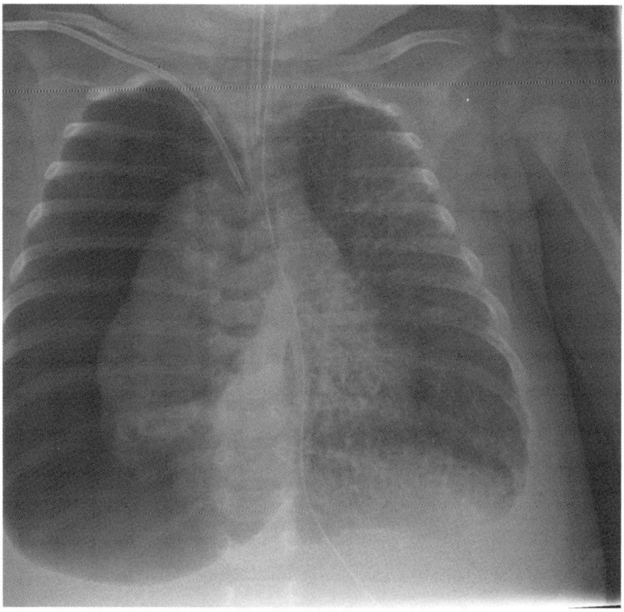

Figure 11.12. Tension pneumothorax in a child. Large right-sided pneumothorax with collapse of the right lung and mediastinal displacement and depression of the ipsilateral hemidiaphragm.

enhanced the utility of ultrasound scanning, supporting its expanding role in the ICU setting [13]. Other advantages include lack of ionising radiation allowing repeatability, easy availability, economy, absence of consumables and reduced risks to patients from transport out of the ICU. Procedures such as drainage and line placement can be performed easily and more safely under ultrasound scanning guidance.

Applications of ultrasound in the ICU include common clinical conditions, including assessment of pleural fluid, renal failure, hydronephrosis, biliary disease, abdominal and pelvic fluid collections, abdominal aortic aneurysm and procedural guidance.

11.3.1 *Thoracic ultrasound*

The most common indication for thoracic imaging in the ICU is the identification and assessment of pleural fluid, volume estimation and guidance of

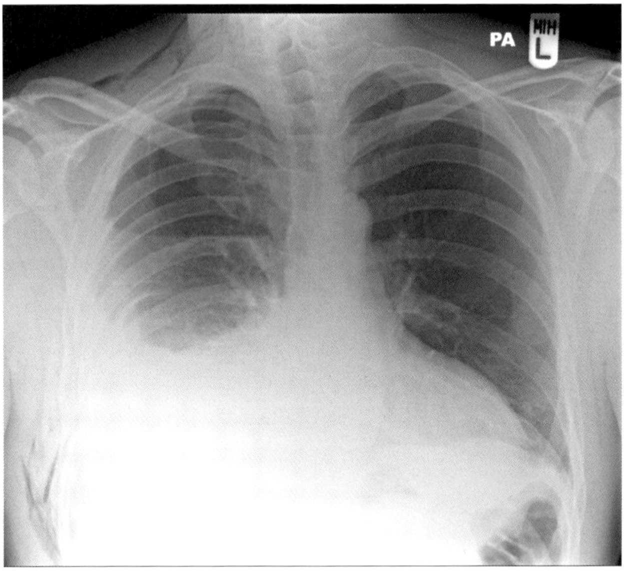

Figure 11.13. Right hydro-pneumothorax and surgical emphysema following a pneumonectomy.

pleural aspiration or drainage. Other indications of thoracic ultrasound in the ICU include identification of pulmonary consolidation, distinction of abnormal lung from pleural disease and identification of pericardial effusions [14].

Optimal upright or lateral decubitus positioning of the patient for optimal quality chest radiographs in the ICU may be difficult. CT provides the gold standard for diagnosis of thoracic disease, but has drawbacks including patient transportation, irradiation and contrast agent exposure. Ultrasound scanning can detect pleural effusions with a sensitivity and specificity of 93% when CT is used as a gold standard.

A pleural effusion is depicted as an anechoic or hypoechoic layer between two pleural layers (Fig. 11.14). The sonographic patterns of pleural effusions are also useful in differentiating a transudate from an exudate: a transudate is almost always echo-free usually, whereas swirling or floating echoes indicate the presence of cells, fibrin, protein or blood particles in an exudate. Exudates can have an anechoic, complex (either complex, septated, or complex, nonseptated), or echogenic appearance [15].

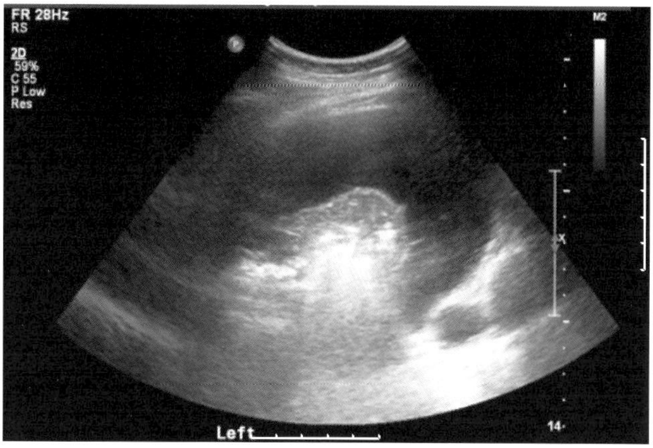

Figure 11.14. Pleural fluid — an anechoic layer between the two layers of pleura with atelectasis of the underlying lung.

Ultrasound scanning can be utilised at the bedside as a real-time imaging technique for thoracocentesis and the placement of pleural drainage catheters. This is especially useful in circumstances where the potential risk for pneumothorax or other complications is high, as in patients on a high level of positive end-expiratory pressure, or those with a small effusion [16]. In the ICU setting, the patient is usually positioned supine or on their side. The operator must check for the absence of interposition of lung, heart, liver or spleen during the respiratory cycle to avoid damage to these organs. Optimally, the patient should remain in the exact same position in which the ultrasound was performed and the drainage procedure should be done straightaway after the marking. Ultrasound scanning can be used to confirm correct positioning of the catheter.

A pneumothorax can be diagnosed by the absence of breath-related movement of the visceral pleura and underlying lung (the 'sliding lung' sign) and specific artefacts ('comet-tail' artefacts) produced by the interface between the pleural layers [17,18]. Stationary reverberation artefacts from the pleura–air interface replacing the normal parietal–visceral pleura interface are another important sign [19].

The most common clinical indication in ICU for assessment of the pericardial space is suspected tamponade. Identification of significant pericardial effusions prior to formal echocardiographic assessment in the ICU setting is a very useful skill [20]. The presence of fluid in this space is detected as an echo-free space. Pericardial fluid is usually easily detected with transthoracic echocardiography; the subcostal view may also be useful in critically ill patients. In addition to assisting in the diagnosis of pericardial effusion and in determining the depth of the effusion, ultrasound can also assist in pericardiocentesis.

11.3.2 *Abdominal ultrasound*

Abdominal ultrasound can assess for global or focal liver, gallbladder, spleen or pancreatic pathology, as well as for appendicitis [21].

Ultrasound scanning is the first-line investigation to diagnose disorders of the gallbladder and biliary tree. Ultrasound scanning has been reported to have a high sensitivity (97–100%), specificity (93.6–100%) and diagnostic accuracy (91–93%) in the diagnosis of gallstones. Gallstones are typically echogenic lesions with posterior acoustic shadowing. In acute cholecystitis, findings may include gallbladder wall thickening, which is considered abnormal when over 3 mm under fasting conditions, mural oedema, mural stratification, pericholecystic fluid, mucosal exfoliation or membranes and the sonographic Murphy's sign. Acalculous cholecystitis shows similar findings in the absence of gallstones (Fig. 11.15). Ultrasound scanning is a good tool for differentiation of obstructive from non-obstructive jaundice, with prediction of the level of biliary obstruction in 80% of cases.

Both diffuse and focal liver diseases can be detected on ultrasound scanning. Ultrasound scanning reveals an irregular surface, coarsened echotexture and decrease in size in cirrhosis. In fatty liver, the parenchyma appears brighter (hyperechoic) than the adjacent right kidney. A liver abscess may appear as a faint hypoechoic solid mass in the initial stages, developing a more mixed echogenicity picture with a central collection of anechoic pus with liquefaction.

An ultrasound scanning examination in ICU may be required for assessment of acute pancreatitis with complications, follow-up of pancreatic pseudocysts, suspected rupture of a pseudocyst or vascular complications including superior mesenteric or portal vein thrombosis and arterial pseudoaneurysms.

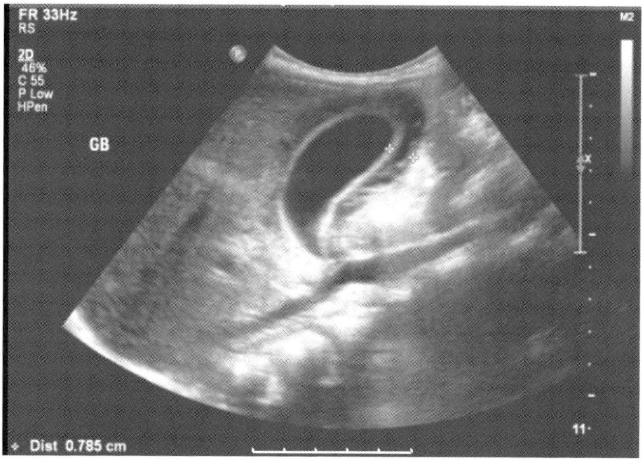

Figure 11.15. Abdominal ultrasound scanning image in a post-operative patient with fever, right upper quadrant (RUQ) pain, leukocytosis and elevation of liver-associated enzymes and bilirubin. There is diffuse thickening of the gallbladder wall in the absence of gallstones, suggestive of acalculous cholecystitis.

The spleen can be evaluated for splenomegaly, commonly seen in cirrhosis, haematological diseases and metabolic diseases. The upper limit of a normal spleen size is reported as 12 cm in long axis. Splenic abscesses are similar in appearance to hepatic abscesses. Multiple hypoechoic nodules in the immunocompromised patient may indicate microabscesses.

Other common indications for ultrasound scanning in the ICU include identification and assessment of abdominal and pelvic fluid collections, differentiating subphrenic from pleural fluid, identification of the cause of abdominal distension, e.g. fluid (see Fig. 11.16), small bowel ileus, bladder distension and masses [22].

Evaluation for intra-abdominal fluid collection or abscess is restricted to areas that are not impeded by gas-filled structures and include the regions around the liver and gallbladder, spleen, kidneys, lateral retroperitoneal areas, lateral gutter and pelvis around the uterus and bladder. Fluid that does not change shape with probe pressure or patient positioning most likely represents a loculated collection (Fig. 11.17). Ultrasound-guided paracentesis can provide a diagnosis when abdominal fluid has an unclear cause [23].

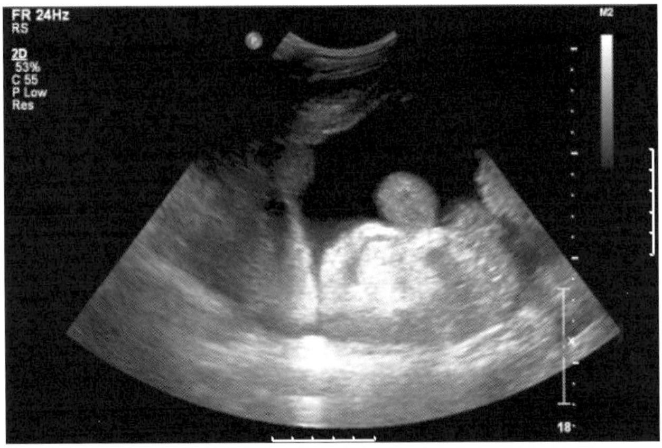

Figure 11.16. Ascites — anechoic fluid in the peritoneal cavity on ultrasound scanning.

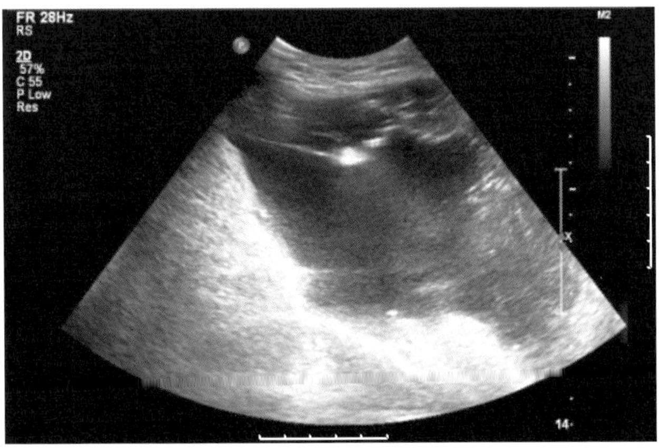

Figure 11.17. A pelvic collection seen as fluid with mobile low-level internal echoes and septations.

The focussed assessment with sonography for trauma (FAST) examination has become routine in the management of blunt abdominal trauma [24]. FAST seeks to determine the presence of fluid in four areas: (i) the subxiphoid region for the pericardial sac, (ii) the right upper quadrant/ Morrison's pouch, (iii) the left upper quadrant in the splenorenal recess, and (iv) the pelvis in the pouch of Douglas or rectovesical space. More novel uses of abdominal sonography include feeding tube placement, diagnosis of pneumoperitoneum, and determination of prandial status.

11.3.3 *Renal ultrasound*

Ultrasound scanning is often used as the initial imaging procedure to identify the cause of acute renal impairment, particularly hydronephrosis [25].

Ultrasound scanning study of the urinary tract includes greyscale evaluation of the renal parenchyma and upper urinary tract, and colour-Doppler for study of the vascularisation. Bipolar length, ranges from 9 to 12 cm and parenchymal thickness between 1.5 and 1.8 cm. Scars appear as outline depressions with rounded angles in a different anatomical distribution from foetal lobulation. Hyperechogenicity of the renal parenchyma, compared with the adjacent hepatic and splenic parenchyma indicates a diffuse parenchymal pathology. In the presence of hydronephrosis, the collecting system becomes visible. Calculi are detected as echogenic structures with characteristic acoustic shadowing.

Renal pathology is frequently associated with changes in parenchymal perfusion, assessed by colour-Doppler vascular renal map, power-Doppler perfusion map, waveform analysis of the intra-renal vessels and venous flow spectral analysis. The most significant semi-quantitative variable to evaluate is the resistive index (RI), given by the ratio between systolic peak velocity — diastolic peak velocity:systolic peak velocity). Values greater than 0.70 are considered abnormal, although major clinical significance is associated with values above 0.80. Acute tubular necrosis, the most common cause of acute renal failure (ARF) results in an increase in the RI.

Assessment of urinary bladder volume can also be very helpful in the evaluation of oligoanuric patients with suspected post renal aetiology.

11.3.4 *Central line placement*

Central venous catheterisation is frequently performed in critically ill patients. Complications related to central venous line placement are most often mechanical (arterial puncture, local hematoma, haemothorax, pneumothorax), infectious (catheter colonisation and related bloodstream infection), and thrombotic.

The use of ultrasound scanning guidance during central venous catheterisation has been well demonstrated to minimise complications, improve the rapidity of catheter placement and decrease the number of failed attempts [26]. Indirect ultrasound guidance uses ultrasound scanning for defining the anatomy, patency and adequacy of the size of the vein before the puncture and needle insertion. Direct ultrasound scanning guidance visualises the needle in real-time throughout the puncture process [27].

11.4 Cranial Imaging in the ICU Patient

11.4.1 *Head injury*

The ability of CT to demonstrate rapidly a surgically correctable lesion, acute bony injury and subarachnoid haemorrhage makes it the modality of choice in the evaluation of acute head injury [28]. Magnetic resonance imaging (MRI) is more sensitive in the detection of diffuse axonal injury and non-haemorrhagic contusions and is the modality of choice in subacute and chronic stages of head injury [29].

11.4.1.1 *Fractures*

Fractures may involve the skull vault, base or both. Depressed fractures can usually be identified with CT (Fig. 11.18). Delineation of a depressed fracture is important as it may be associated with significant injury to the underlying brain (Fig. 11.19). Intracranial air usually indicates traumatic injury to the sinuses or mastoids or a penetrating injury. A fluid level in the paranasal sinuses or mastoid air cells may be the only sign suggesting a basilar skull fracture.

11.4.1.2 *Intracerebral haematoma*

Intracerebral haematomas are differentiated from haemorrhagic contusions in that they are homogenously hyperdense, sharply marginated and surrounded by a rim of decreased density [30]. Considerable mass effect may be present. There may be associated rupture of the haematoma into the ventricular system (Fig. 11.20). Enhancement within or around the haematoma may be evident with intravenous contrast.

11.4.1.3 *Epidural haematoma (EDH)*

Damage to the middle meningeal artery is responsible for most epidural haematoma which are therefore commonly temporo-parietal. Fracture of

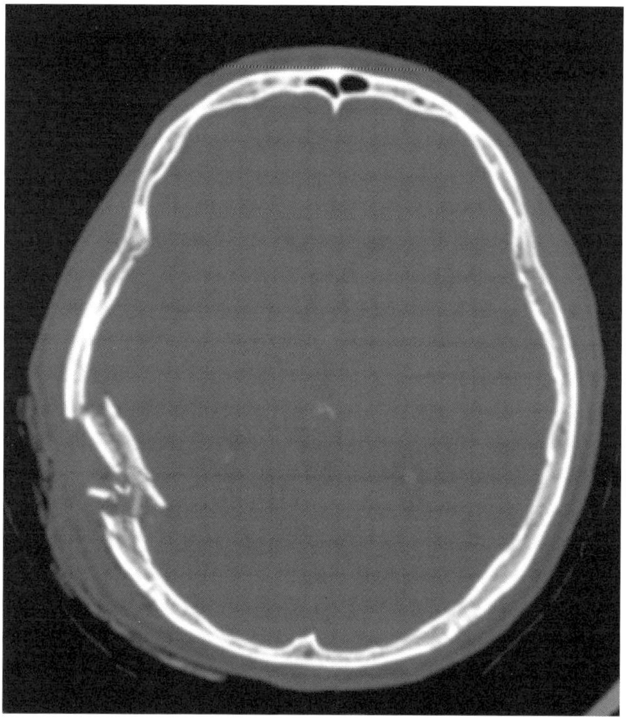

Figure 11.18. Depressed fracture of the right temporal bone.

the adjacent bone is common. EDH are characteristically biconvex or lentiform [31]. An acute EDH is heterogeneous, containing areas of hyperdense blood and isodense serum. Subacute EDH are homogenously hyperdense, consisting of solid blood clot. Chronic EDH are heterogeneous or show decreased attenuation and characteristic enhancing membranes.

Associated mass effect and midline shift are clinically significant. There is often significant mass effect with compression of the ipsilateral lateral ventricle and dilatation of the opposite lateral ventricle due to obstruction of the foramen of Munro. The basal cisterns may be effaced. Transtentorial herniation (the uncus of the temporal lobe is often the first structure to herniate downwards) may be well demonstrated in the coronal plane.

CT and MRI cannot measure the intracranial pressure and can only suggest that the pressure is likely to be raised. A normal brain radiological examination does not exclude raised intracranial pressure, for example

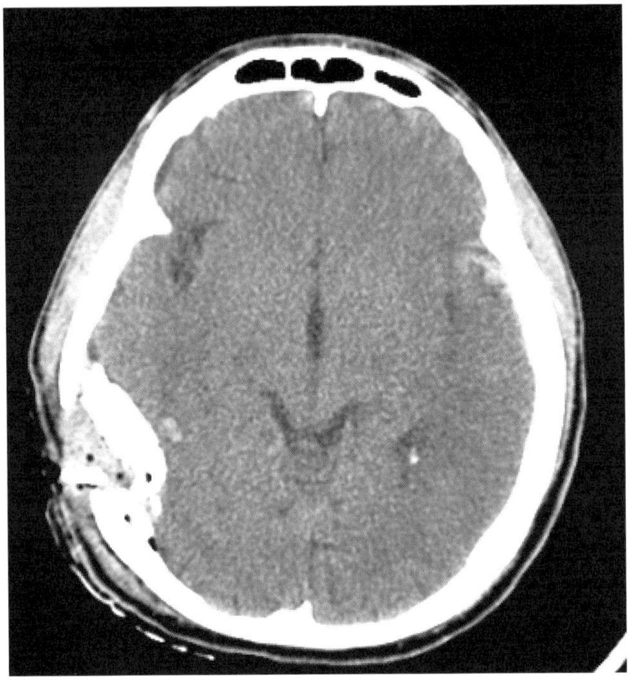

Figure 11.19. The depressed fracture of the right temporal bone shown in Fig. 11.18 is associated with an extra-axial bleed and a haemorrhagic contusion. A subarachnoid bleed in the left Sylvian fissure is also present.

when lumbar puncture is planned, and radiology should be used in conjunction with other clinical features.

11.4.1.4 *Subdural haematoma (SDH)*

Subdural haematoma are most commonly caused by shear forces that result in tearing of the bridging veins. Unlike an epidural haematoma, which is focal, an SDH is diffuse and may overlie an entire cerebral hemisphere. Underlying brain injuries, such as haemorrhagic contusion and oedema, are more frequently associated with SDH. The degree of mass effect may be out of proportion to the size of the SDH and is due to the associated brain oedema and contusions.

The typical appearance of an acute SDH is a hyperdense crescent-shaped collection with a convex lateral border and a concave medial border overlying

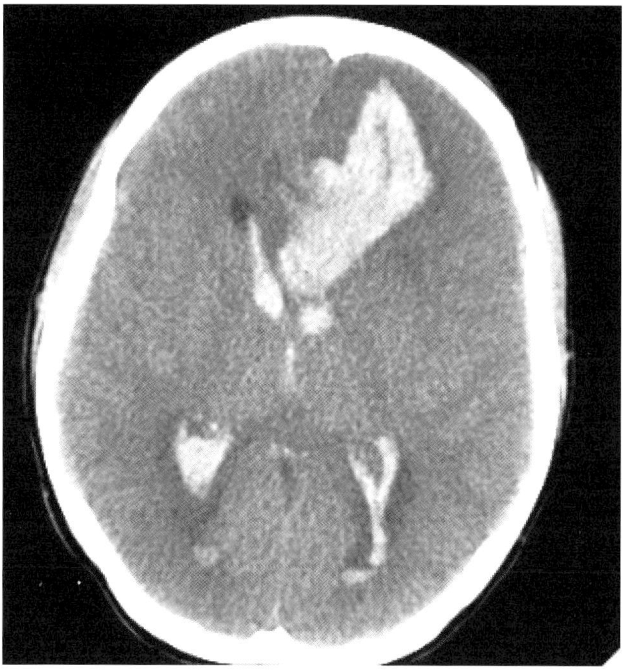

Figure 11.20. Intraparenchymal haematoma in the left frontal lobe with extension of the bleed into the ventricles seen as high attenuation fluid layering in a dependent location.

the cerebral convexity (Fig. 11.21). Effacement of cortical sulci over the cerebral convexity and mass effect on the ventricular system or midline shift indicate the presence of an isodense SDH. SDH may be adjacent to the tentorium cerebelli, in the posterior or anterior interhemispheric fissures.

Chronic SDH are most commonly hypodense on CT. A chronic SDH may appear hyperdense from acute haemorrhage, simulating an acute process. Fluid–fluid levels may be seen as blood products settle in the dependent aspect of the subdural collection.

11.4.1.5 *Subarachnoid haemorrhage (SAH)*

Hyperdensity representing acute haemorrhage is visualised in the sulci overlying the cerebral convexities (Fig. 11.22), in the Sylvian fissures, basal cisterns (Fig. 11.23) and interhemispheric fissure [32]. Contusions appear as areas of heterogeneous increased density mixed with or surrounded by

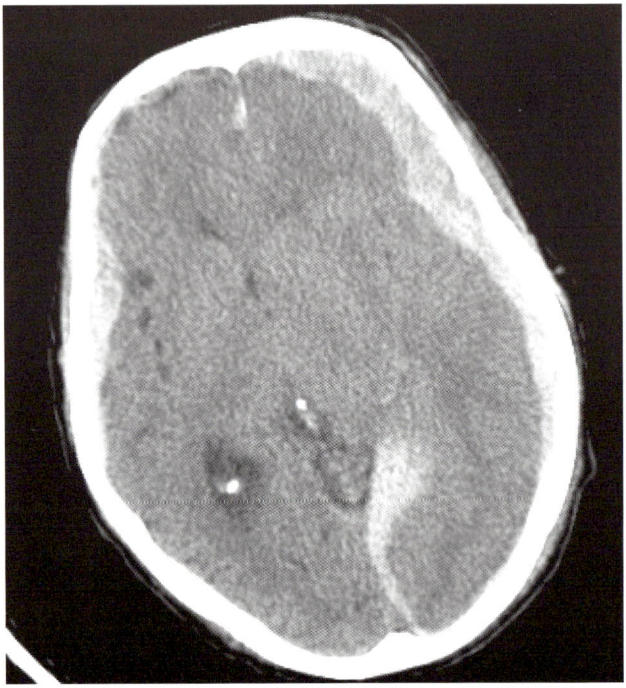

Figure 11.21. Bilateral acute subdural haematomas — concavo-convex, extra-axial high-attenuation areas representing blood subjacent to the skull bones. Extension into the falx cerebelli and mass effect in the form of effacement of the lateral ventricles and midline shift are present.

areas of decreased or normal density (Fig. 11.24). The frontal convexity and the lateral temporal areas are common sites for contrecoup injury. Inferior surface of the frontal and temporal lobes are common sites of contrecoup injuries. MRI studies are more sensitive than CT in the detection of non-haemorrhagic contusions.

11.4.1.6 *Diffuse axonal injury (DAI)*

New MRI techniques are more sensitive than CT in the detection of diffuse axonal injury, but less suited to the acute setting than CT. CT findings include diffuse cerebral swelling, corpus callosal haemorrhage, SAH and intraventricular haemorrhage. Fine petechial haemorrhages at the grey–white matter

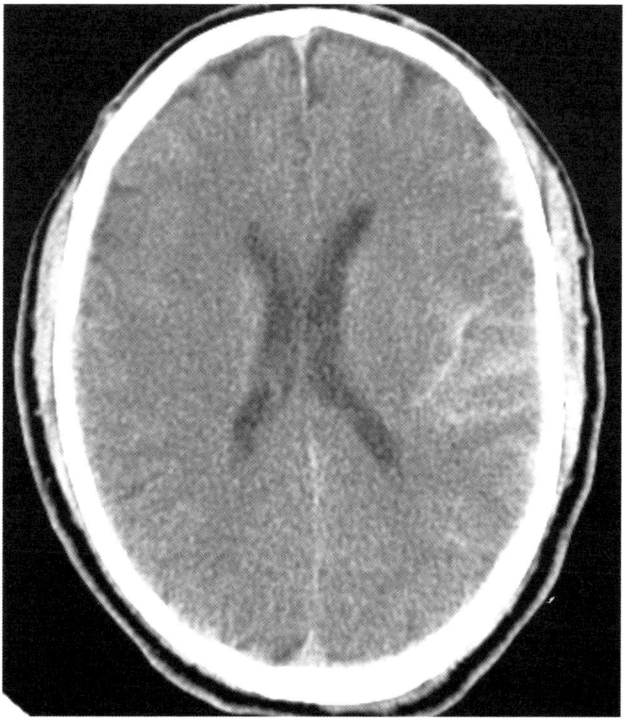

Figure 11.22. Acute subarachnoid haemorrhage -- high attenuation in the left-sided sulci.

junction can sometimes be seen on CT. MRI may show characteristic lesions, in increasing order of injury severity, in the cerebral white matter and grey–white matter junction, corpus callosum, particularly the splenium, and dorsal upper brain stem and cerebellum [33].

11.4.1.7 *Brain swelling and oedema*

Brain swelling and oedema occur commonly in patients with head trauma and are a cause of raised intracranial pressure. Brain swelling is observed more commonly in children. CT findings consist of compression of the lateral and third ventricles and basal cisterns with an associated increase in density of the white matter from transient hyperaemia. Brain oedema is evident as decreased density within and surrounding areas of contusion and intraparenchymal haematoma.

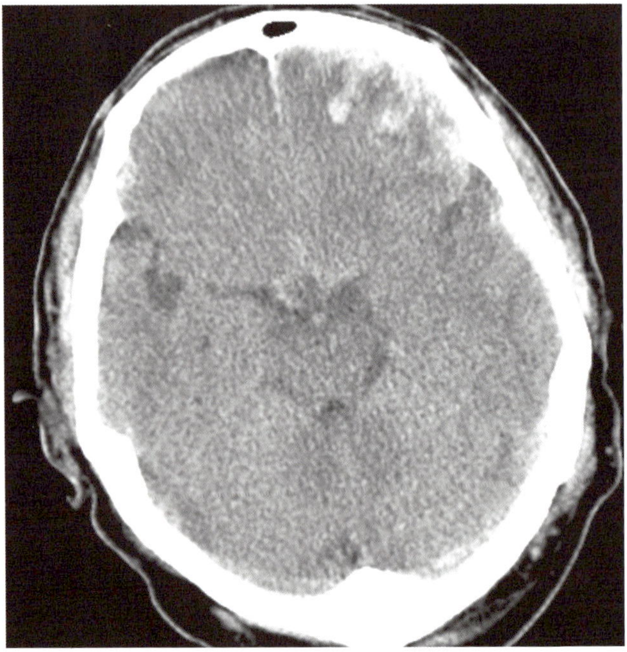

Figure 11.23. Acute subarachnoid haemorrhage seen as high attenuation in the left-sided frontal sulci and in the suprasellar cistern.

11.4.1.8 *MRI in head injury*

Limited availability in acute trauma setting, sensitivity to patient motion, longer imaging time and incompatibility with various medical devices limit the utility of MRI in ICU.

While CT is indicated for detecting injuries requiring a change in treatment, superior depiction of nonsurgical lesions with MRI may affect medical management and predict the degree of neurological recovery.

The soft tissue detail offered by MRI is superior to that from CT for depicting non-haemorrhagic primary lesions such as contusions, for secondary effects of trauma such as oedema and for imaging DAI. Diffusion sequences improve detection of acute infarction associated with head injury. MRI is sensitive for detecting and characterising subacute and chronic haemorrhage.

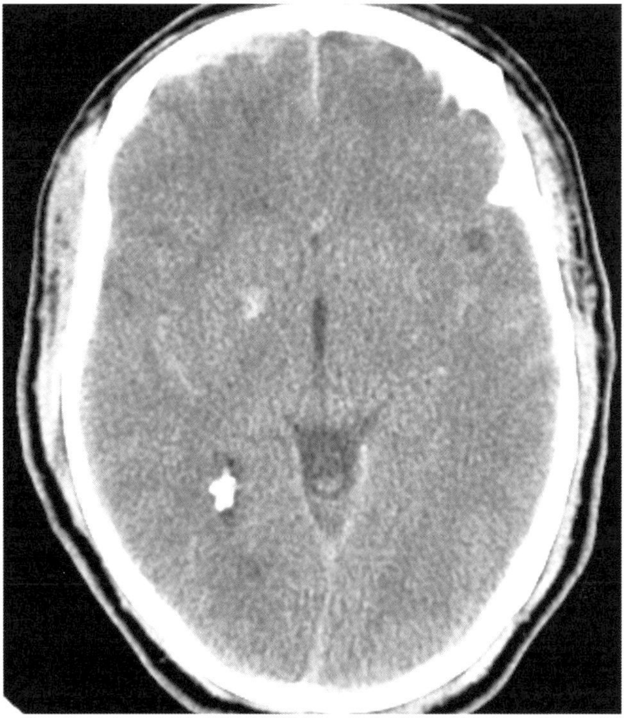

Figure 11.24. A haemorrhagic contusion resulting in an area of increased density in the right basal ganglion. Acute subarachnoid haemorrhage is also present.

11.4.2 *Intracranial infection*

CT and MRI are the modalities of choice in the evaluation of intracranial infection, such as meningitis, encephalitis, ventriculitis, subdural effusion, subdural empyema, epidural empyema and brain abscess [34].

11.4.2.1 *Meningitis*

The role of neuroimaging in meningitis is in the detection of complications such as hydrocephalus, subdural effusion, brain abscess or cerebral infarction [35].

CT is usually normal in uncomplicated meningitis. Unenhanced CT may show obliteration of basal cisterns. Contrast-enhanced CT may show meningeal enhancement in the basal cisterns and Sylvian fissures. MRI may also show obliteration of basal cisterns and is more sensitive for meningeal enhancement. Enhancement can also be seen along the tentorium, falx and convexities, which can be better appreciated with MRI due to its greater contrast resolution.

On CT, a subdural empyema appears as a hypodense or isodense crescentic area adjacent to the inner table of the skull. Enhancement of the medial rim may be seen on contrast-enhanced scan. Empyemas are better visualised with MRI than with CT. Occasionally, gyriform enhancement of the subjacent cortex may be seen, suggesting the presence of concomitant cerebritis.

Epidural empyema is seen as a lentiform hypodense or isodense collection. Contrast enhanced CT or MRI show the inflamed dura in an epidural empyema as a well-demarcated rim of enhancement.

The distinctive feature of a brain abscess is the presence of smooth, thin, uniform capsule which shows enhancement with intravenous contrast with a moderate amount of surrounding cerebral oedema [36]. The enhancement pattern is similar on CT and MRI (Fig. 11.25).

Ventriculitis or ependymitis is indicated by uniform thin ependymal enhancement on contrast-enhanced CT and MRI. Inflammatory debris may be seen within the ventricles.

11.4.2.2 *Encephalitis*

Herpes simplex Type I encephalitis is the most common cause of sporadic encephalitis in adults and characteristically involves the temporal and frontal lobes. CT studies show minimal changes. Unenhanced CT may show hypodense areas with mass effect in both temporal and frontal lobes. Sparing of the lentiform nucleus is said to be characteristic. Streaky linear enhancement may be seen in the region of the Sylvian fissures.

MRI is more sensitive than CT and shows hypointensity on longitudinal-relaxation-time-weighted (T1W) images and hyperintensity on transverse-relaxation-time-weighted (T2W) images [37].

Lack of basal ganglia involvement despite involvement of the adjacent internal capsule is common and may be one means of distinguishing Herpes simplex 1 encephalitis from other entities (e.g. infarction) and

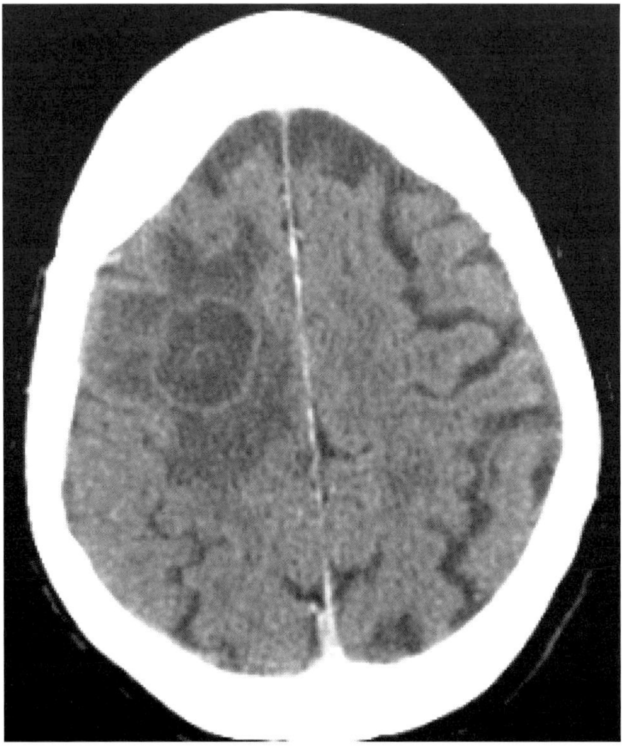

Figure 11.25. A brain abscess — a ring-enhancing lesion on CT with low-attenuation in the white matter representing perilesional oedema.

other forms of encephalitis. Herpes simplex 1 encephalitis can further be distinguished from infarction because encephalitis frequently involves both the medial and lateral aspects of the temporal lobe and involves territory supplied by both the middle cerebral artery and the posterior cerebral artery.

11.4.3 *Stroke and other conditions*

Although MRI is more sensitive than CT in the setting of acute stroke, CT is widely available and likely to remain the most commonly used investigation for hyperacute stroke [38]. An urgent CT is needed to differentiate between ischaemic and primary intracerebral haemorrhagic stroke.

11.4.3.1 *Ischaemic stroke*

Early CT signs of ischaemic stroke include hyperattenuation of an artery which represents acute thrombus within a segment of a cerebral vessel, hypoattenuation in the involved territory, loss of grey–white matter differentiation, loss of the insular ribbon, obscuration of the lentiform nucleus, hypoattenuation of basal ganglia and cortical sulcal effacement [39].

Diffusion-weighted imaging (DWI) on MRI has the highest sensitivity and specificity for acute cerebral infarction. Restricted diffusion in acute infarction returns high signal on DWI and appears dark on the apparent diffusion coefficient (ADC) maps.

11.4.3.2 *Hypertensive bleed*

Hypertensive haemorrhage is the most common cause of nontraumatic intracerebral haemorrhage in adults. Typical hypertensive haemorrhages are found in the basal ganglia and appear as hyperdense foci with surrounding hypodense oedema. Differential diagnosis includes haemorrhage within a tumour, haemorrhagic transformation of an infarct and bleeding from a vascular malformation. Marked enhancement and peritumoural oedema are seen in haemorrhage within a tumour. Contrast enhanced scans show the vessels in an arteriovenous malformation (AVM).

11.4.3.3 *Venous thrombosis*

Occlusion of venous structures may lead to focal cerebral infarction, the location and extent of which are much more variable compared with strokes from arterial occlusion. Haemorrhage is frequently associated with venous infarction and is frequently cortical or subcortical in location.

The most frequent cerebral vein to thrombose is the sagittal sinus. Unenhanced CT may show a strongly hyperdense triangle in the area of the sinus (dense triangle sign). The empty delta sign (an unenhanced central portion of the affected sinus after administration of contrast material) is the best and most frequently seen CT sign of sagittal sinus thrombosis. Thrombosed cortical veins may be seen as linear hyperintense areas (cord sign). CT venography and magnetic resonance (MR) venography offer greater sensitivity and specificity than routine contrast-enhanced CT in the diagnosis of dural sinus thrombosis. Advantages of CT venography include easier patient monitoring in critically ill patients and shorter time to diagnosis in the initial work up of the patient.

11.4.3.4 *Posterior reversible encephalopathy syndrome (PRES)*

This syndrome is known by other names such as hypertensive encephalopathy and reversible posterior leukoencephalopathy syndrome [40]. The syndrome typically occurs in acute elevation of systemic blood pressure, in preeclampsia or eclampsia, or after treatment with a variety of immunosuppressive agents (e.g., cyclosporin A, cisplatin, FK-501, and tacrolimus).

Various neurological conditions, like stroke, intracranial haemorrhage, venous thrombosis and encephalitis, can mimic hypertensive encephalopathy.

Characteristic findings include areas of reversible hypodensity on CT and increased signal on T2W MR images, usually localised to the cortex and subcortical white matter in the occipital lobes. Non-specific imaging features include diffuse or focal oedema in the supratentorial white matter.

11.4.3.5 *Central pontine myelinolysis (CPM)*

Most patients with this disorder have a history of alcoholism associated with hyponatremia. Although CT may show central pontine hypodensity, MRI is much more sensitive [41]. A low-intensity lesion in the central pons on T1W images and a triangle or trident shaped, central pontine hyperintensity on T2W images is characteristic.

11.5 Computed Tomography of the Chest in the ICU Patient

CT body scanning is increasingly being used in diagnosis and for therapeutic procedures in the critically ill. CT is extremely helpful in patients whose clinical course is not explained by the available information or whose chest radiographs are difficult to interpret [42]. Clinical indications for CT in this setting include characterisation of pulmonary parenchymal and pleural disease, mediastinal abnormalities including mediastinitis, mediastinal abscess, abnormal or unusual fluid or air collections, pulmonary embolism and tube-malpositioning. CT may also be used for increased precision in percutaneous drainage and aspiration for loculated or otherwise difficult pneumothoraces or fluid collections [43].

11.5.1 *Intrathoracic sepsis*

CT may be useful in ICU patients with sepsis of unknown origin, identifying the source of fever within the thorax or abdomen in nearly 20% of patients. Chest CT has proven particularly effective in documenting the nature of suppurative lung disease [44]. The differentiation between lung abscess and empyema has important therapeutic consequences. Cross-sectional images demonstrate abscesses as round, thick-walled cavities in areas of destroyed lung. Bronchi and pulmonary vessels terminate abruptly at the advancing wall of an abscess. Abscesses have an irregular luminal width and irregular luminal margins. Empyemas usually have obtuse angles with the chest wall, lenticular shape and uniform wall characteristics and compress the adjacent lung. The most reliable radiographic feature of an empyema is the 'split pleura sign', namely thickened, separated visceral and parietal pleural surfaces which show contrast enhancement of the thickened, hypervascular pleural surfaces.

11.5.2 *Pleural effusion and empyema*

Upright or lateral decubitus positioning of the patient for optimal quality chest radiographs in the ICU may be difficult. The supine chest radiograph is only moderately sensitive and specific for the detection of pleural fluid. Ultrasound remains the first line for further investigation of pleural fluid collections with the advantage of being rapidly available at the bedside.

However, CT provides a superior modality [45] in circumstances where ultrasound is not easily performed (for example, patients with multiple dressings or open wounds), or when the presence of effusions is one of several diagnostic questions, in the presence of complex pleuro-parenchymal disease, or to define the location and extent of loculated pleural collections (Fig. 11.26).

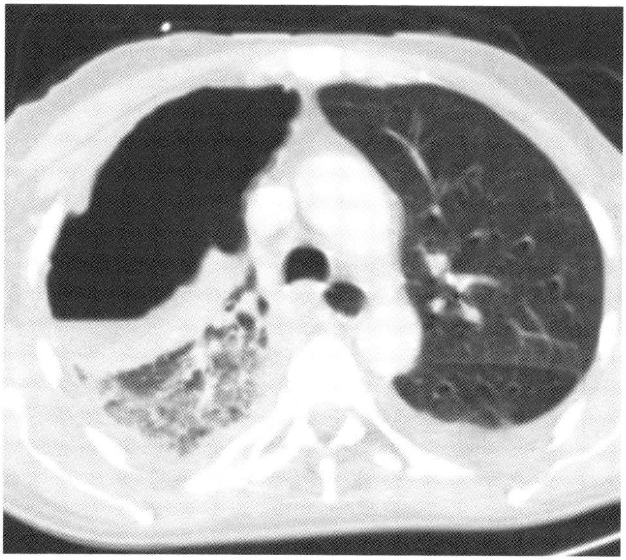

Figure 11.26. Loculated pneumothorax in the right upper chest (lung window settings).

Pleural enhancement with intravenous contrast medium suggests an exudative process, such as haemorrhage, empyema, or tumour [46]. Furthermore, CT is far superior in quantifying effusions as compared with the chest radiograph. Fluid collections are considered loculated if CT shows pleural adhesions, a convex inner margin, a nondependent collection, or a collection that did not conform to the normal crescentic shape of the pleural space. CT provides a more accurate evaluation of the size and location of pleural effusions and is extremely helpful in the guidance of catheters into loculated fluid collections.

11.5.3 *Septic pulmonary emboli*

Another form of thoracic infection that should be considered in ICU patients is septic pulmonary emboli. ICU patients are at risk due to indwelling vascular catheters. Although chest radiographic characteristics of septic pulmonary emboli have been well documented, most findings are non-specific or equivocal. CT findings include patchy subpleural alveolar or nodular opacities with a tendency for cavitation (Fig. 11.27), the 'feeding vessel sign' and pleural effusions [47,48].

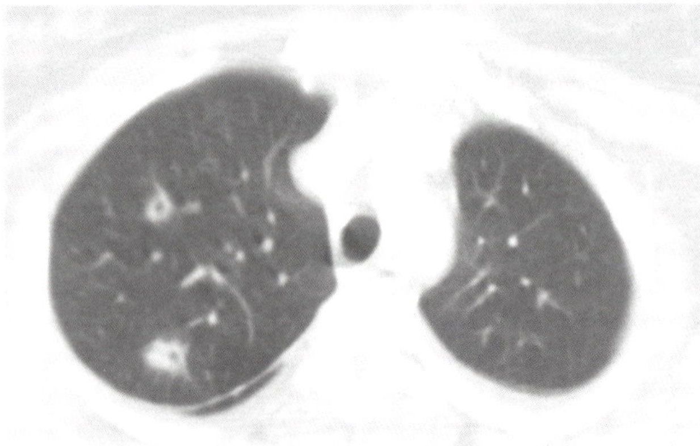

Figure 11.27. Septic emboli — multiple cavitating lesions in an intravenous-drug user.

11.5.4 *Chest trauma*

Injuries to the thoracic cage may be complicated by pneumothorax, pulmonary contusion, pneumomediastinum, mediastinal emphysema, pneumopericardium or mediastinal haemorrhage.

Pulmonary contusion appears as patchy, non-segmental consolidation. Pulmonary lacerations may appear as round thin-walled cystic spaces, which may show a fluid level.

Pneumomediastinum (Fig. 11.28), the presence of air between the tissue planes of the mediastinum, may occur as a result of pulmonary interstitial emphysema, perforation of the trachea, bronchus, oesophagus, or penetrating chest injury. In pneumopericardium, gas does not extend beyond the aortic root or beyond the main pulmonary artery.

The commonest radiographic findings of acute aortic rupture are widening of the mediastinum and obscuration of the aortic knuckle. CT has a very high negative predictive value for aortic rupture.

11.5.5 *Pneumothorax*

Pneumothorax is a frequent complication in patients with severe respiratory disease being ventilated mechanically. CT is the reference standard for the detection of pneumothoraces, because it is the most sensitive and specific modality in this clinical setting. The CT criteria for a diagnosis of

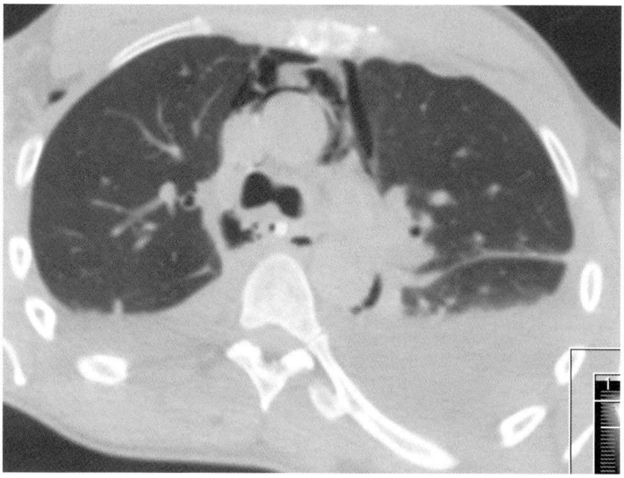

Figure 11.28. Streaks of air in the mediastinum typical of pneumomediastinum.

pneumothorax include any air collections that are displacing the visceral pleura from the chest wall (Fig. 11.29). CT may be indicated in the diagnosis and management of loculated pneumothoraces. In patients with minimal pulmonary reserve, even a small pneumothorax can have adverse haemodynamic effects. The most common locations for loculated pneumothoraces are anteromedial and subpulmonic.

CT-guided percutaneous catheter drainage provides accurate, safe and effective treatment for loculated thoracic air collections and obviates surgical intervention in critically ill, high-risk patients.

11.5.6 *Post-sternotomy complications*

CT has an integral role as an aid in evaluating and characterising post-sternotomy complications, classified by compartment as presternal, sternal, and retrosternal. CT can reveal the extent and depth of infection, which influences whether treatment is surgical or medical, and, if surgical, the type of surgery to be performed [49].

Infection in the presternal compartment manifests as stranding, sinus tracts or frank abscess. CT can help detect sternal complications such as dehiscence, paramedian sternotomy, and osteomyelitis. CT findings of

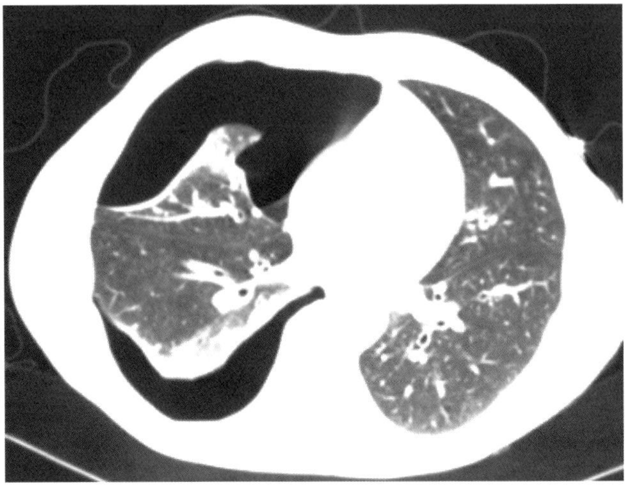

Figure 11.29. Tension pneumothorax. Large pneumothorax (with collapse of the underlying lung which shows crowding of bronchovascular markings) and mediastinal shift.

dehiscence include displaced sternal wires and progressive widening of the incisional gap. Retrosternal complications include mediastinitis, mediastinal abscess, pericardial effusion, hematoma, loculated effusion, and empyema.

Obliteration of mediastinal fat planes and diffuse soft-tissue infiltration with or without gas collections are suggestive of mediastinitis (Fig. 11.30). Frank abscesses are usually of low density and may contain gas.

11.5.7 *Pulmonary embolism*

CT pulmonary angiography (CTPA) is now an established test in the diagnosis of suspected PE [50]. Acute PE is principally diagnosed by visualising a low attenuation filling defect within a well-opacified pulmonary artery (Fig. 11.31). Other CT findings include the 'railway track sign', the vessel cut-off sign and the rim sign, where there is a filling defect due to thrombus with a rim of contrast around it (Fig. 11.32). Ancillary findings include pleural effusions, atelectasis and pulmonary infarcts.

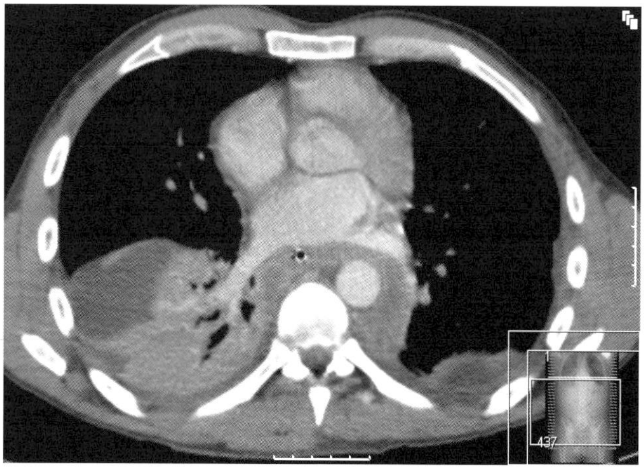

Figure 11.30. Mediastinal collection along with bilateral pleural fluid and right-sided consolidation.

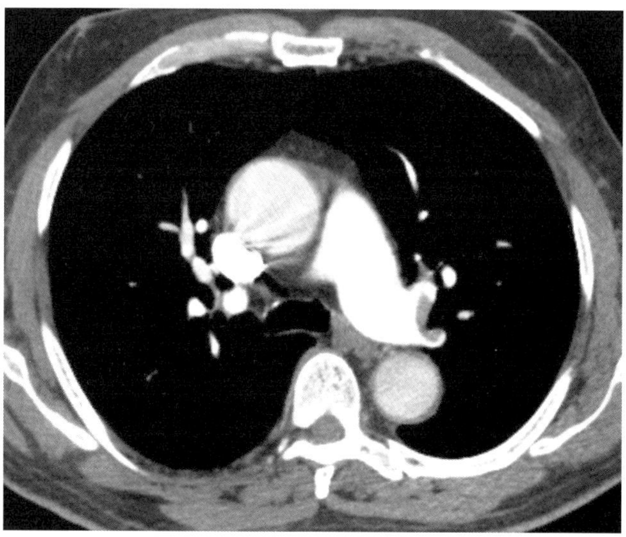

Figure 11.31. Acute pulmonary embolism seen as filling defect in the left pulmonary artery with extension into the left upper lobe pulmonary artery.

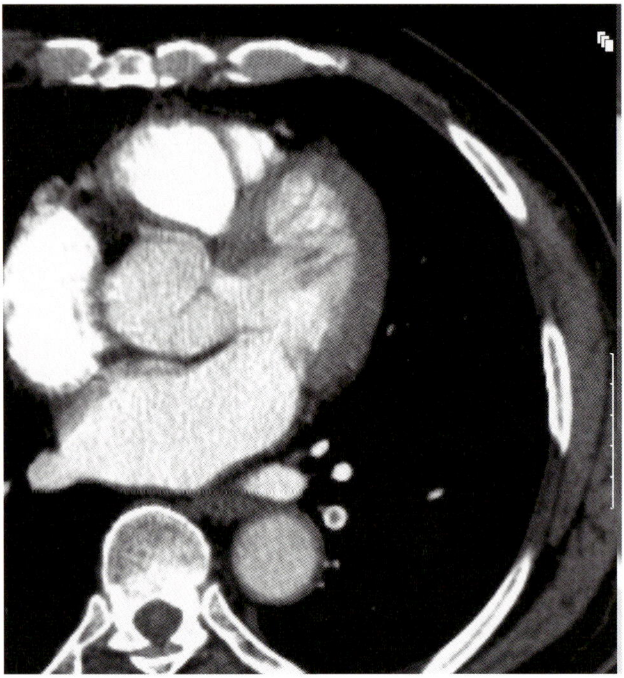

Figure 11.32. Acute pulmonary embolism — central filling defect 'rim sign' in a segmental left lower lobe pulmonary artery.

11.5.8 *Aortic dissection*

CT in acute non-cardiac chest pain is usually requested to diagnose aortic dissection but a spectrum of other cardiovascular diseases may simulate this [51]. These include acute intramural aortic haematoma, leaking aortic aneurysm, atherosclerotic ulcer, pericarditis and pulmonary embolus.

The CT characteristics of classic acute dissection are a double lumen with intervening intimal flap (70%) (Fig. 11.33), internal displacement of calcified intima (17%), compression or distortion of the true lumen and haematoma within the pericardium, mediastinum or pleural space. Dissection originates at sites of maximum intimal stress. Approximately two-thirds arise on the anterior wall of the ascending aorta within 4 cm of the aortic valve.

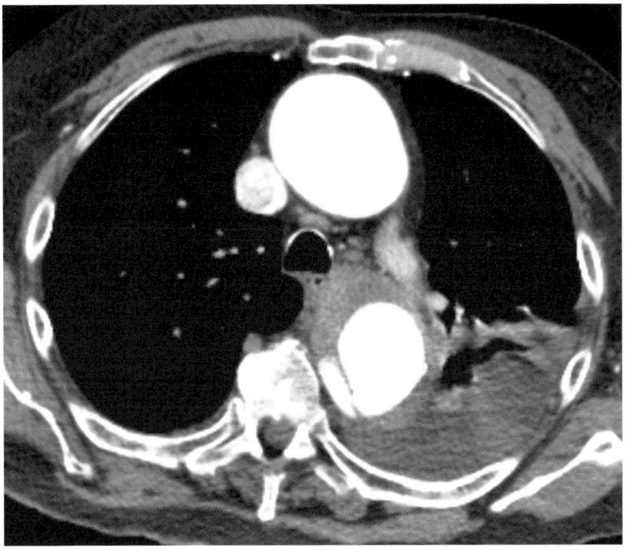

Figure 11.33. Aortic dissection seen as a double lumen with intervening intimal flap, compression or distortion of the true lumen and an associated left pleural effusion.

11.5.9 *Acute respiratory distress syndrome*

CT is useful in patients with ARDS who are not improving or are deteriorating clinically, by identifying pleural effusions, lung abscess, lobar atelectasis, barotrauma (interstitial pulmonary emphysema, pneumothorax, pneumomediastinum, pneumopericardium and subcutaneous emphysema) secondary to mechanical ventilation and malpositioned lines and tubes, [52], all more accurately than chest radiographs. Ground glass opacity, consolidation and a reticular pattern are hallmarks of ARDS on CT. A ventral to dorsal gradient of lung attenuation is typical (Fig. 11.34), with the anterior or most non-dependent lung being normal or near normal, the mid-third of the lung in the ventral to dorsal direction showing ground glass in attenuation and consolidation in the most dependent lung.

11.5.10 *Acute interstitial pneumonitis*

Acute interstitial pneumonitis should be suspected in patients diagnosed initially with severe diffuse bilateral community-acquired pneumonia that does not respond to antibiotics and from whom no infectious organism is

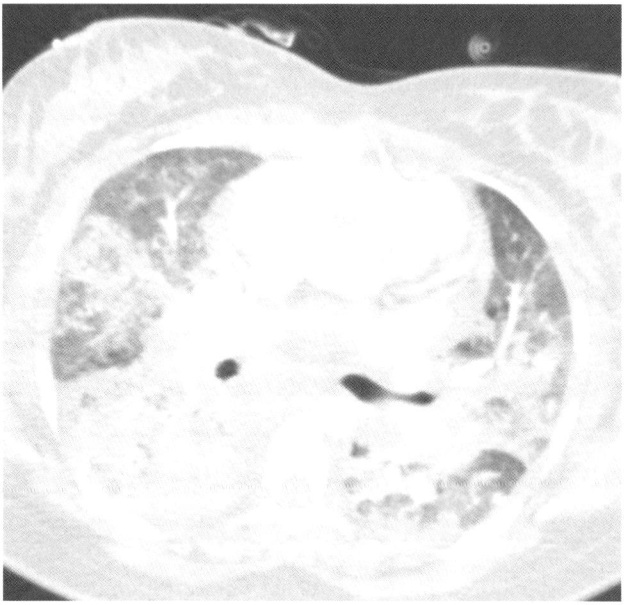

Figure 11.34. Diffuse ground-glass change and consolidation in a patient with ARDS.

isolated. Absence of a known cause and absence of systemic involvement distinguish it from ARDS. CT shows bilateral areas of ground glass opacity and air space consolidation with traction bronchiectasis and honeycombing in patients with prolonged disease.

11.5.11 *Chest tube malposition*

A chest tube may be placed into the pleural space for various pleural disorders including pneumothorax, penetrating chest injuries, haemothorax, empyema and bronchopleural fistula. CT is indicated when a chest tube does not drain adequately and the chest radiograph is non-contributory. CT is extremely accurate in evaluating the position of a malpositioned chest tube [53].

In an intraparenchymal location, the tube is seen traversing the lung and there may be associated haematomas due to lung laceration. Intrafissural tube placement is identified with the tube located in the region of a fissure without areas of parenchymal opacity around it. When a tube tip is positioned outside the parietal pleura, it is considered to be in the chest wall. A chest tube inserted too far may be seen abutting the mediastinum (mediastinal tube placement) (Fig. 11.35) with potential complications including perforation of the heart, pulmonary artery and oesophagus [54]. Extrathoracic placements of a chest tube can also be visualised on CT.

CT scanning for ICU patients generally requires transportation to the radiology department with the logistical difficulties of maintaining life support systems during transportation. Mobile or portable CT scanners are available and offer the potential to image patients without removing them from the ICU environment with a modest but acceptable sacrifice in image quality. Portable CT scanners are currently not capable of performing fast CT angiographic examinations, as required for suspected pulmonary embolism or vascular emergencies.

11.6 Computed Tomography of the Abdomen in the ICU Patient

CT is widely used for the evaluation and follow-up of a variety of intra-abdominal conditions and complications that may be encountered in the intensive care unit setting.

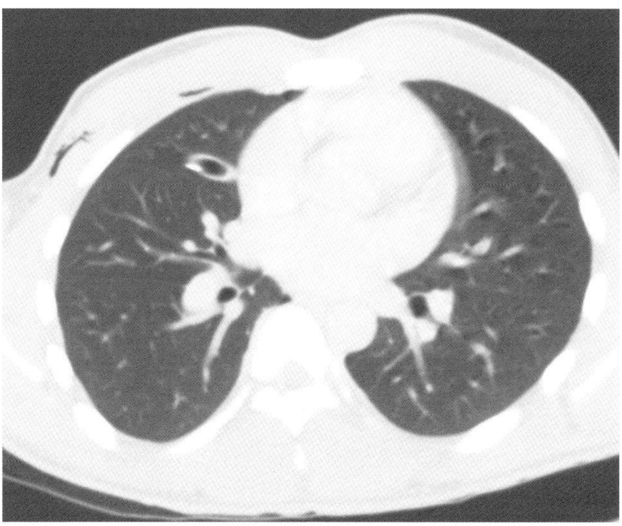

Figure 11.35. Malpositioned chest drain within 1 cm of the mediastinum posing a risk of injury to mediastinal structures.

11.6.1 *Acute pancreatitis*

Contrast-enhanced CT is the imaging procedure of choice in the initial evaluation and follow-up of patients with suspected pancreatitis [55].

CT findings in uncomplicated acute pancreatitis include a generalised or focal increase in the size of the pancreas, and an irregular contour with peripancreatic inflammatory fat stranding. As pancreatitis progresses, fluid collections can accumulate within the pancreas or around the gland. Many collections spontaneously resolve, but some develop into pseudocysts, which may be intrapancreatic or peripancreatic. The capsule of the pseudocyst can show significant enhancement following intravenous contrast. CT is valuable in helping determine the optimal pathway for pseudocyst drainage where appropriate [56].

11.6.1.1 *CT grading of acute pancreatitis*

Grade A: normal pancreas.

Grade B: focal or diffuse enlargement of the pancreas (including contour irregularities, non homogeneous attenuation of the gland, dilatation of the pancreatic duct, and foci of small fluid collections within the gland).

Grade C: intrinsic pancreatic abnormalities associated with haziness and streaky densities representing inflammatory changes in the peripancreatic fat (Fig. 11.36).

Grade D: single, ill-defined fluid collection (phlegmon) (Fig. 11.37).

Grade E: two or more poorly-defined fluid collections, or presence of gas in or adjacent to the pancreas.

11.6.1.2 *CT severity index of acute pancreatitis*

Management of patients with acute pancreatitis is based on the initial assessment of disease severity. The CT severity index (Table 11.1) [57], which combines the CT grading of acute pancreatitis with the degree of pancreatic necrosis, has shown an excellent correlation with the development of local complications and the incidence of death in this population.

Severe acute pancreatitis (necrotising pancreatitis) occurs in about 20–30% of all patients with acute pancreatitis, and is characterised by a

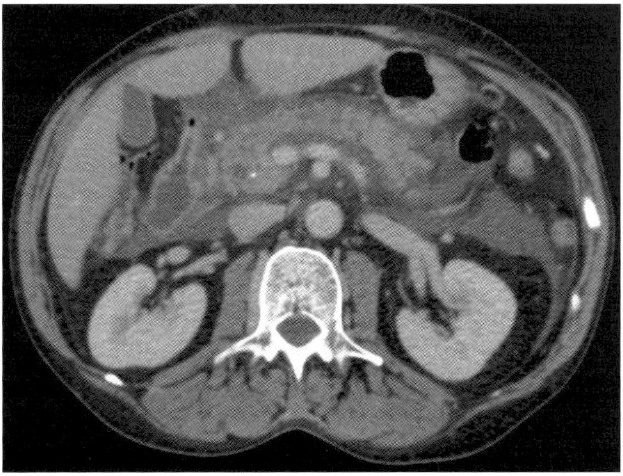

Figure 11.36. Intrinsic pancreatic abnormalities (diffuse enlargement of the pancreas with dilatation of the pancreatic duct, and foci of calcification along with inflammatory changes in the peripancreatic fat.

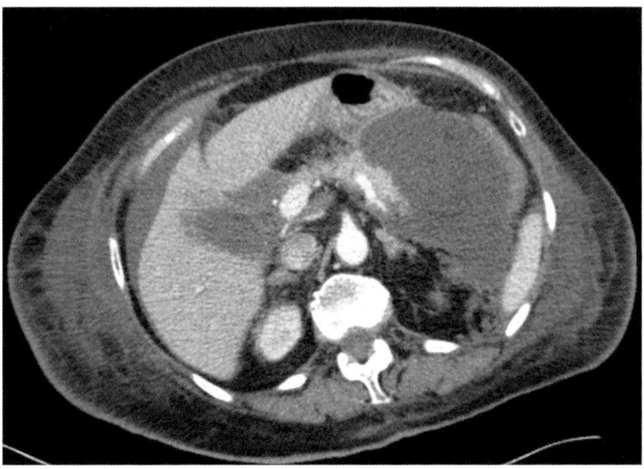

Figure 11.37. Single, ill-defined fluid collection (phlegmon) in the pancreatic tail in acute pancreatitis.

Table 11.1. CT severity index.

CT Grade	Points	Necrosis %	Additional points	CTseverity index*
A	0	0	0	0
B	1	0	0	1
C	2	<30	2	4
D	3	30–50	4	7
E	4	>50	6	10

*CT grade points are added to points assigned for percentage of necrosis.

protracted clinical course, a high incidence of local complications and a high mortality rate. Moreover, virtually all life-threatening complications occur in patients with necrotising pancreatitis.

Accepted criteria for the CT diagnosis of pancreatic necrosis have been defined as focal or diffuse zones of non-enhancing pancreatic parenchyma during contrast-enhanced CT.

11.6.2 *Biliary tract sepsis*

In the absence of sepsis, ultrasound scanning is the procedure of choice in screening for biliary colic and may direct further studies including endoscopic retrograde cholangio-pancreatography (ERCP) and magnetic resonance cholangio-pancreatography (MRCP).

The diagnosis of acute cholangitis is mainly based on symptoms, physical findings and laboratory data. Imaging studies, such as ultrasound scanning or CT, [58] are used for evaluation of the site and cause of biliary obstruction, the degree of biliary dilatation and the presence or absence of hepatic abscess (Fig. 11.38) to plan precise treatment.

Dilated ducts are seen as multiple, branching, tubular round or oval low-density structures which course towards the porta hepatis. A diameter of the common bile duct in excess of 8 mm is suggestive of obstruction. Patients who have had cholecystectomy may have a common bile duct diameter in excess of 8 mm in the absence of obstruction.

Early inhomogenous enhancement of the liver is frequently seen in patients with acute cholangitis in the early phase on dynamic CT, and this finding is no longer present after treatment.

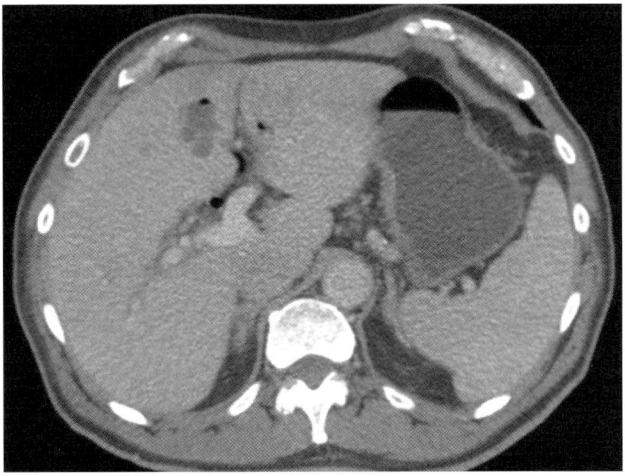

Figure 11.38. Contrast-enhanced CT shows air within the biliary tree (pneumobilia) and an irregular collection with intralesional air and enhancing walls in the left lobe. The findings are suggestive of ascending cholangitis with liver abscess formation in this septic patient.

11.6.3 *Acute pyelonephritis*

Imaging may be required for complicated pyelonephritis to investigate the possibility of an abscess or obstruction. Ultrasound scanning or CT may be suitable, although generally ultrasound scanning is less sensitive than CT.

In severe pyelonephritis, CT may show a diffuse or focal enlargement of the kidney with abnormal enhancement, with a striated nephrogram (Fig. 11.39) seen as wedge-and-band-shaped areas of reduced enhancement. Associated inflammatory stranding in the perinephric fat planes is usually present. Complications include subcapsular or perinephric abscess formation (Fig. 11.40).

Emphysematous pyelonephritis (EPN) occurs almost exclusively in patients with diabetes mellitus, but occasionally in patients without diabetes mellitus with urinary tract obstruction. With the more extensive use of CT in the evaluation of patients with signs and symptoms of sepsis or complicated urinary tract obstruction, more cases of emphysematous pyelonephritis are being recognised.

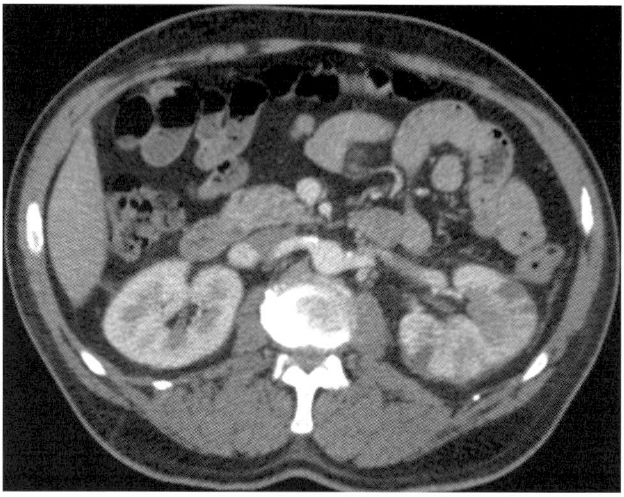

Figure 11.39. Focal pyelonephritis with a striated nephrogram seen as wedge and band shaped areas of reduced enhancement.

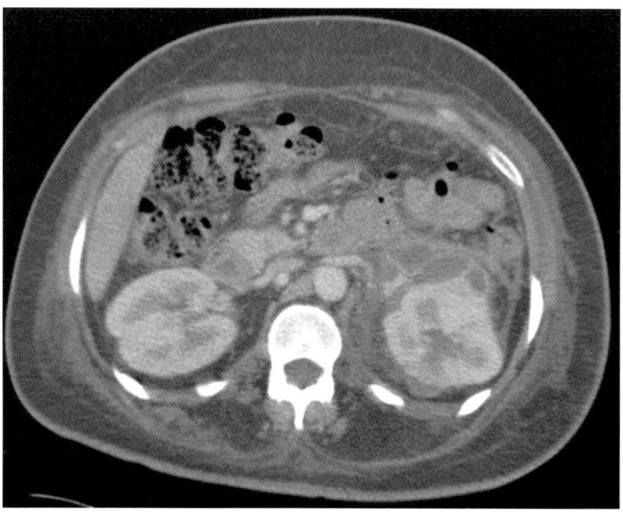

Figure 11.40. Anterior and posterior subcapsular collections and thickening of surrounding fasciae in pyelonephritis.

CT may show localised EPN with gas in the collecting system only or gas in the renal parenchyma (Fig. 11.41). Extensive EPN is seen as extension of gas or abscess to the extrarenal space, bilateral EPN or EPN in a solitary kidney. Imaging may be used for percutaneous catheter drainage for localised EPN or in extensive EPN in low-risk patients.

11.6.4 *Urinary tract obstruction*

Unenhanced spiral CT is the technique of choice in the investigation of ureteric colic. A ureteric calculus is diagnosed as a high-attenuation focus on CT. Calculi are localised as either renal, or proximal-, middle- or distal ureteric, and their maximum diameter can be measured in millimetres. Essentially all urinary tract calculi are radio-opaque.

Hydronephrosis is a frequent, but not invariable, accompaniment to urinary tract obstruction. Perirenal and periureteric stranding is often present. CT may be used in percutaneous drainage of the obstructed urinary tract.

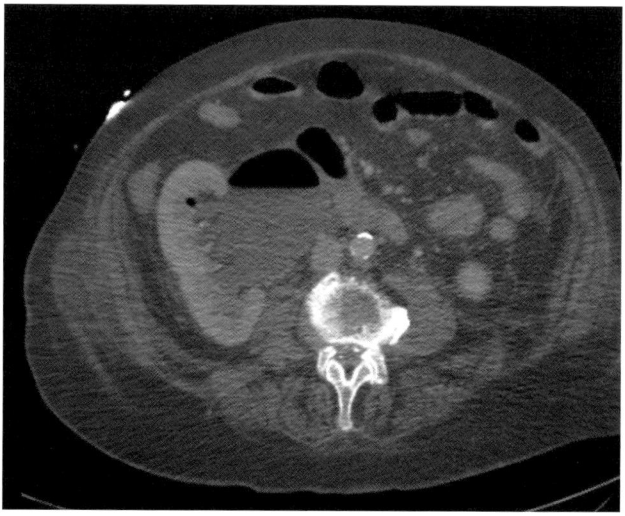

Figure 11.41. Emphysematous pyelonephritis with dependent, layering debris and an air-debris level within a dilated pelvis.

11.6.5 *Appendicitis*

CT has high accuracy for the non-invasive assessment of patients with suspected appendicitis [59].

One of the CT hallmarks of acute appendicitis is appendiceal enlargement (outer-wall to outer-wall transverse diameter greater than 6 mm) (Fig. 11.42). Additional appendiceal signs include appendiceal wall thickening (wall ≥3 mm), appendiceal wall hyperenhancement, mural stratification of the appendiceal wall, appendicolith and intramural gas. Associated findings on CT include caecal thickening and periappendiceal fat stranding.

Complications include perforation (Fig. 11.43), periappendiceal abscess, phlegmon, peritonitis and bowel obstruction, which can also be evaluated with CT.

11.6.6 *Bowel obstruction*

A number of studies have demonstrated the superiority of CT in revealing the site, level and cause of obstruction and in demonstrating signs of lack of bowel viability.

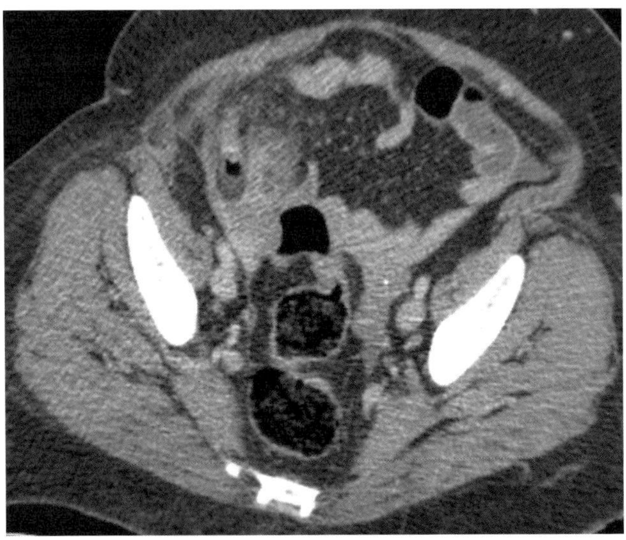

Figure 11.42. Example of an inflamed, thickened appendix.

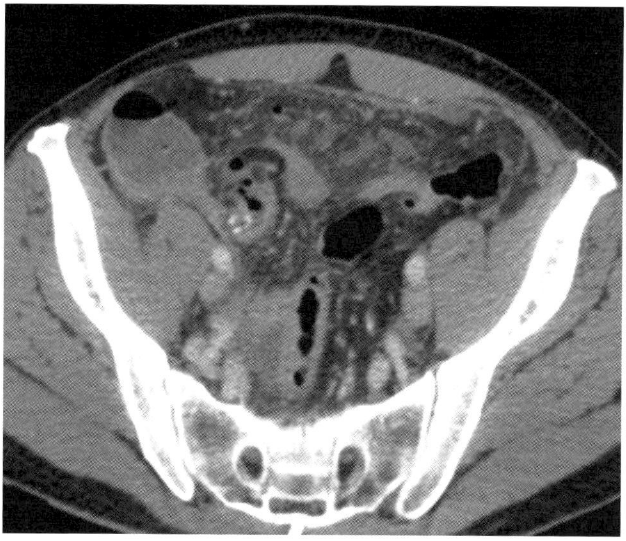

Figure 11.43. Perforated inflamed appendix seen with appendicoliths and small amount of extraluminal air.

CT diagnosis of obstruction (Figs 11.44 and 11.45) is based on dilated small bowel and a corresponding transition point where calibre abruptly decreases. CT has proved useful in characterising small bowel obstruction from extrinsic causes (adhesions, closed loop, strangulation, hernia, extrinsic masses), intrinsic causes (adenocarcinoma, Crohn's disease, tuberculosis, radiation enteropathy, intramural haemorrhage, intussusception), intraluminal causes (e.g., gallstone ileus (Fig. 11.46), bezoars), or intestinal malrotation. CT is useful in depicting the precise site and type of hernia and its contents, including spigelian, obturator, lumbar and ventral hernias.

The diagnosis of small bowel obstruction due to adhesions is made when all other causes of obstruction have been ruled out at CT.

11.6.7 *Computed iomography imaging in colitis*

11.6.7.1 *Ulcerative colitis*

Approximately 10–15% of patients with ulcerative colitis present with acute, fulminating colitis and are at risk of colonic perforation and death.

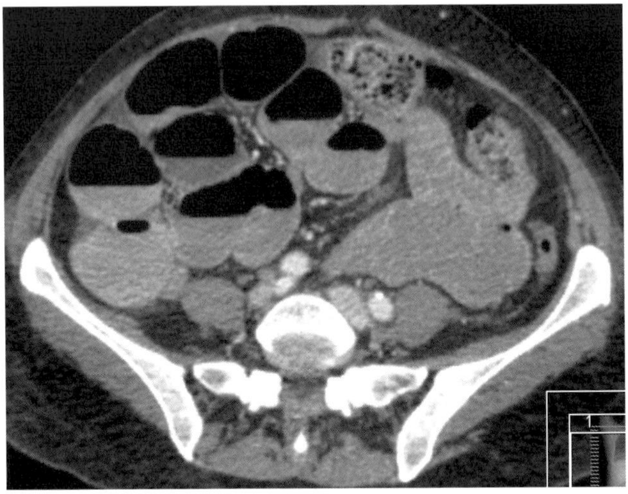

Figure 11.44. Multiple dilated fluid-filled loops of small bowel with a point of transition in small bowel obstruction.

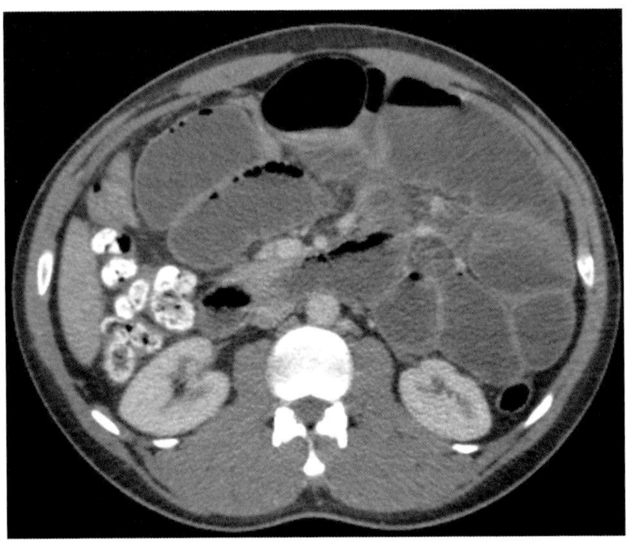

Figure 11.45. Multiple dilated fluid-filled loops of small bowel with air-bubbles trapped in a non-dependent location giving a string of beads appearance in small bowel obstruction.

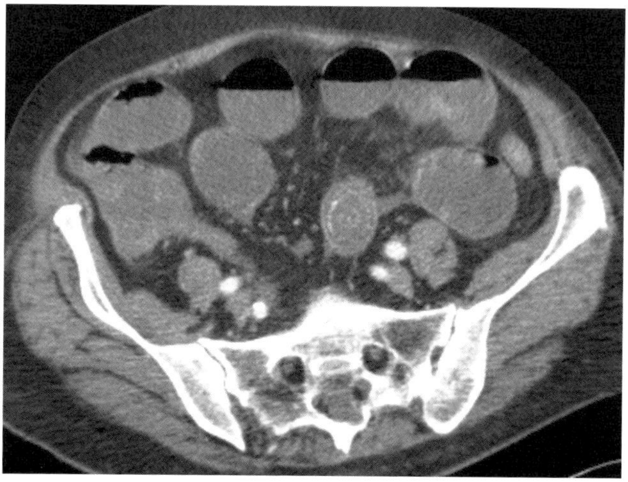

Figure 11.46. Small bowel obstruction due to an obstructing gallstone which had migrated into the small bowel following fistulation into the duodenum.

CT is useful in the rapid assessment of disease extent and severity of acute colitis [60,61]. In total colitis, increased thickness of the colonic wall, irregularity of the mucosa, loss of haustral clefts and absence of any formed faeces (empty colon) are recognised radiological features. Acute toxic dilatation/toxic megacolon is diagnosed when transverse colonic diameter exceeds 5.5 cm (Fig. 11.47). Haustration is lost and oedematous mucosal remnants, 'mucosal islands', indicate the very extensive nature of the ulceration. Toxic megacolon also complicates Crohn's disease, infectious colitis and some other types of colitis.

11.6.7.2 *Pseudomembranous colitis*

Common CT findings in pseudomembranous colitis include wall thickening, low-attenuation mural thickening corresponding to mucosal and submucosal oedema (Fig. 11.48), the 'accordion sign', the 'target sign' ('double halo sign'), pericolonic stranding and ascites [60,62]. The appearance of the colon may resemble that of an accordion, caused by trapping of positive contrast material (if given) between thickened haustral folds, but this sign is not specific. The 'target sign' consists of two or three concentric rings of

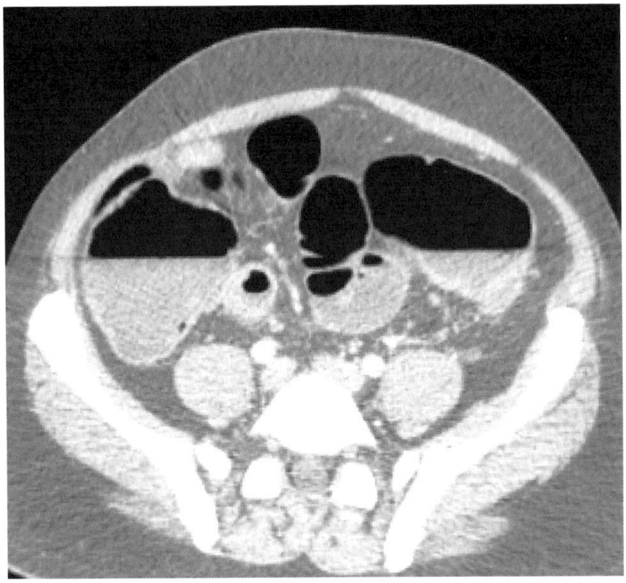

Figure 11.47. CT shows dilated large bowel (more than 5.5 cm) and the presence of air-fluid levels in this patient with ulcerative colitis suggesting toxic megacolon.

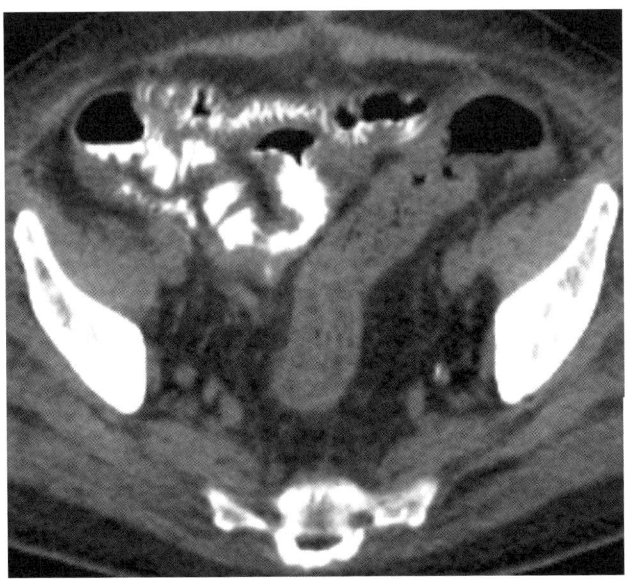

Figure 11.48. Thickened, oedematous sigmoid with stranding of the surrounding fat in a patient with pseudomembranous colitis

different attenuation and indicates mucosal hyperaemia and submucosal oedema or inflammation.

Colonic intramural gas or pneumatosis coli with or without air in the intrahepatic portal vein may be seen in severe cases. Complications of untreated pseudomembranous colitis include toxic megacolon and intestinal perforation.

11.6.7.3 *Neutropaenic colitis*

Fever and abdominal pain in the setting of neutropenia warrant attention to the possibility of neutropenic colitis, usually manifested as a right-sided colitic process. Plain films are non-specific and demonstrate ileocaecal dilatation. CT is the method of choice due to the risk of bowel perforation with colonoscopy or contrast enema examination.

CT may be useful by demonstrating thickening of the caecum, ascending colon and terminal ileum. CT can detect complications such as pneumatosis when there is bowel wall necrosis or pnemoperitoneum when there is a silent perforation.

11.6.7.4 *Diverticulitis*

It is estimated that approximately 15–30% of patients with diverticular disease develop symptomatic diverticulitis at some point in the natural history of the condition, often requiring medical and/or surgical therapy. The CT hallmark of diverticulitis is diverticular change with associated 'fat stranding' in the pericolic fat [63]. Fluid may track down the root of the sigmoid mesentery. In more severe cases, phlegmon or frank abscess formation can occur.

CT allows detection of complications of diverticulitis such as diverticular abscess, colovesical fistula and perforation. CT-guided percutaneous drainage of an abscess can eliminate the need for emergency surgery.

Diverticulitis may be classified as 'mild' if there is minimal wall thickening (4–5 mm) and inflammatory changes only in the pericolic fat; 'moderate' if there is abscess formation (Fig. 11.49); and 'severe' if there is significant wall thickening with evidence of either free perforation, a large (>5 cm) abscess or inflammatory extension into the pelvis.

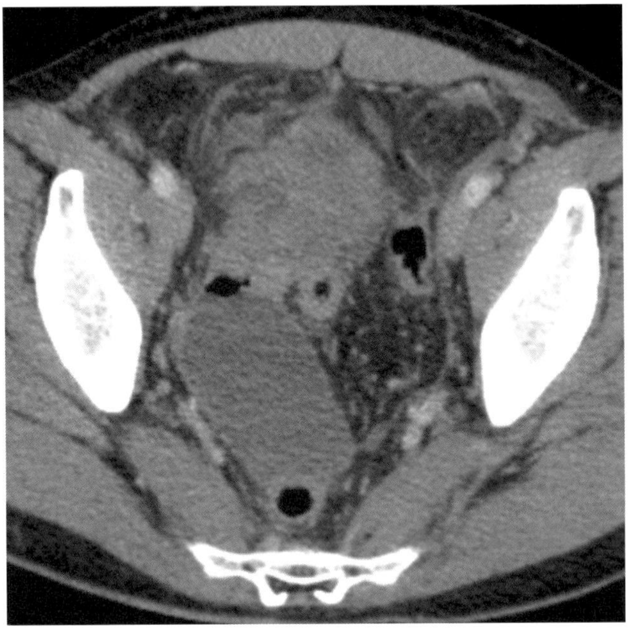

Figure 11.49. A pelvic fluid collection containing a locule of air following diverticulitis.

11.6.8 *Abdominopelvic abscess and perforation*

A frequent indication for CT in the ICU setting is to exclude abdominopelvic abscess in the septic patient. CT, ideally contrast-enhanced, is usually definitive in evaluating the abdomen for abscess, even in the complex, post-operative patient. Ultrasound scanning is generally insensitive due to difficulty detecting interloop and retroperitoneal collections.

Abscesses appear as non-tubular fluid collections with an enhancing rim, which are distinguished from adjacent bowel by their focal, non-continuous nature (Fig. 11.50). In difficult cases, enteral contrast may be required to tag the adjacent bowel structures.

The majority of abdominopelvic abscesses can be accessed with CT guidance for percutaneous drainage, if clinically appropriate (Figs 11.51–11.53). Introducer systems are available for deep-seated or otherwise difficult abscesses. Some collections deep in the pelvis or surrounded by bowel loops may not be accessible, however. Percutaneous drainage is generally ineffective in immature or heavily septated collections.

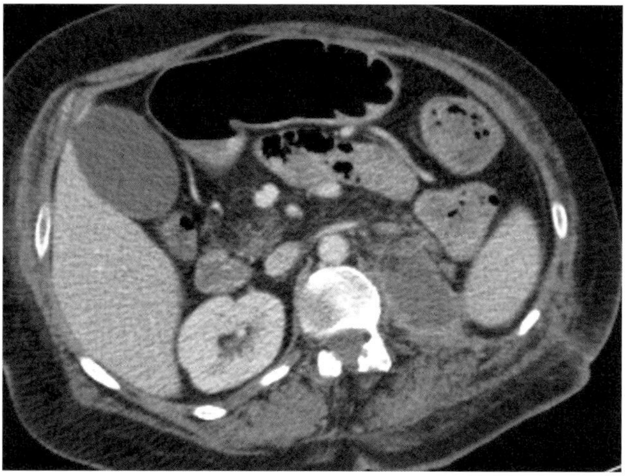

Figure 11.50. Fluid collection with well-defined enhancing walls in left nephrectomy bed.

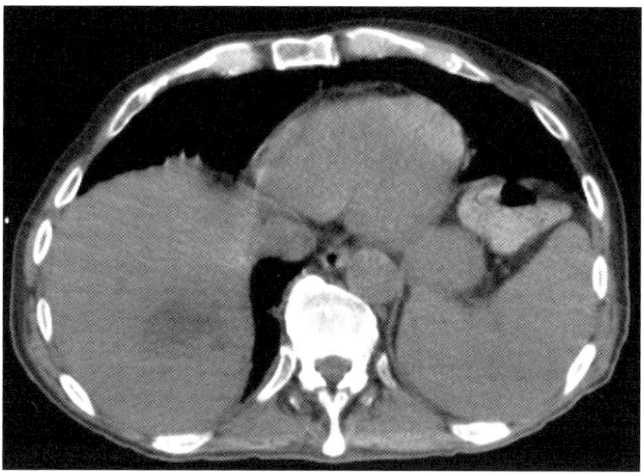

Figure 11.51. Liver abscess — an ill-defined area of reduced enhancement in the right lobe of the liver.

CT remains the procedure of choice to exclude a perforation; as little as 1 ml of free air can be detected. Free perforation is recognised by the presence of intraperitoneal gas (Fig, 11.54) but sealed perforations cannot reliably be detected from CT or plain radiographs.

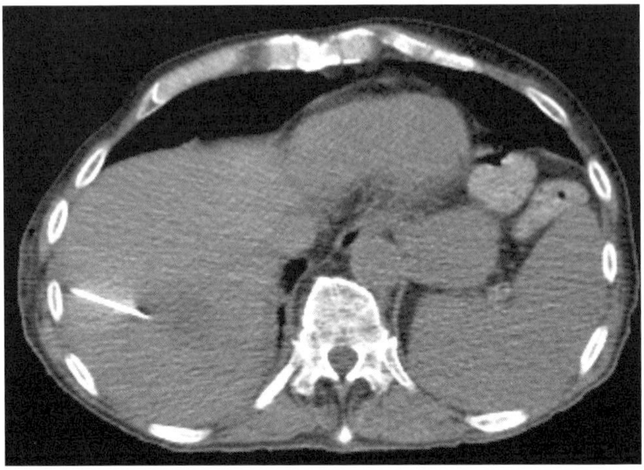

Figure 11.52. CT guided drainage of the liver abscess.

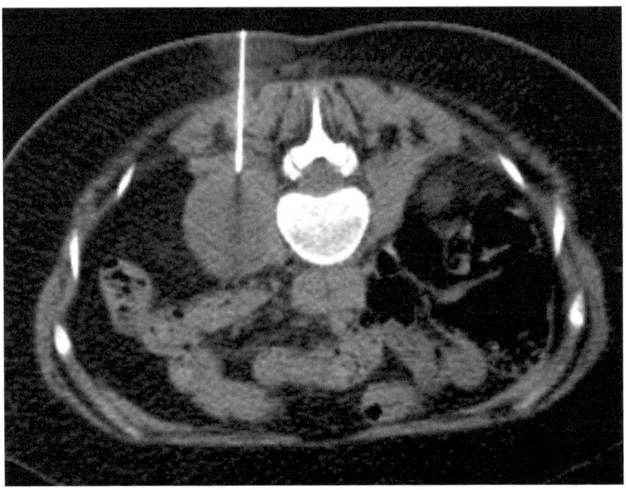

Figure 11.53. CT guided drainage of a psoas abscess.

11.6.9 *Acute mesenteric ischaemia*

Acute mesenteric ischemia (AMI) is a life-threatening condition with mortality rates ranging from 59% to 93% reported in the literature.

Biphasic CT with mesenteric CT angiography [64] is effective in the diagnosis of AMI, and shows a sensitivity of 96% and a specificity of 94% by

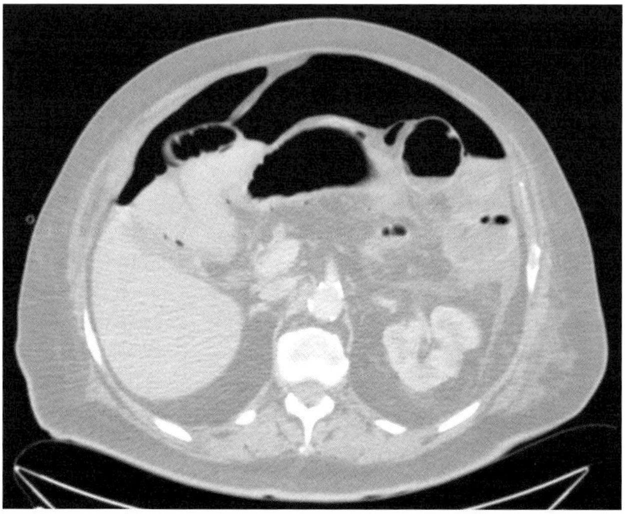

Figure 11.54. Free air in the peritoneal cavity in case of a duodenal perforation.

using any one of the following criteria: pneumatosis intestinalis (Fig. 11.55), venous gas, superior mesenteric artery (SMA) occlusion, celiac and inferior mesenteric artery (IMA) arterial occlusion with distal SMA disease or arterial embolism, or, alternatively, bowel wall thickening combined with any one finding of focal lack of bowel wall enhancement, solid organ infarction or venous thrombosis.

Hallmark angiographic findings such as narrowing of multiple branch vessels of the SMA, small-vessel spasm, or impaired filling of intramural vessels would be more difficult to appreciate on CT scans relative to catheter angiography, which also offers the option of therapy with papaverine. A disadvantage of CT angiography is that it depicts the vessels at a single point in time, and the temporal changes in vascular filling that are seen on catheter angiographic images cannot be appreciated.

11.6.10 *Ruptured abdominal aortic aneurysm*

The use of CT angiography has become routine for imaging of a suspected abdominal aortic aneurysm (AAA) rupture in haemodynamically stable patients and to exclude any other possible causes of abdominal pain.

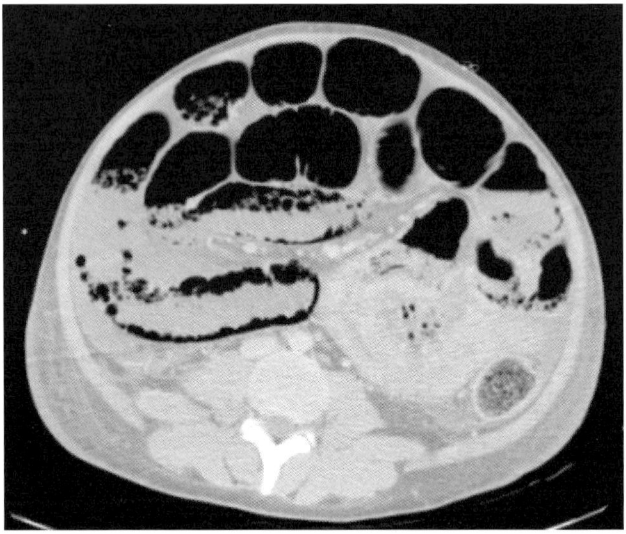

Figure 11.55. CT shows pneumatosis intestinalis as bubbly lucencies within the bowel wall in this patient with multi-system failure suggesting small bowel ischaemia.

The CT diagnosis of AAA rupture [65] is based on the detection of extraluminal haemorrhage, usually retroperitoneal, in patients with abdominal pain and large AAAs. Discontinuity of the aortic wall or a focal gap in otherwise continuous circumferential wall calcifications may point to the location of a rupture.

Imaging features suggestive of instability or impending rupture [66] include increased aneurysm size, a low thrombus to lumen ratio and haemorrhage into a mural thrombus. The crescent sign, a well-defined peripheral crescent of increased attenuation within the thrombus of a large abdominal aortic aneurysm, is a CT sign of acute or impending rupture. Draping of the posterior aspect of an aneurysmal aorta (the draped aorta sign) over the vertebrae is associated with a contained rupture.

References

[1] Hunter, T.B., Taljanovic, M.S., Tsau, P.H. *et al.* (2004). Medical devices of the chest, *Radiographics*, **24**, 1725–1746.

[2] Goodman, L.R., Conrardy, P.A., Laing, F. *et al.* (1976). Radiographic evaluation of endotracheal tube position, *Am J Roentgenol*, **127**, 433–434.

[3] Pillai, J.P., Vegas, A. and Brister, S. (2005). Thoracic complications of nasogastric tube: review of safe practice, *Interact Cardio Vasc Thorac Surg*, **4**, 429–433.
[4] Goodman, L.R. (1980). Postoperative chest radiograph: II. alterations after major intrathoracic surgery, *Am J Roentenol*, **134**, 803–813.
[5] Goodman, L.R. (1980). Postoperative chest radiograph: I. alterations after abdominal surgery, *Am J Roentenol*, **134**, 533–541.
[6] Franquet, T., Giménez, A., Rosón, N. *et al.* (2000). Aspiration diseases: findings, pitfalls, and differential diagnosis, *Radiographics*, **20**, 673–685.
[7] Desai, S.R. (2002). Acute respiratory distress syndrome: imaging of the injured lung, *Clinl Radiol*, **57**, 8–17.
[8] Forbes, K.P.N., Reid, J.H. and Murchison, J.T. (2000). Do preliminary chest x-ray findings define the optimum role of pulmonary scintigraphy in suspected pulmonary embolism? *Clin Radiol*, **56**, 397–400.
[9] Eliott, C.G., Goldhaber, S.Z, Visani, L. *et al.* (2000). Chest radiographs in acute pulmonary embolism, *Chest*, **118**, 33–38.
[10] Woodring, J.H. (1984). Recognition of pleural effusion on supine radiographs: how much fluid is required? *Am J Roentgenol*, **142**, 59–64.
[11] Paramasivam, E. and Bodenham, A. (2007). Pleural fluid collections in critically ill patients, *Contin Educ Anaesth Crit Care Pain*, **7**, 10–14.
[12] Chae, E.J., Seo, J.B., Kim, S.Y. *et al.* (2006). Radiographic and CT findings of thoracic complications after pneumonectomy, *RadioGraphics*, **26**, 1449–1467.
[13] Fox, J.C. and Irwin, Z. (2008). Emergency and critical care imaging, *Emerg Med Clin North Am*, **26**, 787–812.
[14] Beaulieu, Y. and Marik, P.E. (2005). Bedside ultrasonography in the ICU: part 1, *Chest*, **128**, 881–895.
[15] Pneumatikos, I. and Bouros, D. (2008). Pleural effusions in critically ill patients, *Respiration*, **76**, 241–248.
[16] Lichtenstein, D., Hulot, J.S. and Rabiller, A. (1999). Feasibility and safety of ultrasound-aided thoracentesis in mechanically ventilated patients, *Intens Care Med*, **25**, 955–958.
[17] Lichtenstein, D.A. and Menu, Y. (1995). A bedside ultrasound sign ruling out pneumothorax in the critically ill: lung sliding, *Chest*, **108**, 1345–1348.
[18] Lichtenstein, D., Meziere, G., Biderman, P. *et al.* (1999). The comet-tail artefact: an ultrasound sign ruling out pneumothorax, *Intens Care Med*, **25**, 383–388.
[19] Lichtenstein, D., Meziere, G., Biderman, P. *et al.* (2000). The 'lung point': an ultrasound sign specific to pneumothorax, *Intens Care Med*, **26**, 1434–1440.
[20] Beaulieu, Y. (2007). Bedside echocardiography in the assessment of the critically ill, *Crit Care Med*, **35** (Suppl. 5), S235–S249.

[21] Wang, H.P. and Chen, S.C. (2007). Upper abdominal ultrasound in the critically ill, *Crit Care Med*, **35** (Suppl. 5), S208–S215.

[22] Lee, S.Y. and Frankel, H.L. (2000). Ultrasound and other imaging technologies in the intensive care unit, *Surg Clin North Am*, **80**, 975–1003.

[23] Nazeer, S.R., Dewbre, H. and Miller, A.H. (2005). Ultrasound-assisted paracentesis performed by emergency physicians vs the traditional technique: a prospective, randomized study, *Am J Emerg Med*, **23**, 363–367.

[24] Helling, T.S., Wilson, J. and Augustosky, K. (2007). The utility of focused abdominal ultrasound in blunt abdominal trauma: a reappraisal, *Am J Surg*, **194**, 728–733.

[25] Barozzi, L., Valentino, M., Santoro, A. *et al.* (2007). Renal ultrasonography in critically ill patients, *Crit Care Med*, **35** (Suppl. 5), S198–S205.

[26] McGee, D.C. and Gould, M.K. (2003). Preventing complications of central venous catheterization, *N Engl J Med*, **348**, 1123–1133.

[27] Maecken, T. and Thomas, G. (2007). Ultrasound imaging in vascular access, *Crit Care Med*, **35** (Suppl. 5), S178–S185.

[28] Kon, A.H. and LaRoque, R.L. (1977). Evaluation of head trauma by computed tomography, *Radiology*, **123**, 345–350.

[29] Zimmerman, R.A., Bilaniuk, L.T., Hackney, D.B. *et al.* (1986). Head injury: early results of comparing CT and high-field MR, *AJR Am J Roentgenol*, **147**, 1215–1222.

[30] Dublin, B., French, B.N. and Rennick, J.M. (1977). Computed tomography in head trauma, *Radiology*, **122**, 365–369.

[31] Zimmerman, R.A. and Bilaniuk, L.T. (1982). Computed tomographic staging of traumatic epidural bleeding, *Radiology*, **144**, 809–812.

[32] Davis, P.C. (2007). Head trauma, *Am J Neuroradiol*, **28**, 1619–1621.

[33] Parizel, P.M., Ozsarlak, O., Van Goethem, J.W. *et al.* (1998). Imaging findings in diffuse axonal injury after closed head trauma, *Eur Radiol*, **8**, 960–965.

[34] James, M. (2000). CT and MR Imaging of nontraumatic neurologic emergencies, *AJR Am J Roentgenol*, **174**, 289–299.

[35] Whelan, M.A. and Hilal, S.K. (1980). Computed tomography as a guide in the diagnosis and follow-up of brain abscesses, *Radiology*, **135**, 663–671.

[36] Haimes, A.B., Zimmerman, R.D., Morgello, S. *et al.* (1989). MR imaging of brain abscesses, *AJR Am J Roentgenol*, **152**, 1073–1085.

[37] Damaerel, P., Wilms, G., Robberecht, W. *et al.* (1992). MRI of herpes simplex encephalitis, *Neuroradiology*, **34**, 490–493.

[38] Srinivasan, A., Goyal, M., Al Azri, F. *et al.* (2006). State-of-the-art imaging of acute stroke. *Radiographics*, **26** (Suppl. 1), 75–95.

[39] Burdette, J.H. and Elster, A.D. (2006). Cerebral infarction diagnosis by computerized tomography: analysis and evaluation of findings — How far have we really come? *AJR Am J Roentgenol*, **186**, 611–612.

[40] Ay, H., Buonanno, F.S., Schaefer, P.W. *et al.* (1998). Posterior leukoencephalopathy without severe hypertension: utility of diffusion-weighted MRI, *Neurology*, **51**, 1369–1376.

[41] Laubenberger, J., Scheneider, B., Ansorge, O. *et al.* (1996). Central pontine myelionolysis: clinical presentation and radiologic findings, *Eur Radiol*, **6**, 177–183.

[42] Snow, N., Bergin, K.T. and Horrigan, T.P. (1990). Thoracic CT scanning in critically ill patients, Information obtained frequently alters management, *Chest*, **97**, 1467–1470.

[43] Gross, B.H. and Spizarny, D.L. (1994). Computed tomography of the chest in the intensive care unit, *Crit Care Clin*, **10**, 267–275.

[44] Wallace, T. Miller, W.T., Tino, G. *et al.* (1998). Thoracic CT in the intensive care unit: assessment of clinical usefulness, *Radiology*, **209**, 491–498.

[45] Pneumatikos, I. and Bouros, D. (2008). Pleural effusions in critically ill patients, Respiration, **76**, 241–248.

[46] Start, D.D., Federal, M.P., Goodman, P.C. *et al.* (1983). Differentiating lung abscess and empyema: radiography and computed tomography, *AJR Am J Roentgenol*, **141**, 163–167.

[47] Kuhlman, J.E., Fishman, E.K., Teigen, C. (1990). Pulmonary septic emboli: diagnosis with CT, *Radiology*, **174**, 211–213.

[48] Iwasaki, Y., Nagata, K., Nakanishi, M. *et al.* (2001). Spiral CT findings in septic pulmonary emboli, *Eur J Radiol*, **37**, 190–194.

[49] Li, A.E. and Fishman, E.K. (2003). Evaluation of complications after sternotomy using single- and multidetector CT with three-dimensional volume rendering, *AJR Am J Roentgenol*, **181**, 1065–1070.

[50] Moores, L.K. and Holley, A.B. (2008). Computed tomography pulmonary angiography and venography: diagnostic and prognostic properties, *Semin Respir Crit Care Med*, **29**, 3–14.

[51] Hayter, R.G., Rhea, J.T., Small, A. *et al.* (2006). Suspected aortic dissection and other aortic disorders: multi–detector row CT in 373 cases in the emergency setting, *Radiology*, **238**, 841–852.

[52] Gayer, G., Rozenman, J., Hoffman, C. *et al.* (2000). CT diagnosis of malpositioned chest tubes, *Br J Radiol*, **73**, 786–790.

[53] Lim, K.E., Chan, C.Y., Hsu, Y.Y. *et al.* (2005). Diagnosis of malpositioned chest tubes after emergency tube thoracostomy: is computed tomography more accurate than chest radiograph? *Clin Imaging*, **29**, 401–405.

[54] Baldt, M.M., Bankier, A.A., Germann, P.S. *et al.* (1995). Complications after emergency tube thoracostomy: assessment with CT, *Radiology*, **195**, 539–543.
[55] Balthazar, E.J., Robinson, D.L., Megibow, A.J. *et al.* (1990). Acute pancreatitis: value of CT in establishing prognosis, *Radiology*, **174**, 331–336.
[56] Lee, M.J., Rattner, D.W., Legemate, D.A. *et al.* (1992). Acute complicated pancreatitis: Redefining the role of interventional radiology, *Radiology*, **183**, 171–174.
[57] Balthazar, E.J. (2002). Acute pancreatitis: assessment of severity with clinical and CT evaluation, *Radiology*, **223**, 603–613.
[58] Arai, K., Kawai, K., Kohda, W. *et al.* (2003). Dynamic CT of acute cholangitis: early inhomogeneous enhancement of the liver, *AJR Am J Roentgenol*, **181**, 115–118.
[59] Leite, N.P., Pereira, J.M., Cunha, R *et al.* (2005). CT evaluation of appendicitis and its complications: imaging techniques and key diagnostic findings, *AJR Am J Roentgenol*, **185**, 406–417.
[60] Thoeni, R.F. and Cello, J.P. (2006). CT imaging of colitis, *Radiology*, **240**, 623–638.
[61] Horton, K.M., Corl, F.M. and Fishman, E.K. (2000). CT evaluation of the colon: inflammatory disease, *Radiographics*, **20**, 399–418.
[62] Kawamoto, S., Horton, K.M. and Fishman, E.K. (1999). Pseudomembranous colitis: spectrum of imaging findings with clinical and pathologic correlation, *Radiographics*, **19**, 887–897.
[63] Lawrimore, T. and Rhea, J.T. (2004). Computed tomography evaluation of diverticulitis, *J Intensive Care Med*, **19**, 194–204.
[64] Kirkpatrick, I.D.C., Kroeker, M.A. and Greenberg, H.M. (2003). Biphasic CT with mesenteric CT angiography in the evaluation of acute mesenteric ischaemia: initial experience, *Radiology*, **229**, 91–98.
[65] Seigel, C.L., Cohan, R.H., Korobkin, M. *et al.* (1994). Abdominal aortic aneurysm morphology: CT features in patients with ruptured and nonruptured aneurysms, *AJR Am J Roentgenol*, **163**, 1123–1129.
[66] Rakita, D., Newatia, A., Hines, J.J. *et al.* (2007). Spectrum of CT findings in rupture and impending rupture of abdominal aortic aneurysms, *Radiographics*, **27**, 497–507.

12

Biochemistry in Intensive Care

Paul Holloway

12.1 Introduction

Analysing the pathology requests from any intensive care unit (ICU) requires systematic blood sampling for a regular profile of biochemical investigations at least once a day together with intermittent sampling for specific tests as follow-on or to make specific diagnoses. The medical staff need to follow this biochemical testing carefully and the laboratory needs to process these tests rapidly and reliably and provide interpretative support. Review of the 'lab results' is an integral component of the ICU ward round and requesters need to fully understand and interpret these result appropriately in the context of the clinical state, which is often changing rapidly.

12.2 Role in Diagnosis

Beyond clinical and physiological assessments, routine biochemical investigations covering fluid balance, acid–base balance, cardiac, gastrointestinal, hepatic, renal, skeletal (bone and muscle) and general metabolic function are of paramount significance. For most patients these may form the initial baseline investigations, which are helpful in initial diagnosis and prognosis whilst thereon informing on the progress of the patient and alerting to both improvements and set-backs. Although most initial biochemical investigations are for assessment of admission organ dysfunction, the scope needs to be wide enough to allow for succinct diagnostic information. They should be integrated with other admission data to prevent information from being hidden, only to be uncovered at a later stage. A prime example is a not infrequently encountered missed diagnosis of starvation ketoacidosis where early, perhaps pre-ICU admission, ketonuria plus minor hypoglycaemia might have been overlooked. Modern ICU data management systems should facilitate such integration although there is always a human element for some data entry. Together with these components the right biochemistry 'profiles' (see for example Table 12.1) should be established, preferably in conjunction with a clinical biochemist.

12.2.1 *Central laboratory testing and support*

The typical biochemical profile suggested in Table 12.1 is normally requested in an early morning sample with results available for the morning ICU ward round. The pathology laboratory needs to be informed of the ICU requirements and ensure there is a focussed and dedicated process for analysis and delivery of the results. The laboratory may have in place a clinical authorising practice that reviews results outside critical ranges but seldom will it be practical or appropriate for this to be used for ICU results so it will remain the responsibility of the ICU to have in place a system to alert staff of significant results. For many ICUs this is managed through an electronic database but whatever the process it must be effective in informing the key personnel at the bedside.

12.2.2 *Point-of-care testing*

Over the past two decades there has been an increasing shift of biochemical diagnostics for ICU patients towards more point-of-care testing (POCT). The relative need for this will depend on the level of severity of disease in the ICU but this section is aimed at the more complex end of the spectrum with patients requiring ventilatory support and with at least one other organ dysfunction. POCT in the ICU initially suited analytes that are relatively unstable, such as blood gases, but the technology has advanced significantly to allow testing of other parameters considered

Table 12.1. Biochemistry profile for admission and daily monitoring.

Analyte	**Sample**[‡]	**Organ system**	**Role in assessment and monitoring**
Sodium*	S/P	Renal	Fluid balance, acid–base, renal tubular function, cellular integrity, endocrine function
Potassium*	S/P	Renal	Renal tubular function, acid–base, endocrine, cardiac physiology, renal drug effects, replacement monitoring
Chloride*	S/P	Renal/ Gastrointestinal	Fluid balance, acid–base, renal tubular function, gastrointestinal integrity
Bicarbonate*	S/P	Renal/ Gastrointestinal/ Respiratory	Renal tubular function, acid–base, gastrointestinal integrity, respiratory function
Calcium	S/P	Bone/Endocrine	Bone metabolism, endocrine function, cardiac physiology, gastrointestinal absorption, renal tubular function, acid–base
Magnesium	S/P	Renal/ Gastrointestinal	Renal tubular function, gastrointestinal integrity, cardiac functionality, acid–base
Phosphate	S/P	Renal/Bone	Renal tubular function, cellular integrity, gastrointestinal integrity, haemolysis
Bilirubin	S/P	Liver/ Haematological	Hepatic biliary tract integrity, hepatic ion transport, haemolysis
Albumin	S/P	Liver/Renal/ Gastrointestinal	Hepatic protein synthesis, renal glomerular integrity, gastrointestinal integrity, acute phase response
Alanine Transaminase	S/P	Liver	Hepatocellular integrity and function, infective or toxic hepatitis, secondary hepatic failure — e.g. in congestive cardiac failure or sepsis
Alkaline Phosphatase	S/P	Liver/(Bone)	Bile duct membrane transport and enzyme synthesis, cholestasis, (osteoblast activity/rate of bone formation)

(*Continued*)

Table 12.1. (*Continued*)

Analyte	Sample‡	Organ system	Role in assessment and monitoring
Gamma glutamyl transferase	S/P	Liver	Bile duct membrane transport and enzyme synthesis, cholestasis, generalised hepatic pathology, toxin damage or enzyme induction
Creatinine	S/P	Renal	Glomerular filtration rate, hydration
Urea	S/P	Renal	Glomerular filtration rate, hydration, hepatic amino acid metabolism, gastrointestinal protein load (e.g. from haemorrhage)
Glucose*	S/P	Metabolism	Carbohydrate metabolism, endocrine pancreatic function, insulin axis, glycaemic control
Lactate†	S/P	Metabolism	Carbohydrate metabolism, anaerobic glycolytic rate, tissue hypoxia, hepatic function, acid-base
C-Reactive Protein†	S/P	Infection/ Inflammation	Local and systemic inflammation and/or infection, particularly bacterial or fungal
Creatine Kinase†	S/P	Muscle	Myositis, skeletal and cardiac muscle damage or ischaemia
Troponin†	S/P	Cardiac	Cardiac muscle damage and ischaemia
Amylase†	S/P	Pancreas	Exocrine pancreatic damage, acute pancreatitis, parotitis
Osmolality†	S	Fluid balance	Hydration state, extrinsic osmolytes — e.g. alcohols, assessment of plasma sodium abnormalities
Osmolality†	U	Fluid balance	Assessment of plasma sodium abnormalities and fluid balance

* Available as point-of-care test. † Optional for specific cases or types of ICU (e.g. surgical, cardiac).
‡ S = serum; P = plasma.

essential for regular monitoring. Clearly the bulk of the analytical process in this situation becomes the full responsibility of the ICU clinicians and the role of the central laboratory is usually restricted to analyser maintenance and overseeing the quality assurance process.

With the primary emphasis on maximising the efficiency of ventilatory support the regular monitoring of blood 'gases' — partial pressure of oxygen and partial pressure of carbon dioxide — is considered essential and with pH measurements and derived parameters, such as base excess and bicarbonate, this process is now well supported at the point-of-care. Other parameters considered essential for assessment of acid–base status — electrolytes sodium, potassium, calcium (ionised) and chloride as well as the metabolite lactate and measured haemoglobin — are now all available on blood gas analysers. The quality of these measurements is now adequately similar to that of those from the central laboratory and can thus be relied upon, assuming that the point-of-care analyser quality control procedures are adequately monitored.

In the ICU over recent years some have advocated a policy of aiming for tight glycaemic control (TGC), with blood glucose levels targeted to the normal range. This has focussed point-of-care analysis on this metabolite. Blood gas analysers are able to measure this accurately across a wide range of concentrations and in the context of fluctuating arterial oxygen tensions and haematocrit. Until recently specific point-of-care blood glucose devices have proven to have inadequate sensitivity in extremes of critical care and thus are considered too inaccurate to support this policy. This analytical deficiency may not have influenced the results of a recent global study that demonstrated the risk of applying this in standard ICUs that do not have the focussed resources and level of care to the protocol that were available in the original study centres [1]. Nevertheless it is considered advisable that blood glucose measurements in the ICU are carried out on blood gas machines.

Other point-of-care biochemical analytes available for use in the ICU include blood urea, creatinine and bilirubin, and one manufacturer provides ionised magnesium. Data is limited on the influence that measurement of these additional parameters have on patient outcome and the preference for these at point-of-care rather than in the central laboratory is currently questionable. As in all diagnostic testing, questions need to be raised as to what is the optimal interval between testing, the speed of provision of the results for clinical decision making (therapeutic turnaround time) and the cost:benefit ratio of point-of-care provision. The underlying issue may in some circumstances be assessing if there is an analytical accuracy disadvantage in POCT for a specific analyte compared with the slower but perhaps more accurate central laboratory result. The laboratory is best placed to advise on the quality differences.

12.3 The Role of the Chemical Pathologist/Clinical Scientist

ICUs must expect to be served by high-quality clinical laboratories within reasonable proximity and providing at least the essential range of analytical tests with rapid turnaround. The analytical repertoire must be agreed with the laboratory service, including such components as minimum turnaround time and connectivity, but the laboratory must also provide a clinical interpretative and advisory service. Intensive care patients, by the nature of their dependence and potential for complications, including tissue ischaemia and sepsis, tend to have multiple and overlapping pathologies and thus can benefit from objective interpretation of their biochemical data at the laboratory. This covers both the diagnostic and monitoring roles for which the biochemical testing is required and includes the evaluation of potential analytical interferences from treatments (e.g. hyperlipidaemia, antibiotic use) or from the effect of disease processes (e.g. hypoalbuminaemia, acidosis). Laboratory advice may be sought for a spectrum well beyond the apparently mundane organ function assessment and include identifying unmeasured anions in a metabolic acidosis, endocrine causes for an electrolyte imbalance and toxicology. One typical example would be in overriding the misinterpretation of a rising plasma bilirubin assumed to be a manifestation of worsening hepatic function but in fact caused by an increasing degree of haemolysis from a retroperitoneal haematoma. In such a situation the rest of the liver function test profile does not concur with the assumed diagnosis although there may be increases in transaminases, particularly aspartate transaminase (AST), released from adjacent tissues. There are endless other typical situations where specialist biochemical knowledge informs clinical decision-making and management. It is therefore essential that chemical pathologists (laboratory medical consultants) and clinical scientists include intensive care medicine as part of their training.

12.4 Specific Clinical Areas

12.4.1 *Sodium, potassium, hydrogen, calcium and other electrolytes*

Electrolyte assessment is essential in intensive care management and forms a crucial component of biochemical monitoring. Although many electrolyte disorders are the direct consequence of disease processes, a recent review [2] highlights the influence of many commonly prescribed medications on electrolyte imbalances in critically ill patients.

12.4.1.1 *Sodium and fluid management*

Assessment of circulating volume and hydration, to which serum sodium makes an important contribution, is of paramount importance in intensive care. The high incidence of water and sodium disorders (dysnatremias), the difficulty of distinguishing between syndrome of inappropriate antidiuretic hormone (SIADH) and adrenal insufficiency and many other permutations in the susceptible patient, particularly in those with cardiac or renal incapacity, requires viable assessment of volume status. This is now of greater significance with the emergence of antidiuretic hormone (ADH) receptor inhibitors to treat correctly diagnosed SIADH. Sodium and water movement across cell membranes is influenced by alterations in vasopressin release or renal tubular aquaporin response as well as by changing renal, cardiac, respiratory and hepatic pathology and by drugs. The role of sodium in the corrective process of a metabolic acidosis may also necessitate its regular monitoring together with chloride.

Disorders of sodium balance, reflecting therefore water balance and plasma tonicity, are extremely common in intensive care patients (see Figs 12.1 and 12.2) and carry significant risk [3]. The majority of dysnatraemias occur whilst the patient is in the ICU although some patients may be referred to ICU to assist in the sodium management or are admitted when the dysnatraemia is a coincidental pathology. Most studies of dysnatraemia in hospital patients are retrospective and uncontrolled but they confirm the mortality risks from both extremes of electrolyte disorder (Fig. 12.4).

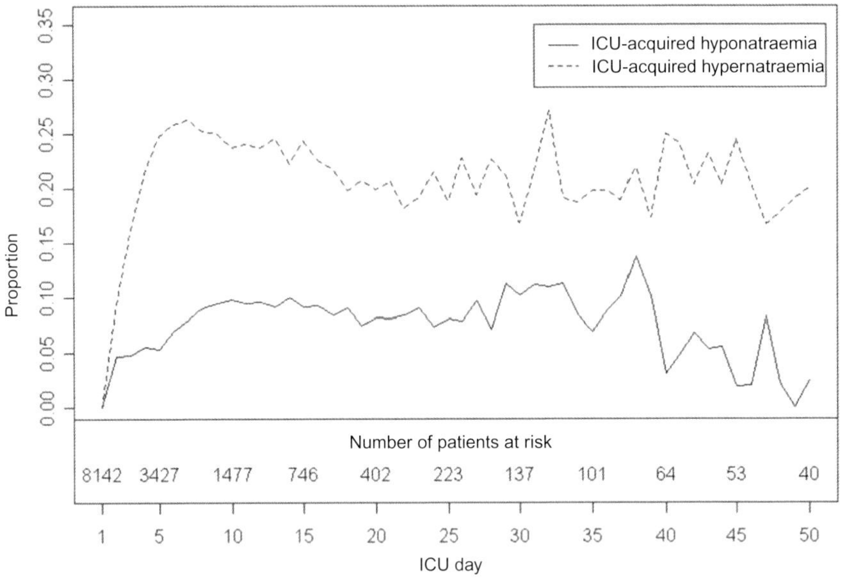

Figure 12.1. Proportion of intensive care patients with serum sodium values outside the normal range during the first 50 days of ICU stay.

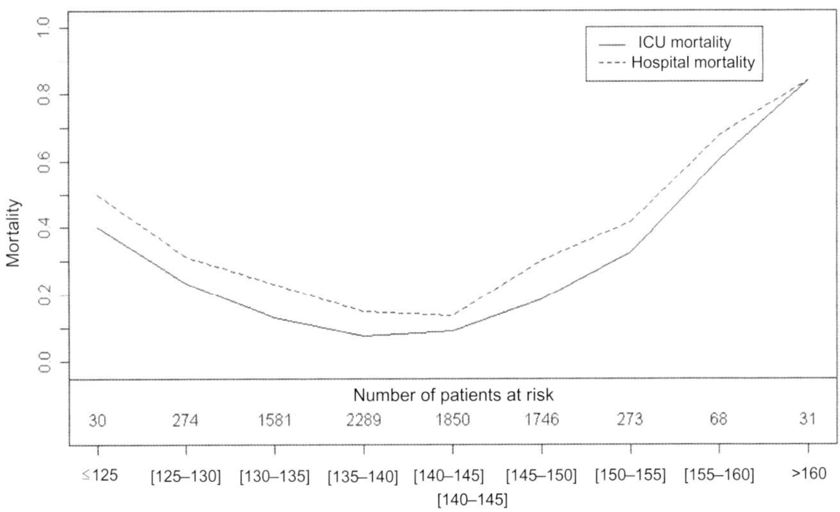

Figure 12.2. Maximum deviation of serum sodium from normal range during ICU admission and patient mortality [4].

12.4.1.1.1 Hypernatraemia

Regardless of the cause, hypernatremia has been shown to be associated with increased morbidity and mortality, and outcome appears to be related to the degree of correction [3,4]. Several recent studies have highlighted the link between hypernatraemia, predominantly ICU-acquired, and increasing mortality or delay to ICU discharge [5,6].

Although the clinician is more readily aware of the risks of hyponatraemia and fluid overload, identifying the cause of and then correcting hypernatraemia is often complex. There is some evidence that hypernatraemia develops in the ICU as a result of fluid loss being either under-replaced or over-replaced with hypertonic fluids [7]. For fluid management to be meaningful and effective, regular serum, and ideally urine, sodium measurements at the point of care are essential [8]. In a study of 130 ICU patients with hypernatraemia (93% with ICU-acquired hypernatraemia), likely contributory factors to the development of this condition were recorded (see Table 12.2) [7]. Of these patients 62% were in negative fluid balance, the remaining 38% in positive fluid balance and the risk factors equally distributed between these groups except for those with renal failure which was more common in those with negative fluid balance (Fig. 12.3).

12.4.1.1.2 Hyponatraemia

Hyponatraemia is usually defined as a plasma/serum sodium of less than the lower limit of the reference interval — usually 135 mmol/l — but in the context of critical care may reasonably also be classified on the basis of a significant decline (e.g. change of > 2 mmol/l over a short period). However defined this is a very common finding in critically ill patients. A recent retrospective study of > 53,000 patients over seven years [9] studied independent associations of community-acquired, hospital-aggravated and hospital-acquired hyponatraemia with in-hospital mortality, length of stay and patient disposition. The study showed not only that hospital-acquired hyponatraemia was very common but that all forms of hyponatraemia were independently associated with in-hospital mortality, the strength of association being related to hyponatraemia severity. Hyponatraemia also increased care costs. In the context of the ICU the same prognostic risk occurs with hyponatraemia [5,10].

Table 12.2. Potential factors contributing to hypernatraemia in intensive care from matched case-controlled study [7].

Mechanisms	Observed causes	Cases (%)	Controls (%)	p value
Concentrating defect	Diseases associated with cranial diabetes insipidus (CDI)	7	5	0.3
	Drugs associated with nephrogenic diabetes insipidus (NDI)	22	15	0.08
	Hypokalaemia (≤ 3.5 mmol/l)	53	34	<0.001
	Hypercalcaemia (Cai (ionised calcium) ≥ 1.29)	17	5	0.001
	Loop diuretics	22	25	0.4
	Renal dysfunction (creatinine ≥ reference interval (RI))	53	13	<0.001
Osmotic diuresis	Mannitol	10	1	0.001
	Hyperglycaemia (> 10 mmol/l)	43	31	0.04
Shift of water	Hypoalbuminaemia (< 35 g/l)	91	55	<0.001
Sodium gain	Sodium bicarbonate use	23	0.4	<0.001
Non-renal water loss	Lactulose	11	7	0.2

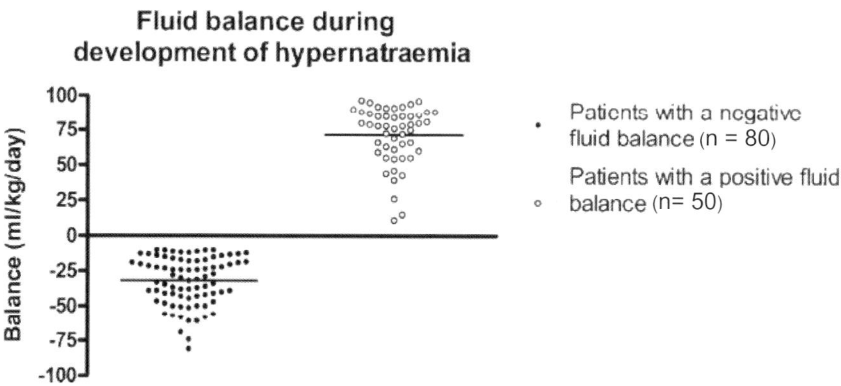

Figure 12.3. Fluid balance during the development of hypernatraemia. Fluid balances were calculated during the development of hypernatraemia using all input (intravenous fluids, oral intake, nutrition, blood products) and output (24-hour urine, insensible and enteral losses, blood loss and wound drains) values [7].

12.4.1.2 *Potassium*

A significant symptom of acute hypokalaemia is muscle weakness which, in addition to potential respiratory compromise, carries a risk of cardiac dysrhythmia when severe. Although the development of hypokalaemia can be gradual, for example as a result of increased urinary losses associated with diuretic administration or excessive gastrointestinal losses it can also develop rapidly within an hour or so. The typical example of this is as a result of sudden lowering of partial pressure of arterial CO_2 in a compensated respiratory acidosis which will cause acute alkalosis with subsequent acute shift of potassium into cells. This process may be further influenced by endocrine changes (e.g., both glucocorticoid and mineralocorticoid) and by pharmacological interventions (e.g., low-dose hydrocortisone and thiazide diuretics). Abnormalities in renal tubular function such as renal tubular acidosis are recognised complications in critically ill patients (e.g.,

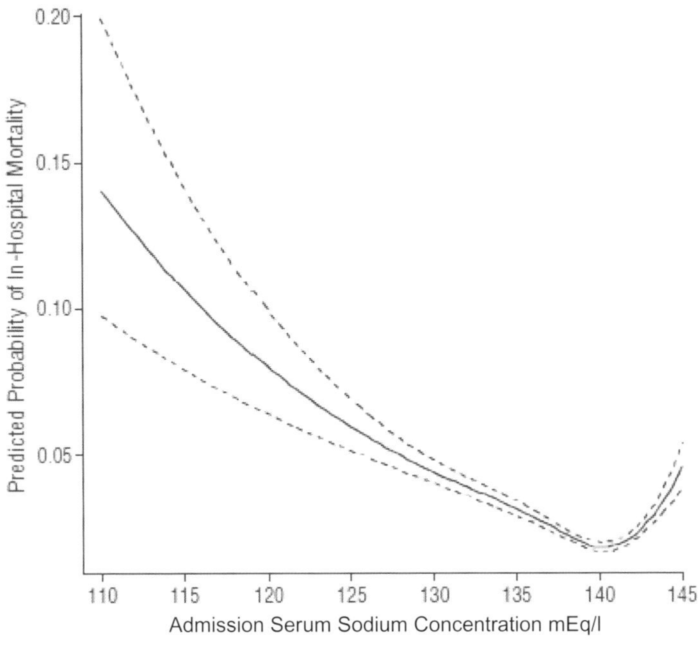

Figure 12.4. Restrictive cubic spline depicting the unadjusted relationship between hospital admission sodium concentrations and in-hospital mortality. Dashed lines represent the 95% confidence interval.

drug-induced, as a complication of diabetic ketoacidosis or from acute tubular necrosis), and this should encourage the intensivist to evaluate urine electrolytes, pH and anion gap carefully. Although these are difficult to evaluate at the point of care, the delays from remote analysis are one of the reasons why these tests are often neglected. Access to rapid urine analysis at the point of care would enhance electrolyte and acid–base assessment and would seem a high priority for development. Serum potassium concentrations can fall from 4.0 to 2.5 mEq/l (4.0 to 2.5 mmol/l) within two hours in extreme cases, and this is a well-recognised cause of cardiac arrhythmia and cardiac arrest.

Hyperkalaemia is also common in ICU patients, both due to movement of potassium from within the cells in exchange for hydrogen ions during acidosis and because of reduced renal excretion of potassium due to renal impairment. Severe hyperkalaemia carries a risk of cardiac arrhythmia and cardiac arrest. Administration of insulin and glucose, either as part of intensive control of blood glucose (see Section 12.4.2.1) or for correction of acidosis, will drive potassium back into the cells and may result in a rapid fall in extracellular potassium. Renal replacement therapies such as hemofiltration also correct acidosis and will remove extracellular potassium. Thus, sudden changes in extracellular potassium concentrations are not uncommon in ICU patients and require regular monitoring of blood potassium, and in some circumstances results need to be available within in a few minutes.

12.4.1.3 *Other electrolytes*

12.4.1.3.1 Chloride

Chloride measurements are now available in most point-of-care testing blood gas analysers [11]. The slow change to the use of these analysers means that for many ICUs chloride is still only available from the central laboratory (usually on a venous sample), assessed once a day and not matched directly to an arterial gas result. Its measurement is essential for derivations such as anion gap $((Na^+ + K^+) — (Cl^- + HCO3^-))$ that help to assess the contribution of unmeasured anions to a metabolic acidosis [12,13]. As discussed later in the context of strong ion difference (Section 12.4.1.3.4) the role of chloride derived from sodium chloride infusions in regular use following surgical procedures or in the treatment of metabolic alkalosis requires that this ion be monitored regularly in ICU patients. The influence of chloride-containing fluids in the resuscitation of patients with diabetic ketoacidosis is well recognised [14,15]. Recent work suggests that restricting chloride-rich fluids in intensive care patients significantly influences acid–base status [16].

12.4.1.3.2 Calcium

A number of factors, including therapeutic interventions such as giving citrated blood products, electrolyte, colloid and drug therapy as well as renal, gastrointestinal, nutritional, metabolic and endocrine changes are likely to significantly affect calcium homeostasis [17]. The most significant clinical effect of hypocalcaemia is cardiac dysrhythmia and risk of cardiac arrest and this is easily treatable once diagnosed [18–20]. Other effects of hypocalcaemia yet to be evaluated clinically include the role in modulating cytokine activation. A high proportion of ICU patients require renal replacement therapy, usually haemofiltration, at some stage. The assessment of ionised calcium is of paramount importance for this process, particularly in the assessment of buffer correction and for when citrate is used as an anticoagulant. Hypocalcaemia is a recognised complication of acute pancreatitis and may provide early indication of multiple organ failure in this group of patients [21] as well as help to identify the condition when secondary to shock [22]. The calculation of 'corrected' or 'adjusted' calcium, on the traditional basis of adjustment for changes in serum albumin concentration, is likely to be unreliable in ICU patients, who will invariably have serum albumin concentrations in the range where analytical precision of serum albumin is poor at low levels and when other calcium-binding proteins such as globulins may be abnormal [23]. In addition, the effects of acid–base disturbance are not taken into account in the routine laboratory measurement of total calcium. Hypocalcaemia may develop in patients following massive transfusion of blood and some blood products and has been shown to be associated with a poor outcome in such patients [24]. Current clinical concerns about the effects of vitamin D deficiency have included the influence of this highly prevalent condition on outcome in critical illness although to date there is no clear indication of the benefit from assessment and correction in general ICU patients [25].

12.4.1.3.3 Magnesium

Serum magnesium is lowered, with a prevalence of as high as 65%, in critical illness as a result of the high metabolic demand, decreased absorption and renal and gastrointestinal loss [26–28]. The most common cause of hypomagnesaemia in ICU is from renal loss, magnesuria enhanced in metabolic acidoses, diuresis and drug therapy affecting renal tubular function such as amphotericin and cyclosporine [29]. Traditionally serum total magnesium is measured daily and low levels are considered a sufficient marker of depleted total body magnesium to instigate magnesium replacement. In general this probably suffices as there are no convincing studies to show that hypomagnesaemia causes major complications in ICUs although it must be assumed at the least to compromise electrical conduction and contractility in cardiac muscle [30]. The most practical method of assessing total body magnesium status is by measuring the excretion of a magnesium load and this can be achieved in ICU patients providing they have adequate renal function. The hypoproteinaemia present almost universally in ICU patients adds a further complication to this and if profound may lead to misinterpretation of the serum total magnesium level, as approximately 30% of serum magnesium is albumin-bound with 10% complexed to anions. The most likely value in the assessment of ionised magnesium will be in patients with renal failure requiring haemofiltration or dialysis [31]. There is however no evidence to suggest that the measurement of serum ionised magnesium is a better reflection of total body levels as less than 1% is in extracellular fluids.

12.4.1.3.4 Hydrogen/acid–base

Simultaneous measurement of arterial carbon dioxide and hydrogen ion concentration (pH) gives an indication of how well the lungs are removing carbon dioxide and the effect this is having on the net balance of acid production and removal. For example, in a patient with poor gas exchange and carbon dioxide retention for 24 hours or more, the initial excess of hydrogen ions due to formation of carbonic acid is normally corrected by renal synthesis (recycling) of additional bicarbonate. Patients with non-respiratory acidosis due, for example, to diabetic ketoacidosis will tend to hyperventilate, thereby lowering their pCO_2 and restoring their extracellular fluid (ECF) hydrogen ion concentration to normal. The effectiveness of this compensation can be assessed by measurement of arterial H^+ (pH) and pCO_2. Acid–base status can change extremely rapidly in the critically ill patient. For example, a patient suffering a cardiopulmonary arrest will develop a mixed respiratory and non-respiratory acidosis within two minutes. Assuming that resuscitation is effective and cardiac and lung function are restored, the patient's acidosis will generally clear within 30 to 60 minutes. Failure of acidosis to resolve within this period indicates further complications, and the patient may require inotropic support, bicarbonate infusion and alterations in ventilation. The calculated parameter of base excess (or deficit) is used as a way of assessing the degree of non-respiratory or metabolic acid–base disturbance. This parameter, if abnormal, does not give an indication of the cause of the metabolic disturbance, but it is common to rely on this as a barometer of change (e.g. base deficit in a metabolic acidosis). Current concepts of acid–base include not only the traditional buffer base Henderson–Hasselbach equation but also the electroneutrality concept described by Stewart [32,33,34].

In all aqueous systems, the balance of anions and cations must retain electrical neutrality. There are only three major independent determinants that control acid–base balance: pCO_2, weak acids (albumin and phosphate) and the strong ion difference (SID). In practice, the SID describes the mathematical difference between plasma Na^+, K^+, Ca^+ and Mg^+ (strong cations) and Cl^- and $lactate^-$ (strong anions) and is normally between 38 and 42 mEq/l (38 and 42 mmol/l). If one of these ions increases in concentration (e.g., Cl^-), then the SID will be reduced. To retain electrical neutrality, more hydrogen ions dissociate from water and the hydrogen ion concentration increases, the pH falls and the patient becomes acidaemic. However, the change in hydrogen ion concentration is in the nanomolar range and is insufficient to maintain electrical neutrality when the chloride rises by millimoles; thus, the plasma proteins play the major role in restoring electrical neutrality. The reverse happens in patients with a chloride deficit, such as might arise with loss of nasogastric aspirate from the upper gastrointestinal tract. This leads to a decrease in the chloride:sodium ratio, an increase in the SID, and thus a decrease in water dissociation and a fall in hydrogen ion activity (hypochloraemic alkalosis). Thus assessment of chloride, and in particular the chloride:sodium ratio, becomes of real value in determining the acid–base disturbance and assessing treatment in critically ill patients [33–37]. Assessment of SID can be used as a quantitative guideline for chloride (NaCl or KCl) replacement. The practical implications of this concept as an influence on patient outcome have been studied in trauma and ICU settings and most commentators acknowledge the added value from the principles involved [38,39] although there is no convincing evidence to make significant alterations to fluid replacement regimes based on the data from the Stewart approach [40]. It has revived awareness that chloride is an essential contributor to acid–base balance in the ICU and confirms that this parameter needs to be available from POCT [41].

Diagnosis and treatment of metabolic acidosis must include an assessment of unmeasured anions. Although lactate is usually available on POCT blood gas analysers, unmeasured anions include phosphate, sulphate and hippurate in renal failure, and ketones in starvation and diabetic ketoacidosis, as well as other anions involved in intermediary metabolism in sepsis [42–44] and those after poisoning (e.g. formic acid from methanol). Careful inspection of the anion gap may suggest a significant contribution from these unmeasured anions. For example, starvation ketoacidosis is frequently a significant problem in ICU patients, yet can easily be missed or ignored [45,46]. Some recent studies have evaluated the comparative values of the strong ion gap and 'albumin-corrected' anion gap (AG(corr)), where AG is adjusted for serum albumin, and have produced strong evidence in support of the use of this derived parameter [44,47,48]. Measurement of blood ketones (ideally the predominant ketoacid hydroxybutyrate) should be considered a high priority in the assessment of a metabolic acidosis and is now widely included in diabetes ketoacidosis management protocols which can be facilitated by hand-held ketone meters [49–53].

12.4.1.3.5 Phosphate

Of the ions of potential value for clinical purposes the phosphate anion, with its prime involvement in acid–base balance and cellular energetics, would seem a prime candidate for development as a point-of-care analyte. Phosphorylation is such a key component of cell signalling and metabolic processes that it would not be unreasonable to assume it to be important that the blood's inorganic phosphorus concentration should be maintained within normal limits. Serum 'phosphate' measurements are made routinely as part of the daily biochemistry profile but little is often done in response to the significant falls that are seen during the ICU stay. One significant reason for this reticence is that interpretation of serum phosphate levels in ICU patients is not straightforward. Most patients, particularly in the early post-operative phase, remain on limited nutritional support for the first few days in the ICU whilst there may be a considerable increase in metabolic demands during this period. Apart from gastrointestinal losses and renal proximal tubular losses in some patients there is a recognised disturbance in calcium homeostasis in many ICU patients, in part stimulated by the increased production of calcitonin precursors such as procalcitonin in severe inflammation and particularly sepsis, and this will affect phosphate turnover [54]. Other factors influencing serum phosphate in this situation are likely to include cytokines and other inflammatory mediators [55]. Recent work has suggested that high ventilatory rates might play a significant role in inducing hypophosphataemia in ICU patients [56,57]. Drug treatments and fluid replacement regimes will also influence serum phosphate and increased metabolic phosphorylation requirements may mask the ensuing phosphate retention in patients with severe renal failure. Hypophosphataemia is a recognised complication during the management of diabetic ketoacidosis and although there is limited literature to support it phosphate replacement is usually given empirically in this situation (although occasionally it can have severe consequences [58–61]. Critical illness has profound effects on muscle bulk and activity, reflected in serum phosphate changes [62,63].

The question that is as relevant for phosphate as it is for other potential point-of-care analytes in ICU is whether there is a clinical need for regular and fast turnaround measurements of body fluid phosphate concentration that cannot be adequately provided by a central laboratory.

Over the last few years greater understanding of the control mechanisms of phosphate handling by the kidney have emerged, particularly the relationship between phosphate and vitamin D and also the defective processes that occur in acute kidney injury (AKI), a common pathology in intensive care patients. A key player in this process is the phosphatonin fibroblast growth factor 23 (FGF-23) and its membrane receptor co-factor Klotho [64,65]. Recent work has also suggested that measurement of serum C-terminal FGF-23 levels can predict outcome from AKI and need for renal replacement therapy [66].

The ICU dietician will note the serum phosphate in the daily profile as part of the nutritional assessment but will not usually be involved in the management of severe hypophosphataemia in acute situations. The metabolic physician would reasonably argue that phosphate measurements should coincide in real-time with blood gas, other electrolyte and metabolite concentrations as part of the metabolic profile and thus would need to be available at point-of-care. Clearly studies are needed to evaluate this concept before such an inclusion in the POCT repertoire could be contemplated.

12.4.2 *Metabolites*

12.4.2.1 *Glucose*

The critically ill patient's ability to maintain blood glucose concentrations within the limits defined for normal subjects is often impaired. Moderate hyperglycaemia is frequently found following an acute inflammatory stimulus (e.g. surgery, myocardial infarction, sepsis, trauma or burns) and is attributed to release of glucocorticoids and catecholamines, which stimulate gluconeogenesis. Hyperglycaemia can worsen a hyperosmotic state such as uraemia and may predispose a patient to infection. Several studies in recent years have revealed an association with hyperglycaemia and increased morbidity and mortality in intensive care patients although there is still some disagreement on the degree of significance [67–71]. Hyperglycaemia in sepsis is also a poor predictor in noncritical-care hospitalised patients and there have been recent guidelines suggesting point-of-care glucose in all hyperglycaemic hospitalised patients, whether diabetic or not [70].

A more serious risk in critically ill patients is hypoglycaemia, which if untreated can cause brain damage and death. In a healthy fasting subject, the glycogen reserves in the liver and muscle will provide glucose (glucose-6-phosphate in muscle) for about 24 hours, after which the glucose supply is derived from gluconeogenesis. In contrast, a critically ill patient who is hypercatabolic will use up the glycogen stores within a few hours and risk becoming hypoglycaemic if gluconeogenic pathways cannot meet the increased glucose demand. This is particularly true in neonates.

Concerns about risks from hypoglycaemia, combined with the lack of information to suggest an 'ideal' blood glucose level in critical illness and concerns about the accuracy of glucose stick tests have always cautioned against aggressive control of blood glucose. In 2001, a large randomised controlled study that compared conventional glucose control (144–198 mg/dl (8–11.0 mmol/l)) with intensive control (72–99 mg/dl (4–5.5 mmol/l)) was stopped following an interim assessment when it was demonstrated that there was significantly lower mortality in the intensive treatment group [72]. This study, which did not demonstrate an increased risk from hypoglycaemia in the intensive treatment group, had an immediate global effect on the management of blood glucose in ICU patients, and the intensive control target values were widely, but not universally, adopted. There is not a clear understanding of the mechanism for the influence on mortality, but it seems likely that the major influence comes from the insulin treatment and the complex metabolic and endocrine effects that it induces rather than from the normalisation of blood glucose itself. Since the original wave of enthusiasm to adopt this intensive insulin therapy (IIT) there have been many studies in a variety of patient groups in both surgical and medical ICUs. There have been conflicting results and the relative merits, as well as pragmatic issues, of the protocol have been hotly debated. The variable quality and compatibility of POCT glucose methodologies, particularly hand-held devices, inevitably raised concerns regarding the risk of hypoglycaemia and these concerns have been endorsed by the Normoglycaemia in Intensive Care Evaluation Survival Using Glucose Algorithm Regulation (NICE-SUGAR) international randomised study which found increased mortality in the IIT group and concluded that the hypoglycaemic risks are too severe to justify such a tight level of glycaemic control [73]. The safe use of IIT has, however, been shown to reduce ICU costs [74]. For this regime to be effective and safe, accurate measurements of blood glucose must be a high priority for point-of-care analysis, and these are usually now provided by a blood gas analyser with integral metabolite electrodes. As intravenous infusions of dextrose and insulin can produce rapid alterations in blood glucose, normoglycaemia in the critically ill patient can only be maintained by frequent monitoring, with results being rapidly available, and these results need to be accurate for the critical care patient whose deranged physiology may interfere with some POCT glucose techniques. There is some further interest in continuous glucose monitoring and, with better technology, options for this interesting development appear to be emerging [75]. Recent work suggests that diabetes mellitus does not increase mortality but may indeed improve outcome from a critical illness, thus confounding further the issue of the potential benefit from IIT [76].

12.4.2.2 *Lactate*

Since the appearance of blood lactate measurement integrated with blood gas analysis the value of blood lactate measurement in the management of the intensive care patient has become widely recognised, although it is also acknowledged that in most instances except in specific cases of defined lactic acidosis the biomarker lacks direct specificity for almost any clinical condition. Blood or serum lactate measurements are of comparative specific value in the management of conditions such as congenital organic acidaemias, some toxic states (e.g. alcohols), although there can be analytical interference with some alcohols and POCT lactate measurements [76], as well as some infective conditions, most notably severe *falciparum* malaria [78–80]. Nevertheless, most of these acidotic states with multiple organ failure are accompanied by increased unmeasured anions that may be quantified using a calculation of the strong ion gap (SIG) [81]. The argument that the knowledge of an elevated blood lactate level may not directly influence general patient management has been promoted for many years but in the ICU the need for focussed, informed management weakens this argument considerably. Recent studies have highlighted the prognostic value of elevated lactate in a variety of critical care situations [82–86], most notably severe sepsis and poor tissue oxygenation [87,88]. The implication of the lactate ion in the generation of a significant base deficit, with its recognised poor prognosis, may lead to an acceleration in therapy of the acid–base defect in many circumstances. Part of the reason why lactic acidaemia, defined here as any metabolic acidaemia with an elevated blood lactate concentration, carries such a stigma is that the condition arises when production exceeds clearance and that is mostly encountered at the later stages of multiple organ failure where other treatment regimes may be of limited benefit. In the conditions where lactate is defining the degree of decreased oxygen delivery it must be understood that this will, in most circumstances, imply global rather than local dysfunctions. Attempts to assess local hypoxia, such as that of the splanchnic bed which pre-empts the onset of multiple organ failure and lactic acidaemia, have included much recent work from measurements of gastric tonometry measuring the relative (lactic) acidosis of the splanchnic vascular [89]. Lactic acidaemia is a severe condition because there is limited specific therapy for the condition and also because acidaemia itself is responsible for cardiac dysfunction and is putatively the ultimate cause of death.

In the author's clinical experience, the introduction of regular blood lactate measurements in ICU, particularly in patients with metabolic acidaemia and significant base deficit, leads to a surprising change in insight of the pathophysiology of many conditions encountered in the intensive care unit. Thus, lactate was often suggested to be the offending anion in an unexplained metabolic acidosis but often subsequently found that this was not the case and that other anions, usually related to unrecognised renal dysfunction (i.e. phosphate, sulphate and hippurate) or to fasting (i.e. ketones) are implicated. Similarly significant elevations in blood lactate are found in many conditions where the acid–base disturbance is not clearly apparent as a result of compensatory mechanisms and from the interference in the respiratory component. In other words, the clinician needs to be wary of the interpretation of elevated blood lactate unless a condition such as severe cardiovascular shock, sepsis or severe malaria is the main clinical presentation. Interpretation has to be carried out computing the information available on oxygen delivery, cardiac, respiratory and hepatic function as well as clinical variables. Even in sepsis the interpretation of elevated blood lactate is compromised by a lack of understanding of the mechanisms responsible for the elevation [90,91] and is further complicated by the metabolic effects of inotrope therapy [92,93]. The effects of epinephrine and norepinephrine can be profound in certain circumstances [94], and are probably mediated by effects on hepatic gluconeogenesis rather than via tissue hypoperfusion. Traditional teaching has been based on studies demonstrating the mechanism of lactic acidosis in sepsis as secondary to an increased metabolic rate and decreased peripheral oxygen delivery. Recent work has suggested that peripheral oxygen consumption is relatively normal and that the balance of lactate metabolism is disturbed by an increased lactate production by tissues such as the lung, particularly when heavily infiltrated by lymphocytes, which have a high capacity for lactate production [95,96]. This is further compromised by a decrease in liver lactate clearance as a result of the effects on intermediary metabolism by the mediators of the inflammatory response, which may themselves be influenced by tissue hypoxia or washout following reperfusion.

12.4.3 *Organ dysfunction/function*

12.4.3.1 *Cardiac function*

Cardiac function is clearly one of the most critical of the organ systems in the ICU patient. The use of specific cardiac biomarkers has an important additional role and when cardiac troponins emerged into routine clinical practice in the 1990s it became clear that these could not only add additional information for evaluating cardiac ischaemia and damage but that the incidence of these conditions may be more common than was previously realised. In this study in patients in a mixed medical and respiratory ICU, 15% of patients were found to have evidence of cardiac damage based on cardiac troponin I elevations but in two-thirds of these patients the myocardial damage had not been detected by conventional monitoring — 'silent myocardial ischaemia'. The suggestion at that stage in the evolution of the troponin biomarkers — troponin I and troponin T — was that these biomarkers could more specifically diagnose undetected myocardial damage in critically ill patients and that their usage could influence outcome. Since then more information has emerged on the specificity and sensitivity of these markers in critically ill patients as well as on analytical aspects of the assays. In a study looking at the prevalence, incidence and outcomes from elevated cardiac troponins in critically ill patients, Lim *et al.* [97] found a prevalence of a raised troponin within the first 48 hours of ICU admission of 42% with approximately 50% of these having a myocardial infarction (MI) and the remainder having raised troponin alone. The incidence of elevated troponin after 48 hours was lower at 12% and again half of these patients demonstrated MI. In the literature the prevalence of raised troponin levels in general ICU patients ranges from 15% to 70% and in patients with sepsis or septic shock this increased to 31% to 80%. Clearly abnormal troponin levels are seen with high frequency in ICU patients with no evidence of coronary artery disease, and such conditions include shock associated with trauma or sepsis, pulmonary embolism, stroke, renal failure and pulmonary disease. The prognostic value of raised troponin in ICU patents can therefore be uncertain (Fig. 12.5). In a more recent study of 103 admissions the picture was similar with 50% of patients presenting with elevated troponin, in half of whom the cause was MI but 18% having sepsis, 12% renal failure and 16% other causes. In this study the mortality in the patients with MI was 23% compared with 39% in those with elevated troponin not due to MI and 2% in those with no troponin elevation. Interestingly therefore a troponin elevation not due to an MI was somewhat predictive of increased hospital mortality. In another study looking at the significance of raised troponin levels in critically ill patients with acute respiratory disease an independent association was found between raised troponin levels and in-hospital, short-term and long-term mortality, even after adjustment for severity of disease using APACHE III prognostic parameters, cardiovascular comorbidities and risk factors [98]. The independent association remained after accounting for MI or renal failure.

Thus, although cardiac troponin has become a critical component in the evaluation of patients with acute coronary syndromes (ACS), its diagnostic specificity is significantly diminished in critically ill patients.

In many of these conditions the troponin rise may not reach the diagnostic cut-off for clinically discriminating an MI (e.g. for troponin $T \geq 0.1$ ng/ml) and in patients with chronic renal failure it has long been realised that the diagnostic sensitivity of troponin for ACS is diminished. There are clearly specific difficulties in interpretation of raised troponin levels in patients with renal impairment. In some studies as many as 80% of patients with low glomerular filtration rate (GFR) have been found to have elevated troponin values whilst in others the association is not as

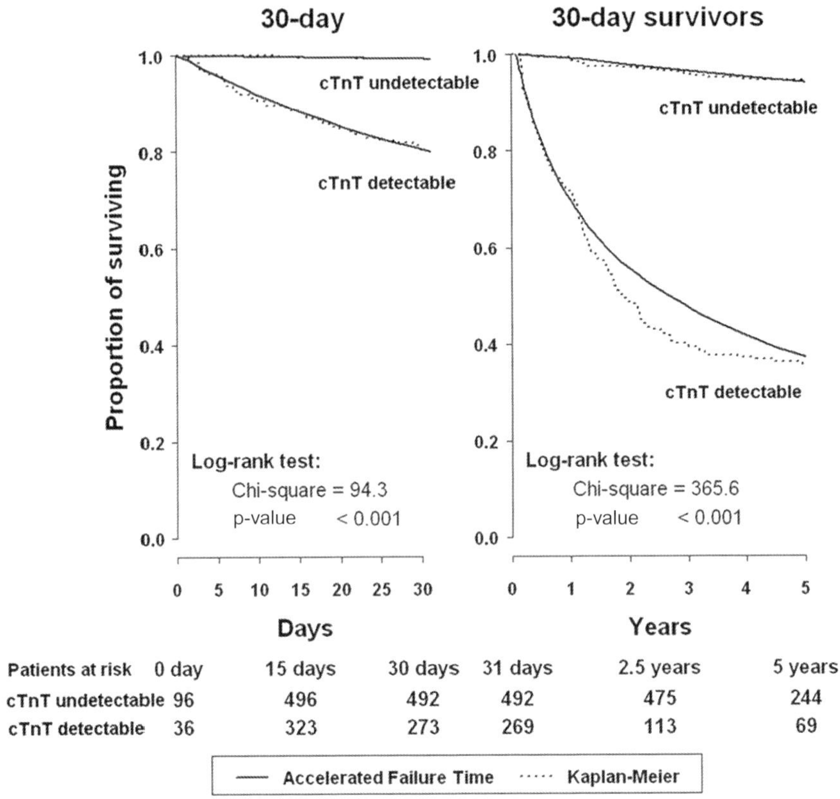

Figure 12.5. Expected probability of death according to the admission troponin T level. cTnT, cardiac troponin T (from [98]).

strong. The current data supports the concept that elevations in troponin so widely seen in these patients can represent relative accumulation of the troponins rather than just a reflection of the extent of any myocardial injury. In patients with renal failure undergoing dialysis or other renal replacement therapies measurement of troponin should ideally be timed for just before the onset of replacement therapy as dialysis will itself affect troponin levels. There is however general agreement that elevated troponin levels in patients with renal failure carries a poor prognosis that may partly reflect the recognised link between renal and cardiovascular disease.

12.4.3.2 *Renal function*

For most purposes routine central laboratory analysis of renal function, performed by daily serum electrolyte, urea and creatinine measurements, provide adequate assessment of renal function fluid management. More regular assessment of glomerular function should be promoted in patients with multiple organ failure particularly as part of the assessment and monitoring of renal replacement therapies. Early prediction of development of acute renal failure is clearly useful, and existing parameters for this, including assessment of free water clearance, fractional excretion of sodium, urine/serum osmolality and tubular reabsorption of phosphate, should be measured regularly; this could be simplified by POCT. Although many POCT blood gas analysers now measure urea (urea nitrogen), and some measure creatinine, accurate urine analysis of many parameters is not well supported by POCT. Estimated GFR, based on serum creatinine concentration, is now widely calculated in relatively stable individuals as a means of grading renal function but this calculation is not secure in critically ill patients and for these formal creatinine clearance measurements are cumbersome and impractical.

In acutely ill ICU patients plasma creatinine rises occur relatively late, typically two to three days, after the trigger of AKI. Thus even regular monitoring of plasma creatinine can be insufficient as an early warning system for detecting AKI [97]. There has therefore recently been an extensive search for better biomarkers that enable early detection of this condition. Indeed a number of biomarkers have emerged over the last decade (Fig. 12.6) and several show considerable promise as a result of functional genomic and proteonomic studies, although none have yet emerged that are confidently classified as an ideal marker there is considerable optimism [99–104]. One of the most promising markers is urine neutrophil gelatinase-associated lipocalin (NGAL) in a variety of clinical settings including sepsis [105].

These studies are immensely complicated to perform with many variables including timing of sampling, baseline estimates of GFR and variable urine output as well as treatment variables. More work is required to establish the optimal marker or panel of markers for this function.

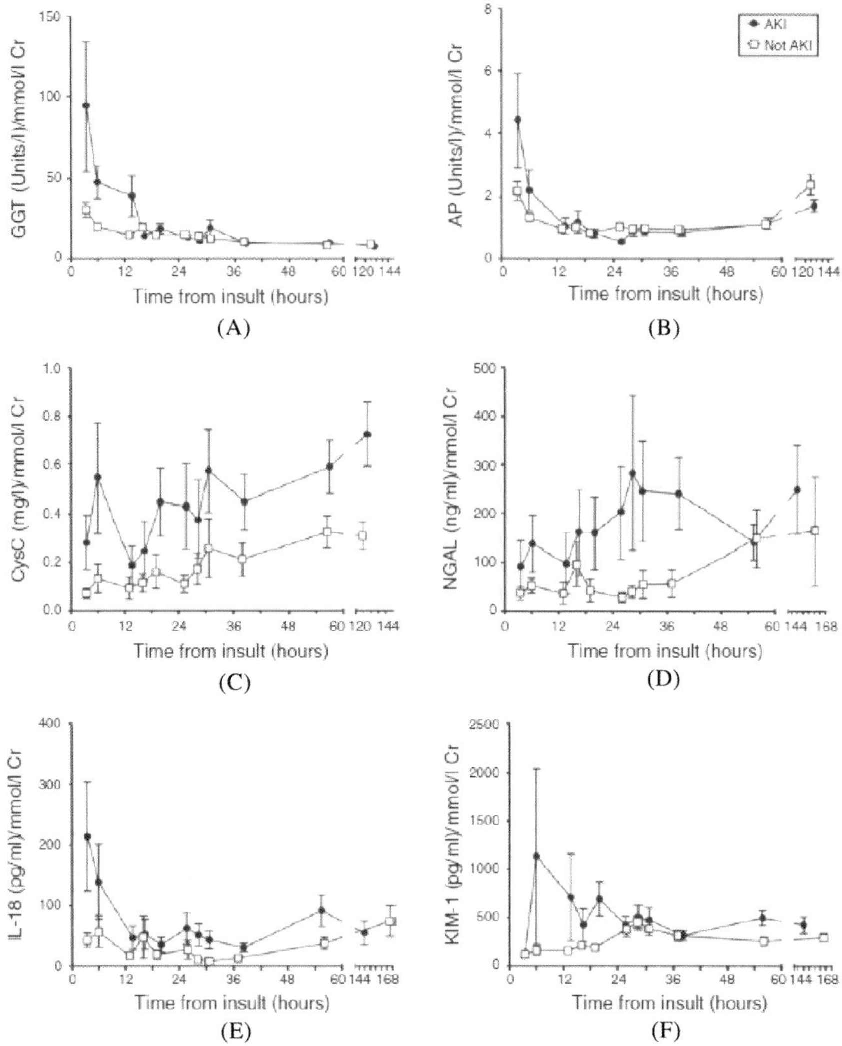

Figure 12.6. Time course of urinary biomarkers from a putative insult — (A) γ Glutamyl transferase (GGT), (B) Alkaline phosphatase (AP), (C) Cystatin C (CysC), (D) Neutrophil gelatinase-associated lipocalin (NGAL), (E) Interleukin-18 (IL-18) and (F) Kidney injury molecule-1 (KIM-1). AKI is AKI on entry and AKIN48 is AKI at any time within 48 hours of entry to the ICU. Mean ± standard error of the mean. Approximately 50 measures at each time point for the AKI group [105].

12.4.4 *Infection and sepsis*

The term sepsis in ICU patients generally refers to the patient response to a severe inflammatory stimulus, which can be caused by insults such as trauma, surgery, ischaemia–reperfusion injury or bacterial infection. The clinical features include pyrexia, confusion or loss of consciousness, with hypotension, tachycardia and vasodilatation with either a rapid fall or rapid increase in white cell count outside the reference range. This combination of symptoms has been defined as the systemic inflammatory response syndrome (SIRS), and carries an increased risk of organ failure and death. Although the clinical features are fairly consistent, the initiating cause of inflammation may not be obvious. Studies of ICU patients with SIRS have failed to identify an infective organism in about 40% of cases, which has supported the concept that many cases of SIRS are due to non-infective inflammatory processes. There is an alternative view, which is that most patients with SIRS are suffering from an infection, but that laboratory investigations have failed to identify an infective organism. However, in order to treat patients effectively, it is important to differentiate between infective and non-infective causes of SIRS. For this reason, there has been a search for more sensitive and specific markers of bacterial sepsis. Much information has emerged from genomics and functional genomics studies, which has shed light on the balance of inflammatory and subsequent anti-inflammatory (immunosuppressive) components of the host response to infection [106].

The most widely used marker of inflammation is C-reactive protein (CRP) but the specificity of this marker is not considered adequate for regular use in ICU patients who in most cases have multiple inflammatory stimulants, especially in the post-operative state [107,108]. Procalcitonin is a 14-kDa protein encoded by the *Calc-1* gene along with calcitonin and katacalcin, which is elevated in patients with sepsis and severe infections. In a study of 123 consecutive ICU patients with SIRS, Bell *et al.* found that procalcitonin was ten times higher in those with positive blood cultures, when combined with CRP was more sensitive than either test alone, and differentiated between patients who died in the hospital or survived [109]. In a comparison of procalcitonin with interleukin (IL)-2 and IL-8 in 33 patients with sepsis or septic shock, all three markers increased in parallel with illness severity. However procalcitonin exhibited the greatest sensitivity (85%) and specificity (91%) in differentiating patients with SIRS from those with sepsis. The authors suggested that daily determination of procalcitonin may be helpful in the follow-up of critically ill patients. In 116 neonates and children up to 12 years old with sepsis, Enguix *et al.* compared procalcitonin with CRP and serum amyloid A on admission or when a bacterial sepsis was suspected [110]. In critically ill neonates, procalcitonin, CRP, and amyloid A all had similar diagnostic efficiency as markers of sepsis, but procalcitonin concentration > 8.1 ng/ml identified all children with bacterial sepsis. In 101 consecutive patients admitted to a medical ICU, serum procalcitonin concentration was a more sensitive and specific marker of sepsis, compared with serum CRP, IL-6 and lactate levels [111]. Finally, a follow-up of 405 trauma patients suggested that procalcitonin is a sensitive predictor of post-trauma complications such as severe sepsis and organ failure [112].

These studies suggest that procalcitonin is a more specific marker for bacterial sepsis than serum CRP or pro-inflammatory cytokines such as IL-2, IL-6, or tumour necrosis factor. Over the last few years the role of procalcitonin measurements in influencing the use of antibiotics in septic patients has been extensively studied and algorithms have been developed that have demonstrated good cost:benefit ratios from the use of this sepsis marker in this context [113–115]. The algorithm requires quantitative testing but this is not yet available for POCT and a semi-quantitative POCT method seems to be restricted to a few paediatric intensive care units to support diagnosis and management of neonatal sepsis. In the author's experience the current demand for POCT is in complex cases where a stronger indication of a bacterial rather than viral source of infection would help manage a case where the diagnosis has become complicated and unproven by other means. The evidence base for such single rather than sequential usage of POCT is however still inadequate except for low-risk infections [116] and a good correlation has been shown between admission POCT levels and positive blood cultures in patients admitted with community-acquired pneumonia.

Sepsis markers can be used at different stages of the infective process and the huge range of potential candidates may be used to target the very early stages (e.g. cytokines), host-response processes within hours (acute phase reactants with variable time of onset and peak levels) and more delayed and sustained markers. None of these, other than lactate with its relatively low specificity, are widely available for POCT at present.

References

[1] Finfer, S., Chittock. D.R., Su, S.Y. *et al.* (2009). Intensive versus conventional glucose control in critically ill patients, *N Engl J Med*, **360**, 1283–1297.

[2] Buckley, M.S., Leblanc, J.M. and Cawley, M.J. (2010). Electrolyte disturbances associated with commonly prescribed medications in the intensive care unit, *Crit Care Med*, **38** (Suppl. 6), S253–S264.

[3] Moritz, M.L. and Ayus J.C. (2004). Dysnatremias in the critical care setting, *Contrib Nephrol*, **144**, 132–157.

[4] Funk, G.C., Lindner, G., Druml, W. *et al.* (2010). Incidence and prognosis of dysnatremias present on ICU admission, *Intens Care Med*, **36**, 304–311.

[5] Luu, J.L., Wendtland, C.L., Gross, M.F. *et al.* (2011). Three-percent saline administration during pediatric critical care transport, *Pediatr Emerg Care*, **27**, 1113–1117.

[6] O'Donoghue, S.D., Dulhunty, J.M., Bandeshe, H.K. *et al.* (2009). Acquired hypernatraemia is an independent predictor of mortality in critically ill patients, *Anaesthesia*, **64**, 514–520.

[7] Hoorn, E.J., Betjes, M.G., Weigel, J. *et al.* (2008). Hypernatraemia in critically ill patients: too little water and too much salt, *Nephrol Dial Transplant*, **23**, 1562–1568.

[8] Rosner, M.H. and Ronco C. (2010). Dysnatremias in the intensive care unit. *Contrib Nephrol*, **165**: 292–298.

[9] Wald, R., Jaber, B.L., Price, L.L. *et al.* (2010). Impact of hospital-associated hyponatremia on selected outcomes, *Arch Intern Med*, **170**, 294–302.

[10] Palmer, B.F. (2009). Hyponatremia in the intensive care unit, *Semin Nephrol*, **29**, 257–270.

[11] Koch, S.M. and Taylor R.W. (1992). Chloride ion in intensive care medicine, *Crit Care Med*, **20**, 227–240.

[12] Ishihara, K. and Szerlip, H.M. (1998). Anion gap acidosis, *Semin Nephrol*, **18**, 83–97.

[13] Yunos, N.M., Kim, I.B., Bellomo, R, *et al.* (2011). The biochemical effects of restricting chloride-rich fluids in intensive care, *Crit Care Med*, **39**, 2419–2424.

[14] Taylor, D., Durward, A., Tibby, S.M. *et al.* (2006). The influence of hyperchloraemia on acid base interpretation in diabetic ketoacidosis, *Intens Care Med*, **32**, 295–301.

[15] Mrozik, L.T. and Yung M. (2009). Hyperchloraemic metabolic acidosis slows recovery in children with diabetic ketoacidosis: a retrospective audit, *Aust Crit Care*, **22**, 172–177.

[16] Yunos, N.M., Bellomo, R., Story, D. *et al.* (2010). Bench-to-bedside review: Chloride in critical illness, *Crit Care*, **14**, 226.

[17] Lind, L., Carlstedt, F., Rastad, J. *et al.* (2000). Hypocalcemia and parathyroid hormone secretion in critically ill patients, *Crit Care Med*, **28**, 93–99.

[18] Kost, G.J. (1993). The significance of ionized calcium in cardiac and critical care. Availability and critical limits at US medical centers and children's hospitals, *Arch Pathol Lab Med*, **117**, 890–896.

[19] Zaloga, G.P. (1992). Hypocalcemia in critically ill patients, *Crit Care Med*, **20**, 251–262.

[20] Jankowski, S. and Vincent, J.L. (1995). Calcium administration for cardiovascular support in critically ill patients: when is it indicated? *J Intensive Care Med*, **10**, 91–100.

[21] Kawa, S., Mukawa, K, Kiyosawa, K. (2000). Hypocalcemia < 7.5 mg/dl: early predictive marker for multisystem organ failure in severe acute necrotizing pancreatitis, proposed by the study analyzing post-ERCP pancreatitis, *Am J Gastroenterol*, **95**, 1096–1097.

[22] Kovacs, J., Gurzu, S., Jung, J. *et al.* (2012). Clinico-pathological particularities of the shock-related pancreatitis, *Pathol Oncol Res*, **18**, 977–981.

[23] Byrnes, M.C., Huynh, K., Helmer, S.D. *et al.* (2005). A comparison of corrected serum calcium levels to ionized calcium levels among critically ill surgical patients, *Am J Surg*, **189**, 310–314.

[24] Ho, K.M. and Leonard A.D. (2011). Concentration-dependent effect of hypocalcaemia on mortality of patients with critical bleeding requiring massive transfusion: a cohort study, *Anaesth Intensive Care*, **39**, 46–54.

[25] Lee, P., Nair, P., Eisman, J,A. *et al.* (2009). Vitamin D deficiency in the intensive care unit: an invisible accomplice to morbidity and mortality? *Intens Care Med*, **35**, 2028–2032.

[26] Toffaletti, J. (1995). Physiology and regulation. Ionized calcium, magnesium and lactate measurements in critical care settings, *Am J Clin Pathol*, **104** (4, Suppl. 1), S88–S94.

[27] Sanders, G.T., Huijgen, H.J. and Sanders, R. (1999). Magnesium in disease: a review with special emphasis on the serum ionized magnesium, *Clin Chem Lab Med*, **37**, 1011–1033.

[28] Escuela, M.P., Guerra, M., Añón, J.M. *et al.* (2005). Total and ionized serum magnesium in critically ill patients, *Intens Care Med*, **31**, 151–156.

[29] Soliman, H.M., Mercan, D., Lobo, S.S. *et al.* (2003). Development of ionized hypomagnesemia is associated with higher mortality rates, *Crit Care Med*, **31**, 1082–1087.

[30] Yurvati, A.H., Sanders, S.P., Dullye, L.J. *et al.* (1992). Antiarrhythmic response to intravenously administered magnesium after cardiac surgery, *South Med J*, **85**, 714–717.

[31] Pedrozzi, N.E., Truttmann, A.C., Faraone, R. *et al.* (1998). Circulating ionized and total magnesium in end-stage kidney disease, *Nephron*, **79**, 288–292.

[32] Stewart, P.A. (1978). Independent and dependent variables of acid-base control, *Respir Physiol*, **33**, 9–26.

[33] Stewart, P.A. (1983). Modern quantitative acid–base chemistry, *Can J Physiol Pharmacol*, **61**, 1444–1461.

[34] Story, D.A., Morimatsu, H. and Bellomo, R. (2004). Strong ions, weak acids and base excess, a simplified Fencl-Stewart approach to clinical acid-base disorders, *Br J Anaesth*, **92**, 54–60.

[35] Morgan, T.J. (2009). The Stewart approach — one clinician's perspective, *Clin Biochem Rev*, **30**, 41–54.

[36] Nagaoka, D., Nassar Junior, A.P., Maciel, A.T. *et al.* (2010). The use of sodium-chloride difference and chloride-sodium ratio as strong ion difference surrogates in the evaluation of metabolic acidosis in critically ill patients, *J Crit Care*, **25**, 525–531.

[37] Kurt, A., Ecevit, A. Ozkiraz, S. *et al.* (2012). The use of chloride-sodium ratio in the evaluation of metabolic acidosis in critically ill neonates, *Eur J Pediatr*, **171**, 963–969.

[38] Zehtabchi, S., Soghoian, S. and Sinert, R. (2007). Utility of Stewart's strong ion difference as a predictor of major injury after trauma in the ED, *Am J Emerg Med*, **25**, 938–941.

[39] Kaplan, L.J. and Kellum, J.A. (2008). Comparison of acid-base models for prediction of hospital mortality after trauma, *Shock*, **29**, 662–666.

[40] Guidet, B., Soni, N., Della Rocca, G. *et al.* (2010). A balanced view of balanced solutions, *Crit Care*, **14**, 325.

[41] Berend, K., van Hulsteijn, L.H. and Gans R,O. (2012). Chloride, the queen of electrolytes? *Eur J Intern Med*, **23**, 203–211.

[42] Moviat, M., Terpstra, A.M., Ruitenbeek, W. *et al.* (2008). Contribution of various metabolites to the unmeasured anions in critically ill patients with metabolic acidosis, *Crit Care Med*, **36**, 752–758.

[43] Mao, H., Wang, H., Wang, B. *et al.* (2009). Systemic metabolic changes of traumatic critically ill patients revealed by an NMR-based metabonomic approach, *J Proteome Res*, **8**, 5423–5430.
[44] Mallat, J., Michel, D., Salaun, P. *et al.* (2012). Defining metabolic acidosis in patients with septic shock using Stewart approach, *Am J Emerg Med*, **30**, 391–398.
[45] Patel, A., Felstead, D., Doraiswami, M. *et al.* (2011). Acute starvation in pregnancy, a cause of severe metabolic acidosis, *Int J Obstet Anesth*, **20**, 253–256.
[46] Scholte, J.B. and Boer, W.E. (2012). A case of nondiabetic ketoacidosis in third term twin pregnancy, *J Clin Endocrinol Metab*, **97**, 3021–3024.
[47] Dubin, A., Menises, M.M., Masevicius, F.D. *et al.* (2007). Comparison of three different methods of evaluation of metabolic acid–base disorders, *Crit Care Med*, **35**, 1264–1270.
[48] Chawla, L.S., Shih, S., Davison, D. *et al.* (2008). Anion gap, anion gap corrected for albumin, base deficit and unmeasured anions in critically ill patients, implications on the assessment of metabolic acidosis and the diagnosis of hyperlactatemia, *BMC Emerg Med*, **8**, 18.
[49] Wallace, T.M., Meston, N.M., Gardner, S.G. *et al.* (2001). The hospital and home use of a 30-second hand-held blood ketone meter, guidelines for clinical practice, *Diabet Med*, **18**, 640–645.
[50] Vanelli, M., Chiari, G. and Capuano, C. (2003). Cost effectiveness of the direct measurement of 3-β-hydroxybutyrate in the management of diabetic ketoacidosis in children, *Diabetes Care*, **26**, 959.
[51] Vanelli, M., Chiari, G., Capuano, C. *et al.* (2003). The direct measurement of 3-beta-hydroxy butyrate enhances the management of diabetic ketoacidosis in children and reduces time and costs of treatment, *Diabetes Nutr Metab*, **16**, 312–316.
[52] O'Donohoe, P.B., Kessler, R., Beattie, T.F. (2006). Exploring the clinical utility of blood ketone levels in the emergency department assessment of paediatric patients, *Emerg Med J*, **23**, 783–787.
[53] Charles, R.A., Bee, Y.M., Eng, P.H. *et al.* (2007). Point-of-care blood ketone testing, screening for diabetic ketoacidosis at the emergency department, *Singapore Med J*, **48**, 986–989.
[54] Muller, B., Becker, K.L., Schächinger, H. *et al.* (2000). Calcitonin precursors are reliable markers of sepsis in a medical intensive care unit, *Crit Care Med*, **28**, 977–983.
[55] Barak, V., Schwartz, A., Kalickman, I. *et al.* (1998). Prevalence of hypophosphatemia in sepsis and infection, the role of cytokines, *Am J Med*, **104**, 40–47.

[56] Srinivasagam, D., Seshadri, M.S., Peter, J.V. *et al.* (1992). Prevalence & pathogenesis of hypophosphatemia in ventilated patients, *Indian J Med Res*, **96**, 87–90.

[57] Paleologos, M., Stone, E. and Braude, S. (2000). Persistent, progressive hypophosphataemia after voluntary hyperventilation, *Clin Sci (Lond)*, **98**, 619–625.

[58] Keller, U. and Berger, W. (1980). Prevention of hypophosphatemia by phosphate infusion during treatment of diabetic ketoacidosis and hyperosmolar coma, *Diabetes*, **29**, 87–95.

[59] Berger, W. and Keller, U. (1992). Treatment of diabetic ketoacidosis and non–ketotic hyperosmolar diabetic coma, *Baillieres Clin Endocrin*, **6**, 1–22.

[60] Ditzel, J. and Lervang H.H. (2010). Disturbance of inorganic phosphate metabolism in diabetes mellitus, clinical manifestations of phosphorus-depletion syndrome during recovery from diabetic ketoacidosis, *Diabetes Metab Syndr Obes*, **3**, 319–324.

[61] Liu, P.Y. and Jeng, C.Y. (2004). Severe hypophosphatemia in a patient with diabetic ketoacidosis and acute respiratory failure, *J Chin Med Assoc*, **67**, 355–359.

[62] Fredriksson, K., Hammarqvist, F., Strigård, K. *et al.* (2006). Derangements in mitochondrial metabolism in intercostal and leg muscle of critically ill patients with sepsis–induced multiple organ failure, *Am J Physiol Endocrinol Metab*, **291**, E1044–E1050.

[63] Gamrin, L., Andersson, K. Hultman, E. *et al.* (1997). Longitudinal changes of biochemical parameters in muscle during critical illness, *Metabolism*, **46**, 756–762.

[64] Cheng, C.Y., Kuro-o, M. and Razzaque M.S. (2011). Molecular regulation of phosphate metabolism by fibroblast growth factor-23-klotho system, *Adv Chronic Kidney Dis*, **18**, 91–97.

[65] Cavalli, L., Mazzotta, C. and Brandi, M.L. (2012). Phosphatonins, physiological role and pathological changes, *Clin Cases Miner Bone Metab*, **9**, 9–12.

[66] Leaf, D.E., Wolf, M., Waikar, S.S. *et al.* (2012). FGF-23 levels in patients with AKI and risk of adverse outcomes, *Clin J Am Soc Nephrol*, **7**, 1217–1223.

[67] D'Ancona, G., Bertuzzi, F., Sacchi, L. *et al.* (2011). Iatrogenic hypoglycemia secondary to tight glucose control is an independent determinant for mortality and cardiac morbidity, *Eur J Cardiothorac Surg*, **40**, 360–366.

[68] Godar, D.A., Kumar, D.R., Schmelzer, K.M. *et al.* (2011). The impact of serum glucose on clinical outcomes in patients hospitalized with community–acquired pneumonia, *WMJ*, **110**, 14–20.

[69] Tiruvoipati, R., Chiezey, B., Lewis, D. *et al.* (2012). Stress hyperglycemia may not be harmful in critically ill patients with sepsis, *J Crit Care*, **27**, 153–158.

[70] Wintergerst, K.A., Foster, M.B., Sullivan, J.E. *et al.* (2012). Association of hyperglycemia, glucocorticoids, and insulin use with morbidity and mortality in the pediatric intensive care unit, *J Diabetes Sci Technol*, **6**, 5–14.

[71] Schuetz, P., Kennedy, M., Lucas, J.M. *et al.* (2012). Initial management of septic patients with hyperglycemia in the noncritical care inpatient setting, *Am J Med*, **125**, 670–678.

[72] Van den Berghe, G., Wouters, P., Weekers, F. *et al.* (2001). Intensive insulin therapy in critically ill patients, *N Engl J Med*, **345**, 1359–1367.

[73] Van den Berghe, G., Schetz, M., Vlasselaers, D. *et al.* (2009). Clinical review, Intensive insulin therapy in critically ill patients, NICE-SUGAR or Leuven blood glucose target? *J Clin Endocrinol Metab*, **94**, 3163–3170.

[74] Krinsley, J.S. and Jones, R.L. (2006). Cost analysis of intensive glycemic control in critically ill adult patients, *Chest*, **129**, 644–650.

[75] Wolfsdorf, J.I. (2009). How effective is continuous glucose monitoring in intensively treated type 1 diabetes mellitus? *Nat Clin Pract Endocrinol Metab*, **5**, 134–135.

[76] Schlussel, A.T., Holt, D.B., Crawley, E.A. *et al.* (2011). Effect of diabetes mellitus on outcomes of hyperglycemia in a mixed medical surgical intensive care unit, *J Diabetes Sci Technol*, **5**, 731–740.

[77] Sandberg, Y., Rood, P.P., Russcher, H. *et al.* (2010). Falsely elevated lactate in severe ethylene glycol intoxication, *Neth J Med*, **68**, 320–323.

[78] Krishna, S., Waller, D.W., ter Kuile, F. *et al.* (1994). Lactic acidosis and hypoglycaemia in children with severe malaria, pathophysiological and prognostic significance, *Trans R Soc Trop Med Hyg*, **88**, 67–73.

[79] Day, N.P., Phu, N.H., Mai, N.T. *et al.* (2000). The pathophysiologic and prognostic significance of acidosis in severe adult malaria, *Crit Care Med*, **28**, 1833–1840.

[80] Planche, T. and Krishna S. (2006). Severe malaria, metabolic complications, *Curr Mol Med*, **6**, 141–153.

[81] von Seidlein, L., Olaosebikan, R., Hendriksen, I.C. *et al.* (2012). Predicting the clinical outcome of severe falciparum malaria in African children, findings from a large randomized trial, *Clin Infect Dis*, **54**, 1080–1090.

[82] Vincent, J.L. (1995). Lactate levels in critically ill patients, *Acta Anaesthesiol Scand Suppl*, **107**, 261–266.

[83] Pittard, A.J. (1999). Does blood lactate measurement have a role in the management of the critically ill patient? *Ann Clin Biochem*, **36**, 401–407.

[84] Jansen, T.C., van Bommel, J., Woodward, R. *et al.* (2009). Association between blood lactate levels, Sequential Organ Failure Assessment subscores, and 28-day mortality during early and late intensive care unit stay, a retrospective observational study, *Crit Care Med*, **37**, 2369–2374.

[85] van Beest, P.A., Mulder, P.J., Oetomo, S.B. *et al.* (2009). Measurement of lactate in a prehospital setting is related to outcome, *Eur J Emerg Med*, **16**, 318–322.

[86] Okorie, O.N. and Dellinger P. (2011). Lactate, biomarker and potential therapeutic target, *Crit Care Clin*, **27**, 299–326.

[87] Trzeciak, S., Dellinger, R.P, Chansky, M.E. *et al.* (2007). Serum lactate as a predictor of mortality in patients with infection, *Intens Care Med*, **33**, 970–977.

[88] Juneja, D., Singh, O. and Dang, R. (2011). Admission hyperlactatemia, causes, incidence, and impact on outcome of patients admitted in a general medical intensive care unit, *J Crit Care*, **26**, 316–320.

[89] Joynt, G.M., Lipman, J., Gomersall, C.D. *et al.* (1997). Gastric intramucosal pH and blood lactate in severe sepsis, *Anaesthesia*, **52**, 726–732.

[90] Bakker, J., Gris, P., Coffernils, M. *et al.* (1996). Serial blood lactate levels can predict the development of multiple organ failure following septic shock, *Am J Surg*, **171**, 221–226.

[91] Rimachi, R., Bruzzi de Carvahlo, F., Orellano-Jimenez, C. *et al.* (2012). Lactate/pyruvate ratio as a marker of tissue hypoxia in circulatory and septic shock, *Anaesth Intensive Care*, **40**, 427–432.

[92] Levy, B. (2005). Bench-to-bedside review, Is there a place for epinephrine in septic shock? *Crit Care*, **9**, 561–565.

[93] Levy, B., Bollaert. P.E., Charpentier, C. *et al.* (1997). Comparison of norepinephrine and dobutamine to epinephrine for hemodynamics, lactate metabolism, and gastric tonometric variables in septic shock, a prospective, randomized study, *Intens Care Med*, **23**, 282–287.

[94] Totaro, R.J. and Raper, R.F. (1997). Epinephrine-induced lactic acidosis following cardiopulmonary bypass, *Crit Care Med*, **25**, 1693–1699.

[95] Kellum, J.A., Kramer, D.J., Lee, K. *et al.* (1997). Release of lactate by the lung in acute lung injury, *Chest*, **111**, 1301–1305.

[96] Haji-Michael, P.G., Ladrière, L., Sener, A. *et al.* (1999). Leukocyte glycolysis and lactate output in animal sepsis and ex vivo human blood, *Metabolism*, **48**, 779–785.

[97] Lim, W., Cook, D.J., Griffith, L.E., *et al.* (2006). *Am J Crit Care*, **15(3)**, 280–8; quiz 289.

[98] Vasile, V.C., Chai, H.S., Khambatta, S. *et al.* (2010). Significance of elevated cardiac troponin T levels in critically ill patients with acute respiratory disease, *Am J Med*, **123**, 1049–1058.

[99] Singbartl, K. and Kellum, J.A. (2012). AKI in the ICU, definition, epidemiology, risk stratification, and outcomes, *Kidney Int*, **81**, 819–825.

[100] Bagshaw, S.M. and Bellomo R. (2010). Urine abnormalities in acute kidney injury and sepsis, *Contrib Nephrol*, **165**, 274–283.

[101] Haase, M., Bellomo, R. and Haase-Fielitz, A. (2010). Neutrophil gelatinase-associated lipocalin, *Curr Opin Crit Care*, **16**, 526–532.

[102] Koyner, J.L., Vaidya, V.S., Bennett, M.R. *et al.* (2010). Urinary biomarkers in the clinical prognosis and early detection of acute kidney injury, *Clin J Am Soc Nephrol*, **5**, 2154–2165.

[103] Moore, E., Bellomo, R. and Nichol, A. (2010). Biomarkers of acute kidney injury in anesthesia, intensive care and major surgery, from the bench to clinical research to clinical practice, *Minerva Anestesiol*, **76**, 425–440.

[104] Endre, Z.H., Pickering, J.W., Walker, R.J. *et al.* (2011). Improved performance of urinary biomarkers of acute kidney injury in the critically ill by stratification for injury duration and baseline renal function, *Kidney Int*, **79**, 1119–1130.

[105] Mårtensson, J., Bell, M., Oldner, A. *et al.* (2010). Neutrophil gelatinase–associated lipocalin in adult septic patients with and without acute kidney injury, *Intens Care Med*, **36**, 1333–1340.

[106] Boomer, J.S., To, K., Chang, K.C. *et al.* (2011). Immunosuppression in patients who die of sepsis and multiple organ failure, *JAMA*, **306**, 2594–2605.

[107] Cicarelli, D.D., Vieira, J.E. and Benseñor, F.E. (2009). C-reactive protein is not a useful indicator for infection in surgical intensive care units, *Sao Paulo Med J*, **127**, 350–354.

[108] Corral, L., Carrió, M.L., Ventura, J.L. *et al.* (2009). Is C–reactive protein a biomarker for immediate clinical outcome after cardiac surgery? *J Cardiothorac Vasc Anesth*, **23**, 166–169.

[109] Bell, K., Wattie, M., Byth, K. *et al.* (2003). Procalcitonin: a marker of bacteraemia in SIRS, *Anaesth Intensive Care*, **31(6)**, 629–636.

[110] Enguix, A., Rey, C., Concha, A. *et al.* (2001). Comparison of procalcitonin with C-reactive protein and serum amyloid for the early diagnosis of bacterial sepsis in critically ill neonates and children, *Intens Care Med*, **27**, 211–215.

[111] Müller, F., Christ-Crain, M., Bregenzer, T. *et al.* (2010). Procalcitonin levels predict bacteremia in patients with community-acquired pneumonia, a prospective cohort trial, *Chest*, **138**, 121–129.

[112] Wanner, G.A., Keel, M., Steckholzer, U. *et al.* (2000). Relationship between procalcitonin plasma levels and severity of injury, sepsis, organ failure, and mortality in injured patients, *Crit Care Med*, **28**, 950–957.

[113] Schuetz, P., Christ-Crain, M., Thomann, R. *et al.* (2009). Effect of procalcitonin-based guidelines vs standard guidelines on antibiotic use in lower respiratory tract infections, the ProHOSP randomized controlled trial, *JAMA*, **302**, 1059–1066.

[114] Bouadma, L., Luyt, C.E., Tubach, F. *et al.* (2010). Use of procalcitonin to reduce patients' exposure to antibiotics in intensive care units (PRORATA trial), a multicentre randomised controlled trial, *Lancet*, **375**, 463–474.

[115] Kollef, M.H. (2010). Will procalcitonin reduce antibiotic use in intensive care? *Lancet*, **375**, 435–436.

[116] Hoeboer, S.H., Alberts, E., van den Hul, I. *et al.* (2012). Old and new biomarkers for predicting high and low risk microbial infection in critically ill patients with new onset fever, a case for procalcitonin, *J Infect*, **64**, 484–493.

13

Haematology in Intensive Care

Lesley Kay

13.1 Introduction

The complex, usually post-surgical or trauma patient seen in intensive care unit (ICU) presents numerous haematological challenges, especially to haemostasis, with bleeding and thrombosis as ever-present risks. Management of these is covered in various guidelines [1,2]. This review will concentrate on serious haematological complications most likely to be encountered in very ill patients. It will point out where guidelines are not always germane to the extreme problems on the ICU. General haematological problems often seen on the ICU will also be mentioned.

13.2 Haematological Aspects of the ICU Patient

It is very helpful to be aware of the patient's initial blood count and coagulation results, not just on entry to the ICU but on first admission to hospital and beforehand. Was a minor abnormality such as reduced platelet count, raised mean corpuscular volume (MCV) or prolonged activated partial thromboplastin time (APTT) missed at that point? Or has the patient's haematological abnormality been acquired since hospitalisation? If so, what is the timing in relationship to the institution of drug or anticoagulant treatment (particularly heparin); do the changes correlate with onset of fever, a rise in C-reactive protein (CRP) or a fall in fibrinogen? Very sick patients may not increase the neutrophil count for some days after contracting a bacterial infection, and an initial transient fall in neutrophil count may presage an overwhelming septicaemia. Some chronic serious bacterial infections, for example osteomyelitis, may be only intermittently associated with fever. All too often fever, that invaluable marker of infection, is abolished by well-meaning administration of paracetamol or other non-steroidal anti-inflammatory drugs (NSAIDs), although there is much evidence that fever is an adaptive immune response [3]. One recent trial of antipyretic use on ICU had to be stopped early because mortality in the treated group exceeded that in the non-intervention group by seven to one [4].

13.3 Haemostasis

In life, blood must be kept fluid within the circulation and yet clot rapidly at sites of blood vessel damage to prevent exsanguination. The endothelial lining of blood vessels holds the balance between the opposing functions of clotting and fluidity. The plasma contains all the clotting agents (factors I, II, V, VII, VIII, IX, X, XI and XII) and all the natural 'anticoagulants', antithrombin III (ATIII), proteins C and S, together with plasminogen, which is a fibrinolytic agent. All circulate in the inactive form. Whenever a coagulation factor is activated its corresponding inhibitor is also activated, for example when factor V is activated it activates protein C; similarly, thrombin activates plasminogen. Thus there are constant checks and balances in play, both in health and in disease or during surgery. A haemophiliac lacking only factor VIII can sustain a painful knee bleed simply getting up from a chair; similarly, the early high-oestrogen contraceptives caused fatal strokes in young women with ATIII deficiency.

The platelet is the single most important clotting trigger within the circulation. Endothelium is a highly specialised and dynamic organ, forming a smooth interface between blood and tissues. It contains heparinoid anticoagulants, and secretes prostacyclin constantly, which inhibits platelet adherence. When the endothelium is damaged by trauma or toxins these functions cease and, in addition, tissue factor and collagen fibrils in the subendothelium become exposed. The collagen binds circulating Von Willebrand factor, a key mediator of platelet function, which in turn causes these to adhere, become activated, aggregate and change shape to form a binding surface and to activate factors VII, IX and X and prothrombin, resulting in thrombin and fibrin production via the extrinsic pathway. The roughness of the damaged endothelium can activate the intrinsic coagulation mechanism directly via 'contact' factors XII, XI and IX which in turn activate factor X and hence the production of fibrin. This branch of clotting is also intimately associated with the kallikrein–bradykinin system which triggers inflammation and blood vessel dilatation.

13.4 Haemostatic Problems in ICU Patients

Patients who have cardiopulmonary bypass or liver surgery are routinely admitted to ICU. More routine patients who become hypotensive are transferred to ICU. In the latter, failure to secure haemostasis, or, in the era of minimal access (keyhole) surgery, unrecognised perforation of a blood vessel, must be excluded. Full blood count (FBC) and clotting screen should be done urgently. If the prothrombin time (PT), APTT, fibrinogen and platelets are all normal, lack of surgical haemostasis is likely. Early recognition is vital and has led to protocols which diagnose surgical bleeding, for example drain rates of over 150 ml/hour beyond the second post-op hour in coronary artery bypass surgery mean surgical loss [5]. The swift return of such patients to theatre is the best way of curtailing secondary dilutional hypocoagulation.

13.4.1 *Dilutional hypocoagulation*

This is due to the administration of colloids, crystalloids and red cells required to maintain the patient's circulation. If a fluid warmer is used from the outset, deterioration in coagulation enzyme function due to hypothermia is avoided. Dilutional hypocoagulation can be expected once 1.5–2 volumes of blood have been replaced [6, 7]; this will be signalled by an increase in the APTT and PT to around 1.5 times normal and a fall in the fibrinogen. Platelets are also reduced. Critically ill patients may have started with a high fibrinogen due to infection or pregnancy, so a sudden drop of 1–2 g may be significant even if the level is still normal. Formerly it was recommended that for every ten units of blood two of fresh frozen plasma (FFP) should be given to prevent hypocoagulation, but since the identification of blood- transmissible agents such as human immunodeficiency virus (HIV), hepatitis C and variant Creutzfeldt–Jakob disease (vCJD), clinical justification is required. However over-caution concerning transfusion-transmitted infection may allow uncontrollable bleeding to cause hypotension, hypoxia and acidosis at tissue level and lead to true consumption coagulopathy.

13.4.2 *Consumption coagulopathy or disseminated intravascular coagulation (DIC)*

Acquired disorders of haemostasis are signalled by deranged coagulation parameters and FBC post-operatively or during the course of severe infection, despite normal values pre-surgery/admission. Clinical signs include oozing from intravenous puncture sites or the sudden appearance of skin purpura. DIC in obstetric patients occurs due to sepsis or amniotic fluid embolism, or in surgical patients due to sepsis, for example after removal of perforated appendix or gangrenous bowel. Unrecognised puncture of the gut during keyhole surgery may also be a source of sepsis [8]. The coagulation screen will show markedly prolonged APTT, PT, thrombin time (TT) and reduced fibrinogen. The FBC will show reduced platelets. Where associated with infection, the white blood cells (WBC) may show a raised neutrophil count and the CRP will be high (over 80). Cross-linked fibrin degradation products (D-dimers) will be increased significantly. D-dimers are commonly increased by a hundred or so units by surgery or infection, intravascular thrombosis is usually associated with levels of 1,000 or more.

Bleeding due to haemodilution and that due to DIC can be difficult to distinguish, as haemodilution can be followed by DIC. However, clinically DIC occurs in a 'sick' septic or obstetric patient and the fibrin degradation products or D-dimers are well over 1000 ng/ml but usually only moderately raised above normal in haemodilution.

13.4.2.1 *Management of coagulopathy*

Transfusion of FFP is indicated. It is frequently stated that little clinical trial evidence exists to support this, however clinical observation shows that clotting times shorten and bleeding reduces once the FFP is transfused. FFP contains all the constituents of plasma in normal concentrations, therefore relatively large volumes may be needed. An initial dose of four units is commonly given as soon as DIC or haemodilution is recognised. To achieve a meaningful rise in fibrinogen, once the level is below normal (1.5 g/l), cryoprecipitate or fibrinogen concentrate is needed. Cryoprecipitate in a dose of two pools (i.e. ten 'old units') will provide approximately 4 g fibrinogen in 200 ml [1]. It also contains factors VIII, XIII and the Von Willebrand factor. The usual dose of fibrinogen concentrate is 3 g. Note that for ICU patients the trigger for fibrinogen replacement is 1.5 g/l and not 1 g/l as some guidelines say.

Platelet transfusion is required in surgical patients if the level drops below 80×10^9 per litre and medical patients if there is evidence of bleeding or counts below 30×10^9 per litre. As soon as these products have been rapidly transfused venous samples for coagulation studies, fibrin degradation products or D-dimer and FBC should be sent urgently to the lab. A fall in the APTT, PT and increase in fibrinogen show that the situation is coming under control, No change or lengthening of the times dictates further action. Further cryoprecipitate and FFP guided by lab results should be given.

13.5 Thromboelastography

Many ICU departments, especially where there are large cardiothoracic or liver transplant units, have the benefit of near-patient test equipment (thrombolelastography (TEG) or ROTEM) [9–11], which, when used by experienced teams, can guide replacement therapy. Rapid diagnosis of the exact cause of bleeding is afforded by manipulation of the test procedure, and allows rapid correction with a resulting diminution in blood product usage [12–14].

In intractable haemorrhage, a further dose of FFP followed by activated factor VII (recombinant) (rVIIa) [15] at a dose of 90 μg/kg can be very helpful if the APTT and PT are still prolonged. rVIIa is usually held in the hospital pharmacy; it is a freeze-dried product which can be rapidly reconstituted for intravenous bolus injection. rVIIa normally binds locally where tissue factor is exposed by injury, thus it generates small amounts of thrombin to activate platelets. rVIIa in pharmacological doses directly activates factor X present on the surface of activated platelets, resulting in a burst of thrombin production exactly where it is needed [16]. It is indicated only for intractable haemorrhage once acidosis and hypothermia are corrected and adequate FFP replacement has been secured. Giving it before FFP is pointless as the other coagulation factors required for total haemostasis such as factors X and V, prothrombin and fibrinogen will be in short supply [17]. The dose of rVIIa can be repeated after two hours. Expert haematological guidance in the use of this is recommended [18]. Further cryoprecipitate is indicated if the fibrinogen is under 1.5 g/l.

13.6 Drug-Induced Bleeding and how to Prevent it

Patients in the ICU may become over-anticoagulated if they are admitted whilst on warfarin and then receive multiple drug treatments. Patients on full anticoagulation who require invasive procedures are transferred from warfarin to full-dose low-molecular-weight heparin (LMWH) to achieve anticoagulation that will not vary with changes in feeding, antibiotics or liver function. For example for atrial fibrillation daily subcutaneous Dalteparin 200 units per kg per 24 hours can be substituted. For a patient on warfarin for mechanical heart valve or stent then the therapeutic dose should be divided and given 12-hourly e.g. 10,000 units dalteparin 12-hourly for a patient over 80 kg weight. Such regimes afford a smoother control of anticoagulation than traditional unfractionated heparin with the advantages that APTT monitoring is not needed and the danger of heparin-induced thrombocytopenia is ten-fold reduced. If monitoring is required then anti-Xa activity should be assessed at four hours after dose. However there is still controversy on the best regimes for peri-procedure anticoagulation for patients with mechanical heart valves [19]. In the critically ill patient the decision on the best method of anticoagulation should be individualised because of multiple and varying pathologies as well as recent or anticipated surgery [20]. In general, aortic valves are less likely to clot than mitral or tricuspid, and multiple-valve patients need more intensive anticoagulation than those with a single prosthetic valve. If LMWH is used the full anticoagulation dose should be divided into twice- or thrice-daily regimes controlled by anti-Xa activity [21].

It is usually accepted that invasive procedures can be undertaken four to five days from stopping warfarin and between 12 and 24 hours after the last dose of LMWH. It is customary to select the shorter interval for valve patients and the longer one for those on once-a-day dosing or who require epidural anaesthesia or neurosurgery.

Sometimes it is not possible to wait five days for warfarin to disappear and urgent reversal is needed.

To reverse warfarin in the event of bleeding or for a surgical procedure it is preferable to use prothrombin complex concentrates (PCC) such as Beriplex (CSL Behring) or Octaplex (Octapharma) than FFP, as the latter requires large volumes and is relatively low in factor IX. PCC also has the advantage of being a freeze-dried product which can be rapidly reconstituted, avoiding the delay involved in thawing FFP. In most hospitals it is supplied by the pharmacy. PCC contains factors VII, IX, X and prothrombin(II), which are those reduced by warfarin, as well as the natural anticoagulants Protein C and S which are similarly depleted in patients on warfarin. When using either FFP or PCC it is best to administer vitamin K simultaneously, e.g. 5 mg intravenously, if there is a need to maintain normal coagulation in the longer term as they are effective for seven to twelve hours only. Fortunately the effects of vitamin K begin six hours after dose. The effectiveness of the reversal should be checked prior to any invasive procedure. The international normalised ratio (INR) must be 1.5 or less. Vitamin K will be less effective in restoring normal coagulation if the patient has hepatic impairment and further replacement with PCC or FFP therapy at 6 or 12 hourly intervals, respectively, will be needed.

Bleeding due to antiplatelet therapy manifests as post-operative oozing and should be prevented by stopping aspirin two weeks and clopidogrel one week before surgery. If urgent surgery has to be done in such patients, platelet transfusion will compensate for aspirin defect but is less successful in reducing the clopidogrel effect.

13.7 Acquired Inhibitors of Coagulation

This rare cause of bleeding is more likely to be encountered on the ICU than in routine departments because it is most often found in very ill middle-aged patients who have a history of immune impairment, recent surgery multiple antibiotic treatments and transfusion. It also occurs in patients with cancer and non-Hodgkin's lymphoma, again often after immunosuppression, transfusion and infection. The clinical case presented at the end of this chapter demonstrates this rare but potentially fatal condition in a typically complex patient.

Inhibitors are actually auto-antibodies specific to a coagulation factor. They may be triggered by exposure to plasma products, for example inhibitors of factor V and prothrombin have been reported after use of fibrin glue or bovine thrombin [22]. The commonest factors involved are factors VIII and IX. The factor is often severely reduced, resulting in soft-tissue bleeding. Suspect acquired inhibitors in sick patients with soft-tissue bleeds who fail to respond by reduction in APTT to adequate FFP replacement. The diagnosis is made on performing an 'inhibitor screen' which shows that the APTT of a 50:50 mix of the patients and normal plasma fails to be corrected. Once this is confirmed, further tests will show which factor is involved.

Treatment relies on correcting the bleeding by 'bypassing' the antibody using activated factor VII (Novo seven or rVIIa) which activates platelet-bound factors X and V directly, or another product, activated prothrombin complex or factor VIII inhibitor bypassing activator (FEIBA) [23–25]. Both may be needed. The dose of factor VII is 90 μg/kg [26], and, as the half-life is short, the dose may need to be repeated every two to three hours to achieve haemostasis. The dose of FEIBA or a PCC is 50–100 units/kg every 6 to 12 hours as it has a longer half-life. Simultaneously, the production of the auto-antibody must be halted. Several methods are available [27]: steroids, rituximab, which eliminates B-cells, or cyclosporin or mycophenolate mofetil, which suppress T-helper cells. All of the former are immunosuppressive, so in a septic patient it may be preferable to try high-dose gamma globulin which cuts off antibody production by blocking Fcγ receptors on immune cells.

13.8 Anaemia on the ICU Not Due to Bleeding

It is common for patients on the ICU to have a moderate stable reduction in haemoglobin, if only because their nutrition is compromised, they are catabolic and blood sampling is frequent. If the haemoglobin is falling post-surgical loss needs to be excluded. Sites where relatively large volumes of blood can go unnoticed are the psoas and thigh muscles and the pelvic and chest cavities.

Long-term patients may have multiple haematinic deficiency and normal MCV due to the presence of both microcytic and macrocytic cells. Thus the problem will be signalled by a widening of the red cell distribution width (RDW) on the haematology report. B12 folate and iron should be checked and any deficiency remedied. If the MCV is moderately raised, check for raised reticulocytes, lactate dehydrogenase (LDH), conjugated bilirubin and direct antiglobulin test (DAT, also known as direct Coomb's test) to exclude auto-immune haemolysis or a delayed reaction to red-cell transfusion. Check for thyroid deficiency if the raised MCV remains unexplained. In auto-immune haemolysis there may be a history of systemic lupus erythematosus (SLE) or use of heavily immunosuppressive cytotoxic drugs such as Fludarabine. The DAT will show immunoglobulin G on the red cells. Prednisolone (40 mg daily) is usually successful in treating this. If the DAT is negative, a blood film should be inspected to look for red cell fragments, which would indicate mechanical haemolysis or microangiopathic haemolytic anaemia.

13.8.1 *Microangiopathic haemolytic anaemia on the ICU*

This is most commonly caused by a leaking prosthetic cardiac valve. In a patient without a mechanical valve, thrombotic thrombocytopaenic purpura (TTP) or haemolytic uraemic syndrome (HUS) [28] may be considered.

TTP is an acute life threatening condition caused by the development of antibodies to a metalloproteinase enzyme known as a disintegrin and metalloproteinase with thrombospondin motifs (ADAMTS) 13. The antibody is triggered by infection, pregnancy, hormone replacement therapy (HRT) oestrogen and cytotoxic drugs, and HIV or its treatment. Some families may be predisposed to the development of antibodies due to mutations in the ADAMTS 13 genes. The function of ADAMTS 13 is to cleave inactive Von Willebrand factor multimers into smaller molecules, which bind to exposed collagen in damaged blood vessels. Thus they activate platelets only at the site of injury. Lack of ADAMTS 13 allows ultra-large

Von Willebrand multimers to accumulate and unfortunately these cause platelet thrombosis within the microcirculation, resulting in altered conscious level in the brain, anaemia due to mechanical haemolysis and renal impairment. The platelet consumption causes purpura and bleeding.

Around three weeks after a triggering event, the patient presents with fatigue, fever, purpura and confusion. Female to male ratio is 3:1. The laboratory diagnostic features are anaemia with red blood cell fragments on the film, raised reticulocytes, bilirubin and LDH but a negative Coomb's test and uraemia. Platelets are very low (20×10^9 per litre), but APTT, PT, TT and fibrinogen are usually normal. ADAMTS 13 can be tested in specialised labs. Less than 5% of the normal level confirms TTP. Treatment depends on replacing ADAMTS13 by exchange transfusion of FFP [29] and suppression of the antibody production by rituximab infusion. Rituximab eliminates antibody-producing B-lymphocytes [30].

HUS and thrombotic microangiopathies (TMA) are caused by direct endothelial damage by drugs, e.g. chemotherapy, cyclosporine, or toxins, e.g. *Escherichia coli* verotoxin (VTEC) or salmonella toxin. Damage to endothelium hampers its normal function of preventing platelet adherence by secretion of prostacyclin. ADAMTS 13 is usually normal, and supportive treatment with renal replacement and removal of the offending drug allows the endothelium to regenerate and the patient to recover.

13.8.2 *Normochromic anaemia with no obvious cause*

Otherwise unexplained normochromic anaemia may occur on the ICU about four to six weeks after reversal of acute renal failure because of a temporary cessation of erythropoietin production. If this is confirmed by checking the erythropoietin level then it may be appropriate to replace this instead of transfusing more red cells. For erythropoietin to work efficiently there must be good iron reserves and intravenous iron is usually required.

13.9 Platelets, Thrombosis and how to Avoid it

The development of a raised platelet count most commonly accompanies infection, and this will be shown by a raised WBC and the CRP. Raised platelets may also be a response to bleeding or iron deficiency. If the count exceeds 1000×10^9 per litre and bleeding has been excluded, then antiplatelet treatment is indicated. Aspirin (75 mg daily) or, if contraindicated, clopidogrel (75 mg daily) can be used. High platelet counts are common in the immediate period after splenectomy and in addition to aspirin these cases need prophylactic antibiotics to cover against polysaccharide-encapsulated bacteria. The spleen contains dendritic macrophages and specialised T-cells specifically adapted for the recognition and elimination of these bacteria, which include *Neisseria menigitidis* and *Gonococcus*, *Haemophilus influenzae* and *Pneumococcus*. Without lifelong penicillin prophylaxis these patients are at risk of rapid onset of overwhelming post-splenectomy infection (OPSI). Specific vaccination is also needed. Death due to OPSI has been reported even 40 years after splenectomy [31].

Falling platelet counts should be investigated by sending off blood for urgent FBC, blood film, coagulation screen, D-dimer, UsEs (urea and electrolytes), LDH, CRP and heparin-induced thrombocytopenia and thrombosis (HITT) screen.

13.9.1 *Heparin-induced thrombocytopaenia with thrombosis (HITT)*

This syndrome is due to the development of IgG antibodies to heparin-bound platelet factor 4 (PF4) complexes [32]. The Fcγ receptor of the antibody then activates bound platelets by causing release of procoagulant activity, leading to thrombin generation. Patients with such antibodies have a thirty-fold increase in the risk of thrombosis. Typically the antibody is formed three to ten days after heparin is started, signalled by a significant fall in the platelet count, of 30–50% from pre-heparinisation levels [33]. The absolute count may still be in the normal range but is usually around $70–100 \times 10^9/\text{l}$ so bleeding is rare. The thrombosis can be venous, particularly at the sites of injury or surgery, or arterial. Rarely adrenal thrombosis and infarction may occur and lead to adrenal failure. Other rare manifestations are venous gangrene and skin necrosis on administration of warfarin. Thrombosis occurs after or simultaneously with the fall in platelet count in over 50% of cases but in up to 30% it can occur one to seven days before the drop in platelet count.

It is also possible for the thrombotic risk to continue for up to four weeks after the onset of the heparin-induced thrombocytopenia (HIT) antibody response, even after the heparin has been stopped and the platelet count restored.

The risk that HIT antibodies will form is greatest in patients exposed to unfractionated heparin (ten times that with LMWH) [34]. The risk that a patient on LMWH will develop HITT is higher with prior exposure to unfractionated heparin rather than LMWH in the past. Although PF4 antibodies can be detected in patients on Danaparoid or Fondaparinux, which are pentasaccharide derivatives of heparin, HITT is rare with these agents, although as time goes on examples with the newer agents may be reported [35].

Drugs with no similarity to heparin cannot induce HITT antibodies. Examples are recombinant derivatives of the leech enzyme Hirudin such as Lepirudin and bivalirudin and direct thrombin inactivators such as dabigatran.

13.9.1.1 *Prevention and management of HITT*

Vigilance is essential in recognising the development of HITT promptly. It is important to anticipate it as far as possible by taking a good history on admission specifically to check for previous heparin exposure. Orthopaedic patients and those with thrombophilia who travel are increasingly likely to have had exposure to LMWH. Cardiac patients are very likely to have been exposed to unfractionated heparin and it is important that if this has occurred within the previous 100 days the presence of HITT antibodies is screened for so that prolonged re-exposure to heparin is avoided. In such patients the first screening platelet count should be done within the first day of re-exposure to heparin in case there is an immediate catastrophic drop in the platelet count, which denotes immediate activation of platelet-bound heparin by avid pre-existing antibody. Heparin re-exposure is best deferred beyond 100 days in patients with a known history of HITT or with an immediate platelet drop.

For patients at risk of HITT i.e. post cardiac surgery or orthopaedic surgery on unfractionated heparin or LMWH the platelet count should be monitored from days 4 to 14 post-operatively.

Obstetric [36], paediatric [37] haemodialysis [38] and medical patients seem at a relatively low risk of HIT despite exposure to heparin. Platelet counts need not be so frequently monitored in these groups.

Any fall in platelets of 50% or more should lead to suspicion of HITT, a search for thrombosis and screen for HITT antibodies and cessation of heparin. The PF4 screening antibody test result is available within 24 hours. Unfortunately, many patients exposed to heparin make detectable antibody, but not all of them develop HITT. If the PF4 antibody screening test is positive but there is clinical doubt as to the presence of HITT a specific platelet-release assay can be done to assess the activity of the antibody. This test is done in specialised laboratories whereas the HITT antibody screening test is widely available.

HITT should be considered in any patient who develops thrombosis whilst on any type of heparin whether or not the platelet count is low, as in some cases the reduction in count is delayed.

Once HITT is diagnosed heparin must be stopped. The resulting rise in platelet count over the next four or so days helps to confirm the diagnosis, but unfortunately does not mean that the patient is out of danger. An alternative anticoagulant should be prescribed, in full therapeutic dose for patients who have sustained a thrombus. Lepirudin is a good choice for patients with normal renal function without high risk of bleeding, as there is no cross-reaction with heparin antibodies and its effect can be monitored by the APTT which should be kept 1.5–2 times the control level and repeated every four to six hours until anticoagulation is stable, and daily thereafter.

In non-uraemic patients the loading dose is 400 μg/kg, followed by continuous intravenous infusion of 150 μg/kg/hour, with a maximum dose of 16.5 mg/hour. If the patient has renal impairment no loading dose is given and the infusion rate is reduced [39].

If creatinine clearance is less than 50 ml/minute then the loading dose is halved to 200 μg/kg and the infusion rate reduced by 50–85%. Patients on dialysis with HIT have been successfully managed using low-dose lepirudin [40]. Unfortunately although lepirudin cannot interact with anti-heparin antibodies it can and frequently does elicit anti-lepirudin antibody, (30% after a single exposure and 70% following re-exposure). Anaphylaxis due to lepirudin [41] has been reported and makes this drug best reserved for single-use in cases of HITT.

Danaparoid is another anticoagulant frequently used to anticoagulate patients with HIT. In practice clinical problems due to crossreacting antibody are rare. It is given intravenously: a start dose of 2,500 units is given followed by 400 units per hour for two hours then 300 units for a further two hours, reduced thereafter to 200 units per hour for five days. If the creatinine clearance is reduced then the dose must be adjusted according to anti-Xa activity at four hours post dose. With normal renal function no monitoring is needed.

Fondaparinux, like danaparoid, is a synthetic pentasaccharide which inhibits activated factor X. The standard dose is 2.5 mg subcutaneously daily for prophylaxis. For treatment of established thrombosis 7.5 mg subcutaneously for patients weighing 50–100 kg is required daily. In renal impairment with a creatinine clearance of 20–50 ml/min, the daily dose is reduced to 1.5 mg.

Once anticoagulation has been established with the selected alternative to heparin it should be continued until the patient is able to take oral drugs, when warfarin should be slowly introduced without a loading regime, as warfarin-induced skin necrosis is more frequent in HIT patients. The warfarin dose should be no more than 5 mg daily and crossed over with the intravenous/subcutaneous anticoagulant for five days. In future new direct thrombin inhibitors which cannot cross-react with heparin and do not require INR monitoring may become available for long-term use. One such drug is Dabigatran [42]. A potent direct competitive inhibitor of thrombin, it is excreted mainly by the kidneys so that dose adjustment may be needed in uraemic patients. No monitoring is required and the usual dose for therapeutic anticoagulation is 110 mg every 12 hours.

Duration of the oral anticoagulant must be six months in those who have suffered a thrombo-embolism and at least four weeks if none has occurred.

13.10 Other Aspects of Venous Thrombosis on the ICU

All patients on ICU without a specific contraindication are candidates for prophylaxis of thromboembolism. Gunshot wounds even in the young and fit need thromboprophylaxis.

Thromboembolism may occur *de novo* in ICU patients in association with HITT or post major surgery. Infection, pregnancy and carcinoma cause high fibrinogen, shortened APTT and increase the risk.

After pulmonary embolus (PE) ventilation–perfusion mismatch worsens, arterial oxygen is reduced, D-dimers increase and electrocardiogram and echocardiogram can show right heart strain if there is increased right ventricular work due to the increased pulmonary vascular resistance. Computerised tomographic pulmonary angiogram is the best confirmatory test. Patients with massive PE threatening the circulation may be transferred to ICU for resuscitation in preparation for interventional radiology and local thrombolysis. Once this has been done patients should always be fully anticoagulated using intravenous unfractionated heparin and six-hourly APTT control (1.5–3 times control level). Moderate-sized emboli are anticoagulated using LMWH as it is more convenient; evidence of its efficacy is available [43]. Doppler ultrasound can detect the source of emboli in pelvis or limbs.

13.10.1 *The use of inferior vena cava filters to prevent pulmonary embolus (PE)*

If patients with large recent ileo-femoral clots require urgent surgery and heparin must be interrupted, then the placement of an inferior vena cava [44] umbrella filter, preferably temporarily, may be justified.

13.11 Clinical Case

A 67-year-old man was admitted to the ICU following laparotomy for mechanical obstruction of the bowel due to adhesions following previous gastrectomy for volvulus of the stomach some years before. He was also known to suffer from gut motility problems, possibly congenital in origin and had had previous colectomies for megacolon.

Initially he made a good post-op recovery and was returned to the ward. He was on prophylactic augmentin and enoxaparin (40 mg subcutaneously daily). Some days later he became febrile and was found to have an aspiration pneumonia complicated by pleural effusions.

He returned to ICU as he required ventilation and high-dose intravenous antibiotics. It soon became obvious that there was a severe gastroparesis and biliary reflux. After recovery from the chest infection he returned to theatre for exploratory laparotomy and feeding jejunostomy. At operation further adhesions were found together with gross distension of the gastric remnant and colon. The adhesions were divided, a Polya gastrectomy performed and the colon was fixated to prevent volvulus.

The patient returned to ICU, and was noted to have fresh blood issuing from the nasogastric tube. Over a 12-hour period the haemoglobin fell from 10.1 to 7.6 g/dl, the APTT rose from 35 seconds (N) to 50.4 seconds, and the PT from 13 seconds to 18 seconds. Although D-dimer was 3,000 the fibrinogen was stable at over 7. However the platelets had fallen from 330×10^9 per litre to 221×10^9 per litre, the CRP was 200 and the WBC 28×10^9 per litre due to neutrophilia. Wide-spectrum bactericidal antibiotics Teicoplanin and Metronidazole were started for presumed sepsis and incipient DIC. FFP (4 units) and red cells were transfused. Ultrasound showed fluid in the right iliac fossa so a drain was inserted. Over the next several days two litres of blood drained and there was a continual need for FFP and red cell transfusion to maintain haemostasis and haemoglobin. The APTT remained prolonged. A further scan was prompted when liver function showed a cholestatic pattern. This revealed a large haematoma between the stomach and liver. A haematologist was consulted and investigation showed APTT of 61 seconds, inhibitor screen was positive, the factor VIII level was found to be 0.04 kIU/ml (normal range 50–150 kIU/ml). All other coagulation factors were normal and the patient was shown to have developed inhibitors (antibody) to factor VIIIc activity. Once the diagnosis was made he was managed with regular transfusion of FEIBA and activated factor VII (rVIIa Novoseven) with a resultant fall of the APTT to normal and increase in factor VIII levels into the normal range. These were needed over many days, until bleeding ceased. Pharmacological immunosuppression to reduce his production of antibody to factor VIII was contraindicated due to the presence of infection and multiple haematomata at risk of infection. High-dose intravenous gamma globulin was given to suppress endogenous antibody production. He eventually made a complete recovery.

References

[1] British Committee for Standards in Haematology (2006). Guidelines on the management of massive blood loss, *Brit J Haem,* **135**, 634–641.

[2] British Committee for Standards in Haematology (2009). Guidelines for the diagnosis and management of disseminated intravascular coagulation, *Brit J Haem*, **145**, 24–33.

[3] Laupland, K.B. (2009). Fever in the critically ill medical patient, *Crit Care Med*, **37** (Suppl. 7), S273–S278.

[4] Schulman, C.I., Namias, N., Doherty, J. *et al.* (2005). The effect of antipyretic therapy upon outcomes in critically ill patients: a randomized prospective study, *Surgical Infections*, **6**, 369–375.

[5] Michelson, E.L., Torosian, M., Morganroth, J. *et al.* (1980). Early recognition of surgically correctable causes of excessive mediastinal bleeding after coronary artery bypass graft surgery, *Am J Surg*, **139**, 313–317.

[6] Mittermayr, M., Margreiter, J., Velik-Salchner, C. *et al.* (2005). Effects of protamine and heparin can be detected and easily differentiated by modified thromboelastography (ROTEM), an *in vitro* study, *Br J Anaesth*, **95**, 310–316.

[7] Hippala, S.T., Mylyla, G.J. and Valhera, E.M. (1995). Hemostatic factors and replacement of major blood loss with plasma-poor red cell concentrates, *Anesthesia and Analgesia*, **81**, 360–365.

[8] Pappas, T.N, and Jacobs, D.O. (2004). Laparoscopic resection for colon cancer, the end of the beginning? *N Eng J Med*, **350**, 2091–2092.

[9] Sorenson, B., and Ingerslev, J. (2005). Tailoring haemostatic treatment to patient requirements- an update on monitoring haemostatic response using thromboelastography, *Haemophilia*, **11** (Suppl. 1), 1–6.

[10] Savy, C., Quinio, P., Lefevre, F. *et al.* (2005). Manageability and potential for haemostasis monitoring by near patient modified thromboelastometer (Rotem) in intensive care unit, *Ann Fr Anaesth Reanim*, **24**, 607–616 [In French].

[11] Rugeri, L., Levrat, A., David, J.S. *et al.* (2007). Diagnosis of early coagulation abnormalities in trauma patients by rotation elastography, *J Thromb Haemost*, **5**, 289–295.

[12] Coakley, M., Reddy, K., Mackie, I. *et al.* (2006). Transfusion triggers in orthotopic liver transplantation: a comparison of the throboelastometry analyzer the thromboelastogram and conventional coagulation tests, *J Cardiothoracic Vasc Anesth*, **20**, 548–553.

[13] Reiss, R.F. (2000). Hemostatic defects in massive transfusion: rapid diagnosis and management, *Am J Crit Care*, **9**, 158–165.

[14] Anderson, L., Quasim, I., Soutar, R. *et al.* (2006). An audit of red cell and blood product use after the institution of thromboelastometry in a cardiac intensive care unit, *Transfus Med*, **16**, 31–39.

[15] Boehlen, F., Morales, A., Fontana, P. *et al.* (2004). Prolonged treatment of massive post-partum haemorrhage with recombinant factor, VIIa: case report and review of the literature, *Br J Obstet Gynaecol*, **111**, 284–287.

[16] Bishop, C.V., Renwick, W.E., Hogan, C. *et al.* (2006). Recombinant activated factor, VII: treating post operative haemorrhage in cardiac surgery, *Ann Thoracic Surg*, **81**, 875–879.

[17] Lewis, N.R., Bunker, P., Lemire, S.J. *et al.* (2009). Failure of recombinant activated factor seven to correct coagulaopathy in a case of severe post partum haemorrhage, *Transfusion*, **49**, 689–695.

[18] Martinowitz, U. and Michaelson, M. (2005). Guidelines for the use of recombinant activated factor seven (rVIIa) in uncontrolled bleeding; a report by the multidisciplinary rVIIa task force, *J Thromb Haem*, **3**, 640–648.

[19] Schlebak, A. and Malik, J. (2009). Managing anticoagulation with heparin in patients with prosthetic heart valves: balancing the risk, *Heart*, **95**, 1643–1645.

[20] Daniels, P.R., McBane, R.D., Lilin, S.C. *et al.* (2009). Peri-procedural anticoagulation management of mechanical prosthetic valve patients, *Thromb Res*, **124**, 300–305.

[21] Spyropoulos, A.C., Turpie, A.S., Dunn, A. *et al.* (2006). Clinical outcomes with unfractionated heparin or low-molecular-weight heparin as bridging therapy in patients on long-term oral anticoagulation: the REGIMEN registry, *J Thromb Hemost*, **4**, 1246–1252.

[22] Zehnder, J.L. and Leung, L.L. (1990). Development of antibodies to thrombin and factor five with recurrent bleeding in a patient exposed to bovine thrombin, *Blood*, **76**, 2011–2016.

[23] Delgado, J. (2003). Acquired haemophilia; Review and meta-analysis focused on therapy and prognostic factors, *Brit J Haem*, **121**, 21–35.

[24] Sallah, S. (2004). Treatment of acquired haemophilia with factor eight inhibitor bypassing activity, *Haemophilia*, **10**, 169–173.

[25] Hay, C.R., Negrier, C. and Ludlam, C.A. (1997). The treatment of bleeding in acquired haemophilia with recombinant factor, VIIa: a multicentre study, *Thromb Haemost*, **78**, 1463–1467.

[26] Roberts, H.R. (2001). Recombinant factor VIIa (Novoseven) and the safety of treatment, *Semin Hematol*, **38**, 48–50.

[27] Holme, P.A. (2005). Acquired haemophilia: management of bleeds and immune therapy to eradicate autoantibodies, *Haemophilia*, **11**, 510–515.

[28] Moake, J.L. (2002). Thrombotic microangiopathies, *New Engl J Med*, **347**, 589–600.

[29] Rock, G.A. (2001). Management of thrombotic thrombocytopenic purpura, *Brit J Haematol*, **109**, 496–507.

[30] Scully, M., Cohen, H., Cavanagh, J. *et al.* (2007). Remission in acute refractory and relapsing thrombotic thrombocytopenic purpura following rituximab is associated with a reduction in IgG antibodies to, ADAMTS 13, *Brit J Haematol*, **136**, 451–461.

[31] Evans, D.I.K. (1985). Post splenectomy sepsis 10 or more years after operation, *J Clin Pathol*, **38**, 309–311.

[32] Warkentin, T.E. and Sheppard, J. (2009). Studies of the immune response in heparin-induced thrombocytopenia, *Blood*, **113**, 4963–4969.

[33] Warkentin, T.E. and Kelton, J.G, (2001). Temporal aspects of heparin induced thrombocytopenia, *N Engl J Med*, **344**, 1286–1292.

[34] American College of Chest Physicians (2008). Treatment and prevention of heparin induced thrombocytopenia, *Chest*, **133** (Suppl. 6), 3405–3805.

[35] Warkentin, T.E., Maurer, B.T. and Aster, R.H. (2007). Heparin associated thrombocytopenia and Fondaparinux, *N Engl J Med*, **356**, 2653–2655.

[36] Faussett, M.B., Vogtlander, M., Lee, R.M. *et al.* (2001). Heparin-induced thrombocytopenia is rare in pregnancy, *Am J Obstet Gynecol*, **185**, 148–152.

[37] Klenner, A.F., Lubenow, N., Raschke, R. *et al.* (2004). Heparin induced thrombocytopenia in children 12 new cases and a review of the literature, *Thromb Haemost*, **91**, 719–724.

[38] O'Shea, S.L., Sands, J.J., Nudo, S.A. *et al.* (2002). Frequency of anti — heparin platelet factor 4 antibodies in haemodialysis patients, *Am J Hematol*, **69**, 72–73.

[39] Shantsila, E., Lip, G.Y.H. and Chong, B.H. (2009). Heparin induced thrombocytopenia, a contemporary clinical approach to diagnosis and management, *Chest*, **135**, 1651–1664.

[40] Tardy-Poncet, B., Charier, D., Diconne, E. *et al.* (2009). Extremely low doses of lepirudin in a patient with heparin-induced thrombocytopenia, high bleeding risk and renal insufficiency, *Brit J Haem*, **146**, 456–457.

[41] Greinacher, A., Lubenow, N. and Eichler, P. (2003). Anaphylxis and anaphylactoid reactions associated with lepirudin in patients with heparin induced thrombocytopenia, *Circulation*, **108**, 2062–2065.

[42] Connolly, S.J., Ezekowitz, M.D., Yusuf, S. *et al.* (2009). Dabigatran versus warfarin in patients with atrial fibrillation, *N Engl J Med*, **361**, 1139–1151.
[43] Hirsh, J., Guyatt, G., Albers, G. *et al.* (2008). American college of chest physicians evidence based clinical practice guidelines on anticoagulation and thrombolysis, *Chest*, **133** (Suppl. 6), 71s–109s.
[44] Baglin, T.P., Bush, J. and Streff, M. (2006). British Committee on standards in haematology guidelines on use of vena cava filters, *Brit J Haem*, **134**, 590–595.

14
Peri-Operative Intensive Care Medicine

S. Ramani Moonesinghe and Michael G. Mythen

14.1 Surgery and Resources: A Global Health Problem

Over 234 million major surgical procedures are estimated to occur worldwide each year. The countries which spend the least on healthcare per head of population undertake only 3.5% of operations worldwide, despite accounting for nearly 35% of the global population. These statistics highlight inequality in the provision of surgical services across the world that is an increasing priority on the public health agenda [1]. We know from clinical experience that, even in the developed world, implementation of evidence-based practice aimed at improving surgical outcomes is hindered by inconsistencies in the literature and availability of resources.

There is increasing evidence that issues related to process and use of resources in healthcare may have significant impact on the population outcomes of surgical patients. A number of cross-sectional studies show that volume is related to outcome in surgery: that is, the more operations that a particular surgeon or institute conducts, the better the outcome for the cohort [2]. While this may not seem surprising, longitudinal studies do not confirm a 'practice makes perfect' explanation for these observations, implying that there are fixed differences between high- and low-volume hospitals in terms of quality and standards of care [3,4]. Another study of over 180,000 non-emergency cases in the USA found a significant increase in 30-day mortality for the population of patients who had their elective surgery performed on a Friday as opposed to those who were operated on between Monday and Wednesday [5]. Investigation of such issues will gain momentum in the future as healthcare systems worldwide focus on quality of care with increasing interest.

The reader will observe that much of the evidence-based guidance in this chapter refers to studies that show improvement in morbidity rather than mortality. For some, this may not be enough of an incentive to invest the time and effort required to practice these recommendations. It is tempting to draw a line under a surgical patient 'episode' when the patient leaves the critical care unit, or the hospital, or even at 30 days. However, a study looking at long-term outcomes in a cohort of over 100,000 surgical patients, suggests that the development of seemingly benign complications such as wound infections, after relatively benign procedures such as laparoscopic cholecystectomy, has an effect on long-term mortality [6]. It has been found that independent of pre-operative risk, the occurrence of any one of a list of 22 different complications within 30 days of surgery reduces median survival by 69%. The effect on long-term survival is worse with increasing severity of complication — myocardial infarction and pneumonia have the most significant effect — however, even wound and urinary tract infections affected mortality. The implication is that the development of post-operative morbidity may begin an inflammatory (or other) response that adversely affects long-term survival. Evidence such as this re-affirms the duty of the peri-operative physician: to ensure that the high-risk surgical patient is identified and optimised in the most robust evidence-guided manner possible, in order to minimise their risk of any complication — the long-term impact of not doing so may be considerably more significant than it seems.

14.2 The High-Risk Surgical Population

Audit data from the 2003 National Confidential Enquiry into Perioperative Deaths reveal that increasing surgical complexity, patient age and numbers of comorbidities are associated with increased risk of adverse outcomes in patients undergoing major surgery [7]. Recent work has shown that the relatively small proportion of patients that fall into this 'high-risk population'

Table 14.1. ASA with population mortalities adapted from wolters *et al* [9].

ASA-PS	I	II	III	IV
Number of patients (%)	1133 (18)	2685 (42.6)	2181 (34.6)	290 (4.6)
Intraoperative blood loss (ml)	78	105	293	1548
Intensive care Stay (days)	0.2	0.8	1.9	5.4
Cardiac complications (%)	0.1	1.5	5.5	18
Bronchopulmonary infections (%)	0.5	2.2	5.2	12.1
Study Mortality (%)	0.1	0.7	3.5	18.3

(approximately 12%) account for the majority of post-operative mortality (approximately 80%) [8].

Various scoring systems have been developed to help clinicians identify high-risk patient populations and assist in comparative audit and the appropriate allocation of healthcare resources. These range from very simple and general scores such as the American Society of Anaesthesiologists' Physical Status score (ASA) [9,10] (Table 14.1) to more complex systems such as the Physiological and Operative Severity Score for the Enumeration of Mortality and Morbidity (POSSUM) [11–13], and surgery specific tools such as the European system for Cardiac Operative Risk Score (EUROSCORE) [14]. These systems are primarily used to stratify patients according to their risk of peri-operative mortality; most of them are not validated for prediction of morbidity [15–18]. The exception to this is the POSSUM score and its various derivatives, which have been validated for risk stratification of both mortality and morbidity in specific surgical specialities [16,19–24]. Such risk-stratification systems are used primarily for comparative audit between different surgical teams and institutions.

14.3 The High-Risk Surgical Patient

No universally agreed definition exists for the 'high-risk surgical patient', and clinical equipoise remains over which methods are most effective at identifying them. Central to this issue is the interaction between the type of surgery that a patient is undergoing and that patient's cardiorespiratory reserve. The direct relationship between surgical complexity and patient risk seems obvious; however it is only relatively recently that attention has turned to addressing the primary cause of this association: the uncoupling of oxygen supply/demand dynamics caused by the surgical insult. Major abdominal surgery, for example, causes an increase in oxygen demand of 40% or more [25]; patients who are physiologically unable to rise to this challenge may be at risk of peri-operative complications.

14.3.1 *Procedure-related risk factors*

Although the definition of 'major surgery' is somewhat arbitrary, the concept of 'surgery-specific risk' is not new. Both the type of surgery and its degree of urgency may influence outcome (see Table 14.2) [26].

It is interesting to note that for many of the operations listed, although they are associated with significant mortality and morbidity, critical care admission after surgery is not a standard of care; however, in the case of cardiac surgery, which has a relatively low risk by comparison, post-operative admission to critical care is routine [27]. Furthermore, there is evidence that within the highest-risk surgical population, only a small proportion of the patients who die are ever admitted to the intensive care

Table 14.2. Mortality of different surgical procedures.

Type of surgery	Mortality (%)	Reference
Abdominal aortic aneurysm repair:		Hadjianastassian *et al.* [28]
Elective	9.6	
Emergency	46.9	
Surgery for colorectal cancer:		Tekkis *et al.* [29]
Elective	5	
Emergency	19.5	
Elective surgery for gastric cancer	10	McCulloch *et al.* [30]
Elective surgery for oesophageal cancer	13.8	
Surgery for fractured neck of femur	4–31 (age is the predominant risk factor for worse outcome)	Roberts and Goldacre [31]
Elective coronary artery bypass grafting	2.3	Shroyer *et al.* [27]

unit, even after they develop post-operative complications [8]. This highlights a deficiency not only in our recognition of the high-risk peri-operative patient, but also in the subsequent management and allocation of resources to these individuals, even when complications have set in.

In some circumstances, it may be possible to modify operative technique so as to reduce the pathophysiological insult of surgery. Endovascular abdominal aortic aneurism repair, for example, is less invasive than open repair, and can be conducted under regional anaesthesia only; improvement in peri-operative outcomes has been demonstrated, although it should be noted that mortality benefit lasts for only two years post-procedure [32]. Most of the time, therefore, it remains the responsibility of the peri-operative physician to physiologically manipulate and optimise the patient with the aim of minimising their risk.

14.3.2 *Demographic risk factors*

Peri-operative risk rises as patients get older; age-related functional deterioration of all organ systems is well acknowledged. However, to assume that age alone is a reliable indicator of peri-operative risk is to underestimate the complexity of the problem. People physiologically age at different rates, and so while age might be a reasonable indicator of population risk, it cannot be relied upon as a sole discriminator of individual patient risk [33].

Obesity is an escalating problem for healthcare services, with a rising number of obese patients attending for surgery. Much emphasis is placed in anaesthetic practice on the potential risks associated with the obese patient, including potential difficulty in airway management and increased incidence of obstructive sleep apnoea. There are also particular problems associated with the peri-operative care of the obese parturient, including increased incidence of pregnancy-induced hypertension, thrombo-embolic complications and wound infection [34,35]. However, although non-pregnant obese patients may be at risk of peri-operative complications as a result of poor functional capacity due to inactivity, as well as comorbidities such as diabetes, ischaemic heart disease and hypertension [36], obesity in itself is not a risk factor for poor peri-operative outcome [37–40].

Table 14.3. Clinical risk factors for peri-operative cardiac events based on the Lee Revised Cardiac Risk Index and adapted from the American College of Cardiology (ACC)/ American Heart Association (AHA) 2007 guidelines.

High risk predictors	Intermediate risk predictors	Minor predictors
Unstable coronary heart disease Decompensated heart failure Significant arrhythmias Severe valvular disease	History of ischaemic heart disease History of decompensated or prior heart failure History of cerebrovascular disease Diabetes mellitus Renal insufficiency	Age greater than 70 years Abnormal electrocardiogram (Left ventricular hypertrophy, left bundle branch block, ST-T abnormalities Cardiac rhythm other than sinus Uncontrolled systemic hypertension

14.3.3 *Risks associated with ischaemic heart disease*

Traditional cardiovascular pre-operative screening tools such as electrocardiography, stress echocardiography and exercise electrocardiogram testing, focus predominantly on ischaemic heart disease as a risk factor for poor outcome from major surgery. However, while the negative predictive value of these tests for predicting peri-operative ischaemic complications is good (> 95%), their positive predictive value is poor (20–30%) [41]. Composite scoring systems such as the Lee Revised Cardiac Risk Index attempt to classify patients' clinical risk of a peri-operative cardiac event based on clinical assessment and history of diabetes, renal dysfunction, cardiac or cerebrovascular disease (see Table 14.3) [42].

14.3.3.1 *Which patients to investigate and which tests are useful?*

The key factor in deciding which patients merit pre-operative investigation of ischaemic heart disease is whether a positive result will change management — that is, whether prophylactic coronary revascularisation will be of benefit. Patient groups in whom coronary revascularisation would be useful before undergoing elective non-cardiac surgery include those with:

- Stable angina and left main stem disease.
- Stable angina and three-vessel disease.

- Stable angina and two-vessel disease including proximal left anterior descending coronary artery stenosis and either an ejection fraction less than 50% or demonstrable ischaemia on non-invasive testing.
- Ongoing unstable angina or acute myocardial infarction [26].

However, there is no evidence to support prophylactic coronary revascularisation in patients with stable coronary artery disease, simply on the basis of positive dobutamine stress echocardiography [43]. Exercise testing reveals an inverse continuum between peri-operative risk and the level of work intensity at which ischaemic changes occur [26]. Stress nuclear myocardial perfusion imaging detects patients at risk of peri-operative cardiac events with high sensitivity but low specificity [26]. The evidence suggests that the most 'significant' coronary stenoses may not necessarily be the ones that are responsible for peri-operative cardiac events, so negating the requirement for prophylactic surgical treatment [43]. Thus, before planning prophylactic coronary revascularisation prior to elective non-cardiac surgery, one should consider carefully the balance of the procedural risks associated with both the cardiac intervention and the non-cardiac surgery, and the patient's functional capacity and overall prognosis. Pre-operative testing for ischaemic heart disease should be restricted to selected patients, based on their clinical risk factors and functional capacity, in order to avoid unnecessary and potentially harmful interventions.

14.3.4 *Risk associated with impaired functional capacity*

Perhaps of more importance in pre-operative risk assessment than the presence or otherwise of coronary artery disease, is the patient's functional capacity. Patients who are unable to meet the increased oxygen demands of the peri-operative period may be at risk of complications. The most recent ACC/AHA guidelines [26] recommend a stepwise approach to peri-operative cardiac assessment based on the degree of surgical urgency, the surgical risk of the procedure itself, the patient's cardiac risk factors and their functional capacity as assessed by the Duke Activity Status Index [44]. This questionnaire grades levels of exertion according to the metabolic equivalent (MET) of oxygen consumption required to achieve the task. One MET corresponds to the resting oxygen consumption of a 70 kg male, that is, 3.5 ml/kg/minute; metabolic expenditure during different physical activities can then be estimated using this as a multiplication factor: simple housework uses 2–4 METs, walking up a hill or strenuous housework up to 6 METs, strenuous competitive sport over 10 METs. Patient questioning about exercise tolerance in this way is helpful, especially in the emergency situation when there is no opportunity for more robust investigation; however it is a subjective assessment and therefore may not be reliable [45]. In institutions where it is available, a more objective assessment of functional capacity may be obtained by cardiopulmonary exercise (CPX) testing.

CPX testing requires the patient to cycle on a bicycle ergometer at gradually increasing intensity during a 'ramp' exercise protocol. The 'ramp' protocol uses increments of work that are so gradual as to be almost imperceptible to the patient; this gradual increase in workload results in a linear relationship between work rate and oxygen consumption [46,47]. Respiratory gas analysis at the mouth, with a non-rebreathing valve connected to a metabolic cart, allows calculation of oxygen consumption, carbon dioxide production and minute ventilation. Non-invasive blood pressure, pulse oximetry and continuous electrocardiogram monitoring are recorded concurrently.

Ventricular function can be assessed by measurement of aerobic capacity, as denoted by the maximum oxygen consumption (VO_2 peak) during the exercise. VO_2 peak is a reproducible index of cardiorespiratory fitness, and when divided by 3.5 ml/kg/minUTE is converted to METs. It is affected both by age (with an approximately 10% reduction per decade in non-trained individuals and 5% in athletes) and by sex: VO_2 peak is between 10% and 20% higher in men than women, as a result of higher stroke volumes, haemoglobin concentrations and muscle mass [48]. VO_2 peak measured during a CPX test is compared with tables of predicted values that have been determined based on age, sex and height [49,50].

CPX testing also measures the anaerobic threshold (AT). This is the point during exercise at which anaerobic metabolism starts to increase significantly as oxygen delivery to muscles is surpassed by the metabolic demands placed by exercise [51]. It is defined as the highest VO_2 value before there is a sustained increased in lactate production and lactate–pyruvate ratio — both of these are hallmarks of anaerobic metabolism. Anaerobic threshold occurs at between 47% and 64% of VO_2 peak in untrained healthy volunteers, and at a higher level in trained athletes [51–53]. This is of importance as it means that AT is attained before the patient begins to fatigue, and so removes the subjectivity of VO_2 peak measurement in patients who are less motivated. An AT of 11 ml/kg/minute is thought to be the value below which a peri-operative patient may be deemed 'high risk' [54,55].

CPX testing can be used to help risk stratify individual patients and inform them of their peri-operative risk and also helps to select out the high-risk individuals for whom a goal-directed peri-operative management strategy may be beneficial.

14.4 Peri-Operative Monitoring and Management of High-Risk Surgical Patients

14.4.1 *Goal-directed therapy in the peri-operative period*

The role of optimisation of patients in the peri-operative period with fluid and inotropic therapy remains one of the most controversial areas of anaesthetic practice. More than 25 randomised controlled trials have been conducted since interest in this area was ignited by the work of Shoemaker [56–58]. One of the problems with establishing and implementing optimisation guidelines is the heterogeneity of the studies contributing to the literature on this subject:

- How to measure the goal (pulmonary artery catheterisation versus less invasive methods).
- Which goal to use (for example, oxygen delivery versus measures of flow such as cardiac output).
- What target to aim for (normalisation versus supra-normalisation).
- How to achieve the goal (fluids and inotropes versus fluid alone).
- When to do the optimisation (pre-, intra- or post-operatively).

Nonetheless, there is convincing evidence that measures of flow or oxygen delivery are superior predictors of mortality than traditional measures of pressure such as blood pressure and central venous pressure, or other vital signs such as oxygen saturation, haemoglobin concentration or temperature: survivors of high-risk surgery have higher values for oxygen delivery and flow than non-survivors [59–61]. False reassurance may be given by monitors showing that a patient has a 'normal' arterial or central venous pressure, as these values are poor surrogates for both global and local tissue blood flow [62,63]. While it is true that a minimum mean arterial pressure is required for organ perfusion, the target pressure varies between individuals, and strategies to ensure maintenance of this pressure are not necessarily sufficient to maintain tissue perfusion throughout the body.

14.4.1.1 *Which measurement device?*

Early work in this field centred on the use of pulmonary artery catheters (PACs) and targeted the measurements that they could provide, such as cardiac output, systemic vascular resistance and pulmonary artery occlusion pressure, which is an indirect measure of left ventricular end-diastolic pressure [57,64–66]. Shoemaker's trial targeting supra-normal values for oxygen delivery, cardiac index and oxygen consumption was the first to show a statistically significant improvement in mortality, complications and resource-utilisation markers such as length of hospital and ICU stay [57]; positive results have since been seen in cardiac surgical patients in whom mixed venous oxygen saturations were targeted [67]. However, several more recent studies have not been able to show an improvement in outcome with PAC-directed therapy [64,66]. Several systematic reviews of the literature have been conducted regarding the use of PACs in high-risk surgical patients; these generally favour the use of PACs [68–70], but were all conducted before the publication of the largest randomised controlled trial (RCT) in this field in 2003 [71]. This study found no improvement in mortality or morbidity with PAC-guided therapy and a significantly higher incidence of pulmonary embolus in the protocol group; however, it should be stated that this study has been heavily criticised, as many of the patients in the treatment arm did not achieve predefined haemodynamic targets until some time into the post-operative period. Nevertheless, a number of large studies have failed to show the PAC to be clinically effective or to improve resource utilisation in a number of different settings [72–74], and clinical experience shows that it is largely being replaced by newer, less invasive devices.

Newer techniques include measurement of the cardiac output and aortic flow time using the oesophageal Doppler, and estimation of pulse-pressure variation (PPV) either via arterial cannulae using transpulmonary thermodilution calibration or less invasively with lithium-dilution calibration. All of these methods have certain limitations, despite their degree of accuracy when compared with pulmonary artery thermodilution; a comparison of them is given in Chapter 5.

The strongest body of evidence for peri-operative haemodynamic management favours the use of oesophageal Doppler. Randomised controlled trials are heterogeneous in their choice of targets and methods for optimisation; however, Doppler-guided fluid resuscitation has consistently been demonstrated to show improvement in outcomes related to both morbidity and resource use. These outcomes include rate of post-operative recovery and length of hospital stay in high-risk orthopaedic surgery [75,76] and complication rates, return to normal gut function and length of hospital stay in major abdominal surgery [77–81]. While the available evidence dictates that we should use oesophageal Doppler technology for peri-operative haemodynamic optimisation, one should consider that the method and timing of optimisation must surely be of more significance than the technology used to facilitate it.

14.4.1.2 *When and how to optimise?*

14.4.1.2.1 Pre-operative

Shoemaker's original study of peri-operative optimisation targeted supra-normal oxygen delivery (600 ml/min/m^2) in pre-operative patients using the PAC, and demonstrated a dramatic decrease in morbidity and mortality in a high-risk surgical population [57]. More recent studies using the PAC for pre-operative supra-normal optimisation, have re-affirmed improvements in morbidity and mortality, when targeting cardiac output [82] and again, oxygen delivery [83]. All of these studies used both fluid and vasoactive agents in a physician-led protocol to achieve their targets; this, in conjunction with the resources associated with pre-operative critical care admission, has meant that these strategies have not been widely adopted. It is worth noting however, that when cost-effectiveness has been specifically examined, the improvement in process measures afforded by pre-operative optimisation gives financial support to pre-operative critical care admission for optimisation in high-risk patients [83,84]. Nevertheless, it is often practically difficult to admit patients to critical care pre-operatively, and so more recent work has focussed on intra- and post-operative goal-directed therapy.

14.4.1.2.2 Intra-operative

Trials looking at intra-operative optimisation, using the PAC [85] oesophageal Doppler [76–79] and pulse contour analysis [86] to guide fluid and inotropic therapy have also shown positive results; the findings of oesophageal-Doppler-based trials have been discussed previously. Pulse-contour-analysis-guided therapy leads to improvement in resource use (mechanical ventilation days, ICU and hospital length of stay) as well as post-operative complications and a mortality reduction was demonstrated in a trial using dobutamine and fluid support targeting supra-normal oxygen delivery using the PAC [85].

14.4.1.2.3 Post-operative

More recently, evidence has started to emerge that goal-directed therapy started in the post-operative period may be of benefit. Studies have been conducted in cardiac surgical patients, using oesophageal Doppler to target stroke index > 35 ml/m^2 [87] or the PAC to target mixed venous oxygen saturation (S_VO_2) > 70% and lactate < 2 mmol/l [67]; in the high-risk general surgical population, lithium-dilution-calibrated pulse contour analysis has been used to target an oxygen delivery of > 600 ml/min/m^2 [88]. All these studies used both fluids and inotropes to achieve their targets where required. Whereas the cardiac surgery studies were only able to show an improvement in length of hospital stay, the more recent trial in general surgical patients also demonstrated a significant reduction in complications. A key point of this study was that a goal-directed protocol was applied for only the first eight hours post-operatively; thus, it may be that targeted therapy early in the post-operative period may be a practicable method by which the critical care physician can optimise the high-risk surgical patient.

14.4.1.3 *Summary*

In light of this evidence, and with the advantage that ICU patients are intensively nursed, thereby facilitating nurse-led protocol-based optimisation, the critical care team in the post-operative period can play an important role leading to improvement in both resource-based and clinical outcomes. The evidence favours targeting of supra-normal values for oxygen delivery, cardiac index or stroke volume, initially using fluid optimisation, followed by inotropic therapy if required. No significant benefit is derived from pre-operative ICU admission for optimisation using the PAC; intra- or post-operative goal-directed therapy seems to confer similar benefit, with less imposition on ICU resources. The ideal monitoring device is still a matter for debate; what is clear, however, is that algorithms based on flow measurements such as oxygen delivery and stroke volume are preferable to pressure (arterial or venous)-guided fluid and inotropic support.

14.4.2 *Modifying the neuro-humoral response to surgery*

14.4.2.1 *Regional anaesthesia*

The use of regional anaesthesia is probably the single most investigated peri-operative intervention that may lead to improvement in surgical outcome, as a result of improved analgesia, reduction in respiratory complications and the modification of the neuro-humoral response. At a cellular level, epidural analgesia is thought to cause sympatholysis, resulting in improved oxygen consumption/supply dynamics, reduction in cortisol secretion and reduction in hyperglycaemia by efferent neural blockade of the adrenal medulla and liver [89,90]. Although the addition of an opiate to epidural local anaesthetic infusions provides superior pain relief, the opiate does not confer any additional physiological benefit.

The evidence for benefit of peri-operative epidural analgesia on outcome is somewhat contradictory. The most recent meta-analysis on this subject looked at 141 trials involving nearly 10,000 patients, across a wide variety of specialities including general, urological, vascular and orthopaedic surgery [91]. In patients who received neuroaxial blockade, a reduction in mortality of one-third was demonstrated; this did not significantly differ across type of surgery, type of blockade (spinal or epidural) or whether or not the regional technique was combined with general anaesthesia. There were also improvements in peri-operative morbidity, including rates of respiratory depression, renal failure, thromboembolic disease and myocardial infarction. Since then, however, an international randomised controlled trial found no effect on mortality, and only very modest improvement in morbidity with epidural analgesia, although this study was criticised as being inadequately powered to be able to discern a mortality reduction [92]. The most recent major publication in this field, a retrospective propensity score matched-cohort study of nearly 260,000 patients, found a marginal improvement in 30-day mortality with epidural anaesthesia [93]. However the magnitude of this improvement was small, with number needed to treat of 477; thus the authors were unable to conclude that there was compelling evidence for epidural anaesthesia improving outcome after major surgery. The jury is still out on this subject, although there is little doubt that epidural analgesia provides superior pain relief and reduces post-operative respiratory complications, as a result of the analgesic effect and the avoidance of systemic opioids [91,92,94].

14.4.2.2 *Systemic analgesics*

While opiates have been shown to modify the neuro-humoral response to surgery by suppressing hypothalamic and pituitary hormone secretion in both lower-abdominal [95] and cardiac surgery [96], this is not the case with upper abdominal surgery; furthermore, no convincing effect on outcome has been demonstrated [97]. Similarly, the alpha-2 agonist clonidine, which has both anti-hypertensive and analgesic properties, is known to modify the stress response by providing sympatholysis, haemodynamic stability and analgesia [98]. One RCT has looked at the effect of peri-operative systemic clonidine administration (commenced the night before surgery and continued for four days) in patients at risk of coronary artery disease, and found that clonidine improved peri-operative cardiovascular morbidity and long-term mortality [99].

14.4.2.3 *Normothermia*

Prevention of hypothermia in the peri-operative period is an important and easily facilitated intervention that reduces sympathetic stimulation, prevents unpredictable changes in drug pharmacokinetics and dynamics, and improves outcomes such as wound infection rates, cardiac morbidity and peri-operative blood loss [100–102].

14.4.2.4 *Glycaemic control*

Much work been conducted on the role of using insulin to attain tight glycaemic control (TGC) in the peri-operative and critical care settings. Insulin has been shown to have anti-inflammatory properties in other circumstances, including severe trauma and burns [103]. The original and most famous study looking at TGC in surgical patients was conducted in a single centre and published in 2001, showing impressive reductions in mortality and morbidity with a target blood glucose range of 4.1–6.0 mmol/l, when compared with 10–11 mmol/l [104]. This study has been criticised however, for, amongst other reasons, having an unexpectedly high mortality in the control group. Furthermore, a recent meta-analysis was unable to show any difference in mortality in either the general critical care population, or the surgical ICU population, between patients managed with very tight glycaemic control (target blood glucose < 6.1 mmol/l), moderately tight control (< 8.1 mmol/l) and 'usual' glycaemic control (around 11 mmol/l, in accordance with the original TGC study) [105]. This meta-analysis also showed a significantly increased risk of hypoglycaemia with TGC; thus, as well as not proving TGC to be of benefit, based on the results of this study, one cannot exclude the possibility that TGC may actually cause harm.

Table 14.4. A summary of the most recent guidelines on surgical thromboprophylaxis. Based on [102].

Type of surgery	Recommended agent	Grade of recommendation	Comments
Major abdominal	Low-molecular-weight heparin (LMWH)	1A	
	Low-dose unfractionated heparin (LDUFH)	1A	
	Fondaparinux	1A	
Major gynaecological or open urological	LMWH	1A	IPC as an adjunct to pharmacological therapy
	LDUFH	1A	
	Fondaparinux	1A	
	Intermittent pneumatic compression (IPC)	1A	
Hip fracture surgery	Fondaparinux	1A	Target INR for vitamin K antagonists: 2.5
	LMWH	1B	
	LDUFH	1B	
	Vitamin K antagonist	1B	

14.4.2.5 *Thromboprophylaxis*

In common with other critical care patients, the evidence for pharmacological thromboprophylaxis in the surgical population is consistent and robust [106]. A summary of the most recent guidelines on surgical thromboprophylaxis is tabulated below (see Table 14.4). For patients undergoing hip or knee arthroplasty or hip fracture surgery, continuation of thromboprophylaxis is recommended for a minimum of ten days and up to 35 days post-procedure.

14.4.3 *Modifying peri-operative risk in patients with cardiac disease*

Much attention in this chapter has been focussed on optimisation of patients with poor cardiorespiratory reserve due to any cause. In patients with known cardiac disease, precautions can be taken in the peri-operative period to reduce their risk of ischaemic or other cardiac events. A full description of these measures is beyond the scope of this chapter; however, the American College of Cardiology/American Heart Association consensus statements offer concise, evidence-based guidance on this subject [26,107]. Of particular note is guidance regarding peri-operative beta-blockade, as this has been the subject of much debate in the light of the results of the Perioperative Ischemic Evaluation Study (POISE) [108]. This large, placebo-controlled RCT looked at the peri-operative *de novo* administration of extended-release metoprolol, and found that while the incidence of combined end-points of cardiac death, non-fatal myocardial infarction and non-fatal cardiac arrest was reduced in the beta blockade group, the overall mortality and risk of stroke were higher. The evidence would seem to suggest that beta-blockade may have a role in selected patients, but we have yet to identify precisely which ones. In the meantime, while there is a grade I recommendation that beta-blockade be continued in patients already established on it, the current evidence suggests that commencement of beta-blockade in the peri-operative period cannot be recommended.

14.4.4 *Transfusion guidelines for peri-operative patients*

Current red cell transfusion guidelines for the peri-operative period recommend a transfusion trigger of 7 g/dl, and target haemoglobin of 7–10 g/dl; they also state that transfusion of patients with haemoglobin concentrations of greater than 10 g/dl is unjustified [109,110]. This guidance is based on studies which show no increased benefit for higher haemoglobin concentrations, amid increasing pressure to reduce allogenic transfusion because of the associated risks and constant concern over blood bank reserves. However, there are several points to consider on this issue. First, it is worth noting that all of the studies informing this policy were conducted before leucocyte depletion of packed red cells became routine, thus reducing the risk of various complications, including transfusion-related acute lung injury. Secondly, none of these trials were conducted specifically in peri-operative patients, and moreover, high-risk surgical patients. Finally, the risk of transmission of viral or bacterial infection via red-cell transfusion is vanishingly low, although it must be acknowledged that the risk of transmission of prion diseases is unknown. Given that haemoglobin concentration is an important part of oxygen flux, and the evidence to support supra-normal oxygen delivery in surgical patients as discussed above, it may be worth the peri-operative physician considering a higher transfusion trigger than that of the general critical care population.

14.5 The Multi-Modal Approach to Peri-Operative Care

In recent years, the traditional approach to peri-operative management has been challenged by advocates of enhanced recovery or 'fast-track' surgical programmes. Such programmes implement a multi-modal, multidisciplinary approach to post-operative care in a variety of surgical specialities, with the aim of reducing morbidity, mortality and duration of hospital stay, while improving patient satisfaction and speed of recovery. General measures not already mentioned include the avoidance of nasogastric tubes, in order to reduce pulmonary morbidity in gastric [111], hepatic [112] and aortic surgery [113] and the avoidance of bowel preparation before colonic surgery [114]. Many of the standards of care already discussed in this chapter are also integral parts of an enhanced recovery programme, including neuroaxial blockade, alpha-2 agonists, thromboprophylaxis, and peri-operative goal-directed therapy to optimise stroke volume and/or oxygen delivery. Interestingly, minimally invasive surgery in the context of an enhanced recovery programme has not been shown to be of benefit over open procedures in studies of abdominal or hip-replacement surgery [115,116]; nevertheless, proponents of fast-track surgery continue to support the use of minimal-access surgery where possible [117].

The most consistently demonstrated advantage of enhanced recovery programmes is a reduction in length of hospital stay and post-operative morbidity, across a wide variety of surgical specialities [117,118]. However, no studies have yet been conducted looking at high-risk emergency surgical patients.

14.6 Conclusion

Care of the high-risk peri-operative patient begins some time before the operating theatre, with investigations to identify and quantify risk. Goal-directed therapy, and appropriate analgesia and monitoring will help to optimise oxygen supply/demand dynamics in the peri-operative period.

As with all aspects of critical care, a multidisciplinary approach is recommended. Although most of the studies conducted in the peri-operative outcomes field have failed to show improvements in mortality with specific interventions, improvements in morbidity have been demonstrated with goal-directed therapy, neuroaxial analgesia and enhanced recovery programmes. A huge number of patients undergo surgical procedures each year, with the risk of peri-operative morbidity which may lead to a reduction in long-term survival. The appropriate allocation of Level 2 and 3 facilities to manage these patients should therefore be a priority for the critical care physician.

References

[1] Weiser, T.G., Regenbogen, S.E., Thompson, K.D. *et al.* (2008). An estimation of the global volume of surgery: a modelling strategy based on available data, *Lancet*, **372**, 139–144.

[2] Halm, E.A., Lee, C. and Chassin, M.R. (2002). Is volume related to outcome in health care? A systematic review and methodologic critique of the literature, *Ann Intern Med*, **137**, 511–520.

[3] Hamilton, B.H. and Ho, V. (1998). Does practice make perfect? Examining the relationship between hospital surgical volume and outcomes for hip fracture patients in Quebec, *Med Care*, **36**, 892–903.

[4] Khuri, S.F. and Henderson, W.G. (2005). The case against volume as a measure of quality of surgical care, *World J Surg*, **29**, 1222–1229.

[5] Zare, M.M., Itani, K.M., Schifftner, T.L. *et al.* (2007). Mortality after nonemergent major surgery performed on Friday versus Monday through Wednesday, *Ann Surg*, **246**, 866–874.

[6] Khuri, S.F., Henderson, W.G., DePalma, R.G. *et al.* (2005). Determinants of long-term survival after major surgery and the adverse effect of postoperative complications, *Ann Surg*, **242**, 326–341.

[7] Cullinane, M., Gray, A.J.G., Hargraves, C.M.K. *et al.* (2003). *National Confidential Enquiry into Perioperative Deaths,* National Confidential Enquiry into Patient Outcome and Deaths (NCEPOD), London.

[8] Pearse, R.M., Harrison, D.A., James, P. *et al.* (2006). Identification and characterisation of the high-risk surgical population in the United Kingdom, *Crit Care*, **10**, R81.

[9] Wolters, U., Wolf, T., Stutzer, H. *et al.* (1996). ASA classification and perioperative variables as predictors of postoperative outcome, *Br J Anaesth*, **77**, 217–222.

[10] Davenport, D.L., Bowe, E.A., Henderson, W.G. *et al.* (2006). National Surgical Quality Improvement Program (NSQIP) risk factors can be used to validate American, Society of Anesthesiologists Physical Status Classification (ASA PS) levels, *Ann Surg*, **243**, 636–641.

[11] Copeland, G.P., Jones, D. and Walters, M. (1991). POSSUM: a scoring system for surgical audit, *Br J Surg*, **78**, 355–360.

[12] McIlroy, B.S. and Copeland, G.P. (1996). An evaluation of the POSSUM surgical scoring system, *Br J Surg*, **83**, 1483–1484.

[13] Copeland, G.P. (2002). The POSSUM system of surgical audit, *Arch Surg*, **137**, 15–19.

[14] Nilsson, J., Algotsson, L., Hoglund, P. *et al.* (2006). Comparison of 19 preoperative risk stratification models in open-heart surgery, *Eur Heart J*, **27**, 867–874.

[15] Valenti, V., Hernandez-Lizoain, J.L., Baixauli, J. *et al.* (2009). Analysis of POSSUM score and postoperative morbidity in patients with rectal cancer undergoing surgery, *Langenbecks Arch Surg*, **394**, 55–63.

[16] Al-Homoud, S., Purkayastha, S., Aziz, O. *et al.* (2004). Evaluating operative risk in colorectal cancer surgery: ASA and POSSUM-based predictive models, *Surg Oncol*, **13**, 83–92.

[17] Rohrig, R., Junger, A., Hartmann, B. *et al.* (2004). The incidence and prediction of automatically detected intraoperative cardiovascular events in noncardiac surgery, *Anesth Analg*, **98**, 569–577.

[18] de Cassia Braga, R.K. and Kowalski, L.P. (2003). APACHE II., POSSUM and ASA scores and the risk of perioperative complications in patients with oral or oropharyngeal cancer, *Arch Otolaryngol Head Neck Surg*, **129**, 739–745.

[19] Copeland, G.P., Jones, D., Wilcox, A. *et al.* (1993). Comparative vascular audit using the POSSUM scoring system, *Ann R Coll Surg Engl*, **75**, 175–177.

[20] Tekkis, P., Trotter, G. and South, L.M. (1999). Comparison of POSSUM and the Portsmouth predictor equation for predicting death following vascular surgery, *Br J Surg*, **86**, 713–714.

[21] Tekkis, P.P., Kocher, H.M., Bentley, A.J. *et al.* (2000). Operative mortality rates among surgeons: comparison of POSSUM and p-POSSUM scoring systems in gastrointestinal surgery, *Dis Colon Rectum*, **43**, 1528–1532. Discussion 1532–1534.

[22] Constantinides, V.A., Tekkis, P.P. and Senapati, A. (2006). Comparison of POSSUM scoring systems and the surgical risk scale in patients undergoing surgery for complicated diverticular disease, *Dis Colon Rectum*, **49**, 1322–1331.

[23] Valenti, V., Hernandez-Lizoain, J.L., Baixauli, J. *et al.* (2009). Analysis of POSSUM score and postoperative morbidity in patients with rectal cancer undergoing surgery, *Langenbecks Arch Surg*, **394**, 55–63.

[24] Wright, D.M., Blanckley, S., Stewart, G.J. *et al.* (2008). The use of orthopaedic POSSUM as an audit tool for fractured neck of femur, *Injury*, **39**, 430–435.

[25] Older, P. and Smith, R. (1988). Experience with the preoperative invasive measurement of haemodynamic, respiratory and renal function in 100 elderly patients scheduled for major abdominal surgery, *Anaesth Intensive Care*, **16**, 389–395.

[26] Fleisher, L.A., Beckman, J.A., Brown, K.A. *et al.* (2007). ACC/AHA 2007 guidelines on perioperative cardiovascular evaluation and care for noncardiac surgery: A report of the American College of Cardiology/American Heart Association Task Force on Practice Guidelines (Writing Committee to Revise the 2002, Guidelines on Perioperative Cardiovascular Evaluation for Noncardiac Surgery): Developed in collaboration with the American Society of Echocardiography, American Society of Nuclear Cardiology, Heart Rhythm Society, Society of Cardiovascular Anesthesiologists, Society for Cardiovascular Angiography and Interventions, Society for Vascular Medicine and Biology and Society for Vascular Surgery, *Circulation*, **116**, e418–e499.

[27] Shroyer, A.L., McDonald, G.O., Wagner, B.D. *et al.* (2008). Improving quality of care in cardiac surgery: evaluating risk factors processes of care, structures of care and outcomes, *Semin Cardiothorac Vasc Anesth*, **12**, 140–152.

[28] Hadjianastassiou, V.G., Tekkis, P.P., Goldhill, D.R. *et al.* (2005). Quantification of mortality risk after abdominal aortic aneurysm repair, *Br J Surg*, **92**, 1092–1098.

[29] Tekkis, P.P., Poloniecki, J.D., Thompson, M,R. *et al.* (2003). Operative mortality in colorectal cancer: prospective national study, *BMJ*, **327**, 1196–1201.

[30] McCulloch, P., Ward, J. and Tekkis, P.P. (2003). Mortality and morbidity in gastro-oesophageal cancer surgery: initial results of ASCOT multicentre prospective cohort study, *BMJ*, **327**, 1192–1197.

[31] Roberts, S.E. and Goldacre, M.J. (2003). Time trends and demography of mortality after fractured neck of femur in an English population, 1968–98: database study, *BMJ* **327**, 771–775.

[32] Wilt, T.J, Lederle FA, Macdonald R, *et al.* (2006). Comparison of endovascular and open surgical repairs for abdominal aortic aneurysm, *Evid Rep Technol Assess* (*Full Rep*), **144**, 1–113.

[33] Wasserman, K. (1993). Preoperative evaluation of cardiovascular reserve in the elderly, *Chest*, **104**, 663–664.

[34] Robinson, H.E., O.'Connell, C.M., Joseph, K.S. *et al.* (2005). Maternal outcomes in pregnancies complicated by obesity, *Obstet Gynecol*, **106**, 1357–1364.

[35] Satpathy, H.K., Fleming, A., Frey, D. *et al.* (2008). Maternal obesity and pregnancy, *Postgrad Med*, **120**, E01–E09.

[36] Bamgbade, O.A., Rutter, T.W., Nafiu, O.O. *et al.* (2007). Postoperative complications in obese and nonobese patients, *World J Surg*, **31**, 556–560.

[37] Dindo, D., Muller, M.K., Weber, M. *et al.* (2003). Obesity in general elective surgery, *Lancet*, **361**, 2032–2035.

[38] Kaafarani, H.M., Itani, K.M., Thornby, J. *et al.* (2004). Thirty-day and one-year predictors of death in noncardiac major surgical procedures, *Am J Surg*, **188**, 495–499.

[39] Leykin, Y., Pellis, T., Del, M.E. *et al.* (2006). Anesthetic management of morbidly obese and super-morbidly obese patients undergoing bariatric operations: hospital course and outcomes, *Obes Surg*, **16**, 1563–1569.

[40] Klasen, Junger, A., Hartmann, B. *et al.* (2004). Increased body mass index and peri-operative risk in patients undergoing non-cardiac surgery, *Obes Surg*, **14**, 275–281.

[41] Older, P. and Hall, A. (2004). Clinical review: how to identify high-risk surgical patients, *Crit Care*, **8**, 369–372.

[42] Lee, T.H., Marcantonio, E.R., Mangione, C.M. *et al.* (1999). Derivation and prospective validation of a simple index for prediction of cardiac risk of major noncardiac surgery, *Circulation*, **100**, 1043–1049.

[43] Landesberg, G. (2003). The pathophysiology of perioperative myocardial infarction: facts and perspectives, *J Cardiothorac Vasc Anesth*, **17**, 90–100.

[44] Hlatky, M.A., Boineau, R.E., Higginbotham, M.B. *et al.* (1989). A brief self-administered questionnaire to determine functional capacity (the Duke Activity Status Index), *Am J Cardiol*, **64**, 651–654.

[45] Wiklund, R.A., Stein, H.D., Rosenbaum, S.H. (2001). Activities of daily living and cardiovascular complications following elective, noncardiac surgery, *Yale J Biol Med*, **74**, 75–87.

[46] Milani, R.V., Lavie, C.J., Mehra, M.R., *et al.* (2006). Understanding the basics of cardiopulmonary exercise testing, *Mayo Clin Proc*, **81**, 1603–1611.

[47] Myers, J., Buchanan, N., Walsh, D. *et al.* (1991). Comparison of the ramp versus standard exercise protocols, *J Am Coll Cardiol*, **17**, 1334–1342.

[48] Fleg, J.L., Pina, I.L., Balady, G.J. *et al.* (2000). Assessment of functional capacity in clinical and research applications: An advisory from the Committee on Exercise Rehabilitation and Prevention, Council on Clinical Cardiology, American Heart Association, *Circulation*, **102**, 1591–1597.

[49] Ross, R.M. (2003). ATS/ACCP statement on cardiopulmonary exercise testing, *Am J Respir Crit Care Med*, **167**, 1451.

[50] Hansen, J.E., Sue, D.Y. and Wasserman, K. (1984). Predicted values for clinical exercise testing, *Am Rev Respir Dis*, **129**, S49–S55.

[51] Milani, R.V., Lavie, C.J. and Mehra, M.R. (2004). Cardiopulmonary exercise testing: how do we differentiate the cause of dyspnea? *Circulation*, **110**, e27–e31.

[52] Shimizu, M., Myers, J., Buchanan, N. *et al.* (1991). The ventilatory threshold: method: protototocol, and evaluator agreement, *Am Heart J*, **122**, 509–516.

[53] Neuberg, G.W., Friedman, S.H., Weiss, M.B. *et al.* (1988). Cardiopulmonary exercise testing. The clinical value of gas exchange data, *Arch Intern Med*, **148**, 2221–2226.

[54] Older, P., Hall, A. and Hader, R. (1999). Cardiopulmonary exercise testing as a screening test for perioperative management of major surgery in the elderly, *Chest*, **116**, 355–362.

[55] Older, P., Smith, R., Courtney, P. *et al.* (1993). Preoperative evaluation of cardiac failure and ischemia in elderly patients by cardiopulmonary exercise testing, *Chest*, **104**, 701–704.

[56] Shoemaker, W.C., Appel, P. and Bland, R. (1983). Use of physiologic monitoring to predict outcome and to assist in clinical decisions in critically ill postoperative patients, *Am J Surg*, **146**, 43–50.

[57] Shoemaker, W.C., Appel, P.L., Kram, H.B. *et al.* (1988). Prospective trial of supranormal values of survivors as therapeutic goals in high-risk surgical patients, *Chest*, **94**, 1176–1186.

[58] Shoemaker, W.C., Appel, P.L. and Kram, H.B. (1993). Hemodynamic and oxygen transport responses in survivors and nonsurvivors of high-risk surgery, *Crit Care Med*, **21**, 977–990.

[59] Shoemaker, W.C., Chang, P., Bland, R. *et al.* (1979). Cardiorespiratory monitoring in postoperative patients: II. Quantitative therapeutic indices as guides to therapy, *Crit Care Med*, **7**, 243–249.

[60] Shoemaker, W.C. and Czer, L.S. (1979). Evaluation of the biologic importance of various hemodynamic and oxygen transport variables: which

variables should be monitored in postoperative shock? *Crit Care Med*, **7**, 424–431.

[61] Shoemaker, W.C., Appel, P.L. and Kram, H.B. (1993). Hemodynamic and oxygen transport responses in survivors and nonsurvivors of high-risk surgery, *Crit Care Med*, **21**, 977–990.

[62] Grocott, M.P., Mythen, M.G. and Gan, T.J. (2005). Perioperative fluid management and clinical outcomes in adults, *Anesth Analg*, **100**, 1093–1106.

[63] Hamilton-Davies, C., Mythen, M.G., Salmon, J.B. *et al.* (1997). Comparison of commonly used clinical indicators of hypovolaemia with gastrointestinal tonometry, *Intens Care Med*, **23**, 276–281.

[64] Bender, J.S., Smith-Meek, M.A. and Jones, C.E. (1997). Routine pulmonary artery catheterization does not reduce morbidity and mortality of elective vascular surgery: results of a prospective, randomized trial, *Ann Surg*, **226**, 229–236.

[65] Berlauk, J.F., Abrams, J.H., Gilmour, I.J. *et al.* (1991). Preoperative optimization of cardiovascular hemodynamics improves outcome in peripheral vascular surgery, A. prospective, randomized clinical trial, *Ann Surg*, **214**, 289–297.

[66] Valentine, R.J., Duke, M.L., Inman, M.H. *et al.* (1998). Effectiveness of pulmonary artery catheters in aortic surgery: a randomized trial, *J Vasc Surg*, **27**, 203–211.

[67] Polonen, P., Ruokonen, E., Hippelainen, M. *et al.* (2000). A prospective, randomized study of goal-oriented hemodynamic therapy in cardiac surgical patients, *Anesth Analg*, **90**, 1052–1059.

[68] Ivanov, R.I., Allen, J., Sandham, J.D. *et al.* (1997). Pulmonary artery catheterization: a narrative and systematic critique of randomized controlled trials and recommendations for the future, *New Horiz*, **5**, 268–276.

[69] Heyland, D.K., Cook, D.J., King, D. *et al.* (1996). Maximizing oxygen delivery in critically ill patients: a methodologic appraisal of the evidence, *Crit Care Med*, **24**, 517–524.

[70] Kern, J.W. and Shoemaker, W.C. (2002). Meta-analysis of hemodynamic optimization in high-risk patients, *Crit Care Med*, **30**, 1686–1692.

[71] Sandham, J.D., Hull, R.D., Brant, R.F. *et al.* (2003). A randomized, controlled trial of the use of pulmonary-artery catheters in high-risk surgical patients, *N Engl J Med*, **348**, 5–14.

[72] Harvey, S.E., Welch, C.A., Harrison, D.A. *et al.* (2008). Post hoc insights from, PAC-Man–the, U.K. pulmonary artery catheter trial, *Crit Care Med*, **36**, 1714–1721.

[73] Harvey, S., Stevens, K., Harrison, D. *et al.* (2006). An evaluation of the clinical and cost-effectiveness of pulmonary artery catheters in patient management in intensive care: a systematic review and a randomised controlled trial, *Health Technol Assess*, **10** (iii–xi), 1–133.

[74] Harvey, S., Harrison, D.A., Singer, M. *et al.* (2005). Assessment of the clinical effectiveness of pulmonary artery catheters in management of patients in intensive care (PAC-Man): a randomised controlled trial, *Lancet*, **366**, 472–477.

[75] Venn, R., Steele, A. and Richardson, P. (2002). Randomized controlled trial to investigate influence of the fluid challenge on duration of hospital stay and perioperative morbidity in patients with hip fractures, *Br J Anaesth*, **88**, 65–71.

[76] Sinclair, S., James, S. and Singer, M. (1997). Intraoperative intravascular volume optimisation and length of hospital stay after repair of proximal femoral fracture: randomised controlled trial, *BMJ*, **315**, 909–912.

[77] Noblett, S.E., Snowden, C.P., Shenton, B.K. *et al.* (2006). Randomized clinical trial assessing the effect of Doppler-optimized fluid management on outcome after elective colorectal resection, *Br J Surg*, **93**, 1069–1076.

[78] Wakeling, H.G., McFall, M.R., Jenkins, C.S. *et al.* (2005). Intraoperative oesophageal, Doppler guided fluid management shortens postoperative hospital stay after major bowel surgery, *Br J Anaesth*, **95**, 634–642.

[79] Walsh, S.R., Tang, T., Bass, S. *et al.* (2008). Doppler-guided intra-operative fluid management during major abdominal surgery: systematic review and meta-analysis, *Int J Clin Pract*, **62**, 466–470.

[80] Abbas, S.M. and Hill, A.G. (2008). Systematic review of the literature for the use of oesophageal, Doppler monitor for fluid replacement in major abdominal surgery, *Anaesthesia*, **63**, 44–51.

[81] Mythen, M.G. and Webb, A.R. (1995). Perioperative plasma volume expansion reduces the incidence of gut mucosal hypoperfusion during cardiac surgery, *Arch Surg*, **130**, 423–429.

[82] Boyd, O., Grounds, R.M. and Bennett, E.D. (1993). A randomized clinical trial of the effect of deliberate perioperative increase of oxygen delivery on mortality in high-risk surgical patients, *JAMA*, **270**, 2699–2707.

[83] Wilson, J., Woods, I., Fawcett, J. *et al.* (1999). Reducing the risk of major elective surgery: randomised controlled trial of preoperative optimisation of oxygen delivery, *BMJ*, **318**, 1099–1103.

[84] Fenwick, E., Wilson, J., Sculpher, M., *et al.* (2002). Pre-operative optimisation employing dopexamine or adrenaline for patients undergoing

major elective surgery: a cost-effectiveness analysis, *Intens Care Med*, **28**, 599–608.

[85] Lobo, S.M., Salgado, P.F., Castillo, V.G. *et al.* (2000). Effects of maximizing oxygen delivery on morbidity and mortality in high-risk surgical patients, *Crit Care Med*, **28**, 3396–3404.

[86] Lopes, M.R., Oliveira, M.A., Pereira, V.O. *et al.* (2007). Goal-directed fluid management based on pulse pressure variation monitoring during high-risk surgery: a pilot randomized controlled trial, *Crit Care*, **11**, R100.

[87] McKendry, M., McGloin, H., Saberi, D. *et al.* (2004). Randomised controlled trial assessing the impact of a nurse delivered, flow monitored protocol for optimisation of circulatory status after cardiac surgery, *BMJ*, **329**, 258.

[88] Pearse, R., Dawson, D., Fawcett, J. *et al.* (2005). Early goal-directed therapy after major surgery reduces complications and duration of hospital stay, a randomised, controlled trial [ISRCTN38797445], *Crit Care*, **9**, R687–R693.

[89] Moore, C.M., Cross, M.H., Desborough, J.P. *et al.* (1995). Hormonal effects of thoracic extradural analgesia for cardiac surgery, *Br J Anaesth*, **75**, 387–393.

[90] Yardeni, I.Z., Shavit, Y., Bessler, H. *et al.* (2007). Comparison of postoperative pain management techniques on endocrine response to surgery: a randomised controlled trial, *Int J Surg*, **5**, 239–243.

[91] Rodgers, A., Walker, N., Schug, S. *et al.* (2000). Reduction of postoperative mortality and morbidity with epidural or spinal anaesthesia: results from overview of randomised trials, *BMJ*, **321**, 1493.

[92] Rigg, J.R., Jamrozik, K., Myles, P.S. *et al.* (2002). Epidural anaesthesia and analgesia and outcome of major surgery: a randomised trial, *Lancet*, **359**, 1276–1282.

[93] Wijeysundera, D.N., Scott Beattie, W., Austin, P.C. *et al.* (2008). Epidural anaesthesia and survival after intermediate-to-high risk non-cardiac surgery: a population based cohort study, *Lancet*, **372**, 562–570.

[94] Ballantyne, J.C., Carr, D.B., deFerranti, S. *et al.* (1998). The comparative effects of postoperative analgesic therapies on pulmonary outcome: cumulative meta-analyses of randomized, controlled trials, *Anesth Analg*, **86**, 598–612.

[95] Hall, G.M., Young, C., Holdcroft, A. *et al.* (1978). Substrate mobilisation during surgery. A comparison between halothane and fentanyl anaesthesia, *Anaesthesia*, **33**, 924–930.

[96] Desborough, J.P., Hall, G.M., Hart, G.R. *et al.* (1990). Hormonal responses to cardiac surgery: effects of sufentanil, somatostatin and ganglion block, *Br J Anaesth*, **64**, 688–695.

[97] Desborough, J.P. (2000). The stress response to trauma and surgery, *Br J Anaesth*, **85**, 109–117.
[98] Aantaa, R. and Scheinin, M. (1993). Alpha 2-adrenergic agents in anaesthesia, *Acta Anaesthesiol Scand*, **37**, 433–448.
[99] Wallace, A.W., Galindez, D., Salahieh, A. *et al.* (2004). Effect of clonidine on cardiovascular morbidity and mortality after noncardiac surgery, *Anesthesiology*, **101**, 284–293.
[100] Rajagopalan, S., Mascha, E., Na, J. *et al.* (2008). The effects of mild perioperative hypothermia on blood loss and transfusion requirement, *Anesthesiology*, **108**, 71–77.
[101] Sessler, D.I. (2001). Complications and treatment of mild hypothermia, *Anesthesiology*, **95**, 531–543.
[102] Wong, P.F., Kumar, S., Bohra, A. *et al.* (2007). Randomized clinical trial of perioperative systemic warming in major elective abdominal surgery, *Br J Surg*, **94**, 421–426.
[103] Jeschke, M.G., Klein, D. and Herndon, D.N. (2004). Insulin treatment improves the systemic inflammatory reaction to severe trauma, *Ann Surg*, **239**, 553–560.
[104] Van den, B.G., Wouters, P., Weekers, F. *et al.* (2001). Intensive insulin therapy in the critically ill patients, *N Engl J Med*, **345**, 1359–1367.
[105] Wiener, R.S., Wiener, D.C. and Larson, R.J. (2008). Benefits and risks of tight glucose control in critically ill adults: a meta-analysis, *JAMA*, **300**, 933–944.
[106] Geerts, W.H., Bergqvist, D., Pineo, G.F. *et al.* (2008). Prevention of venous thromboembolism: American College of Chest Physicians Evidence-Based, Clinical Practice Guidelines (eighth edition), *Chest*, **133**, 381S–453S.
[107] Fleisher, L.A., Beckman, J.A., Brown, K.A. *et al.* (2007). ACC/AHA, 2007 Guidelines on Perioperative Cardiovascular Evaluation and Care for Noncardiac Surgery: Executive Summary: A Report of the American College of Cardiology/American Heart Association Task Force on Practice Guidelines (Writing Committee to Revise the 2002 Guidelines on Perioperative Cardiovascular Evaluation for Noncardiac Surgery, *Circulation*, **116**, 1971–1996.
[108] Devereaux, P.J., Yang, H., Yusuf, S. *et al.* (2008). Effects of extended-release metoprolol succinate in patients undergoing non-cardiac surgery (POISE trial): a randomised controlled trial, *Lancet*, **371**, 1839–1847.
[109] Association of Anaesthetists of Great Britain and Ireland (2008). Blood transfusion and the anaesthestist, Red Cell Transfusion 2.

[110] Scottish Intercollegiate Guidelines Network (2001). *Peri-operative Blood Transfusion for Elective Surgery,* Guideline 54, Scottish Intercollegiate Guidelines Network, Edinburgh.
[111] Nelson, R., Edwards, S. and Tse, B. (2007). Prophylactic nasogastric decompression after abdominal surgery, *Cochrane Database Syst Rev*, CD004929.
[112] Pessaux, P., Regimbeau, J.M., Dondero, F. *et al.* (2007). Randomized clinical trial evaluating the need for routine nasogastric decompression after elective hepatic resection, *Br J Surg*, **94**, 297–303.
[113] Goueffic, Y., Rozec, B., Sonnard, A. *et al.* (2005). Evidence for early nasogastric tube removal after infrarenal aortic surgery: a randomized trial, *J Vasc Surg*, **42**, 654–659.
[114] Jung, B., Pahlman, L., Nystrom, P.O. *et al.* (2007). Multicentre randomized clinical trial of mechanical bowel preparation in elective colonic resection, *Br J Surg*, **94**, 689–695.
[115] Basse, L., Jakobsen, D.H., Bardram, L. *et al.* (2005). Functional recovery after open versus laparoscopic colonic resection: a randomized, blinded study, *Ann Surg*, **241**, 416–423.
[116] Ogonda, L., Wilson, R., Archbold, P. *et al.* (2005). A minimal-incision technique in total hip arthroplasty does not improve early postoperative outcomes. A prospective, randomized, controlled trial, *J Bone Joint Surg Am*, **87**, 701–710.
[117] Kehlet, H. and Wilmore, D.W. (2008). Evidence-based surgical care and the evolution of fast-track surgery, *Ann Surg*, **248**, 189–198.
[118] Wind, J., Polle, S.W., Fung Kon Jin, P.H. *et al.* (2006). Systematic review of enhanced recovery programmes in colonic surgery, *Br J Surg*, **93**, 800–809.

15

Post-Operative Intensive Care

Umeer Waheed and Mark G. A. Palazzo

15.1 Introduction

For many intensive care units (ICUs) the immediate management of patients following complex surgery accounts for the majority of their workload. Increasingly, patients, surgeons and their relatives expect a high-quality service following interventions, while critical care specialists recognise that even simple procedures in the progressively aging and debilitated population carry a higher risk of early morbidity and mortality. It has taken some time to recognise these risks, which seem to have coincided with some adverse changes in medical and nursing working patterns and the breakdown of traditional ward operational structures. Indeed it has been such changes which have provoked the development of outreach teams and medical alert systems to provide safety nets for patients who prove to be too sick for the location within which they are being cared for.

Post-operative admission to a critical care unit should ensure adequate monitoring for potential complications. Complications in the first 24 hours are often related to a surgical problem but their manifestations are usually heralded by disturbances in vital function revealed by hypovolaemia, hypotension, tachyarrhythmias, tachypneoa and the consequences of a fall in cardiac output such as oliguria and metabolic acidosis. Late complications are more often related to the intrinsic ability of a patient to withstand a normal surgical insult or iatrogenicity. Delayed management of complications can readily lead to organ dysfunction and local problems such as wound infection, wound dehiscence or even anastomotic breakdown if viability was marginal.

Admission to ICU for appropriate supportive management and discharge to step down wards capable of continuing the care of at-risk patients maximises the chance of good outcome [1].

The majority of deaths related to surgery are at least three days into the post-operative period. Some have extended the logic of ICU admission practice and suggest that those patients at most risk post-operatively should be admitted pre-operatively and 'optimised' to reduce risk of mortality. After several years of exploring the haemodynamic profiles of survivors of surgery, Shoemaker showed in a prospective randomised controlled study that patients that were pre-optimised to supra-normal cardiac indices with fluids and inotropes (goal-directed therapy) gained a major benefit in terms of morbidity and mortality [2]. This work was supported by subsequent studies [3]. However the wisdom of such an approach for the elderly and frail was challenged by studies which applied the same approach to a mixed ICU population and noted no benefit and even suggested an adverse effect [4,5].

More recent studies, however, continue to suggest that early haemodynamic support for emergency patients and in the pre-operative period for elective surgical patients is beneficial [6,7]. However, the York study [7] received some criticism because it revealed an unexpectedly high mortality in control patients and therefore exaggerated the benefit of pre-optimisation. Consequently, the question remains: given sufficient resources, would high risk patients benefit from pre-operative admission to critical care units? In reality, awareness amongst anaesthetists of the influence of haemodynamic volume status on outcome has gone a long way towards resolving this problem and has reduced the need for such an approach.

Effective patient management in the post-operative period requires an understanding of the normal physiological response to uncomplicated surgery, anticipation of potential problems related to specific interventions and vigilance for perturbations likely to arise from patient comorbidity.

15.2 Stress Response to Surgery

The normal response to surgery or injury is a systemic reaction or 'stress response' which results in significantly upregulated neuroendocrine and immune–haematological activity. The response classically has two phases; the acute ebb or shock phase and the flow phase. The shock phase is transient and characterised by a hypodynamic and hypometabolic state. The opposite is true of the flow phase which results in a hyperdynamic state and may last for several days or longer depending on the type and duration of surgical insult. The flow phase is typified by an increase in metabolic rate, enzyme modulation, reconstitution of blood volume and stimulation of the immune system (Table 15.1).

15.2.1 *Neuro-endocrine response*

This is characterised by increased secretion of pituitary hormones and activation of the sympathetic nervous system [8].

The initial physiological response following injury is directed towards mechanisms which lead to avid retention of salt and water in order to maintain circulating volume and cardiovascular homeostasis, compensating for cytokine mediated capillary fluid sequestration.

In addition the hormonal changes facilitate mobilisation of substrates via catabolism, which make energy sources available for the repair process.

15.2.2 *Sympathoadrenal response*

Activation of the sympathetic autonomic nervous system results in increased secretion of catecholamines from the adrenal medulla and release of noradrenaline from presynaptic nerve terminals. The plasma levels increase immediately after injury and peak between 24 and 48 hours

Table 15.1. Systemic response to surgery.

- Sympathetic nervous system activation
- Endocrine 'stress response'
  - Pituitary hormone secretion
  - Insulin resistance
- Immunological, haematological changes
  - Cytokine production
  - Acute phase reaction
  - Neutrophil leucocytosis
  - Lymphocyte proliferation

Table 15.2. Hormonal response to surgery.

Endocrine gland	Hormones	Change
Anterior pituitary	Adrenocorticotropic hormone	Increases
	Growth hormone	Increases
	Thyroid-stimulating hormone	Increases/decreases
	Follicle-stimulating hormone and luteinising hormone	Increases/decreases
Posterior pituitary	Arginine vasopressin	Increases
Adrenal cortex	Cortisol	Increases
	Aldosterone	Increases
Pancreas	Insulin	Decreases
	Glucagon	Increases
Thyroid	Thyroxine	Decreases
	Triiodothyronine	Decreases

later, depending upon the severity of the insult. This leads to tachycardia, hypertension and the modification of function of several visceral organs, including the liver, pancreas and kidney.

15.2.3 *Hypothalamic–pituitary–adrenal axis*

The stress response is typically associated with increased hypothalamic–pituitary–adrenal activity (Table 15.2). Adrenocorticotrophic hormone (ACTH), growth hormone (GH) and prolactin are secreted in increased amounts from the anterior pituitary, however, concentrations of the other anterior pituitary hormones do not change markedly.

ACTH is a peptide produced from pro-opiomelanocortin, stimulating the adrenal cortical secretion of glucocorticoids and hence increasing the level of cortisol. Cortisol secretion increases rapidly following a surgical insult. Baseline values around 350–400 nmol/l can rise to more than 1500 nmol/l within six hours. The metabolic effects are complex and involve carbohydrate, fat and protein changes which are directed to overcome the stressful state. Like GH, ACTH facilitates increased concentrations of plasma glucose by inhibiting cell usage and promoting gluconeogenesis. It promotes protein breakdown and lipolysis, which increases the production of gluconeogenic precursors. Cortisol also has significant anti-inflammatory effects, it does this by inhibiting the accumulation of macrophages and neutrophils into areas of inflammation and interfering with inflammatory mediators.

GH is a protein of 131 amino acids, its secretion increases in response to surgery and is related to the severity of the injury. GH actions are mediated through secondary messengers, namely insulin-like growth factors (IGFs). During the stress response GH stimulates protein synthesis (unlike cortisol) and inhibits protein breakdown, promotes lipolysis and glycogenolysis and has an anti-insulin effect by inhibiting glucose uptake and usage by cells.

The net effect of the neuro-endocrine response is an increased secretion of catabolic hormones, hence providing food substrates from the breakdown of carbohydrate, fat and protein.

A number of hormonal changes occur which influence sodium chloride and water metabolism, and support the preservation of body fluid volumes.

Arginine vasopressin promotes water retention and the production of concentrated urine by direct action on the kidney. Depending on the injury or development of complications, vasopressin release may continue for up to five days. As a result of sympathetic efferent stimulation, renin is released from the juxtaglomerular cells of the kidney resulting in the production of angiotensin II. This, in addition to ACTH, stimulates the release of aldosterone, which in turn leads to sodium and water reabsorption from the distal tubules of the kidney.

The stresses listed in the table above are well tolerated by normal healthy individuals but those admitted to the ICU usually have significant comorbidities and the associated stresses could well lead to life-threatening complications.

There has been considerable interest in methods to modify the stress response with the aim of improving surgical outcome, particularly amongst patients with significant comorbidities. Modification may begin pre-operatively with simple measures e.g. alleviation of anxiety premedication. Intra-operative considerations aimed at modifying stress response include the type of general anaesthetic [9], type and quantity of fluid administration [10] and analgesia [11]. Many measures have been shown to have positive effects upon the stress response and the achievement of homeostasis.

15.3 Analgesia and Sedation

Critically ill patients requiring mechanical ventilation are frequently managed with sedatives and analgesics. One question often arising is whether sedation in ICUs is used only to allow tolerance of an endotracheal tube. In the main the answer is yes; however, reducing discomfort, distress and, more importantly, anxiety also help attenuate the stress response. Protocols and practices vary widely, which may have much to do with institutional bias but also because sedation requirements vary from patient to patient. While many post-operative patients do not require ventilation and hence sedation, all patients require adequate analgesia.

Pain following surgery is common in intensive care in spite of seemingly appropriate analgesic dosing. Preventing pain is more effective than treating established pain. In 1990, the Royal College of Surgeons (England) report 'Pain after Surgery' found that up to 70% of patients suffered moderate or severe pain after surgery [12]. Analgesics should be administered on a continuous or scheduled intermittent basis, with supplemental bolus doses given as required [13].

Failure to manage pain adequately often leads to excessive administration of sedative agents and hence their adverse effects.

What are the factors affecting post-operative pain?

- Surgical procedure:
  - Incision — muscle splitting or cutting.
  - Size of the wound — amount of tissue damage.
  - Operative technique — open/laparoscopic, type of stitch (tension sutures are worse).
  - Wound retraction.
  - Oedema in a confined space (shoulder/knee replacement).
- Therapeutic devices:
  - Chest/abdominal drains.
  - Intravenous lines.
  - Orthopaedic traction devices (external fixators).

- Patient factors:
  - Age, sex, emotional state, cognitive processes.
  - Cultural attitude to/experience of illness and pain.
  - Nausea, insomnia and environmental factors (noise).

The undesired effects of inadequate analgesia with respect to the stress response include tachycardia, increased myocardial oxygen consumption, hypercoagulability and immunosuppression. Inadequate analgesia is often accompanied by disorientation, agitation and exhaustion. Effective analgesia promotes patient cooperation with physiotherapy aimed at reducing lung atelectasis and earlier mobilisation [14].

There are also potential organisational benefits from effective pain management, which facilitates early discharge and reduce the length of stay [15].

A pain management plan and goals should be established for each patient and re-evaluated as the clinical condition changes.

What are the reasons for pain management failure? Suboptimal use of conventional drugs is the commonest cause of failure of analgesia [16]. Other factors which adversely influence pain management include:

- Staff factors:
  - Staff difficulties with pain assessment.
  - Staffs fear of complications from potent analgesics.
  - Concern that analgesics might obscure a diagnosis.
  - Occurrence of an adverse effect.
  - Fear of patient drug addiction.
- Patient factors:
  - *De novo* expectations and pain threshold differences.
  - Prior experiences of illness, treatment and pain.
  - Variance in emotional response can confound assessment.
  - Cognitive processes.

In normal circumstances, assessment of pain relies heavily on the reports of subjective patients. However, critically ill patients are often unable to communicate their level of pain due to the effects of sedation or type of surgery incurred. Behavioural and physiological indicators have been advocated (Table 15.3).

Table 15.3. Behavioural and physiological indicators of pain.

Verbal report		
Numerical rating scale (NRS)/Verbal rating scale (VRS)		
Pain-related behaviours		
Movements	**Facial indicators**	**Posture**
None	Grimacing	Rigid
Slow/decreased	Frowning	
Restlessness	Tears	**Splinting**
Attention seeking	Wrinkling of forehead	Tense
Vocalisation		
Physiological Indicators		
Hypertension/hypotension		
Tachypnoea/hypoventilation		
Perspiration		
Palor		

Pain therapy can be divided into non-pharmacological and pharmacological methods.

Non-pharmacological methods include:

- Attention to positioning.
- Stabilisation of fractures.
- Reducing irritating stimuli:
  - Tracheal tubes/urinary catheters.
  - Environmental factors:
    - Appropriate lighting.
    - Unpleasant auditory stimuli.
    - Supportive staff, explanations, high bedside presence.

Pharmacological methods include an array of agents. Certain drug attributes are desirable especially in the post-operative patient. These include: rapid onset and offset with ease of titration (short context-sensitive half-life), metabolism within the circulation, with the absence of active metabolites or accumulation and excretion independent of renal/biliary systems. The ideal drug should have minimal pharmacodynamic effects on organ systems, particularly respiratory, cardiovascular and gastrointestinal.

In the initial post-operative period, analgesics are best given intravenously, which guarantees 100% bioavailability. Enteral administration is limited when patients are strictly nil-by-mouth, have gastric stasis or suffer with nausea and vomiting. Even if the gastrointestinal tract is stable, drug bioavailability can be variable, often depending on factors such as gastric pH which may have been modified by other drugs. Intramuscular analgesic administration is contraindicated in patients receiving anticoagulants or those who are haemodynamically unstable. The latter have erratic perfusion states which can result in variable plasma concentrations.

Analgesic administration by intravenous infusion is common practice; however, it is important to give a loading dose at the outset otherwise steady-state levels are only reached after approximately four half-lives when an infusion is used alone. In certain groups (e.g. the noncritically ill), patient-controlled analgesia (PCA) has been shown to result in stable drug concentrations, less sedation, less opioid consumption and hence reduced adverse effects (respiratory depression) in comparison to standard therapy [15]. However the equipment for PCA is expensive and the patient needs to be shown what to do and be emotionally and physically able to use the device. Transdermal patches in most post-operative ICU settings are not used frequently. They provide unreliable drug delivery due to post-operative tissue oedema, temperature and perfusion changes.

Epidural analgesia is commonly provided as part of the anaesthetic technique and is continued in the critical care unit for post-operative pain management. Insertion of epidural catheters in the post-operative period in the critical care unit is less well described.

Combinations of opioids and local anaesthetics act synergistically to produce improved analgesia with fewer side effects [17]. Epidurals potentially allow for early mobilisation and better patient cooperation with staff. There is evidence to suggest that epidural analgesia is associated with improved respiratory, renal and myocardial function, reduced incidence of embolic events and patient mortality [18]. The association between neural blockade and inhibition of the stress response has been well described in literature. Evidence suggests that neural blockade leads to improvements in physiological variables in a number of organs [19].

Although the analgesia provided by effectively working epidurals is superior to many other forms of analgesia, the effects of high-thoracic epidurals on the cardiovascular system can be problematic. Epidurals inserted with blocks above thoracic vertebra T4 have significant hypotensive effects often resistant to fluid administration and might require inotropes to maintain adequate mean arterial pressures. This could, and indeed does, delay discharge from ICU if adequate analgesia by this method is imperative. Occasionally epidurals may be so effective that important adverse events, e.g. haematomas and neural compression, may not be recognised in a timely manner [20].

15.3.1 *Analgesia and sedation available in the ICU*

Although comparative trials have not been performed in the critical care setting, opioids are considered the initial analgesic of choice. The type of opioid used depends largely upon the patient, type of surgery, expected course of recovery, drug pharmacology and adverse effects. Some of the commonly used opioids are listed in Table 15.4.

Desirable attributes of an opioid include rapid onset, ease of titration, lack of accumulation of the parent drug or its metabolites and low cost. Fentanyl has a rapid onset with a short duration, but repeated dosing leads to accumulation and prolonged effects. Morphine has a longer duration of action and may even be given intermittently, but is associated with hypotension and has potent active metabolites (morphine 6 glucuronide, morphine 3 glucuronide) which may prolong its effects in the presence of renal failure.

Renal and hepatic insufficiency alters opioid and metabolite elimination, therefore titration to the desired response and assessment of the drugs' prolonged effects are required. The elderly population may have reduced opioid requirements [21].

Adverse effects occur frequently and are commonly associated with respiratory, cardiovascular, gastrointestinal and neurological systems. Respiratory depression, though often a positive effect (for tube tolerance) can cause concern in patients breathing spontaneously or for those depending on self-initiated non-invasive ventilation. Hypotension may occur in haemodynamically unstable patients or those with elevated sympathetic tone [22]. Opioid-induced hypotension in normovolaemic patients is a result of sympatholysis, bradycardia and histamine release.

Table 15.4. Opioids used in the ICU.

Agent	Metabolism	Excretion	Active metabolites	Clinical Importance
Morphine	Glucuronidation Up to 80% first pass metabolism	Renal 90% Faeces 10%	Morphine 3 glucuronide Morphine 6 glucuronide (M-6-G)	Parent drug not removed by dialysis. Drug is 20 times more potent than parent drug
Fentanyl	Hydroxylation N-dealkylation	Renal 10%	None	Not removed by dialysis; drug accumulates
Alfentanil	N-dealkylation Glucuronidation	Renal 90%	None	Not removed by dialysis
Remifentanil	Ester hydrolysis	Not available	Carboxylic acid	Metabolite 300–1000 times less potent
Pethidine	N-demethylation Hydrolysis	Renal 1–25%	Norpethidine	Metabolite has 50% potency of parent. Proconvulsant in renal failure

Gastric retention and ileus is common in the post-operative phase and is exacerbated by opioid use [23]. Opioids can exaggerate depression of consciousness and hallucinations and increase agitation.

There has been much interest in remifentanil, which was initially used as an adjunct to anaesthesia and sedation. It benefits from a short duration of action regardless of the duration of infusion (short context-sensitive half-life). It is safe and easy to administer with minimal changes in intracranial and cerebral perfusion pressure. Its cardiovascular effects are minimal (bradycardia has been noted on initiation of infusion) and it is unaffected by hepatic or renal failure due to its metabolism in plasma from serum esterases. In many neurosurgical critical care units it has become the agent of choice. Of all the opioids mentioned, remifentanil is the nearest to the ideal agent and may reduce the requirement of extra sedative agents [24].

Non-steroidal anti-inflammatory drugs (NSAIDs), though commonly used outside the ICU setting, are used sparingly in ICU due to their adverse effects. These include gastrointestinal bleeding secondary to mucosal ulceration and platelet inhibition, bronchoconstriction and the potential for provoking glomerular vasoconstriction and acute renal failure. Risk factors for acute renal failure associated with NSAIDs include: age, hypotension, hypovolaemia, chronic renal and liver failure, hypertension with vascular disease and diabetes, conditions which are common in ICU [25].

Paracetamol (acetaminophen), a non-narcotic analgesic and antipyretic, is used to manage mild-to-moderate pain and unlike the NSAIDs has no anti-inflammatory effects. Its use is associated with few adverse effects, although post-administration hypotension has been noted [26]. As a sole agent paracetamol lacks potency, though in combination with opioids it works synergistically and has been shown to be opioid-sparing. The recent development of an intravenous formulation has reduced the need for enteral and *per rectum* use and the associated variable bioavailabilities with these routes. Care must be taken to avoid excessive and potentially hepatotoxic doses, as patients with depleted glutathione stores are more susceptible and should be maintained on reduced doses [27].

Clonidine and dexmedetomidine, both alpha-2 agonists, have been used as adjuncts to traditional agents of sedation and analgesia. They augment the effects of opioids and are used to treat withdrawal syndromes. Their role in the immediate post-operative phase is yet to be determined.

Dexmedetomidine is a highly selective alpha-2 agonist with a receptor affinity eight times that of clonidine. In addition to its analgesic effects it has potent sedative and anxiolytic effects similar to benzodiazepines and is used as the sole agent for sedation and analgesia in many centres across North America. Rapid administration is associated with a biphasic cardiovascular response, initial hypertension followed by a more sustained hypotension.

The indications for sedative agents are not well defined. Sedatives are common adjuncts for the treatment of anxiety and agitation. Agitation is common, occurring at least once in 71% of patients in a medical-surgical unit [28]. Agitation has deleterious effects and can contribute to ventilator dysynchrony, increased oxygen consumption and unintentional removal of drains and catheters. Sedatives have been shown to modify the stress response, and to facilitate physiological and metabolic stabilisation of patients [29]. An analgesic should be the initial line of therapy when pain is the suspected cause of agitation; however, despite having sedative effects many analgesics do not diminish awareness nor provide amnesia from stressful events.

The choice of agent used for sedation depends upon a number of factors, including patient age, comorbidities, presence of hepatic/renal failure, type of surgery and expected duration of stay in the ICU. Table 15.5 shows commonly used sedations and their properties.

Table 15.5. Commonly used sedation agents.

Agent	Speed of onset	Half-life	Metabolism	Active metabolites	Clinical importance
Diazepam	2–5 minutes	20–120 hours	Demethylation Hydroxylation	Yes	Phlebitis
Lorazepam	5–20 minutes	8–15 hours	Glucuronidation	None	Solvent related acidosis/renal failure in high doses
Midazolam	2–5 minutes	3–11 hours	Oxidation	Yes	Prolonged sedation in renal failure
Propofol	1–2 minutes	26–32 hours	Oxidation	None	Triglyceridaemia

Acute agitation has a number of causes, including pain, and, while a short-acting opioid may provide relief, immediate sedation and comfort, there have not been any controlled trials comparing opioids with other sedatives in the post-operative setting. Commonly, agitation is managed with the benzodiazapine midazolam, which has a rapid onset. An alternative is the anaesthetic-induction agent propofol; however, both are associated with hypotension. Hypotension due to propofol, particularly on initiation of an infusion or a bolus, sometimes results in support with inotropes.

Numerous comparisons have been made between agents, focussing on measures which include speed of onset, ability to maintain a target level of sedation, adverse effects and the time required to awakening.

The majority of trials for short-term duration (<24 hours) of sedation have compared midazolam with propofol. Awakening times for patients on propofol ranged from 1 to 105 minutes compared with 1 to 405 minutes for patients on midazolam infusions. Times to extubation following <24 hours infusion were found to be similar [30].

With longer infusion (1–3 days) patients receiving propofol were shown to have more predictable awakening times when the agent was compared with midazolam; however, the difference was not statistically significant and there was no difference in time to ICU discharge [31]. A three-way comparison of midazolam, propofol and lorazepam in surgical ICU patients found lorazepam to be the preferred agent of choice in this population [32]. These three agents provided similar levels of sedation, achieved adequate sedation in similar times and needed a similar number of dose adjustments. However midazolam was shown to produce adequate sedation for a greater percentage of time, while propofol was associated with undersedation and lorazepam with oversedation. Equivalent doses of opioids were provided in these patients.

For patients needing intubation for longer than 72 hours due to specific surgical procedures, repeat procedures or complications (e.g. sepsis or systemic inflammatory response syndrome (SIRS)), studies have shown that propofol consistently produced more rapid awakening than midazolam. Patients receiving propofol were extubated in 0.24–4 hours compared with midazolam where time to extubation was up to 49 hours [31]. When lorazepam and midazolam were compared, both showed similar times to awakening and extubation although lorazepam appeared to be more predictable.

Recommendations from the American College of Critical Care Medicine [33] suggest:

(i) Midazolam should be used for rapid sedation of acutely agitated patients.
(ii) Propofol is the preferred sedative when rapid awakening is important.
(iii) Midazolam is recommended for short-term use only, as it is associated with unpredictable awakening and time to extubations with infusions longer than 72 hours.
(iv) Lorazepam is recommended for the sedation of most patients via intermittent or continuous infusion.
(v) The use of sedation guidelines/algorithms is recommended in all clinical settings.

Time to extubation, as seen previously, varies from one agent to another and clearly depends upon the duration of infusion. In practice, clinicians become familiar with a small range of drugs and manage to tailor these sometimes quite imperfect agents to provide the desired waking up time without detriment to patient discharge times. In the critically ill, consciousness does not equate to readiness for extubation. Furthermore, extubation does not equate with readiness for discharge from critical care. Consequently, apparent pharmacodynamic gains based on pharmacokinetics are not always realised, so the choice of agents does not necessarily need to follow logic.

15.4 Post-Operative Respiratory Management

The goal of post-operative respiratory management is to achieve timely extubation and consequently avoid the common problems of atelectasis and nosocomial pneumonia while ensuring the conditions for self-ventilation. For the majority this can be achieved by techniques which facilitate deep breathing and provide adequate pain control. Patients who are elderly, have chronic underlying pulmonary disease, smoke or are obese are at risk of post-operative pulmonary complications and weaning problems [34].

The timing of extubation is guided by a combination of rules regarding blood gases, consciousness and measures of ventilatory effort and a clinician's experience. An optimal reintubation rate should be zero, but it has been postulated that when in the region of 5–10% a balance is achieved between failed extubation rate and undue cautiousness which would lead to delayed appropriate extubations [35].

Delays in extubation have been associated with increased complication rates, including ventilator-associated pneumonia, airway trauma, increased hospital costs and mortality. Assessment of the appropriate time for extubation is based on the patients' overall condition i.e. whether they are improving from their surgery, evidence of haemodynamic stability, adequacy of gas exchange and neurological status. Objective ventilation parameters include partial pressure of oxygen in arterial blood (PaO_2): fraction of inspired oxygen (FiO_2) ratio, level of positive end-expiratory pressure (PEEP), FiO_2 and acid–base status.

Although it might seem reasonable to use such parameters, individuals vary significantly in their ability to wean and become extubated. Table 15.6 lists many of the extubation parameters used today. Studies have shown that, despite relatively high sensitivity (78–100%), these parameters were plagued with low specificity and in many cases are so conservative as to contribute to prevention of extubation in patients who were otherwise able to breathe independently [36].

There is evidence to suggest that spontaneous breathing trials (SBT) have a role in successful extubation; however, controversy lies with the

Table 15.6. Extubation parameters.

Parameter	**Desired value**
Respiratory rate	Less than 30 breaths per minute
Tidal volume	4–6 ml/kg
Minute ventilation	10–15 l/min
Max inspiratory pressure	−15 to −30 cm H_2O
Rapid shallow breathing index	60–105
Rapid shallow breathing index rate	<20%
CROP (compliance, rate, oxygenation, pressure) score	13

type of SBT [37]. Whether continuous positive airway pressure (CPAP) of 5 cm H_2O versus T piece for one hour, or T piece versus a CPAP of 7 cm H_2O or SBT of 30 minutes versus 120 minutes, is more beneficial is yet to be proven; however, all methods have their advocates.

It has been suggested that the optimal way of interpreting SBT is to combine objective with subjective indicators of intolerance or failure of SBT. These indicators would include parameters of inadequate gas exchange, increased work of breathing, haemodynamic instability and altered mental state. The rapid shallow breathing index (RSBI) rate or change of RSBI (respiratory rate/tidal volume) over time has been recently shown to be more predictive. The rate is calculated as follows:

$$\text{RSBI Rate} = [(\text{RSBI } 2 - \text{RSBI } 1)/\text{RSBI } 1] \times 100, \qquad (15.1)$$

where RSBI 1 = initial value at time 0 and RSBI 2 = a specified time, e.g. 30, 60, 120 min.

An RSBI rate of less than 20% has been shown to be 90% sensitive and 100% specific for predicting success.

Reintubation, which when it occurs does so in the first 72 hours for 25% of patients, is a relevant consequence of respiratory failure after extubation. Common reasons for failure include absence of a patent airway, inability to consistently protect the airway, inability to clear secretions, poor cough, altered mental state, apnoea, severe pain and cardiovascular instability. Reintubation is a risk factor for nosocomial pneumonia, mortality and increased hospital stay as well as a marker for increased severity of illness.

Non-invasive ventilation is used by many clinicians to bridge a period after extubation and normal independent ventilation among patients who would otherwise become reintubated. However, there remains controversy; some evidence suggests that outcome [38] and reintubation rate is not improved by the use of non-invasive methods post failed extubation. These observations are confounded by evidence that suggests that non-invasive ventilation should be used immediately post extubation and not brought in at the last minute when ventilation has already failed [39]. Patients with known chronic obstructive airways disease have been shown to benefit from non-invasive ventilation [38].

15.5 Sepsis and the Systemic Inflammatory Response Syndrome

The development of sepsis or SIRS is another condition which may prevent early discharge of the post-operative patient from the ICU. Confusion between the two conditions is common, and physicians often diagnose sepsis or a septic state when there is only an inflammatory response present. The main difference is the presence or absence of an infectious agent (Table 15.7).

Infection and sepsis cause a significant morbidity and mortality on critical care units. The number of patients who develop an episode of sepsis is high: 40–60% depending on the ICU. It is the leading cause of multiple organ failure, with prognosis deteriorating with age, unresolved hyperlactataemia, leucopoenia, low systemic vascular resistance and increasing number of organ failures. Mortality due to septic shock lies between 40% and 60% [40].

The body has two defence mechanisms against infection: the innate system and adaptive immune system. The innate system comprises phagocytes (macrophages, neutrophils and dendritic cells), mast cells, basophils, eosinophils and natural killer cells. It defends the body by reacting in a non-specific manner to foreign material that enters the body and also activates the adaptive immune system via T and B lymphocytes. The adaptive

Table 15.7. Inflammation/sepsis.

Infection	Invasion of sterile host tissue by microorganisms
Bacteraemia	Viable bacteria in the blood
SIRS	Inflammatory response to infective/non infective conditions; more than two out of four criteria: Temperature >38 or <36 Heart rate >90 beats/min Respiratory rate >20/min or partial pressure of arterial CO_2 ($PaCO_2$) <4.3kPa White cell count >12000 or <4000 cells/mm^3
Sepsis	SIRS due to infection
Septic shock	Sepsis with features of shock: Hypotension Inadequate organ perfusion

immune response is more specific — it recognises specific pathogens and generates immunity to them by antibodies. The two mechanisms effectively combat moderate infections. Three processes are involved in sepsis:

(i) Recognition of microbial material as a foreign body.
(ii) Release of inflammatory mediators causing vasodilatation and attracting neutrophils.
(iii) Leucocytes and other cells lyse and destroy foreign material eliminating the infectious challenge.

If these processes are overwhelmed, or the organism is particularly virulent or treatment is inadequate, persistent inflammation and sepsis occur.

Sepsis and septic shock are due to cytokine-mediated hyperpermeability, fluid sequestration, abnormal microcirculatory flow, intravascular coagulopathy and ultimately poor organ perfusion leading to dysfunction. The vascular abnormality is characterised by vasodilatation and vascular hyporeactivity which are the result of excess nitric oxide production, activation of potassium channels and low circulating levels of endogenous vasopressin.

In septic shock peripheral vascular impairment is often associated with a modest degree of myocardial depression, which may contribute to hypotension unresponsive to fluid therapy. The potential sources of infection in post-operative patients may or may not be directly related to a complication of surgery e.g. the breakdown of anastomosis or abscess formation post laparotomy.

Management is geared towards identifying and treating the provoking cause of sepsis. Investigations should include both general (C-reactive protein, white cell count and differential, procalcitonin, coagulation profile, cultures of blood sputum urine and pus (prior to starting antibiotics)) and arterial blood gases. More specific investigations, such as X-rays, ultrasound, computed tomography scan and drain-fluid analysis, will depend upon the type of surgery undertaken.

Antibiotic therapy is initially empirical whilst awaiting the results of microbiology cultures to guide therapy. Initial antibiotic therapy is based on an assessment of the most likely causative organism, which, in turn, is influenced by the location of surgery, duration of hospital stay, previous antibiotic administration, resistance patterns of likely organisms in the hospital/unit, and the likelihood of nosocomial infection acquired by horizontal microbial spread from patients in the unit. The factors which increase the risk of nosocomial infections include increasing age, male sex, prolonged post-operative mechanical ventilation, drugs that alter immunocompetence and failure to adhere to infection-control guidelines [41].

Management of sepsis is both specific, which is directed to the causative condition, and usually treated with antibiotics or corrective surgery, and supportive. Supportive management such as fluids, inotropes, ventilation and dialysis are directed to maintaining organ function while buying time for specific therapy.

In early septic shock, widespread vasodilation and fluid sequestration, which are the sequelae of cytokine-mediated inflammatory activity, cause relative hypovolaemia, and hypotension. Furthermore these changes are confounded by microthrombosis and result in global and local redistribution of blood flow, which aims to protect vital organ function at the expense of gut and peripheral perfusion. Adequate fluid administration in the early stages can correct relative hypovolaemia and hypotension and maintain organ perfusion. Left untreated, organ perfusion also becomes compromised.

When treated appropriately peripherally cool patients with sluggish capillary return become warm and dilated. However, early and over-treatment with vasoconstrictors may never allow patients to reach this phase. As the condition progresses, toxic myocarditis impairs myocardial function, reducing cardiac output and response to fluid administration. Excessive fluid administration may cause an increase in the interstitial fluid space leading to oedema, initially in the subcutaneous tissue affecting wound healing and surgical anastomosis and later, if excessive, in the pulmonary interstitium. Note that other than the brain the lungs are the most protected of organs against oedema and peripheral oedema does not necessarily equate with oedema in the lung; the reasons for this have been described as 'Guyton safety factors' [42].

Once fluid administration is deemed sufficient, flow rate at appropriate pressure can be improved by the addition of an inotrope. Numerous studies have compared different inotropes [43], but ultimately whether it is dopamine, dobutamine, adrenaline or noradrenaline or any combination, the important element of this supportive treatment is to provide an adequate cardiac output, which is judged by organ perfusion and function and maintenance of normal acid–base chemistry. The latter, when assessed with mixed venous oxygen saturations and lactate:pyruvate ratios, remain the best surrogates for adequate cellular oxygenation and presumably cellular function.

Better than treatment of sepsis is its prevention. For many patients prevention will be facilitated by clear and precise infection-control protocols, efficient microbiological monitoring, policing of antibiotic usage and, if these fail, benefit is associated with prompt appropriate management.

The management of the post-operative surgical patient in the intensive care setting is both challenging and rewarding. A good understanding of the surgical procedure is vital to appreciate the interactions of the insult with the patient's comorbidities and changes in physiology. Awareness of potential complications and prompt intervention can significantly influence patient morbidity and mortality and use of hospital resources. A good relationship with the primary surgeon is indispensable in achieving this.

15.6 Clinical Case

A 65-year-old retired Caucasian banker was admitted to the ICU following a Whipple's procedure. He had an average daily alcohol intake of three to four units; otherwise he was a non-smoker in good general health. He had no past history of jaundice or abdominal pain but did describe one episode of pyrexia coinciding with a transient period of passing dark urine. The relevant pre-operative laboratory data were: white blood cell count, 8900/mm^3; haemoglobin, 14.2 g/dl; normal clotting screen, C-reactive protein (CRP), <2; total bilirubin, 13 mmol/l; alanine transferase, 197; alkaline phosphatase, 254 IU/l; gamma-glutamyltranspeptidase, 926 IU/l; serum amylase, 65 IU/l; and alpha-fetoprotein, 9 IU/l. Viral hepatitis A, B and C serology was negative. The operation, which lasted seven hours, included a pancreaticogastrostomy, gastrojejunostomy, and choledochojejonostomy reconstruction.

On admission to critical care, the patient was intubated and sedated on propofol and had a blood pressure of 85/40 with heart rate of 115 beats/min. Blood gases revealed a mild metabolic acidosis, pH 7.25, base excess −6, blood lactate 4.1mmol/l and a PaO_2 11 kPa (at 34.5°C) on FiO_2 0.4.

An epidural inserted at thoracic vertebra T7 was running a bupivicaine/fentanyl infusion.

On examination, the patient had cool peripheries with delayed capillary return (five seconds), auscultation of chest and heart were normal. The abdomen was soft with a midline scar and three abdominal drains, each placed in proximity to an anastomosis.

Initial management involved fluid resuscitation with crystalloid at 2 ml/kg/h and further boluses were given based upon urine output target (1–2 ml/kg/h), acid–base status, and superior vena cava venous oxygen saturations (SVO_2) (>70%). The patient was warmed and routine blood samples were taken, all of which were unremarkable, including the coagulation profile. After four hours the patient's temperature had risen to 36 °C and 2 litres of crystalloid/colloid had been infused (maintenance plus fluid boluses). An infusion of noradrenaline was started to reverse the hypotensive effects of the thoracic epidural and maintain adequate renal perfusion (mean arterial pressure (MAP) 70 mmHg).

The patient was extubated six hours after the procedure; he was comfortable and remained haemodynamically stable on noradrenaline (0.08 µg/kg/min). On a FiO_2 of 40% O_2 arterial saturations remained above 95% with a PO_2 of 9.5 kPa (PaO_2:FiO_2 = 23.75). A post-operative chest X-ray revealed bibasal atelectasis but was otherwise unremarkable.

Six hours later, the urine output declined (<0.5 ml/kg/h) despite a positive fluid balance of 2.5 litres and an adequate MAP. The central venous pressure (CVP) was elevated at 19 mmHg, and inspired oxygen requirements increased to 60% in order to keep the PaO_2 above 8.0 kPa (PaO_2/FiO2 = 13.3). CPAP was started to improve oxygenation.

At 24 hours after the procedure, the patient remained oliguric and CPAP-dependant with increasing cardiovascular support (noradrenaline increased from 0.08 to 0.2 µg/kg/min). Arterial blood gases deteriorated with pH 7.27, bicarbonate 22 mmo/l and lactate 6 mmol/l.

The patient became agitated and less tolerant of CPAP, necessitating reintubation. A full blood count revealed a leucocytosis of 19,000/mm^3 and an elevated CRP of 325. Repeat chest X-ray showed further bibasal collapse with small bilateral effusions and interstitial fluid. On examination, he remained peripherally cool and tachycardic at 120 beats per minute. Widespread crepitations were heard throughout both lung fields. The abdomen remained soft with absent bowel sounds. Of the three drains, the pancreatogastrostomy anastomotic drain had produced over 800 ml. Drainage in the other two was minimal. The drain fluid was sent for an urgent amylase which returned at >5000 U/ml. Based upon this a computed tomography scan of the abdomen was performed, which revealed an anastomotic breakdown of the pancreatogastrostomy. The patient returned to theatre where the anastomosis was repaired. Following this the patient made an unremarkable recovery and was discharged to the ward five days after the initial procedure.

15.6.1 *Comment*

The most important part of managing patients in the post-operative period is to be able to differentiate between standard post-operative resuscitation and the patient that fails to respond to standard treatment in the first few hours post surgery. The latter has failed to respond to routine resuscitative measures and subsequently deteriorated. The next step is to ask why. In the majority of cases, if the patient is failing to progress or deteriorating, a complication of the surgical procedure should be suspected. Often complications do not manifest themselves immediately but may arise in subsequent post-operative days. A surgical complication may be highly suspected, as in this case, by continuance of oligoanuria despite fluid loading, worsening respiratory function and increasing circulatory support or it may be more subtle e.g. grumbling pyrexia and pain more difficult to manage than expected. Investigations should always be prompt as any delay could lead to significant morbidity or mortality.

References

[1] Curran, J.E. and Grounds, R.M. (1998). Ward versus intensive care management of high-risk surgical patients, *Br J Surg*, **85**, 956–961.

[2] Shoemaker, W.C., Appel, P.L., Kram, H.B. *et al.* (1988). Prospective trial of supranormal values of survivors as therapeutic goals in high-risk surgical patients, *Chest*, **94**, 1176–1186.

[3] Boyd, O., Grounds, R.M. and Bennett, E.D. (1993). A randomized clinical trial of the effect of deliberate perioperative increase of oxygen delivery on mortality in high-risk surgical patients, *JAMA*, **270**, 2699–2707.

[4] Gattinoni, L., Brazzi, L., Pelosi, P. *et al.* (1995). A trial of goal-oriented hemodynamic therapy in critically ill patients, *N Engl J Med*, **333**, 1025–1032.

[5] Hayes, M.A., Timmins, A.C., Yau, E.H. *et al.* (1994). Elevation of systemic oxygen delivery in the treatment of critically ill patients, *N Engl J Med*, **330**, 1717–1722.

[6] Rivers, E., Nguyen, B., Havstad, S. *et al.* (2001). Early goal-directed therapy in the treatment of severe sepsis and septic shock, *N Engl J Med*, **345**, 1368–1377.

[7] Wilson, J., Woods, I., Fawcett, J. *et al.* (1999). Reducing the risk of major elective surgery: randomised controlled trial of preoperative optimisation of oxygen delivery, *BMJ*, **318**, 1099–1103.

[8] Desborough, J.P. and Hall, G.M. (1993). 'Endocrine response to surgery', in Kaufman, L. (ed.), *Anaestheisa Review*, volume 10, Churchill Livingstone, Edinburgh, pp. 131–148.

[9] McDonald, R.K., Evans, F.T., Weise, V.K. *et al.* (1959). Effect of morphine and nalorphine on plasma hydrocortisone levels in man, *J Pharmacol Exp Ther*, **125**, 241–247.

[10] Velickovic, I., Yan, J. and Grass, J.A. (2002). Modifying the neuroendocrine stress response, *Semin Anaesth Perio M*, **21**, 16–25.

[11] Bromage, P.R., Shibata, H.R. and Willoughby, H.W. (1971). Influence of prolonged epidural blockade on blood sugar and cortisol responses to operations upon the upper part of the abdomen and the thorax, *Surg Gynecol Obstet*, **132**, 1051–1056.

[12] The Royal College of Surgeons of England (1990). *Report of the Working Party on Pain After Surgery*, The Royal College of Surgeons of England, London.

[13] Acute Pain Management Guideline Panel (1992). *Acute Pain Management: Operative or Medical Procedures and Trauma (Clinical Practice Guideline)*, Document number AHCPR.92-0032, Agency for Health Care Policy and Research, Rockville.

[14] Epstein, J. and Breslow, M.J. (1999). The stress response of critical illness, *Crit Care Clin*, **15**, 17–33.
[15] Gust, R., Pecher, S., Gust, A. *et al.* (1999). Effect of patient-controlled analgesia on pulmonary complications after coronary artery bypass grafting, *Crit Care Med*, **27**, 2218–2223.
[16] Whipple, J.K., Lewis, K.S., Quebbeman, E.J. *et al.* (1995). Analysis of pain management in critically ill patients, *Pharmacotherapy*, **15**, 592–599.
[17] Bogra, J., Arora, N. and Srivastava, P. (2005). Synergistic effect of intrathecal fentanyl and bupivacaine in spinal anesthesia for cesarean section, *BMC Anesthesiol*, **5**, 5.
[18] Rodgers, A., Walker, N., Schug, S. *et al.* (2000). Reduction of postoperative mortality and morbidity with epidural or spinal anaesthesia: results from overview of randomised trials, *BMJ*, **321**, 1493.
[19] Norman, J.G. and Fink, G.W. (1997). The effects of epidural anesthesia on the neuroendocrine response to major surgical stress: a randomized prospective trial, *Am Surg*, **63**, 75–80.
[20] Crowe, S. (2001). Diagnosing epidural haematomas, *Anaesthesia*, **56**, 1211.
[21] Wagner, B.K. and O'Hara, D.A. (1997). Pharmacokinetics and pharmacodynamics of sedatives and analgesics in the treatment of agitated critically ill patients, *Clin Pharmacokinet*, **33**, 426–453.
[22] McArdle, P. (1999). Intravenous analgesia, *Crit Care Clin*, **15**, 89–104.
[23] Yuan, C.S., Foss, J.F., O'Connor, M. *et al.* (1998). Effects of low-dose morphine on gastric emptying in healthy volunteers, *J Clin Pharmacol*, **38**, 1017–1020.
[24] Park, G. (2002). Remifentanil in the ICU: a new approach to patient care, *Curr Anaesth Crit Care*, **16**, 313–320.
[25] Schlondorff, D. (1993). Renal complications of nonsteroidal anti-inflammatory drugs, *Kidney Int*, **44**, 643–653.
[26] Boyle, M., Hundy, S. and Torda, T.A. (1997). Paracetamol administration is associated with hypotension in the critically ill, *Aust Crit Care*, **10**, 120–122.
[27] Zimmerman, H.J. and Maddrey, W.C. (1995). Acetaminophen (paracetamol) hepatotoxicity with regular intake of alcohol: analysis of instances of therapeutic misadventure, *Hepatology*, **22**, 767–773.
[28] Fraser, G.L., Prato, B.S., Riker, R.R. *et al.* (2000). Frequency, severity, and treatment of agitation in young versus elderly patients in the ICU, *Pharmacotherapy*, **20**, 75–82.

[29] Stannard, D., Puntillo, K., Miaskowski, C. *et al.* (1996). Clinical judgment and management of postoperative pain in critical care patients, *Am J Crit Care*, **5**, 433–441.

[30] Carrasco, G., Cabre, L., Sobrepere, G. *et al.* (1998). Synergistic sedation with propofol and midazolam in intensive care patients after coronary artery bypass grafting, *Crit Care Med*, **26**, 844–851.

[31] Hall, R.I., Sandham, D., Cardinal, P. *et al.* (2001). Propofol vs midazolam for, ICU sedation: a Canadian multicenter randomized trial, *Chest*, **119**, 1151–1159.

[32] McCollam, J.S., O'Neil, M.G., Norcross, E.D. *et al.* (1999). Continuous infusions of lorazepam, midazolam, and propofol for sedation of the critically ill surgery trauma patient: a prospective, randomized comparison, *Crit Care Med*, **27**, 2454–2458.

[33] Jacobi, J., Fraser, G.L., Coursin, D.B. *et al.* (2002). Clinical practice guidelines for the sustained use of sedatives and analgesics in the critically ill adult, *Crit Care Med*, **30**, 119–141.

[34] Epstein, S.K. (2002). Decision to extubate, *Intens Care Med*, **28**, 535–546.

[35] Esteban, A., Frutos, F., Tobin, M.J. *et al.* (1995). A comparison of four methods of weaning patients from mechanical ventilation, Spanish Lung Failure Collaborative Group, *N Engl J Med*, **332**, 345–350.

[36] Goldstone, J. (2002). The pulmonary physician in critical care, 10: difficult weaning, *Thorax*, **57**, 986–991.

[37] Esteban, A., Alia, I., Gordo, F. *et al.* (1997). Extubation outcome after spontaneous breathing trials with T-tube or pressure support ventilation, The Spanish Lung Failure Collaborative Group, *Am J Respir Crit Care Med*, **156**, 459–465.

[38] Ferrer, M., Valencia, M., Nicolas, J.M. *et al.* (2006). Early noninvasive ventilation averts extubation failure in patients at risk: a randomized trial, *Am J Respir Crit Care Med*, **173**, 164–170.

[39] Jiang, J.S., Kao, S.J. and Wang, S.N. (1999). Effect of early application of biphasic positive airway pressure on the outcome of extubation in ventilator weaning, *Respirology*, **4**, 161–165.

[40] Laterre, P.F., Levy, H., Clermont, G. *et al.* (2004). Hospital mortality and resource use in subgroups of the Recombinant Human Activated Protein C Worldwide, Evaluation in Severe Sepsis (PROWESS) trial, *Crit Care Med*, **32**, 2207–2218.

[41] Tess, B.H., Glenister, H.M., Rodrigues, L.C. *et al.* (1993). Incidence of hospital-acquired infection and length of hospital stay, *Eur J Clin Microbiol Infect Dis*, **12**, 81–86.

[42] Guyton, A.C. (1991). *Textbook of Medical Physiology*, W.B. Saunders Company, Philadelphia.

[43] Lisbon, A. (2003). Dopexamine, dobutamine, and dopamine increase splanchnic blood flow: what is the evidence? *Chest*, **123** (Suppl. 5), 460S–463S.

[44] Bernard, G.R., Vincent, J.L., Laterre, P.F. *et al.* (2001). Efficacy and safety of recombinant human activated protein C for severe sepsis, *N Engl J Med*, **344**, 699–709.

16
Sepsis

Richard Stümpfle

16.1 Introduction

16.1.1 *Definition*

In 1991, the American College of Chest Physicians and the Society of Critical Care Medicine held a Consensus Conference with the aim of agreeing on the definition of sepsis. The conference defined for the first time the criteria for systemic inflammatory response syndrome (SIRS) and established the term sepsis as the development of SIRS in response to infection. Furthermore, a grading system was agreed upon whereby severe sepsis was defined as sepsis associated with organ dysfunction and septic shock as severe sepsis with hypotension refractory to fluid resuscitation [1].

SIRS criteria:

- Temperature >38°C or <36°C.
- Heart rate >90 beats per minute.
- Respiratory rate >20 breaths per minute or partial pressure of carbon dioxide (PCO_2) <4.3kPa.
- White blood cell count >12,000 or <4,000 cells/mm3.

16.1.2 *Incidence*

The incidence of sepsis has been calculated by different studies and other research and governmental bodies using a variety of methodologies and hence there is difficulty in arriving at accurate figures. Hospital discharge data from the USA collected over the last decade has shown a doubling in hospitalisations for sepsis from 326,000 to 727,000 between 2000 and 2008, translating to a calculated rate increase from 11.6 to 24.9 cases per 10,000 of the population per year [2]. Reasons for this increase are speculative but may include an increasingly aged population, advances in the treatment of chronic conditions and worsening patterns of antimicrobial resistance [3]. A study from Finland in 2006 established the prevalence of severe sepsis as 10.5% of intensive care unit (ICU) admissions, whilst a similar study from Germany the same year reported a prevalence of 11%, resulting in a calculated incidence of 3.8 and 11.6 respectively per 10,000 population annually [4,5]. The Extended Prevalence of Infection in Intensive Care (EPIC II) study was conducted in 2007 in 1,265 ICUs across 75 countries. Of the ICUs surveyed, 51% of all ICU admissions were classed as being infected on the day of the study. This study also revealed global differences in prevalence with the highest rates reported in South America (60%) and the lowest rates in Africa (46%) [6].

16.1.3 *Mortality*

As with incidence rates, reported figures for mortality vary according to reporting methods and region. Hospital discharge data from the USA was used to calculate a mortality rate of 17% for patients admitted with sepsis [2] whilst the EPIC II study calculated an ICU mortality of 18.2% and a hospital mortality of 24.2% [6]. The Promoting Global Excellence in Severe Sepsis (PROGRESS) study conducted in 2009 collected data on over 12,000 severely septic patients from 37 countries. The quoted hospital mortality for this group was nearly 50% [7]. The true figure however is likely to be much higher as patient follow-up studies reveal cumulative two-year mortalities of between 45% and 67% [8].

16.1.4 *Costs*

Considerable costs are incurred in the treatment of sepsis. Exact figures are difficult to interpret due to wide global variations in healthcare and accounting. In the USA yearly costs for hospitalisation have risen since 1997 from $4 billion to $14 billion in 2008[9]. Patients hospitalised for sepsis experience lengths of stay 75% longer than those hospitalised for other illnesses [2] and survivors of severe sepsis are more likely to suffer long-term organ dysfunction and lower quality of life relative to other conditions [10]. Most estimates of cost do not include social and rehabilitative care.

16.2 Pathophysiology

Two decades ago, Gram-negative organisms were the predominant pathogens associated with sepsis. More recently, the incidences of Gram-positive and fungal sepsis have increased [13]. Both the EPIC II and PROGRESS studies found 57–62% of positive microbiological isolates to be Gram-negative, 44–47% Gram-positive and 11–19% fungal. Mixed infections constituted the remainder of isolates. The most common sites of infections were lungs (47–64%), abdomen (20–23%), bloodstream (20%) and renal tract (8–14%) [6,7]. Infection rates are more prevalent in patients with multiple comorbidities, longer lengths of ICU stay, those on invasive ventilation or renal replacement therapy or the immunocompromised [6].

Originally, the manifestations of severe sepsis were attributed to an exaggerated cytokine-mediated, pro-inflammatory response to the presence of pathogens — the Lewis Thomas theory [11]. This theory was propagated by the observation that infusions of bacteria and bacterial components resulted in profound release of pro-inflammatory mediators many of which resulted in death. This gave impetus to a number of trials exploring the potential role for anti-inflammatory therapies, most of which failed to demonstrate the expected benefits. This was probably because the true picture is one of mixed inflammatory and anti-inflammatory primary responses. How these mechanisms interact is poorly understood [12,13]. What is clear is that sepsis results from a complex interaction of mechanisms between pathogenic organisms and the host's immune response, vascular endothelium and coagulation system that, in unison, lead to multiple organ failure and death.

16.2.1 *Microbial factors*

Virulence gene acquisition and expression are important in distinguishing pathogenic organisms from commensal flora. Toxins released by pathogenic organisms and the host's response to them account for some of the features of sepsis and septic shock. There are three classes of toxins. Type 1 toxins cause injury to the host extracellularly. Bacterial superantigens fall into this class, binding directly to major histocompatibility complex (MHC) class II molecules and cross-linking to large numbers of T-cells, leading to their activation. Resulting lymphokine and monokine release produce the features of toxic shock syndrome associated with *Staphylococcus aureus* or *Streptococcus pyogenes* infections. Type 2 toxins derive from bacterial cell-wall structures and act by damaging host-cell membranes, allowing intracellular access thus facilitating host tissue invasion and immune response evasion. Haemolysins and phospholipases are examples of these. Type 3 toxin-producers include the well known toxin-producing bacteria such as cholera, anthrax and shigella as well as more common pathogens such as *Staphylococcus aureus, Streptomyces pyogenes* and *Escherichia coli.*

Furthermore, many bacteria posses the ability to detect their population density via genetically mediated mechanisms known as quorum sensing. Through quorum sensing, bacteria are able to switch off virulence genes at times of low populations and thus avoid host detection at times of maximal pathogen vulnerability. When pathogen numbers are more favourable, the same mechanism is able to upregulate virulence genes involved in adhesion, host-cell invasion, immune evasion and antibiotic resistance. In this way, pathogenic organisms are able to maximise their virulence at times when potential host responses are most attenuated [13].

16.2.2 *Host's initial response*

Host defence starts with the physical barriers to potentially pathogenic organisms, comprised of skin, gastrointestinal tract, nasopharyngeal tract, respiratory tract and eyes. These barriers are rich in cells such as mast cells, macrophages, dendritic cells, histiocytes and natural killer (NK) cells, all of which make up the host's innate immunity. These cells react in non-specific ways upon contact with pathogens and damaged host tissue to release chemical mediators that cause local inflammation, recruit more inflammatory cells and trigger responses from the host's adaptive immunity. The adaptive immune system evokes more specific responses from T- and B-lymphocytes, resulting in the proliferation of cytotoxic cells, release of more inflammatory mediators and the development of immunity through antibodies. Together, these mechanisms are designed to isolate and control infection and result in the well-recognised features of localised infection: swelling, erythema and pus. When local defence mechanisms are overwhelmed, the inflammatory response spills out into the systemic circulation producing features of sepsis: pyrexia, tachycardia and flushing which, when severe, lead to hypotension and organ dysfunction.

16.2.3 *Pathogenic recognition and signal transduction*

Pathogen recognition is achieved by the host's immune system's ability to bind to components of cell structures unique to pathogens, known as pathogen-associated molecular patterns (PAMPs). Binding occurs via a limited number of pattern-recognition receptors (PRRs). PRRs are also able to recognise endogenous mediators released by tissue damage incurred by non-infectious means such as trauma or ischaemia, thereby preparing the host for potential infection. These mediators are termed danger-associated molecular patterns (DAMPs).

Among PRRs, the Toll family of receptors play a central role in the initiation of the host's immune response. Toll-like receptors (TLRs) are single-spanning transmembrane proteins that bind to unique and common PAMPs and DAMPs, and can be found both on cell surfaces and intracellularly [13]. Lipopolysaccharide, a major component of Gram-negative bacterial cell walls, for example, interacts with cell surface TLR4. Gram-positive bacterial cell walls have no lipopolysccharide but are rich in lipoteichoic acid, which is recognised by TLR2, also on cell surfaces [14]. Both Gram-negative and Gram-positive bacteria express unmethylated cytosine–guanine nucleotides (CpG DNA), rare in mammalian cells, which, via common intermediate steps, are recognised by intracellular TLR9. Because of this ability to exploit cell components unique and common to a range of pathogenic organisms, as few as ten TLRs are able to detect the majority of known pathogens (Table 16.1) [15].

16.2.4 *Acute inflammatory response*

TLR activation results in a number of intracellular signalling cascades that converge via common pathways resulting in the release of three

Table 16.1. Toll-like receptors and their targets.

Extracellular	
TLR4	Gram-negative lipopolysaccharide
	Rous sarcoma virus fusion protein
TLR1/2/6	Gram-positive lipoteichoic acid
	Fungal zymosan
	Mycoplasma lipoproteins
TLR5	Bacterial flagellin
Intracellular	
TLR3	Viral double-stranded DNA
TLR7/8	Viral single-stranded DNA
TLR9	Unmethylated CpG DNA

transcription factors: nuclear factor-kB (NF-kB), activator protein-1 (AP-1) and interferon response factor-1 (IRF1) [15]. All three drive transcription of a range of pro-inflammatory cytokines, namely tumour necrosis factor (TNF)-α, interleukin (IL)-1, IL-6, IL-12 and IL-8. The pathogen-induced release of pro-inflammatory mediators results in the well-recognised physiological response: pyrexia, neutrophilia, glucone-ogensis, muscle catabolism, altered lipid metabolism and activation of both complement and coagulation pathways [14].

IL-1 and TNF-α induce the release of C-reactive protein (CRP) and serum amyloid A (SAA). IL-6 induces the release of fibrinogen and α2 macroglobulin. There are numerous acute-phase proteins, many of which have not been studied and whose exact roles are not well understood. Some, such as granulocyte colony-stimulating factor (G-CSF), ensure that the bone marrow releases adequate numbers of activated neutrophils, important in mounting an adequate antibacterial response. Others, such as fibrinogen, in conjunction with specific bacteria, result in marked organ damage (Table 16.2) [14].

Cytokine gene polymorphisms have been the subject of interest in sepsis research. A number of cytokines such as TNFα, IL-1β, IL-6 and IL-10 have been shown to correlate with outcome. However, these cytokines all demonstrate a high degree of pleiotropism, meaning that they may show both inflammatory and anti-inflammatory effects depending on pathogen or cell type under investigation [14].

Table 16.2. Acute phase proteins [14].

Classical acute phase proteins	SAA, CRP
Complement components	C3, C4, C4 binding protein, CI inhibitor
Coagulation components	Factor VIII, fibrinogen, plasminogen, prothrombin, Von Willebrand factor
Transport proteins	Haptoglobin, ferritin, ceruloplasmin
Proteases	Kallikrein, phospholipase A2
Protease inhibitors	

16.2.5 *Endothelium, nitric oxide and the clotting cascade*

The endothelium plays an important role in maintaining vascular tone, vascular permeability and coagulation. Vasomotor tone is normally determined by the interplay between endothelium-derived vasodilators, such as nitric oxide (NO) and prostacyclin, and vasoconstrictors, such as endothelin and platelet activating factor (PAF) [16]. In sepsis, NO is the most important of these. Pro-inflammatory cytokines, namely TNF-α and IL-1 lead to inducible nitric oxide production in immune and vascular cells. Additionally, Gram-negative bacteria can, via TLR4 and lipopolysaccharide on their cell walls, trigger the production of interferons that also lead to the production of inducible nitric oxide and further vasodilatation [14]. Vasodilatation slows the flow of blood and provides passing neutrophils an opportunity to adhere.

Pro-inflammatory cytokines also enhance endothelial cell adhesiveness via the expression of molecules such as the selectins (E- and L-selectin), intercellular cell adhesion molecules (ICAM-1, ICAM-2) and vascular cell adhesion molecules (VCAM). TNFα, IL-1, interferon and oxygen free radicals induce endothelial cells to apoptose. Apoptosed endothelial cells release more oxygen free radicals and express more adhesion molecules that amplify neutrophil recruitment [16]. The resulting damage to the endothelial barrier facilitates immune cell migration and cytokine permeability but also results in systemic vascular leakage of intravascular fluid and proteins, namely albumin.

Increased concentrations of pro-thrombotic components such as fibrinogen, high-molecular-weight kininogen and tissue factor (TF) are induced by the acute phase response. TF is a potent initiator of the clotting cascade leading to the activation of the extrinsic coagulation pathway whilst concentrations of natural inhibitors of this pathway, such as plasminogen inhibitor, protein C and antithrombin III, are reduced.

Damage to the endothelium exposes underlying structural cell components, such as the basement membrane, to activated platelets. This results in the build up of platelets and fibrin in the microvasculature. Platelets and the endothelium release kinins from high-molecular-weight kininogen (HMWK) via the activation of factor XII. The resulting microvascular thormboses from disseminated intravascular coagulation lead to endothelial damage, organ hypoperfusion and ultimately, failure [14].

Three main anticoagulant proteins dampen the clotting cascade: tissue-factor-pathway inhibitor (TFPI), antithrombin III (ATIII) and activated protein C (APC). During sepsis, concentrations of all three are reduced, resulting in an overall procoagulant state [13]. APC inhibits the extrinsic coagulation pathway by its capacity to proteolytically inactivate factors Va and VIIa. Additionally, when bound to protein S, neutrophil chemotaxis, NK-kB activation and TF expression are also inhibited, thus attenuating both pro-coagulant and pro-inflammatory effects of sepsis [13,14].

16.2.6 *Immune suppression and apoptosis*

There is much debate regarding the timing and sequence of the pro-inflammatory and anti-inflammatory or immunosuppressive phase in the evolution of sepsis. Some suggest the two phases run concurrently whilst others promote the concept that immunosuppression is an initial feature that precedes the hyper-inflammatory phase [13]. A number of mechanisms involved in dampening the inflammatory response have been studied.

The cholinergic nervous system, via the vagus nerve in particular, inhibits cytokine release by acetycholine's action on $\alpha 7$ receptors on macrophages. Molecules such as MyD88 short, interleukin-1-receptor-associated kinase (IRAK) M and Toll-interacting protein (TOLLIP) are also involved in regulating the potential over-stimulation of the host's inflammatory response. Macrophage migratory inhibitory factor (MIF) is produced by host cells and may be involved in the resolution of sepsis by suppressing natural apoptosis, hence prolonging the pro-inflammatory response phase to the detriment of the host. Glucocorticoids promote the release of MIF, which is also found in high concentrations in septic patients and is associated with increased mortality in laboratory studies [13].

Apoptosis, or programmed cell death, is a mechanism by which cellular damage may be limited in sepsis. Most cells that undergo apoptosis in sepsis are lymphoid in origin, releasing anti-inflammatory cytokines as they die. Immune cell death has been implicated in the immune dysfunction and high mortality associated with severe sepsis. Apoptosis inhibitors have shown promising results in mice, where prevention of apoptosis was shown to improve survival. However, they have not been tested in humans due to concerns regarding cell selectivity and uncontrolled cell growth [13].

16.3 Treatment

In 2002 three critical care organisations, the European Society of Intensive Care Medicine, the Society of Critical Care Medicine, and the International Sepsis Forum, met in Barcelona and agreed on an initiative to recognise and treat sepsis with the aims of reducing mortality by 25% over five years. Thus the Surviving Sepsis Campaign (SSC) was born and in 2004 the first series of guidelines and recommendations was published, each assessed and graded for quality. These were updated in 2008 [17]. Since then, there has been much debate relating to the evidence behind many of their recommendations. This was not helped by questions regarding the involvement of the pharmaceutical industry in their formulation [18]. Nevertheless, the spirit of the SSC continues and many of its recommendations will remain until such time as new evidence dictates otherwise. Key to their successful implementation is early recognition of sepsis and timely and aggressive intervention.

16.3.1 *Fluids*

Early goal-directed therapy remains a cornerstone of therapy during the first six hours after the recognition of sepsis. In Rivers' original paper, patients randomised to the treatment arm were given 500 ml boluses of crystalloid at 30-minute intervals titrated to defined sequential goals as follows:

Central venous pressure (CVP) 8–12 mmHg.
Mean arterial pressure (MAP) ≥60 mmHg.
Central venous oxygen saturation ($ScvO_2$) ≥70%.

Pressors were added after CVP optimisation if MAPs were not achieved, followed by packed red cells to a haematocrit of greater than 30% if $ScvO_2$ was less than 70%. Finally, Dobutamine was added should transfusion still not achieve the desired goal of $ScvO_2 \geq 70\%$. Haemodymanic parameters were monitored, including heart rate and urine output. This simple algorithm translated to a 28-day hospital mortality improvement of 46.5% to 30.5% [19]. The SSC adopted these measures with some modification. A 1000 ml volume of crystalloid or 300–500 ml of colloid should be administered over 30 minutes or less. Filling rates should be reduced or stopped if cardiac filling pressures increase, as evidenced by CVP, without concomitant improvement in haemodynamics. A CVP of 8–12 mmHg should be the initial target, though this may be revised upwards when high ventilatory pressures, decreased ventricular compliance or significant pulmonary hypertension result in physiologically elevated CVP. Caution should be exercised, however. Early goal-directed fluid therapy is just that — early. The original study focussed on the first six hours following recognition of sepsis. Thereafter, current thinking recommends late conservative fluid management. This is based on a number of studies that demonstrate the negative effect that cumulative fluid balance has on mortality [18]. Indeed, in a recent publication from the Vassopressin in Septic Shock Trial (VASST) group, the highest mortality was found in patients with the greatest positive fluid balance at 12 and 72 hours. Their findings suggested that after 12 hours, CVP-guided fluid therapy becomes unreliable [19]. Thus, once adequate resuscitation has taken place early in the course of treatment, an even to negative fluid balance should be pursued.

The type of fluid used in resuscitation has been extensively investigated. Until recently there was no consensus with regard to the choice of fluids between crystalloids and artificial colloids [21]. The Saline versus Albumin Fluid Evaluation (SAFE) study suggested there was a non-statistical benefit in using albumin in septic patients [22] though this was later refuted in the

Sepsis Occurrence in Acutely ill Patients (SOAP) study. This observational study noted, however, that those patients receiving albumin had significantly higher illness severity scores [23]. More recently, a meta-analysis of albumin use in sepsis concluded that there was a statistically significant reduction in mortality with its use over other fluid regimes [24]. Until a study specifically addressing this question is conducted, the choice of resuscitation fluid will remain subject to debate.

16.3.2 *Inotropes and pressors*

Rivers' chosen target of MAP of 65 mmHg was derived from data which showed tissue perfusion to be preserved at that pressure. Below 60 mmHg, auto-regulatory function is lost. This target however may need to be revised according to the patient's normal blood pressure. Hypertensive patients will upregulate their auto-regulatory mechanisms and perfusion of key organs will require higher MAPs.

Despite there being no clear evidence to support the use of any particular pressor or inotrope [25], norepinephrine is the first-choice pressor in sepsis. Dopamine featured in the SSC recommendations together with norepinephrine but a recent meta-analysis comparing the two demonstrated a higher mortality with significantly increased risk of arrhythmias with the use of dopamine [26]. Norepinephrine is a potent α-agonist with minor β-agonist effects. Its main clinical effects result from peripheral vasoconstriction raising the systemic vascular resistance. It has minimal effect on heart rate or myocardial contractility, increasing cardiac output by 10–20%. It is more potent than dopamine and more effective at reversing hypotension resulting from septic shock, though it may cause renal ischaemia if used in hypovolaemia [27]. Excessive peripheral vasoconstriction leads to increased afterload that in some instances may overwhelm the myocardium, leading to low cardiac output despite adequate MAPs. Dobutamine, with its primary action on β_1-adrenoceptors, improves myocardial contractility though it has the propensity to cause arrhythmias and hypotension. Nevertheless, it offers attractive additional support in patients with poor myocardial function resulting in low cardiac output.

Epinephrine exerts its effects by increasing cardiac index and stroke volume, raising systemic vascular resistance and heart rate only modestly.

Its detrimental effects include tachycardia and arrhythmias as well as slower resolution of lactataemia and acidosis resulting from reduced splanchnic blood flow. Myocardial oxygen consumption is also increased, which may lead to ischaemia in susceptible patients. However, its effects on patients who have not responded to fluids or pressors can be dramatic. A study comparing the combination of norepinephrine and dobutamine with epinephrine failed however to demonstrate a mortality or safety difference [28]. As such it should be used as a second line agent for as limited a time as possible [27].

The VASST trial was conceived from the observation that septic patients were deficient in vasopressin and that restoration of plasma levels resulted in improvements in vascular tone and blood pressure. This randomised control trial found no mortality difference using a low-dose regime (0.03 U/min). At this dose there was no difference in adverse events associated with vasopressin (mesenteric ischaemia, digital necrosis, cardiac arrest) between the two groups [29]. Further analysis of this study suggested a synergistic benefit for patients receiving both vasopressin and low-dose corticosteroids [30]. This potential is currently under investigation by the Vasopressin and Corticosteroids in septic Shock (VACS) study group [31].

It is vital to achieve the correct balance between negating the vasoplegic effects of sepsis and the dangers of excessive vasoconstriction with resulting critical reduction in organ perfusion. Clinical examination of the extremities will give clues about peripheral circulation and lactate levels and urine output monitoring will provide a guide to adequacy of blood flow and thus tissue perfusion [17–27]. Currently there are numerous devices that allow monitoring of cardiac output and calculation of systemic vascular resistance with varying degrees of invasiveness and reproducibility. The use of cardiac output monitoring has never been shown to reduce mortality, nor has any one device shown superiority over another. Whichever device is chosen, key to its successful use is the clinician's response to the patient's dynamic measured physiology.

16.3.3 *Source identification*

It is imperative that efforts be made to identify the source of sepsis. This, however, should not be to the detriment of initiating life-saving therapy.

The SSC guidelines recommend that at least two blood cultures be taken from the periphery and, where applicable, from vascular access ports to identify catheter-related bloodstream infections. A septic screen should include urine and sputum samples as well as swabs from any obvious external sources of infection. Screening swabs for methicillin-resistant *Staphylococcus aureus* (MRSA) are also important as they may alter antibiotic choice later in the septic course. The clinical history should guide whether more invasive modes of sampling, such as lumbar puncture, are warranted but should not delay administration of antibiotics [17]. Samples should be processed promptly for maximum yield and should include Gram staining as well as more specialised stains where appropriate.

Deep-seated sites of infection may manifest as collections or abscesses not amenable to easy sampling. In such cases, diagnostic imaging is useful in identifying potential sources of sepsis and to guide sampling and drainage. As with peripheral sampling, this should not delay initiation of therapy. Indeed, transfer of septic patients to appropriate facilities can be dangerous, as monitoring and availability of essential resuscitation equipment may be limited. Patients with haemodynamic instability may respond poorly to transfer and interventional procedures.

Microbiological sampling does not always yield treatment-altering results. Blood cultures, though good at detecting bacteraemias, are prone to low yield in certain conditions such as community-acquired pneumonia. Inherent delays in processing add further limitations to their use. Slow-growing organisms, such as *Mycobacterium tuberculosis*, fastidious organisms, such as *Legionella pneumophilia* or *Chlamydia pneumoniae*, and concomitant use of antibiotics often render blood culture sensitivity low. A number of molecular techniques may greatly speed up the identification process as well as provide fast antibiotic resistance profiling using polymerase chain reaction (PCR) and microarray techniques [32].

Many biomarkers have been investigated for their usefulness in detecting infection. Of these, only procalcitonin has been successfully marketed. A number of trials, however, have failed to demonstrate its usefulness as a predictor and discriminator of infection. Instead, it has proven useful in plotting the course of successful treatment of sepsis and predicting safe de-escalation of antibiotics with resulting reduction in antibiotic exposure and selective pressure [33].

16.3.4 *Source control*

Where the source of infection has been anatomically defined by clinical examination or by imaging techniques, consideration should be given to the confirmation and removal of infected tissues. In cases such as nectrotising fasciitis, faecal or ischemic peritonitis, surgery is warranted where possible. Microbiological sampling at the time of surgery may further help treatment choices. Removal of infected and necrotic tissue will help stem the stimulus for severe sepsis and septic shock. Percutaneours techniques may be more appropriate for abscesses and superficial collections. Although the SSC recommend delayed necrosectomy in cases of peripancreatic necrosis, where infection is suspected, radiological or surgical intervention should be undertaken [17–34]. With all instances of surgical or radiological intervention, samples of tissues or fluid must always be assessed microbiologically.

16.3.5 *Antibiotics*

It has been estimated that for every hour-delay in instituting appropriate antibiotic cover for suspected sepsis there is a 7% increase in mortality [35]. As mentioned above, cultures should be taken before commencing antibiotics where possible. Choice of antibiotics should be guided by likely source and adequate penetration into the presumed site of infection. A suspicion of likely pathogens can be surmised from the clinical history and features, community and hospital pathogen patterns and recent antibiotic use. The immune state of the patient should be taken into account and the possibility of fungal infection should be considered. Initially, broad-spectrum antibiotics are chosen to cover all likely pathogens. Daily review of antibiotics will help to optimise efficacy, prevent resistance, avoid toxicity and reduce costs. De-escalation of antibiotics may follow emerging microbiological data from samples or changing clinical state. Antibiotic courses should continue for seven to ten days; deep infections and/or an immunocompromised host often require longer courses [17].

Dosing and dosing regimes have attracted much interest of late. Numerous studies have consistently demonstrated underestimation of dosing levels. Additionally, there may be benefits from continuous rather than intermittent dosing where bacterial killing is dependent on the proportion of time plasma antibiotic concentrations exceed the minimum inhibitory concentration (MIC). Knowledge of the effective concentration at the site of infection is also of importance as hydrophilic antibiotics (e.g. beta-lactams, aminoglycosides) penetrate deep tissues slowly compared with lipophilic ones (e.g. macrolides, rifampicin, linezolid). Sepsis and septic shock often result in significant alterations in the pharmacokinetic behaviour of drugs. Capillary leak and fluid resuscitation leads to an expansion of the volume of distribution, resulting in a reduction in the plasma concentration following therapeutic loading. Renal function is often affected by sepsis, leading to reduced drug clearance and elimination. This factor has to be reconsidered when renal replacement therapy is instituted. Hypoalbuminaemia is another important factor that can lead to underdosing in highly protein-bound antibiotics (e.g. teicoplanin, ceftriaxone) where high levels of free drug results in greater clearance and elimination when renal function is preserved. Under these circumstances higher dosing may be warranted [36].

16.3.6 *Steroids*

It has long been recognised that sepsis induces a state of relative adrenal insufficiency. This initially led to the widely adopted use of short courses of high-dose steroids in sepsis. Later studies however failed to demonstrate a mortality benefit and highlighted the risk of superinfection. A number of studies looked at longer courses of steroids at lower doses. Some demonstrated a mortality improvement and quicker resolution of sepsis, particularly in patients not responsive to a corticotrophin challenge. The Corticoid Steroid Therapy for Septic Shock (CORTICUS) trial was a large multicentre study looking at patients' response to hydrocortisone (50 mg intravenously every six hours) versus placebo in sepsis. No mortality difference was demonstrated. This finding included patients who did not respond to corticotrophin [37]. More recently, two meta-analyses confirmed the benefits of longer courses of low-dose steroids but highlighted their maximal potential in the more severely septic patients whose haemodynamics were unresponsive to fluids and pressors [38,39]. This observation coincides with the SSC's view that low-dose steroid (hydrocortisone, 50 mg intravenously every six hours) use should be confined to this group irrespective of corticotrophin challenge response [17].

16.3.7 *Activated protein C (APC)*

The close relationship between the inflammatory response and the coagulation cascade has already been alluded to above. Key to regulating the pro-coagulant drivers of sepsis are three anticoagulant proteins, TFPI, ATIII and APC. Of these only APC demonstrated potential benefit in clinical trials, the other two demonstrating no mortality benefit and increased haemorrhage risk [40–42]. In 2001, APC, marketed as Drotrecogin alpha, was tested for efficacy and safety in a large randomised controlled, multi-centre, international study. Patients on the treatment arm presented a 6.1% reduction in absolute risk of death (from 30.8% to 24.7%) and a 20% reduction in relative risk of death after 28 days. The incidence of bleeding was higher in the Drotrecogin alpha group but was not statistically significant ($p=0.06$) [43]. Having been approved by the Food and Drug Administration (FDA), Drotrecogin alpha was then enrolled in two studies, the Extended Evaluation of Recombinant Human Activated Protein C (ENHANCE) and Administration of Drotrecogin Alfa in Early Stage Severe Sepsis (ADDRESS) trials. Both trials demonstrated an increased risk of haemorrhage compared with the original study. The second study was terminated early, on the second interim analysis, due to lack of demonstrable efficacy [44,45]. After these trials, the SSC recommended APC be reserved only for patients at high risk of death with multiple organ failure [17]. Much controversy was fuelled both by the lack of reproducible efficacy and higher than first reported incidences of serious bleeding. Furthermore, the impartiality of the SSC was called into question due to part-funding by the drug manufacturers. In 2007 the European Medicines Agency (EMEA) requested a further trial, funded by the manufacturer, to assess the efficacy of Drotrecogin alpha in patients with severe septic shock and at high risk of death [46]. In October 2011, Drotrecogin alpha was withdrawn from the market by its manufacturer after the Recombinant Human Protein C Worldwide Evaluation in Severe Sepsis (PROWESS)-SHOCK trial failed to show any mortality benefit in its treatment arm [47].

16.3.8 *Supportive measures*

There are numerous general evidence-based measures employed in intensive care that significantly affect patient outcomes, and it goes without saying that these should be adhered to for maximal benefit. There are some, however, that have particular reference to sepsis and thus merit specific mention.

16.3.8.1 *Blood transfusion*

Oxygen delivery is much dependent on oxygen-carrying capacity. Optimisation of haematocrit was an essential component of Rivers' goal-directed therapy aimed at preserving organ perfusion and function. A number of studies, however, have established a correlation between the number of units of blood transfused and risk of developing sepsis in critical illness [48]. A similar correlation has been found with mortality [49], though this has been called into question in subsequent observational studies and analyses [50]. There is no doubt that blood transfusion confers an immunosuppressive effect on the patient and in the with the exception of transfusion for resuscitation, a conservative approach to blood transfusion, as evidenced by the influential Transfusion Requirements in Critical Care (TRICC) study, should be followed [51].

16.3.8.2 *Glycaemic control*

The Leuven Protocol, an intensive insulin therapy regime that targets blood glucose levels between 80–110 mg/dl, was introduced following a single-centre study based on a post-surgical ICU that demonstrated a reduced mortality, particularly in those patients with a septic focus. Other benefits included reductions in septic episodes, renal replacement requirements and incidence of critical illness polyneuropathy [52]. Since then, a number of follow-up studies and reviews have led to conflicting results. In 2008, the Volume Substitution and Insulin Therapy in Severe Sepsis (VISEP) study was stopped early due to excess deaths in the treatment arm. This multi-centre study aimed to look both at the potential benefits of 10% pentastarch as a resuscitation fluid and intensive insulin therapy [53]. Following this, a large multicentre study in 2009 aimed at resolving questions surrounding the benefits if intensive insulin therapy demonstrated an excess mortality in the intensive-insulin arm. This was attributed largely to higher incidences of hypoglycaemia. In conclusion, a more moderate target of 180 mg/dl or less was deemed to be safer [54].

16.3.8.3 *Sedation protocols*

Septic patients often require ventilation and experience numerous invasive and painful interventions during the course of their treatment. To date, there are no specific recommendations regarding choice of sedative agent. A number of studies have demonstrated a relationship between sedation and infection, though it is not clear whether this is a temporal association with the risks of developing infection in critical illness. The immunomodulatory effects of specific sedatives are increasingly the subject of research. Opioids suppress T- and B-lymphocytes, NK cells and IL-2, interferon (IFN), TNF-α and NO production [55]. Benzodiazepines too have been shown to have similar effects on cytokine production. More recently, dexmedetomidine has been the subject of much research. *In-vitro* and animal studies demonstrate dose-dependent suppression of TNF-α, IL-1β, IL-6, IFNγ and inducible nitric oxide synthase [56]. No studies have as yet investigated the potential benefit of different sedative regimes on sepsis outcome. Until such time, eligible patients should undergo daily sedation holds and spontaneous breathing trials with the aim of shortening time to extubation, thereby minimising the associated risks of prolonged sedation and ventilation.

16.3.8.4 *Renal replacement modalities*

Renal replacement is often required in the context of sepsis and multiple organ failure. Numerous studies have investigated the benefits of intermittent versus continuous therapy. Although some studies have demonstrated a benefit with intermittent therapy, a Cochrane review found no benefit when compared against continuous therapy. However, this review noted that many studies excluded patients with hypotension. Furthermore, continuous therapies resulted in improved mean arterial pressures and less pressor support. In keeping with the SSC guidelines, neither holds an advantage over the other, though in patients with haemodynamic instability, continuous therapy may confer advantages [17–57]. Similarly, the dose of renal replacement has also been debated. Inflammatory mediators fall into the middle molecular weight category — that is between 5 and 10 kDa. In sepsis, these are produced at higher rates than they are cleared by standard renal-replacement dosing regimes of 25–30 ml/kg/h. Animal studies indicated the benefits of removing so-called middle molecules from the circulation. Though initial studies demonstrated benefits with high-dose renal replacement therapy (≥30 ml/kg/h), a recent systematic review and meta-analysis failed to show any benefits particularly in the septic population subgroup [58,59].

16.4 Past and Future

The consensus conference that defined sepsis paved the way for a surge in sepsis research. Sadly, many trials that initially showed promise have not translated into clear outcome benefits. Despite good-quality trials using the consensus definitions, variations remain when defining measured features such as organ dysfunction or tissue hypoperfusion. Furthermore, the inclusion of a range of severities of sepsis has led to wide variations in baseline mortality, thereby making any potential benefits more difficult to measure. This is amplified by recruiting patients from a wide time frame of presentation. Patients will exhibit a range of severities and may be at different stages of evolution or resolution if recruited over a greater period. The confounding effects of co-interventions also play a major role in the success of clinical trials. Fluid resuscitation choice, inotrope and pressor choice, therapeutic drug interactions, ventilator settings, time to source identification and control and antibiotic prescribing policy all affect final patient outcomes [60].

Much research currently focuses on a number of aspects of sepsis management. Early identification of septic patients will be facilitated by the development of novel biomarkers. Candidates currently being investigated include Pro-B-type naturetic peptide and matrix metaloproteinases and their inhibitors [61]. Interventions that target specific mechanisms within the inflammatory cascade are also under investigation. Synthetic

TLR4 antagonists may offer protection against severe Gram-negative sepsis in mice [62] but phase II clinical trials have not translated into mortality benefits [63]. As a unifying target for sepsis therapy continues to elude the research community, researchers will continue to look at specific pathways amenable to manipulation. Selecting the right population remains problematic. Genetic polymorphisms relating to sepsis predisposition and survival are also an area of great interest. The future may well lie in selecting individuals early based on their inflammatory response profiles and targeting specific receptor or cell lines in order to rectify their aberrant immune response — immunotherapy [64].

The SSC has managed to bring sepsis research and management to the forefront of intensive care. Individual recommendations have been questioned and debated but one of the successes of the campaign was to introduce the concept of bundles — that is the grouping of a number of interventions common to a disease process. Some of these interventions are a decade old in their design and publication and yet their uptake remains variable, probably owing to doubt about their validity. Much work is being currently undertaken to understand why uptake is low in some instances and how to increase compliance [65]. There is evidence that when taken together, the implementation of a sepsis bundle can have a significant effect on sepsis mortality [66,67]. As more light is shed on the finer points of each intervention, components of bundles will change and their re-evaluation will be necessary.

References

[1] Bone, R.C., Balk, R.A., Cerra, F.B. *et al.* (1992). Definitions for sepsis and organ failure and guidelines for the use of innovative therapies in sepsis. The ACCP/SCCM Consensus Conference Committee. American College of Chest Physicians/Society of Critical care Medicine, *Chest*, **101**, 1644–1655.

[2] Hall, M.J., Williams, S.N., DeFrances C.J. *et al.* (2011). Inpatient care for septicemia or sepsis: a challenge for patients and hospitals, *NCHS data brief*, **62**, 1–8.

[3] Angus, D.C., Linde-Zwirble, W.T., Lidicker, J. *et al.* (2001). Epidemiology of severe sepsis in the United States: analysis of incidence, outcome, and associated costs of care, *Crit Care Med*, **29**, 1303–1310.

[4] Karlsson, S., Varpula, M., Ruokonen, E. *et al.* (2007). Incidence, treatment, and outcomes of severe sepsis in ICU-treated adults in Finland: the Finnsepsis study, *Intens Care Med*, **33**, 435–443.

[5] Engel, C., Brunkhorst, F.M., Bone, H.-G. *et al.* (2007). Epidemiology of sepsis in Germany: results from a national prospective multicenter study, *Intens Care Med*, **33**, 606–618.

[6] Vincent, J.L., Rello, J., Marshall, J. *et al.* (2009). International study of the prevalence and outcomes of infection in intensive care units, *JAMA*, **302**, 2323–2329.

[7] Martin, G., Brunkhorst, F.M., Janes, J.M. *et al.* (2009). The international PROGRESS registry of patients with severe sepsis: drotrecogin alfa (activated) use and patient outcomes, *Crit Care*, **13**, R103.

[8] Karlsson, S., Ruokonen, E., Varpula, T. *et al.* (2009). Long-term outcome and quality-adjusted life years after severe sepsis, *Crit Care Med*, **37**, 1268–1274.

[9] Agency for Healthcare Research and Quality (2010). *HCUP facts and figures: Statistics on hospital based care in the United States, 2008.* Available at: http://www.hcup-us.ahrq.gov/reports/factsandfigures/2008/TOC_2008.jsp [Accessed 5 February 2013].

[10] Iwashyna, T.J., Ely, E.W., Smith, D.M. *et al.* (2010). Long-term cognitive impairment and functional disability among survivors of severe sepsis, *JAMA*, **304**, 1787–1794.

[11] Thomas, L. (1972). Germs, *N Engl J Med*, **287**, 553–555.

[12] Hotchkiss, R.S. and Karl, I.E. (2003). The pathology and treatment of sepsis, *N Engl J Med*, **348**, 138–150.

[13] Van der Poll, T. and Opal, S.M. (2008). Host–pathogen interactions in sepsis, *Lancet Infect Dis*, **8**, 32–32.

[14] Sriskandan, S. and Altmenn, D.M. (2008). The immunology of sepsis, *J Pathol*, **214**, 211–223.

[15] Gao, H., Evans, T.W. and Finney, S.J. (2008). Bench to bedside review: sepsis, severe sepsis and septic shock — does the nature of the infecting organisms matter? *Crit Care*, **12**, 213.

[16] Ait-Oufella, H., Maury, E., Lehoux, S. *et al.* (2010). The endothelium: physiological functions and role in microcirculatory failure during severe sepsis, *Intens Care Med*, **36**, 1286–1298.

[17] Dellinger, R.P., Levy, M.M., Carlet, J.M. *et al.* (2008). Surviving Sepsis Campaign: international guidelines for management of severe sepsis and septic shock: 2008, *Intens Care Med*, **34**, 17–60.

[18] Marik, P.E. (2011). Surviving sepsis: going beyond the guidelines, *Annals of Intensive Care*, **1**, 17.

[19] Rivers, E., Nguyen, B., Havstad, S. *et al.* (2001). Early goal-directed therapy in the treatment of severe sepsis and septic shock, *N Engl J Med*, **345**, 1368–1377.

[20] Boyd, J.H., Forbes, J., Nakada, T. *et al.* (2011). Fluid resuscitation in septic shock: a positive fluid balance and elevated central venous pressure increase mortality, *Crit Care Med*, **39**, 259–265.

[21] Vincent, J.-L. and Gerlach, H. (2004). Fluid resuscitation in severe sepsis and septic shock: an evidence-based review, *Crit Care Med*, **32**, s451–s454.

[22] The SAFE Study Investigators (2004). A comparison of albumin and saline for fluid resuscitation in the intensive care unit, *N Engl J Med*, **350**, 2247–2256.

[23] Vincent, J.L., Sakr, Y., Reinhart, K. *et al.* (2005). Is albumin administration in the acutely ill associated with increased mortality? Results of the SOAP study, *Crit Care*, **9**, R745–R754.

[24] Delaney, A., Arina, D., McCaffrey, J. *et al.* (2011). The role of albumin as a resuscitation fluid for patients with sepsis: a systematic review and meta-analysis, *Crit Care Med*, **39**, 386–391.

[25] Havel, C., Arrich, J., Losert, H. *et al.* (2011). Vasopressors for hypotensive shock, *Cochrane Database of Systematic Reviews*, CD003709.

[26] Vasu, T.S., Cavallazzi, R., Hirani, A. *et al.* (2012). Norepinephrine or dopamine for septic shock: systematic review of randomized clinical trials, *J Intensive Care Med*, **27**, 172–178.

[27] Hollenberg, S.M., Ahrens, T.S., Annane, D. *et al.* (2004). Practice parameters for haemodynamic support of sepsis in adult patients: 2004 update, *Crit Care Med*, **32**, 1928–1948.

[28] Annane, D., Vignon, P., Rebault, A. *et al.* (2007). Norepinephrine plus dobutamine versus epinephrine alone for the management of septic shock: a randomised trial, *Lancet*, **370**, 676–684.

[29] Russell, J.A., Walley, K.R., Singer, J. *et al.* (2008). Vasopressin versus norepinephrine infusion in patients with septic shock, *N Engl J Med*, **358**, 877–887.

[30] Russell, J.A., Walley, K.R., Gordon, A.C. *et al.* (2009). Interaction of vasopressin infusion, corticosteroid treatment, and mortality of septic shock, *Crit Care Med*, **37**, 811–818.

[31] ISRCTN Register (2009). *Vasopressin and Corticosteroid in Septic Shock: an open label randomised controlled trial*, [Online]. Available at: http://www.controlled-trials.com/ISRCTN66727957 [Accessed 5 February 2013].

[32] Peters, R.P.H., van Agtmael, M.A., Danner, S.A. *et al.* (2004). New developments in the diagnosis of bloodstream infections, *Lancet Infect Dis*, **4**, 751–760.

[33] Boudama, L., Luyt, C.-E., Tubach, F. *et al.* (2010). Use of procalcitonin to reduce patients' exposure to antibiotics in intensive care units (PRORATA trial): a multicentre randomized controlled trial, *Lancet*, **375**, 463–474.

[34] Working Party of the British Society of Gastroenterology, Association of Surgeons of Great Britain and Ireland, Pancreatic Society of Great Britain and Ireland *et al.* (2005). UK guidelines for the management of acute pancreatitis. *Gut*, **54**, 1–9.

[35] Kumar, A., Roberts, D., Wood, K.E. *et al.* (2006). Duration of hypotension before initiation of effective antimicrobial therapy is the critical determinant of survival in human septic shock, *Crit Care Med*, **34**, 1589–1596.

[36] Pea, F. and Viale, P. (2009). Bench-to-bedside review: appropriate antibiotic therapy in severe sepsis and septic shock — does the dose matter? *Crit Care*, **13**, 214.

[37] Sprung, C., Annane, D., Keh, D. *et al.* (2008). Hydrocortisone therapy for patients with septic shock, *N Engl J Med*, **358**, 111–124.

[38] Annane, D., Bellissant, E., Bollaert, P.E. *et al.* (2009). Corticosteroids in the treatment of severe sepsis and septic shock in adults: a systematic review, *JAMA*, **301**, 2362–2375.

[39] Minneci, P.C., Deans, K.J., Eichacker, P.Q. *et al.* (2009).The effects of steroids during sepsis depend on dose and severity of illness: an updated meta-analysis, *Clin Microbiol Infect*, **15**, 308–318.

[40] Abraham, E., Reinhart, K., Opal, S. *et al.* (2003). Efficacy and safety of tifacogin (recombinant tissue factor pathway inhibitor) in severe sepsis: a randomized controlled trial, *JAMA*, **290**, 238–247.

[41] Warren, B.L., Eid, A., Singer, P. *et al.* (2001). Caring for the critically ill patient. High-dose antithrombin III in severe sepsis: a randomized controlled trial, *JAMA*, **286**, 1869–1878.

[42] Afshari, A., Wetterslev, J., Brok, J. *et al.* (2007). Antithrombin III in critically ill patients: systematic review with meta-analysis and trial sequential analysis, *BMJ*, **355**, 1248–1251.

[43] Bernard, G.R., Vincent, J.L., Laterre, P.F. *et al.* (2001). Efficacy and safety of recombinant human activated protein C for severe sepsis, *N Engl J. Med*, **344**, 699–709.

[44] Vincent, J.L., Bernard, G.R., Beale, R. *et al.* (2005). Drotrecogin alfa (activated) treatment in severe sepsis from the global open-label trial enhance: further evidence for survival and safety and implications for early treatment. *Crit Care Med*, **33**, 2266–2277.

[45] Abraham, E., Laterre, P.F., Garg, R. *et al.* (2005). Drotrecogin alfa (activated) for adults with severe sepsis and a low risk of death, *N Engl J Med*, **353**, 1332–1341.

[46] Silva, E., de Figueiredo, L.F.P. and Colombari, F. (2010). PROWESS-SHOCK trial: a protocol overview and perspectives, *Shock*, **34**(S1), 48–53.

[47] FDA (2011). *FDA Drug Safety Communication: Voluntary market withdrawal of Xigris [drotrecogin alfa (activated)] due to failure to show a survival benefit,* [Online] Available at: http://www.fda.gov/Drugs/DrugSafety/ucm277114.htm [Accessed 5 February 2013].

[48] Gould, S., Cimino, M.J. and Gerber, D.R. (2007). Packed red blood cell transfusion in the intensive care unit: limitations and consequences, *Am J Crit Care,* **16**, 39–48.

[49] Vincent, J.L., Sakr Y., Sprung, C. *et al.* (2008). Are blood transfusions, associated with greater mortality rates? *Anesthesiology,* **108**, 31–39.

[50] Vincent, J.L., Baron, J.F., Reinhart, K. *et al.* (2002). Anemia and blood transfusion in critically ill patients. *JAMA,* **288**, 1499–1507.

[51] Hébert, P.C., Wells, G., Blajchman, M.A. *et al.* (1999). A multicenter, randomized, controlled clinical trial of transfusion requirements in critical care, *N Engl J Med,* **340**, 409–417.

[52] Van den Berghe, G., Wouters, P., Weekers, F. *et al.* (2001). Intensive insulin therapy in critically ill patients, *N Engl J Med,* **345**, 1359–1367.

[53] Brunckhorst, F.M., Engel, C., Bloos, F. *et al.* (2008). Intensive insulin therapy and pentastarch resuscitation in severe sepsis, *N Engl J Med,* **358**, 125–139.

[54] NICE-SUGAR Study Investigators. (2009). Intensive versus conventional glucose control in critically ill patients, *N Engl J Med,* **360**, 1283–1297.

[55] Nseir, S., Makris, D., Mathieu, D. *et al.* (2010). Intensive care unit-acquired infection as a side effect of sedation, *Crit Care,* **14**, R30.

[56] MacLaren, R. (2009). Immunosedation: a consideration for sepsis, *Crit Care,* **13**, 191.

[57] Rabindranath, K., Adams, J., Macleod, A. *et al.* (2007). Intermittent versus continuous renal replacement therapy for acute renal failure in adults, *Cochrane Database Syst Rev,* CD003773.

[58] Ronco, C., Kellum, J.A., Bellomo, R. *et al.* (2008). Potential interventions in sepsis-related acute kidney injury, *Clin J Am Soc Nephrol,* **3**, 531–544.

[59] Van Wet, R., Friedrich, J.O., Scales, D.C. *et al.* (2010). High-dose renal replacement therapy for acute kidney injury: systematic review and meta-analysis, *Crit Care Med,* **38**, 1360–1369.

[60] Annane, D. (2009). Improving clinical trials in the critically ill: unique challenge — sepsis, *Crit Care Med,* **37**, s117–s128.

[61] Stearns-Kurosawa, D.J., Osuchowski, M.F., Valentine, C. *et al.* (2011). The pathogenesis of sepsis, *Annu Rev Pathol Mech Dis,* **6**, 19–48.

[62] Roger, T., Froidevaux, C., Le Roy, D. *et al.* (2009). Protection from lethal Gram-negative bacterial sepsis by targeting Toll-like receptor 4, *Proc Natl Acad Sci USA,* **106**, 2348–2352.

[63] Tidswell, M., Tillis, W., Larosa, S.P. *et al.* (2010). Phase 2 trial of eritoran tetrasodium (E.5564), a Toll-like receptor 4 antagonist, in patients with severe sepsis, *Crit Care Med*, **38**, 72–83.
[64] Hotchkiss, R.S. and Opal, S. (2010). Immunotherapy for sepsis — a new approach against an ancient foe, *N Engl J Med*, **363**, 87–89.
[65] Stoneking, L., Denningshoff, K., De Luca, L. *et al.* (2011). Sepsis bundles and compliance with clinical guidelines, *J Intensive Care Med*, **26**, 172–182.
[66] Coba V., Whitmill, M., Mooney, R. *et al.* (2011). Resuscitation bundle compliance in severe sepsis and septic shock improves survival, is better late than never, *J Intensive Care Med*, **26**, 304–313.
[67] Cardoso, T., Carneiro, A.H., Ribeiro, O. *et al.* (2010). Reducing mortality in severe sepsis with the implementation of a core 6-hour bundle: results from the Portuguese community-acquired sepsis study (SACiUCI Study), *Crit Care*, **14**, R83.

17

Airway Management in Intensive Care

Virinder S. Sidhu

17.1 Introduction

Airway management in the intensive care unit (ICU) is a hazardous but necessary undertaking. The limited physiological reserve and comorbidities increase the likelihood of complications both during the initial airway intervention but also once the airway has been secured. The need for rapid intubation due to progressive illness, difficulties with airway evaluation, pre-oxygenation, the risk of aspiration and limited access to the patient all compound difficulties. A well-managed airway may be life-saving and a poorly managed airway can lead to a series of events resulting in serious complications [1,2]. Safe airway management requires a suitably trained practitioner, a careful assessment of the patient, skilled assistance, a selection of equipment, close monitoring and back-up plans if difficulty is anticipated. The use of 'intubation bundles' can significantly reduce complication rate [3].

17.2 Prediction of Airway Difficulty

An airway assessment should be performed to ascertain the following:

- Difficult mask ventilation.
- Difficult direct laryngoscopy.

- Difficult endotracheal intubation.
- Difficult surgical airway (cricothyroidotomy or tracheostomy).

Difficult mask ventilation may be due to an inadequate face mask seal or excessive resistance to the ingress of gas. Independent predictors include a body mass index (BMI) > 26, age > 55, the presence of a beard, a lack of teeth, a history of snoring [4] and a history of radiation treatment to the face or neck. Difficult direct laryngoscopy is defined as the inability to visualise the vocal cords (Cormack and Lehane [5] grades III and IV) and difficult intubation may be the result of difficult direct laryngoscopy or due to difficulty in the passage of the tracheal tube. An airway evaluation should look for common predictors of difficult intubation [6–13]. These can be broadly classified anatomically into three groups (see Table 17.1)

Bedside tests are associated with only moderate sensitivity, specificity and positive predictive value. By combining tests, specificity and predictive value may be increased. The combination of Mallampati grade and thyromental distance has been found to have the highest predictive value [14]. However in many cases the ICU patient is unable able to cooperate in the performance of bedside tests. Likewise certain imaging modalities are not practicable but, in some cases, may have been done prior to arrival in the ICU. Abnormal neck anatomy may make surgical rescue techniques more difficult.

Table 17.1. Predictors of difficult intubation and associated tests.

Limited mouth opening	**Limited atlanto-axial (AA) extension**	**Narrowed airway**
Inter-incisor gap < 3 cm	Reduced 'head-nodding'	Difficulty in breathing lying supine. Stridor
Limited jaw protrusion (grades B and C)	*Thyromental distance < 6 cm *Sternomental distance < 12 cm	Nasendoscopy
Limited visibility of uvula (Mallampati grades III and IV)	Absent C1–C2 gap or C0–C1 gap on cervical spine X-ray (lateral, in flexion)	Chest X-ray, computed tomography or magnetic resonance imaging scan

* Indirect measure of atlanto-axial extension.

17.2.1 *Airway equipment and monitoring*

There is a vast array of equipment that is available. It is best to include few familiar items on an airway trolley that relate to the knowledge, training and experience of personnel. Each ICU should develop its own specific trolley checked and stocked on a regular basis. A flexible fibrescope should be available. Patients will require full monitoring including electrocardiogram, pulse-oximetry, arterial pressure and capnography, the latter now considered essential [2]. Suction equipment must be immediately available.

17.3 Conduct of Endotracheal Intubation

Patients in the ICU are often at high risk for aspiration as they may have been fed enterally, have an ileus or a distended abdomen. A rapid-sequence induction (RSI) should be performed in patients at risk of aspiration. If a nasogastric tube is in place this should be aspirated and left *in situ* [15].

17.3.1 *Rapid-sequence induction (RSI)*

The patient should be pre-oxygenated. The efficacy of traditional pre-oxygenation over fast-track oxygenation is supported in the literature [16]. Extending the period of pre-oxygenation from four to eight minutes does not usefully increase the partial pressure of oxygen (PaO_2) in arterial blood in critically ill patients [17]. Although a target end-tidal O_2 of 0.9 is ideal, in some patients baseline PaO_2 may remain; therefore, the risk of severe hypoxemia during intubation is significant. During pre-oxygenation the mask should fit tightly on the face and the oxygen flow should be high (> 10 l/minute). If the patient is receiving continuous positive airway pressure (CPAP) this should be left *in situ* and the inspired oxygen increased to 100%. In obese patients the use of a 25° head-up position during pre-oxygenation increases PaO_2 and prolongs the time to desaturation during apnoea. RSI should entail the application of cricoid pressure 10 N (equivalent to 1 kg) whilst awake and the ability to increase this to 30 N as consciousness is lost using a single-handed technique [18]. In patients with acute lung injury a recruitment manoeuvre applied directly after intubation reduces the incidence of hypoxemia [19].

17.3.2 *Confirmation of endotracheal intubation*

All the clinical signs of successful intubation may be mimicked with oesophageal intubation. On visual confirmation the tube is seen on direct laryngoscopy to lie within the vocal cords or at least superior to the interarytenoid groove. Capnography is the gold standard. The presence of at least six successive CO_2 traces will confirm correct placement.

17.3.3 *Oral or nasal intubation*

The oral route is the usual route. The nasal route offers a more stable position, is better tolerated and offers better oral hygiene. However, it necessitates the use of a smaller diameter tube and may result in nasal haemorrhage, mucosal ulceration, sinus infection and bacteraemia and is contraindicated in the presence of skull-base fracture.

17.3.4 *Endotracheal tube size, length and cuff pressure*

The standard size tube is an internal diameter of 7–8 mm and 8–9 mm in the average female and male patient, respectively. Tubes with larger diameters facilitate tracheobronchial toilet. Uncut tracheal tubes allow a degree of flexibility in the depth of insertion and will accommodate facial swelling (e.g. burns, trauma or anaphylactoid oedema) at the risk of endobronchial intubation. The position of the endotracheal tube at the incisors should be noted and should be 21 cm and 23 cm in the average female and male patient, respectively [20]. The position tip of the tube is confirmed on chest X-ray and should lie between 3 and 5 cm above the carina, i.e. the middle third of the trachea at the level of thoracic vertebrae T3–T4 with the head in the neutral position [21]. The minimal cuff inflation pressure should be used to produce a seal, thereby reducing tracheal mucosal injury [22].

17.3.5 *Exchanging endotracheal tubes*

The most common reason to change an endotracheal tube is the result of cuff leakage or partial occlusion by insipissated secretions. This task should not be underestimated. When any degree of difficulty is anticipated the tube should be exchanged over a bougie or an airway exchange

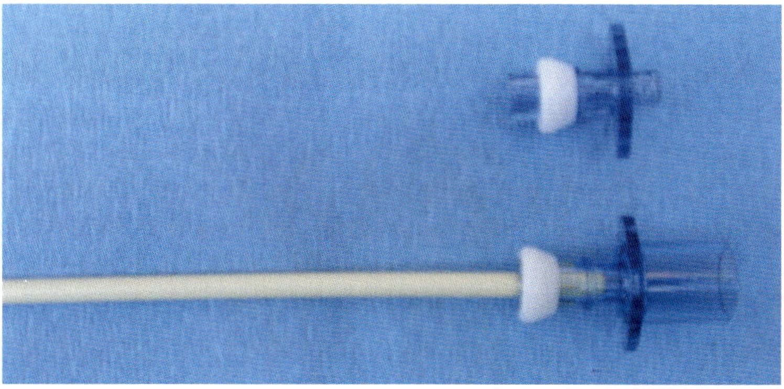

Figure 17.1. Airway exchange catheter with 15 mm connector (below) and Rapi-fit® connector (above).

catheter (Cook Medical®). The catheter is available with two snap-on connectors (Fig. 17.1), a 15 mm connector to provide oxygen by insufflation and a luer-lock Rapi-fit® connector for jet ventilation.

17.4 Induction of Anaesthesia and Choice of Drugs

17.4.1 *Induction agents*

Etomidate is useful in patients who are cardiovascularly unstable although it may inhibit the adrenal axis for at least 24 hours after a single dose [23]. If used, steroid supplementation should be considered. Etomidate should be avoided in patients with septic shock [24]. The use of etomidate has declined in ICU practice. Ketamine, a much underused induction agent, remains an excellent option in cardiovascularly unstable patients, including those with a head injury [25]. Midazolam has a slow response time and a risk of inadequate anaesthesia. Propofol may be used but can result in significant hypotension. Sodium thiopentone has a predictable action, a rapid onset and causes less hypotension than propofol. Opioid-based induction (e.g. fentanyl) allows reduced dosage of induction agents and is ideal in patients who may become cardiovascularly unstable. Titrated dosages of vasopressor (e.g. metaraminol) may offset the vasodilatory and cardiopressant effects of induction agents.

17.4.2 *Muscle-relaxants*

RSI is frequently performed in the critically ill patient. Suxamethonium is the usual drug of choice but has a poor side-effect profile, an alternative is rocuronium if intubation is predicted to be easy. A dose of 0.6 mg/kg can provide intubating conditions within 60 to 90 seconds, and a dose of 1 mg/kg provides conditions comparable to suxamethonium [26,27]. Rocuronium neuromuscular blockade can now be reversed with Sugammadex [28,29]. If RSI is not considered necessary other agents ,such as vecuronium (0.1 mg/kg) or atracurium (0.6 mg/kg), produce intubating conditions within two to three minutes, but it may be prudent to check that the patient can be ventilated by 'bag and mask' prior to administration of the drug.

17.5 Complications of Endotracheal Intubation

Complications include failure to intubate, maintenance of oxygenation, aspiration and localised trauma. Haemodynamic instability should be anticipated after induction of anaesthesia. Hypotension is common, hypovolaemia and the initiation of positive-pressure ventilation with consequent deleterious effects on venous return may aggravate this and can lead to cardiac arrest. Intravenous fluids, vasopressors and inotropic support may become necessary and should be available to be used in unstable patients.

17.6 Unanticipated Failed Intubation

The incidence of difficult intubation in critically ill patients is considered to be 8–10% [1,30], twice as likely as for patients scheduled to undergo general anaesthesia in the operating room. Algorithms for the unanticipated difficult intubation in patients presenting for general anaesthesia [31] have become established and can generally be applied to the ICU situation, although waking the patient is not usually an option.

After an initial failed attempt, senior assistance should be summoned. Further attempts at intubation should only occur after re-oxygenation. Persistent attempts may lead to airway oedema. If difficulty persists a laryngeal mask airway (LMA™) should be inserted. If oxygenation and ventilation are satisfactory and the risk of aspiration low, the LMA™ can be used as a conduit for intubation. If ventilation is difficult using the LMA™ due to leakage of gas, the LMA ProSeal™ or LMA Supreme™ are alternatives. These second-generation supraglotic devices are designed with an oesophageal drainage tube and thus reduce the risk of aspiration. If there is difficulty with ventilation and oxygenation, face mask ventilation should be reinstituted.

17.6.1 *Intubation via the laryngeal mask airway (LMA™)*

The intubating LMA (iLMA™) is the most successful blind intubation technique. Success on the first attempt has been reported as 75% [32]. Using the iLMA™ and a flexible fibrescope success is as high as 95% [33]. A 4 mm fibrescope can be passed through an Aintree intubation catheter (Cook Medical®) and then through a iLMA™ (Fig. 17.2). The fibrescope and iLMA™ are removed, leaving the catheter *in situ* for railroading a tracheal tube [34].

17.6.2 *Alternative laryngoscopy techniques*

In experienced hands a flexible fibrescope or laryngoscopes which does not rely on the alignment of the oral, pharyngeal and laryngeal axis can be

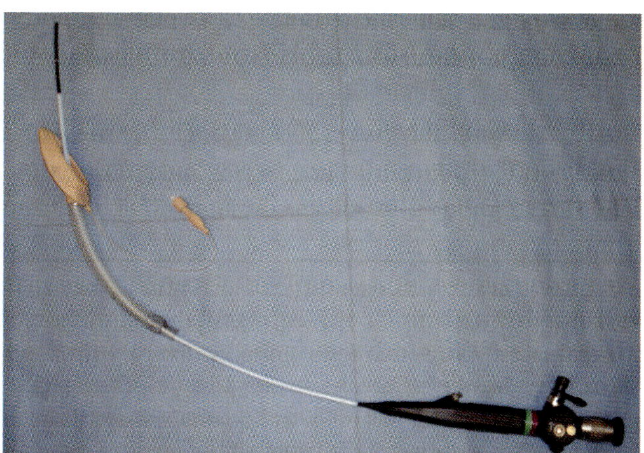

Figure 17.2. Fibrescope loaded with Aintree catheter passed through LMA™.

used. There are a number of video-laryngoscopes that are now available; the GlideScope® is popular in the author's institution. However the presence of blood, secretions and, in the case of the video-laryngoscope, limitation of mouth opening and a small oral cavity, may make these techniques more difficult in the ICU setting.

17.6.3 *Percutaneous tracheostomy*

In the situation where intubation by a senior clinician in the ICU has failed and the airway is satisfactorily controlled with a LMA™, an immediate percutaneous tracheostomy can be considered [35].

17.7 'Can't Intubate, Can't Ventilate' (CICV) Scenario

It is rare to encounter a CICV scenario during elective anaesthesia [36]. However, the process of tracheal intubation in the ICU is more hazardous [1,2,37]. The development of severe hypoxemia is an indication for immediate cricothyroidotomy. The latter is quicker than emergency tracheostomy. The cricothyroid membrane is located 1 cm below the vocal cords. It is superficial, easily located and relatively avascular and has a lower complication rate.

There are three types of cricothyroidotomy techniques:

- Small cannula devices (2–3 mm internal diameter (ID)).
- Large-bore device (4 mm ID or larger).
- Surgical cricothyroidotomy (6 mm ID tracheostomy or endotracheal tube).

17.7.1 *Small cannula devices*

Intravenous cannulae that are prone to kinking are not recommended. The 13 g Ravussin (VBM Medizintechnik, Germany) is a kink-resistant cannula (Fig. 17.3). It requires a high-pressure device (200–400 kPa) such as a Sanders injector or Manujet III (VBM) (Fig. 17.4) to ventilate the patient. Upper airway patency is essential to allow exhalation and avoid barotrauma.

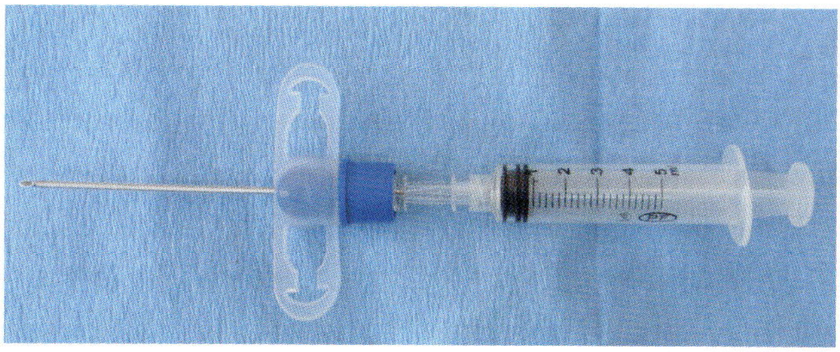

Figure 17.3. Ravussin (VBM) cannulae.

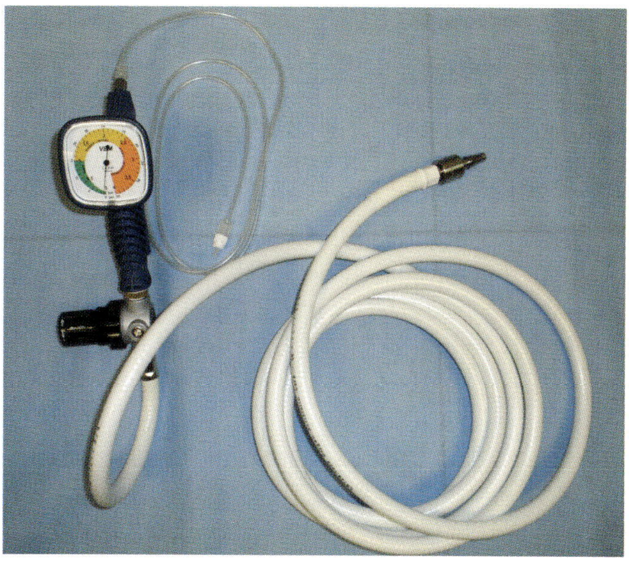

Figure 17.4. Manujet III (VBM).

Technique:

- Position patient (head and neck extended) and identify landmarks.
- Immobilise cricoid between thumb and middle finger of non-dominant hand.
- Puncture lower border of cricothyroid membrane with a jet cannula attached to a 5 ml syringe whilst applying continuous negative pressure.
- Advance cannula in a 45° caudad direction.
- Confirm cannula position by aspirating air into syringe (if time permits partially filled with saline).

- Attach ventilation system to a jet cannula.
- Ensure clear upper airway, single jet initially — verify deflation .
- Commence ventilation — ensure ventilation of lungs and exhalation through upper airway after each breath (watch and palpate rise and fall of chest).
- If ventilation fails, or surgical emphysema develops convert immediately to surgical cricothyroidotomy.

The use of transtracheal jet ventilation has been reported in 23 patients in respiratory failure in a CICV situation in the ICU [37].

17.7.2 *Large-bore devices*

Large-bore devices are designed to allow emergency oxygenation and ventilation through the cricothyroid membrane. With a 4 mm device passive exhalation of 500 ml takes 4 seconds, limiting ventilatory frequency to 10–12 respirations per minute [38]. The Quicktrach II (VBM) is a cuffed 4 mm ID cannula-over-needle device (Fig. 17.5) and the Melker (Cook Medical®) device is a Seldinger (wire-guided) cricothroidotomy airway, the cuffed version is 5 mm ID (Fig. 17.6). There is a learning curve to the use of these devices [39]. In the field, the British Army initially use the Quicktrach II and then convert to the Melker when the patient is well oxygenated [40]. Uncuffed devices leave the airway unprotected and increase the risk of gastric aspiration. Some of the gas will escape through the upper airway and ventilation may be suboptimal. The widely available Portex Mini-Trach® II is a 4 mm ID uncuffed airway designed for tracheobronchial suction and not for emergency ventilation.

17.7.3 *Surgical cricothyroidotomy*

Surgical cricothyroidotomy provides a more definitive airway and is the technique of choice should other methods fail. Reported complication rate can be as high as

40%, including 13% and 6% incidences of misplacement and severe bleeding, respectively [41].

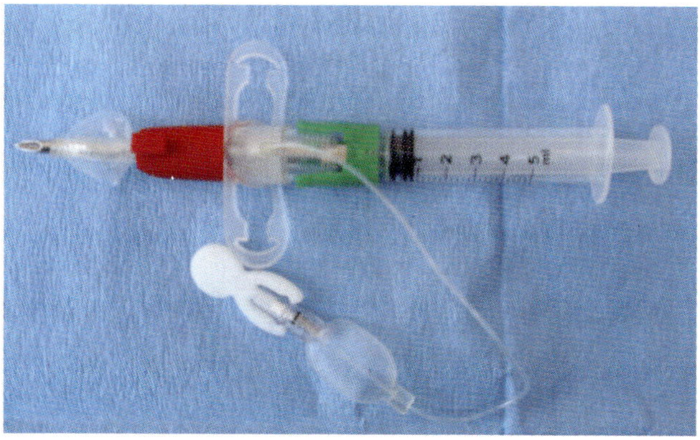

Figure 17.5. Quicktrach II (VBM).

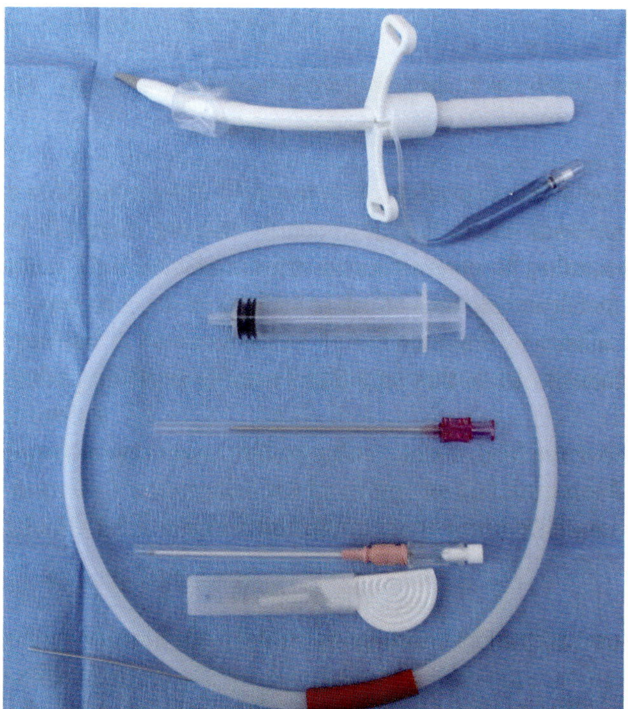

Figure 17.6. Melker cricothyroidotomy set.

Technique [42]:

- Position patient, identify cricothyroid membrane and imobilise trachea.
- Make a horizontal stab incision through skin and membrane (No. 20 scalpel blade). Leave blade *in situ.*
- Perform caudal and ventral traction on cricoid cartilage with tracheal hook and remove blade.
- Insert tube and inflate cuff (6 mm ID tracheostomy tube or endotracheal tube).

A tube loaded over a bougie may ease insertion. Most cases of emergency cricothyroidotomy should proceed to formal dissection tracheostomy in theatre.

17.8 Anticipated Difficult Intubation

17.8.1 *Fibreoptic intubation*

This is the gold standard when direct laryngoscopy is considered difficult [43,44]. However, it may fail if there are excessive secretions or bleeding and is contraindicated in an uncooperative patient, a history of allergy to local anaesthetics and should be used with extreme caution in severe airway obstruction. Complete airway obstruction has been reported secondary to the irritant effects of local anaesthetic [45,46].

The best approach will be with the patient sitting and the operator facing the patent. The nasal route is easier. The oral route requires an intubating airway as a guide [47] (e.g. Berman airway, Vital Signs, USA). Sedation should be avoided if there is airway obstruction.

Technique:

- Premedicate with glycopyrrolate (5 μg/kg intravenously 10 to 15 minutes prior).
- Spray lignocaine (5%) phenylephrine (0.5%) to nasal cavity.
- Nebulise 4–6 ml 4% lignocaine to airway.
- Administer oxygen by face mask.
- Apply lubricant over cuff and entrance to nasal cavity.

- Load a 6 mm ID reinforced endotracheal tube over fibrescope.
- Advance fibrescope through the nasal cavity, identifying the nasal turbinates, soft palate, epiglottis, vocal cords and tracheal rings. If the view becomes obscured wait before advancing until it returns, or withdraw fibrescope until a recognisable structure is identified.
- Rotate tube whilst advancing (i.e. spin through many 360° turns).
- Ensure tracheal rings and carina are visible through fibrescope following intubation.

Alternatively, a 'spray as you go' technique is popular but coughing can be a problem [48]. The smaller diameter tube is better tolerated in unsedated patients. If the nasal passage is narrow it can be dilated with a nasopharyngeal airway or the oral route can be used.

17.9 Special Consideration — 'The Narrowed Airway'

The patient presenting with a narrowed airway presents the most difficult situation. Common causes include tumour, neck haematoma (trauma, post-surgical), infection (cellulitis, retropharyngeal abscess, epiglottitis) and oedema (angioedema, burns). Stridor at rest implies airway narrowing of at least 50%. Heliox (21% oxygen and 79% helium) will reduce the work of breathing [49] and supplementary oxygen will be necessary. Airway oedema may be reduced using nebulised adrenaline (3–5 ml 1:1000) [50]. A nasendoscopy should be performed to assess the upper airway. A computed tomography (CT) or magnetic resonance imaging (MRI) scan will reveal the entire length of the airway i.e. teeth to carina. It will show the lower extent of subglottic tumours and the risk of an incision for a surgical airway entering a tumour. It will allow the narrowest portion of the trachea to be measured. Imaging is, however, contraindicated in acute critical airway narrowing. Once a full airway assessment is done, and discussed with a senior ear nose and throat surgeon, a plan to secure the airway should be made on the basis of the following:

- The type of lesion and severity of the obstruction.
- The anatomical level is the obstruction (supraglottic, subglottic, lower trachea).
- The diameter of the trachea.

- The accessibility of the airway for surgical or fibreoptic access.
- The risk of complete airway obstruction if anaesthetised or if the airway is manipulated if awake.

A secondary and tertiary plan should be made in case the first fails. The back-up plan should be in place and include a surgical airway. The patient should be transferred to the operating theatre. A senior ear, nose and throat (ENT) surgeon should be present and scrubbed. The surgical instrument pack for tracheostomy should be open, checked and ready to use.

17.9.1 *Techniques for securing the 'narrowed airway'*

A number of techniques have been described but all have limitations.

17.9.1.1 *Awake fibreoptic intubation*

This is considered for upper and lower airway obstruction, the patient maintaining their own airway and the endoscopist negotiating the obstruction. However, with critical airway narrowing there may be problems in advancing the endotracheal tube and a risk of complete airway obstruction [51].

17.9.1.2 *Inhalational anaesthesia.*

Sevoflurane inhalational anaesthesia is considered for upper and lower airway obstruction. If obstruction worsens the plane of anaesthesia lightens. However, induction is slow and depth of anaesthesia may be difficult to judge or not attained. A change to halothane if available may be necessary [51]. With loss of upper airway muscle-tone total airway obstruction may occur especially when the patient lies supine. In the initial intubation attempt a narrow, uncut tube should be prepared and loaded on a bougie (e.g. 31 cm Mallincrodt® microlaryngoscopy tube (MLT) 5 or 6 mm ID).

17.9.1.3 *Use of a rigid bronchoscope*

In patients in whom the passage of a tracheal tube is difficult a rigid bronchoscope may help [52]. It will allow jet ventilation [53] and can be used to pass an airway exchange catheter or bougie allowing a tracheal tube to be railroaded [54]. In selected cases of tracheobronchial tumours a rigid bronchoscope may be inserted using a standard intravenous induction technique [55]. It can be a life-saving technique in extensive tracheobronchial lesions [56] and when there is external tracheal compression. For the latter, a tracheal stent can be passed via the bronchoscope. However, insertion of the bronchoscope may be technically difficult in patients with limited mouth opening and restricted cervical spine movements.

17.9.1.4 *Cricothyroidotomy (small cannula, large-bore or surgical)*

These can be used if the initial intubation plan fails. Small cannula cricothyroidotomy can also be done prophylactically in an anticipated difficult airway [57–59].

Jet ventilation may be difficult in severe airway obstruction due to problems with exhalation in which case there is a risk of barotrauma [60]. If cannula cricothyroidotomy is attempted and fails then a surgical cricothyroidotomy should be performed.

17.9.1.5 *Tracheostomy under local anaesthesia*

In patients with marked upper airway obstruction a surgical tracheostomy should be considered. However this requires optimal positioning and will be difficult if the anatomy is difficult. Emergency percutaneous tracheostomy is an option [61–63] but should only be undertaken by an experienced practitioner. It would seem prudent to stabilise the patient with a cricothyroidotomy and then proceed semi-electively with the tracheostomy using a wire guided single-dilatational technique. For lower tracheal lesions it essential to use an extended-length tracheostomy tube and to ensure that the tip of tube extends beyond the obstruction.

17.9.1.6 *Cardiopulmonary bypass*

For extensive tracheobronchial lesions and anterior mediastinal masses facilities for cardiopulmonary bypass should be available [65–67].

When the narrowing exceeds 50% it may be prudent to cannulate the femoral vessels under local anaesthesia, in readiness for cardiopulmonary bypass.

17.10 Extubation

In the more straightforward patient extubation can be protocol-driven, in other patients a trial of extubation may be necessary and the patient extubated directly to non-invasive ventilation or CPAP. Prolonged translaryngeal intubation may lead to subglottic oedema [68]. Dexamethasone given regularly prior to extubation may reduce oedema and reintubation rates [67,68]. In patients who have been intubated for upper airway obstruction, the development of a cuff leak is a useful sign. In high-risk patients the procedure should be performed in the operating theatre with an ENT surgeon in attendance. An airway exchange catheter or a flexible bronchoscope can be used as a conduit for extubation.

17.11 Tracheostomy

Tracheostomy is one of the oldest surgical procedures and is depicted in Egyptian engravings dated to 3600 BC. Asclepiades of Persia was credited as the first person to perform a tracheostomy in 100 BC. Antonio Musa Brassavola, an Italian physician, performed the first documented case of a successful tracheostomy in 1546 on a patient with tonsillar obstruction. Trachesotomies were originally used for the emergency treatment of upper airway obstruction. The former President of the USA, George Washington, died of upper airway obstruction. His physician was reluctant to perform his first tracheostomy on a person of Washington's stature.

17.11.1 *Indications*

The most common indication is to aid weaning from mechanical ventilation (Table 17.2)

Table 17.2. Indications for tracheostomy.

Weaning from intermittent positive-pressure ventilation	Avoidance of injury from prolonged intubation, reduced dead space and resistance, reduced sedation. Patient comfort and cooperation, aids speech and swallowing.
Airway protection	Bulbar palsy
Bronchial toilet	Excessive secretions, inadequate cough.
Airway maintenance	Upper airway obstruction, intubation and extubation difficulties, reduced level of consciousness.

17.11.2 *Timing*

If ventilation is still required at 10 to 14 days a tracheostomy is usually performed. The optimal timing of tracheostomy is unknown. There is a current trend towards earlier tracheostomy to facilitate weaning [69]. A large multicentre trial of early versus late tracheostomy in 2009 reported a reduced requirement of sedation in the early group but no differences in mortality [70].

17.11.3 *Complications*

A tracheostomy is not without risk. Tracheostomy displacement and blockage have been identified as a serious cause of airway-related morbidity and mortality in the ICU [2]. The development of algorithms may reduce the incidence of complications associated with tracheostomies [2].

In general terms, complications may be classified as immediate, early or late:

Immediate complications (<24 hours):

- Hypoxemia, airway obstruction (tip against carina or tracheal wall), decreased minute volume, loss of positive end-expiratory pressure (PEEP).
- Misplacement, pre-tracheal tissue, right main bronchus.
- Haemorrhage, subcutaneous vessels, anterior neck vessels, thyroid vessels.

- Localised injury e.g. oesophagus, recurrent laryngeal nerve.
- Pneumothorax, pneumomediastinum, surgical emphysema.

Early complications (one to seven days):

- Malposition or displacement.
- Obstruction.
- Stoma Infection.

Late complications (>seven days):

- Haemorrhage — tracheoinnominate fistula.
- Tracheoesophageal fistula.
- Tracheomalacia, tracheal stenosis.
- Granulation tissue and scarring.
- Delayed healing of stoma.
- Chronic speech and swallowing deficits.

17.11.4 *Percutaneous or open surgical?*

Although it was first described by an Italian surgeon named Sanctorio Sanctorius in 1626, the American surgeon Pasqual Ciaglia modified and popularised the percutaneous technique in 1985 [71]. The ideal technique of tracheostomy insertion remains undetermined. Percutaneous tracheostomy at the bedside in the ICU is increasingly popular. Compared with the open surgical procedure, the technique is quicker, at least as safe [72,73] and may be associated with reduced rates of infection and bleeding, although the incidence of tracheal ring fracture and posterior wall damage may be higher [74,75]. Major bleeding during the procedure may necessitate the involvement of the surgical team. Ciagalia described an incision site between the cricoid cartilage and the first tracheal ring, this was associated with a higher incidence of tracheal stenosis. Low insertion sites are technically more difficult, increase the risk of erosion of the great vessel, are more uncomfortable and cause difficulty in swallowing.

17.11.5 *Caution and contraindications*

In the absence of airway obstruction the only contraindications to a tracheostomy are severe local sepsis or uncontrollable coagulopathy. Relative cautions and contraindications to percutaneous tracheostomy include:

- Moderate coagulopathy — ensure international normalised ratio <1.5, activated partial thromboplastin time <1.5, platelets >100 (10^9/l).
- Difficult anatomy — e.g. tracheal or thyroid pathology, morbid obesity, restricted neck mobility.
- Difficult gas exchange — e.g. fraction of inspired oxygen (FiO_2) >0.6 and PEEP > 10.
- Cardiovascular instability.
- Proximity to site of recent surgery.

17.11.6 *Percutaneous tracheostomy*

Informed consent should be obtained from the patient or next of kin. Anticoagulation should be discontinued and nasogastric feeding should be stopped a minimum of six hours prior to the procedure. An ultrasound scan of the neck is of value in identifying blood vessels, thyroid and tracheal rings [76]. Bronchoscopic visualisation is advantageous and reduces the risk of complications. It will confirm midline tracheal cannulation, that the tracheostomy tube is correctly sited and that there is no active bleeding. Problems associated with bronchoscopy include impairment of ventilation and damage to the bronchoscope during cannulation. Currently the single-dilator (Fig. 17.7) technique [77] is the most popular in the UK.

Technique (modified from [78]):

Anaesthetic sequence:

- Aspirate nasogastric tube.
- Pre-oxygenate.
- Induce anaesthesia (fentanyl and propofol), paralyse and maintain anaesthesia with a propofol infusion.
- Ventilate with 100% oxygen and adequate PEEP.

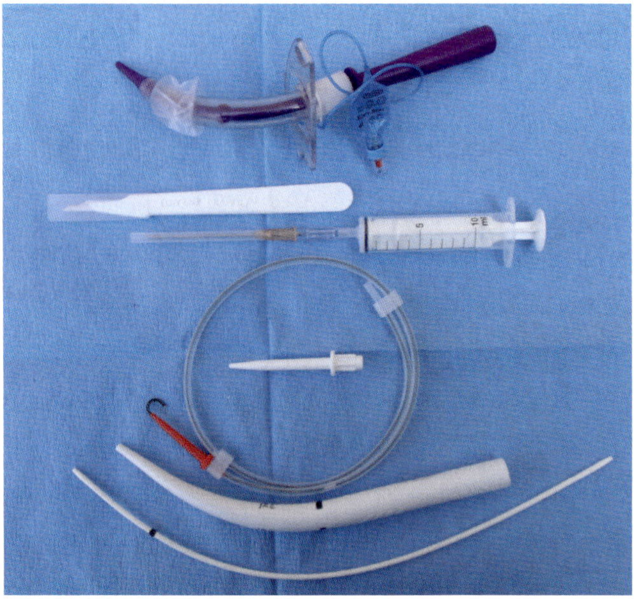

Figure 17.7. Single-dilator tracheostomy set.

- Optimise head position i.e. neck-extension and slightly head-up (to reduce venous bleeding).
- Direct laryngoscopy — aspirate secretions in pharynx and suction trachea, assess difficulty of re-intubation.
- Retract tracheal tube so that the cuff lies just below the vocal cords i.e. the tip is at the level of cricoid cartilage or use LMA™ [79].
- Flexible bronchoscopy — check position of the tip of the tracheal tube and tracheal cannulation; above tracheostomy tube to ensure that the cuff lies within lumen of trachea and through the tracheostomy to ensure no bleeding distally.

Operator sequence:

- Performed under strict asepsis — gloves, gown, mask and eye protection.
- Skin disinfection — 2% chlorhexidine or iodine.
- Apply surgical drapes — ensure anaesthetist has access to airway.
- Check kit correctly laid out ready for use.

- Identify site of insertion, ideally thoracic vertebrae T2–3 (in a normal neck this is usually midway between cricoid cartilage and suprasternal notch).
- Infiltration with lignocaine (2%) with adrenaline 1:200000.
- Superficial transverse skin incision (1–1.5 cm) and blunt dissection of subcutaneous tissue with forceps.
- Needle insertion — a 5 ml syringe with saline with continuous negative pressure, in the midline aiming posterior and slightly caudad. Once the trachea is cannulated air is entrained and the plastic cannula advanced into the trachea followed by the guide-wire. Visualised by bronchoscopy.
- Dilate trachea using 4.5 cm 14 gauge dilator over wire and then remove.
- Insert guiding catheter over wire.
- Advance single dilator over guiding catheter dilating tracheal aperture.
- Remove tracheal dilator and advance tracheostomy tube (loaded onto loading catheter).
- Remove loading catheter, guiding catheter and wire and confirm tracheostomy tube placement and then inflate cuff and connect to the ventilator.

17.11.7 *Types of tracheostomy tube*

Traditionally a single-lumen cuffed tracheostomy tube is used initially. Some patients may be weaned directly from this tube. However in patients in whom weaning is anticipated to be prolonged a double-cannula tube is usually inserted following the acute illness. This aids tracheostomy weaning and is a necessity for the ward. The obturator should be kept at the bedside in the event that reinsertion of the tracheostomy is necessary.

Double- cannula tubes are supplied with an inner tube that can be removed independently of the outer tube. This allows cleaning and reduces the incidence of occlusion. The work of breathing, however, is increased. Some are designed such that the inner tube must be *in situ* to allow connection to 15 mm ventilator tubing. The outer tube of a double-cannula tube may be fenestrated or unfenestrated (Fig. 17.8). With a fenestrated tube *in situ* and the cuff deflated there is maximal flow through the larynx

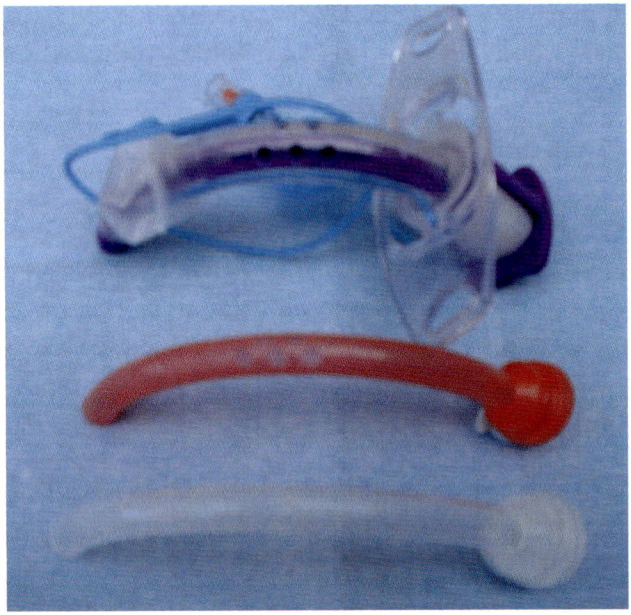

Figure 17.8. Fenestrated outer tube (top) of a double cannula tracheostomy tube. Fenestrated (middle) and unfenestrated (bottom) inner tubes.

and this encourages speech. It also allows assessment of the normal route of air-passage prior to decannulation. If positive-pressure ventilation is required the unfenestrated inner tube must be used to eliminate air leakage. However the risk of surgical emphysema remains [80]. Single- and multiple-fenestrated tubes are available.

Adjustable flange tubes (Fig. 17.9) have a moveable flange that allows adjustment of the distance from the skin surface to the tracheostomy. They are useful where there is a long skin to trachea distance. Some tubes are reinforced, which precludes their use with MRI. Double-cannula lumen tubes with a proximal extension for the 'deep-trachea' and distal extension for a narrowed upper trachea (Fig. 17.10) have become available and are useful in patients likely to need a tube for a more prolonged period.

Uncuffed tubes are reserved for patients requiring long-term tracheostomy who have reasonable bulbar function. Custom-made tubes in silicone or silver are available for long-term or permanent tracheostomy use.

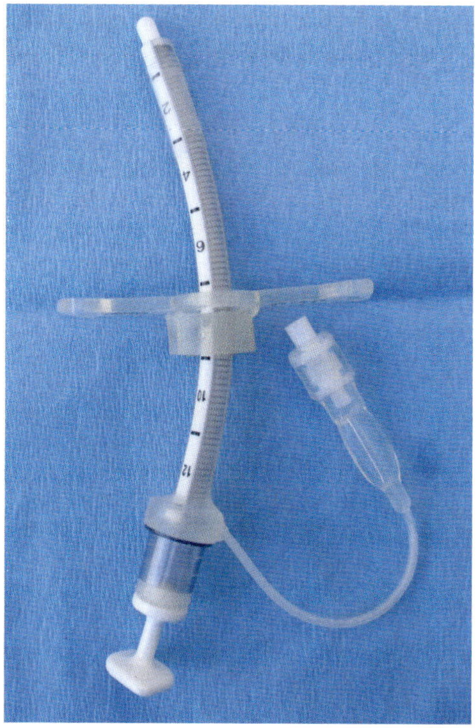

Figure 17.9. Reinforced adjustable flange tube.

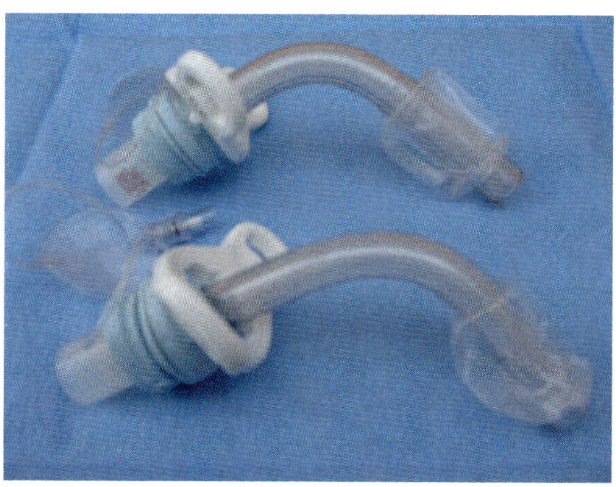

Figure 17.10. Double cannula trachestomy tubes, distal extension (above) and proximal extension (below).

17.11.8 *Tracheostomy tube size, cuff pressure and humidification*

There is usually a compromise between choosing a large ID tube that will reduce the work of breathing and allow easier tracheobronchial toilet and the need to limit the ID to allow airflow through the upper trachea on cuff deflation.

The tracheostomy cuff does not eliminate the risk of aspiration. A recent development is the Portex Blue Line Ultra Suctionaid® tracheostomy tube which incorporates an additional posterior lumen with an opening above the cuff. The cuff is shaped such that pooling of secretions occurs around the opening, thus allowing aspiration of subglottic secretion.

The cuff pressure should be monitored regularly and not exceed 25 cm H_2O [81]. Excessive cuff pressure may be the result of over-inflation due to a small or malpositioned tube. Recent developments include a cuff pressure monitor (Portex Pressure Easy®) that continuously monitors cuff pressure. It has an auto-feedback feature that ensures proper sealing at peak inspiratory pressure. The Bivona® is a foam-cuff tracheostomy tube (Fig. 17.11). The cuff is deflated on insertion and inflates at atmospheric pressure, conforming to the trachea and potentially reducing mucosal injury.

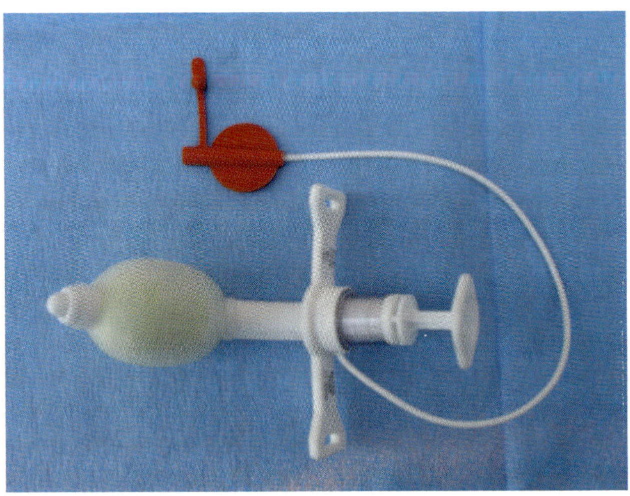

Figure 17.11. Bivona® trachesotomy tube.

The tracheostomy cuff should be deflated to promote swallowing, when a speaking valve or decannulation cap is *in situ*. Humidification is essential to reduce the incidence of tube occlusion. Attention should be paid to the patient's overall state of hydration. The use of a heated hot-water humidifier supplemented with a 0.9% N saline nebuliser and nebulised N-acetylcysteine in ventilated patients with thick secretions is often used. In self-ventilating patents on low O_2 requirements a HME is usually adequate.

17.11.9 *Tracheotomy tube change*

The initial tracheostomy tube change should not be within 72 hours following surgical tracheostomy and not before three to five days (ideally seven to ten days) following a percutaneous tracheostomy. This is because failure to re-cannulate or creation of a false passage may occur. Changing the tube over a bougie or airway exchange catheter is best and a fibrescope will provide confirmation. If the tube change is problematic the patient should be re-intubated by mouth or nose. At ten days the stoma tract is well formed and changing the tube is straightforward. Single-lumen tracheostomy tubes should be changed every 7–14 days and a double-cannula tube should not remain in longer than 30 days.

17.11.10 *Swallowing, weaning and decannulation*

The vast majority of patients are weaned and decannulated once their clinical condition improves. Absolute requirements include patent upper airway, spontaneous cough and ability to swallow secretions. A multidisciplinary team approach improves success. The 'blue dye' test assesses the ability to swallow secretions, however, sensitivity and specificity are low [82]. Assessment by speech and language therapists, the use of videofluroscopy and review by an ENT surgeon in difficult cases is useful.

The standard practice is to deflate the cuff when feeding is attempted. Oral intake may be possible with an inflated or partially inflated cuff but this usually makes swallowing more difficult as a result of oesophageal compression increasing the risk of aspiration. A number of centres advocate feeding trials. This usually involves sips of sterile water and if tolerated without coughing or desaturation or signs of aspiration then thickened fluids may be introduced followed by a soft diet. There is a more modern school of thought which advocates introduction of thickened fluids and soft diet before water.

A number of patients can be weaned simply by deflating the cuff or changing to a smaller or uncuffed tube. Others will require downsizing and the use of a fenestrated tube. The smaller tube will allow more air to pass around the tube on cuff deflation and improves swallowing. Prior to weaning, ventilator dependency and oxygen requirements should be assessed. $FiO_2 > 0.4$, PEEP > 5 cm H_2O and pressure support > 10 cm will negate the use of cuff deflation. In patients with low requirements the cuff is deflated for progressively increasing periods during the day. Laryngeal function is improved by the introduction of a one-way speaking valve. This allows air to be entrained through the tracheostomy tube during inspiration and during expiration it forces air through the vocal cords, thus allowing phonation. Once the cuff deflation period has increased to 24 hours the trachesotomy tube is 'capped off' for at least 12 hours prior to decannulation. Once decannulated the patient should be observed for signs of respiratory distress.

17.12 Non-Invasive Ventilation (NIV)

NIV continues to be developed beyond its traditional use in patients with chronic pulmonary disease presenting with respiratory failure. Early use of NIV may reduce the 'need to intubate' in acute hypoxemic respiratory failure [83] and improves outcome in immunocompromised patients requiring ventilation [84]. NIV has use has been extended to facilitate weaning [85]. It is relatively contraindicated in patients with excessive secretions, high-risk of gastric aspiration or refractory hypoxemia and in patients with reduced level of consciousness.

17.13 Lung Isolation Techniques

Lung isolation techniques may be used to protect one lung from possible contamination from the other diseased lung such as in haemorrhage or pus. The usual technique is to insert a double-lumen endoobronchial tube. Alternatively a bronchus-blocker may be inserted with the aid of a fibrescope to isolate a lung or lobe. In the emergency situation a single lumen tube can be advanced into one lung (e.g. MLT). Independent lung ventilation is used in the management of a bronchopleural fistula. The benefit of a double-lumen tube over a single-lumen tube should be carefully balanced against the risk of losing control of the airway. This is particularly the case in patients dependent on a high-inspired oxygen concentration and PEEP, such as in the case of a severe pneumonia confined to one lung.

17.14 Clinical Case

An elderly man was admitted as an emergency having noticed his tongue had become swollen. His past medical history included hypertension for which he took lisinopril. He was sitting upright, unable to lie down and drooling saliva. There was marked swelling of his tongue. He had difficulty in speaking but there was no stridor. Mallampati was graded IV. He had a 'bull-shaped' neck. A nasendoscopy performed revealed marked supraglottic oedema. He was transferred to the operating theatre. An experienced ENT surgeon and surgical scrub-team were present.

The cricothyroid membrane was infiltrated with lignocaine (2%) adrenaline 1:200000. A jet-ventilation cannula was made ready for use with a Manujet III (VBM) connected to a high-pressure source. The patient's nasal cavity was anaesthetised with lignocaine and phenylephrine and his airway anaesthetised with nebulised lignocaine. A fibrescope loaded with a 6 mm ID flexometallic endotracheal tube was passed through the nose and advanced beyond the vocal cords and the tracheal tube was railroaded into the distal trachea. No sedation was used. A CT scan showed extensive oedema and inflammatory tissue extending from the level of the hyoid bone to the distal trachea (Fig. 17.12), but not beyond the tip of the endotracheal tube. A repeat CT scan on day nine showed some resolution of inflammatory tissue and the tube was changed to an 8.0 mm ID oral tube in the operating theatre. He was extubated on day 11. All investigations including immunology were negative.

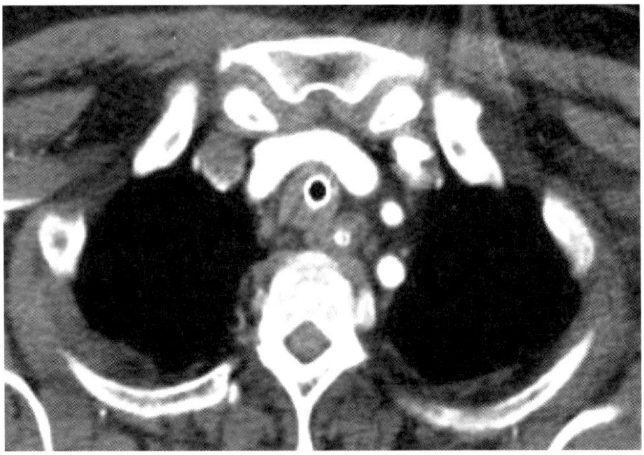

Figure 17.12. CT scan of chest.

17.14.1 *Discussion*

In view of the rapid progression of symptoms it was necessary to secure the airway. As the airway narrowing was judged not to be critical, a fibre-optic intubation was planned with a cricothyroidotomy back-up plan. Inhalational induction was considered as a difficult option given the presenting anatomical features. Fibreoptic intubation allowed the tip of the endotracheal tube to be placed beyond the narrowing. A formal tracheostomy was not performed as it was considered that the oedema would be self-limiting. The cause of his airway obstruction was attributed to lisinopril [86,87].

References

[1] Schwartz, D.E., Matthay, M.A. and Cohen, N.H. (1995). Death and other complications of emergency airway management in critically adults. A prospective investigation of 297 tracheal intubations, *Anesthesiology*, **82**, 367–376.

[2] Cook, T.M., Woodall, N., Harper, J. *et al.* (2011). Major complications of airway management in the, UK: results of the Fourth National Audit Project of the Royal College of Anaesthetists and the Difficult Airway Society. Part 2: intensive care and emergency departments, *Br J Anaesth*, **106**, 632–634.

[3] Jaber, S., Jung, B., Corne, P. *et al.* (2010). An intervention to decrease complications related to endotracheal intubation in the intensive care unit: a prospective, multiple-center study, *Intens Care Medicine*, **36**, 248–255.
[4] Langernon, O., Masso, E., Huraux, C. *et al.* (2000). Prediction of difficult mask ventilation, *Anesthesiology*, **92**, 1229–1236.
[5] Cormack, R.S. and Lehane, J. (1984). Difficult tracheal intubation in obstetrics, *Anaesthesia*, **39**, 1105–1111.
[6] Frek, C.M. (1991). Predicting difficult intubation, *Anaesthesia*, **46**, 1005–1008.
[7] Patil, V.U., Stehling, L.C. and Zauder, H.L. (1983). *Fibreoptic Endoscopy in Anaesthesia*, Year Book Medical Publishers, Chicago.
[8] Wilson, M.E., Spiegehlhalter, D., Robertson, J.A. *et al.* (1998). Predicting difficult intubation, *Br J Anaesth*, **61**, 211–216.
[9] Savva, D. (1994). Prediction of difficult intubation, *Br J Anaesth*, **73**, 149–153.
[10] Mallampati, S.R., Gatt, S.P., Gugino, L.D. *et al.* (1985). A clinical sign to predict difficult tracheal intubation: a prospective study, *Can Anaesth Soc J*, **32**, 429–434.
[11] Samsoon, G.L. and Young, J.R. (1987). Difficult tracheal intubation: a retrospective study, *Anaesthesia*, **42**, 487–490.
[12] Nichol, H.C. and Zuck, D. (1983). Difficult laryngoscopy — The anterior larynx and the atlanto-occipital gap, *Br J Anaesth*, **55**, 141–145.
[13] Calder, I., Calder, J., Crockard, H.A. (1995). Difficult direct laryngoscopy in patients with cervical spine disease, *Anaesthesia*, **50**, 756–763.
[14] Shiga, T., Wajima, Z., Inoue, T. *et al.* (2005). Predicting difficult intubation in apparently normal patients: a meta-analyses of bedside screening test performance, *Anesthesiology*, **103**, 429–437.
[15] Salem, M.R., Joseph, N.J. and Heyman, H.J. (1985). Cricoid compression is effective in obliterating the oesophageal lumen in the presence of a nasogastric tube, *Anesthesiology*, **63**, 443–446.
[16] McCarthy, G., Elliot, P. and Mirakhur, R.K. (1991). A comparison of different pre-oxygenation techniques in the elderly, *Anaesthesia*, **46**, 824–827.
[17] Mort, T.C., Waberski, B.H. and Clive, J. (2009). Extending the preoxygenation period from 4 to 8 min in critically ill patients undergoing emergency intubation, *Cril Care Med*, **37**, 68–71.
[18] Vanner, R.G. (1995). Safe use of cricoid pressure (editorial), *Anaesthesia*, **54**, 1–3.
[19] Constantin, J.M., Futier, E., Cherprenet, A.L. *et al.* (2010). A recruitment maneuver increases oxygenation after intubation of hypoxemic intensive care unit patients: a randomized controlled study, *Crit Care*, **14**, R76.

[20] Owen, R.l. and Cheney, F. (1987). Endobronchial intubation: a preventable complication, *Anesthesiology*, **67**, 255–357.

[21] Conrardy, P., Goodman, L., Laing, F. *et al.* (1976). Alteration of endotracheal tube position. Flexion and extension of the neck, *Crit Care Med*, **4**, 8–12.

[22] Seegobin, R.D. and van Hasselt, G.L. (1984). Endotracheal cuff pressure and tracheal mucosal blood flow: endoscopic study of four large-volume cuffs, *Br Med J*, **288**, 965–968.

[23] Absalom, A., Pledger, D. and Kong, A. (1999). Adrenocortical function in critically ill patients 24 h after a single dose of etomidate, *Anaesthesia*, **54**, 861–867.

[24] Annane, D., Sebille, V. and Bellissant, E. (2003). Corticosteroids for patients with septic shock, *JAMA*, **289**, 43–44.

[25] Morris, C., Perris, A., Klein, J. *et al.* (2009). Anaesthesia in haemodynamically compromised emergency patients: does ketamine represent the best choice of induction agent? *Anaesthesia*, **64**, 532–539.

[26] McCourt, K.C., Salmela, L., Mirakhur, R.K. *et al.* (1998). Comparison of rocuronium and suxamethonium for use during rapid sequence induction of anaesthesia, *Anaesthesia*, **53**, 867–871.

[27] Andrews, J.L., Kumar, N., Van Den Brom, R.G.H. *et al.* (1999). A large simple randomized trial of rocuronium vesus suxamethonium in rapid sequence induction of anaesthesia with propofol, *Acta Anaesthesiologica Scandinavicia*, **43**, 4–8.

[28] Sparr, H., Vermeyen, K., Beaufort, A. *et al.* (2007). Reversal of profound rocuronium induced neuromuscular blockade by sugammadex in a randomized multicenter study: efficacy, safety and pharmacokinetics, *Anesthesiology*, **610**, 935–943.

[29] De Boer, H.D., Driessen, J.J., Marcus, M.A. *et al.* (2007). Reversal of rocuronium induced (1.2mg/kg) profound neuromuscular block by sugammadex: a multicenter, dose-finding and safety study, *Anesthesiology*, **107**, 239–244.

[30] Martin, L.D., Mhyre, J.M., Shanks, A.M. *et al.* (2011). 3423 Emergency tracheal intubations at a University Hospital: airway outcomes and complications, *Anesthesiology*, **114**, 42–48.

[31] Hendersson, J.J., Popat, M.T., Lato, I.P. *et al.* (2004). Difficult Airway Society guidelines for the management of the unanticipated difficult intubation, *Anaesthesia*, **59**, 675–694.

[32] Frezon, D.Z., Rosenblatt, W.H., Johansen, M.J. *et al.* (2001). Use of the intubating LMA in 254 patients with difficult to manage airways, *Anesthesiology*, **95**, 1175–1181.

[33] Silk, J., Hill, H.M. and Calder, I. (1991). Difficult intubation and the laryngeal mask, *Eur J Anaesthesiol Suppl*, **4**, 47–51.

[34] Atherton, D.P., O'Sullivan, E., Lowe, D. *et al.* (1996). A ventilation-exchange bougie for fibreoptic intubation with the laryngeal mask airway, *Anaesthesia*, **51**, 1123–1126.

[35] Divatia, J.V., Kulkarni, A.P., Sinhkar, S. *et al.* (1999). Failed intubation in the Intensive Care Unit managed with a laryngeal mask airway and percutaneous tracheostomy, *Anaesth Intensive Care*, **27**, 409–411.

[36] Benumof, J.L. and Scheller, M.S. (1993). The importance of transtracheal jet ventilation in the management of the difficult airway, *Anesthesiology*, **78**, 769–778.

[37] Patel, R.G. (1999). Percutaneous transtracheal jet ventilation: a safe, quick and temporary way to provide oxygenation and ventilation when conventional methods are unsuccessful, *Chest*, **116**, 1689–1694.

[38] Dworkin, R., Benumof, J.L., Benumof, R. *et al.* (1990). The effective tracheal diameter that causes air trapping during jet ventilation, *J Cardiothorac Anesth*, **40**, 731–736.

[39] Wong, D.T., Prabhu, A.J., Coloma, M. *et al.* (2003). What is the minimum training required for successful cricothyroidotomy? A study in mannequins, *Anesthesiology*, **98**, 349–353.

[40] Milner, S.M. and Bennett, J.M. (1991). Emergency cricothyroidotomy, *J Laryngol Otol*, **105**, 883–885.

[41] McGill, J., Clinton, J.E. and Ruiz, E. (1982). Cricothyroidotomy in the emergency department. *Ann Emerg Med*, **11**, 2008–2011.

[42] Brofeldt, B.T., Panacek, E.A. and Richards, J.R. (1996). An easy cricothyriodotomy approach: The rapid 4-step technique, *Acad Emerg Med*, **3**,1015–1019.

[43] Benumof, J.L. (1991). Management of the difficult adult airway, *Anesthesiology*, **75**, 1087–1110.

[44] American, Society of Anaesthesiologists Task Force on Management of the Difficult Airway (2003). Practice guidelines for the management of the difficult airway. An updated report, *Anesthesiology*, **95**,1269–1277.

[45] McGuire, G. and El-Beheiry, H. (1999). Complete upper airway obstruction during awake fibreoptic intubation in patents with unstable cervical fractures, *Can J Anaesth*, **46**, 176–178.

[46] Shaw, I.C., Welchew, E.A., Harrison, B.J. *et al.* (1997). Complete airway obstruction during awake fibreoptic intubation, *Anaesthesia*, **52**, 576–585.

[47] Randell, T., Valli, H. and Hakala, P. (1997). Comparison of the Ovassapian intubating airway and the Berman intubating airway in fibreoptic intubation, *Eur J Anaesthesiol*, **14**, 380–384.

[48] Sidhu, V.S., Whithead, E.M., Ainsworth, Q.P. *et al.* (1993). A technique of awake fibreoptic intubation. Experience in patients with cervical spine disease, *Anaesthesia*, **48**, 910–913.

[49] Mizrahi, S., Yaari, Y., Lugass, G. *et al.* (1986). Major airway obstruction relieved by helium/oxygen breathing, *Crit Care Med*, **14**, 986–987.

[50] MacDonnel, S.P.J., Timmins, A.C. and Watson, J.D. (1995). Adrenaline administered via nebuliser in adult patients with upper airway obstruction, *Anaesthesia*, **50**, 35–36.

[51] Mason, R., Fielder, C.P. (1999). The obstructed airway in head and neck surgery, *Anaesthesia*, **54**, 625–628.

[52] Chao, Y.K., Liu, Y.H., Hsieh, M.J. *et al.* (2005). Controlling the difficult airway by rigid bronchoscopy-an old but effective method, *Interact Cardio Vasc Thorac Surg*, **4**, 175–179.

[53] Sanders, R.D. (1967). Two ventilating attachments for bronchoscopes, *Delaware Medical Journal*, **39**, 170–175.

[54] Nekhendzy, V. and Simmonds, P.K. (2004). Rigid bronchoscope- assisted endotracheal intubation: yet another use of the gum elastic bougie, *Anesth Analg*, **98**, 545–547.

[55] Sidhu, V.S. and Greenbaum, R. (1995). 'General anaestheisa for laser bronchoscopy', in Hetzel, M.R. (ed.), *Minimally Invasive Techniques in Thoracic Medicine and Surgery*, Chapman & Hall, London, pp. 93–104.

[56] Bittar, D. (1975). Respiratory obstruction associated with induction of general anaesthesia in patients with Hodgkin's disease, *Anaesth Analg*, **54**, 399–403.

[57] Gerig, H.J., Schnider, T. and Heidegger T. (2005). Prophylactic percutaneous transtracheal catheterization in the management of patients with anticipated difficult airways: a case series, *Anaesthesia*, **60**, 801–805.

[58] Chandradeva, K., Palin, C., Ghosh, S.M. *et al.* (2005).Percutaneous transtracheal jet ventilation as a guide to tracheal intubation in severe upper airway obstruction from supraglottic oedema, *Br J Anaesth*, **94**, 683–686.

[59] Wymuller, E.A., Paugh, D., Pavlin, E.G. *et al.* (1987). Management of difficult airways with percutaneous transtracheal ventilation, *Ann Otol Rhinol Laryngol*, **96**, 34–37.

[60] Cook, T.M., Bigwood, B. and Cranshaw, J. (2006). A complication of trans-tracheal jet ventilation and use of the Aintree catheter, *Anaesthesia*, **61**, 692–697.

[61] Dob, D.P., McLure, H.A. and Soni, N. (1998). Failed intubation and emergency percutaneous tracheostomy, *Anaesthesia*, **53**, 72–74.

[62] Mori, M., Fujimito, J., Iwaski, H. *et al.* (2002). Emergency percutaneous dilatational tracheostomy after failed intubation, *Anaesth intensive Care*, **30**, 101–102.

[63] Griggs, W.M., Myburgh J.A. and Worthley, L.I. (1991). Urgent airway access-an indication for percutaneous tracheostomy? *Anaesth Intensive Care*, **19**, 586–587.

[64] Goh, M.H., Liu, X.Y. and Goh, Y.S. (1999). Anterior mediastinal masses: an anesthetic challenge, *Anaesthesia*, **54**, 670–682.

[65] Wilson, R.F., Seiger, Z., Jacobs, J. *et al.* (1984). Temporary partial cardiopulmonary bypass during emergency operative management of near total tracheal occlusion, *Anesthesiology*, **61**, 103–105.

[66] Coles, J.C., Doctor, A., Lefcof, M. *et al.* (1979). A method of anaesthesia for imminent tracheal obstruction, *Surgery*, **80**, 379–380.

[67] Darmon, J.Y., Hamelberg, W. and Ziegler, C.H. (1992). Evaluation of risk factors for laryngeal oedema after tracheal extubation in adults and its prevention by dexamethasone. A placebo controlled, double-blind multicenter study, *Anesthesiology*, **77**, 245–251.

[68] Fan, T., Wang, G., Mao, B. *et al.* (2008). Prophylactic administration of parenteral steroids for preventing airway complications after extubation in adults; meta-analysis of randomized placebo controlled trials, *Br Med J*, **337**, a1841.

[69] Griffiths, J., Barber, V.S., Morgan, L. *et al.* (2005). Systematic review and meta-analyses of studies of the timing of tracheostomy in adult patients undergoing artificial ventilation, *Br Med J*, **330**, 1243–1248.

[70] http://www.tracman.org.uk (accessed, January, 2012).

[71] Ciaglia, P., Firsching, R. and Syniec, C. (1985). Elective percutaneous dilatational tracheostomy, *Chest*, **87**, 715–719.

[72] Freeman, B.D., Isabella, K., Lin, N. *et al.* (2000). A meta-analysis of prospective trials comparing percutaneous and surgical tracheostomy in critically ill patients, *Chest*, **118**, 1412–1418.

[73] Silvester, W., Goldsmith, D., Uchino, S. *et al.* (2006). Percutaneous versus surgical tracheostomy: a randomized controlled study with long-term follow up, *Crit Care Med*, **8**, 2145–2152.

[74] Rana, S., Pendem, S. and Pogodzinski, M.S. *et al.* (2005). Tracheostomy in critically ill patients, *Mayo Clinic Proceedings*, **80**, 1632–1638.

[75] Delaney, A., Bagshaw, S.M. and Nalos, M. (2006). Percutaneous dilatational tracheostomy versus surgical tracheostomy in critically patient: a systematic review and meta-analysis, *Crit Care Med*, **10**, R55.

[76] Muhammad, J., Patton, D.W., Evans, R.M. *et al.* (1999). Percutaneous dilatational tracheostomy under ultrasound guidance, *Br J Oral Maxillofac Surg*, **31**, 309–311.

[77] Bewster, M.S., Adams, A.M., Clarke, C.W. *et al.* (2001). Evaluation of a new percutaneous dilatational tracheostomy set apparatus, *Anaesthesia*, **56**, 859–864.

[78] Intensive Care Society (2008). *Standards for the Care of Adult Patients with a Temporary Tracheostomy*, p. 10. Available online at: http://www.ics.ac.uk/ics-homepage/guidelines-standards. Accessed 17 October 2012.

[79] Tarpey, J.L., Lynch, L. and Hart, S. (1994). The use of the laryngeal mask airway to facilitate insertion of a percutaneous tracheostomy, *Intens Care Med*, **20**, 448–449.

[80] Fikkers, B.G., Van Veen, J.A. and Kooloos, J.G. (2004). Emphysema and pneumothorax after percutaneous tracheostomy. Case reports and an anatomic study, *Chest*, **125**, 1804–1814.

[81] Ching, N. and Nealon, T.F. (1974). Cuff pressure measurements, *Chest*, **66**, 604–605.

[82] Lewarski, J.S. (2005). Long-term care of the patient with a tracheostomy, *Resp Care*, **4**, 534–537.

[83] Caples, S.M. and Gay, P.C. (2005). Non-invasive positive pressure ventilation in the intensive care unit: a concise review, *Crit Care Med*, **33**, 2651–2658.

[84] Hilbert, G., Grugson, D., Vargas, F. *et al.* (2001). Non-invasive ventilation in immunocompromised patients with infiltrates, fever and acute respiratory failure, *New Engl J Med*, **344**, 522–523.

[85] Nava, S., Gregoretti, C. and Fanfulla, F. (2005). Non-invasive ventilation to prevent respiratory failure after extubation in high-risk patients, *Crit Care Med*, **33**, 2464–2470.

[86] Ulmer, J.L. and Garvey, M.J. (1992). Fatal angioedema associated with lisinopril, *Ann Pharmacother*, **26**, 1245–1246.

[87] Rai, R.M., Amen, F. and Idrees, F. (2004). Angiotensin-converting enzyme inhibitor related angioedma and the anaesthetist, *Anaesthesia*, **59**, 283–289.

18
Neurocritical Care

Nicholas Hirsch, Christopher Taylor and Martin Smith

18.1 Introduction

Although many acute neurological emergencies are treated in specialised neurocritical care units, which allow a concentration of expertise, the frequency of such conditions inevitably means that many patients will be cared for in general intensive care units. This chapter discusses the basic principles of the intensive care management of commonly presenting neurological disorders.

18.2 Traumatic Brain Injury

There has been a marked decline in mortality from severe traumatic brain injury (TBI) in adults over the last two decades because of improvements in resuscitation and pre-hospital care [1]. There have also been simultaneous advances in our understanding of the pathophysiology of brain injury and in monitoring techniques that have allowed the development of evidence-based intensive care for patients with TBI [2].

18.2.1 *Pathophysiology*

Head injury is a heterogeneous diagnosis, encompassing a wide range of pathologies including diffuse axonal injury, focal contusions and space-occupying haematomas. If the initial (primary) injury is not immediately fatal, it is usually exacerbated by secondary events that lead to secondary brain injury. This develops over the subsequent minutes, hours and days and has an adverse effect on outcome. The primary injury activates an auto-destructive cascade of ionic, metabolic, inflammatory and immunological changes that render the brain more susceptible to secondary physiological insults and ultimately result in irreversible cell damage or death. Secondary insults arise from both systemic and intracranial changes that initiate or propagate pathophysiological processes and fatally damage neurones already rendered susceptible by the primary injury (Table 18.1).

18.2.2 *Initial Resuscitation and Assessment*

Resuscitation is a crucial stage at which mortality and morbidity can be influenced. In particular, the prevention of secondary brain injury by the correction of systemic hypoxaemia and hypotension, and rapid diagnosis and evacuation of expanding intracranial haematomas, are key determinants of outcome. The Glasgow Coma Scale (GCS) is a reliable and robust method of assessing overall conscious level after TBI (Table 18.2).

Post-resuscitation GCS, in particular its motor component, is a powerful predictor of outcome. Focal signs, such as pupil and limb responses, should also be documented.

The indications for urgent cranial computed tomography (CT) scan and referral to a neurosurgical unit include severe TBI (GCS $\leq$ 8), deterioration in GCS of two or more points, focal neurology or skull-base

Table 18.1. Causes of secondary brain injury.

Intracranial causes

- Expanding intracranial haematoma
- Brain swelling
- Seizures

Extracranial causes

- Hypoxaemia
- Systemic hypotension
- Hypercapnia and hypocapnia
- Hyperthermia
- Hyperglycaemia and hypoglycaemia

Table 18.2. Glasgow Coma Scale.

	1	2	3	4	5	6
Eyes	Does not open eyes	Opens eyes in response to painful stimuli	Opens eyes in response to voice	Opens eyes spontaneously	N/A	N/A
Verbal	Makes no sounds	Incomprehensible sounds	Utters inappropriate words	Confused, disoriented	Oriented, converses normally	N/A
Motor	Makes no movements	Extension to painful stimuli	Abnormal flexion to painful stimuli	Flexion/ Withdrawal to painful stimuli	Localises painful stimuli	Obeys commands

fracture. The cervical spine should be imaged in all unconscious head-injured patients because of the high risk of coincidental injury.

18.2.3 *Monitoring*

Besides close monitoring and assessment of cardiac and respiratory functions common to all critically ill patients, several techniques are now available for global and regional brain monitoring [3].

18.2.3.1 *Intracranial pressure*

Intracranial pressure (ICP) [4] cannot be reliably estimated from any specific clinical feature or CT finding and must actually be measured. A ventricular catheter is the gold standard for ICP monitoring but it is an invasive technique associated with complications such as infection. Miniature solid-state probes that are inserted into brain parenchyma via a small burr hole are effective and safer alternatives. ICP monitoring allows determination of cerebral perfusion pressure (CPP = mean arterial pressure (MAP)–ICP) and detection of abnormal ICP waveforms.

18.2.3.2 *Cerebral oxygenation*

Measurement of jugular venous oxygen saturation ($SjvO_2$), via a jugular bulb catheter, provides a global assessment of the balance between cerebral oxygen supply and demand [5]. Jugular desaturation ($SjvO_2$ <50%) is associated with increased mortality after TBI and worsened outcome in survivors. Because $SjvO_2$ is a global measure it cannot exclude significant regional ischaemia. Focal brain tissue oxygen tension ($PtiO_2$) can now be measured using microprobes. Initial low values of $PtiO_2$ rise over the first 24 hours after injury and the depth and duration of tissue hypoxia are related to outcome.

18.2.3.3 *Brain tissue biochemistry*

Cerebral microdialysis (MD) is being increasingly used as a bedside monitor to provide on-line analysis of brain tissue biochemistry during neurointensive care. MD has the potential to provide early warning of impending cerebral hypoxia/ischaemia [6].

18.2.3.4 *Cerebral blood flow*

Transcranial Doppler (TCD) ultrasonography of blood flow velocity in the middle cerebral artery provides an indirect assessment of cerebral blood flow (CBF), a non-invasive assessment of CPP, cerebral pressure autoregulation and carbon dioxide reactivity and the identification of cerebral vasospasm. An invasive device incorporating thermal diffusion flowmetry (TDF) provides a sensitive, real-time assessment of local CBF.

18.2.3.5 *Multi-modal monitoring*

Individual monitoring techniques provide information about specific aspects of cerebral physiology but all have disadvantages and most suffer from significant artefacts. Monitoring of several variables simultaneously (multi-modal monitoring) allows cross-validation between monitors, artefact rejection and greater confidence in making treatment decisions [3].

18.2.4 *Intensive Care Management*

The intensive care unit (ICU) management of TBI (Table 18.3) has undergone extensive revision as evidence accumulates that longstanding and established practices are not as efficacious or innocuous as previously believed [7]. Traditional therapies such as fluid restriction and hyperventilation have been called into question and are no longer recommended, and newer therapies, such as therapeutic hypothermia and tight glycaemic control, remain controversial. The sole goal of identifying and treating intracranial hypertension has been superseded by a neuroprotective strategy incorporating a systematic, stepwise approach to control of ICP and maintenance of adequate CPP. It is likely that specialist neurointensive care, using protocol-guided therapy, improves outcome in patients with severe TBI [8]. Consensus, expert management guidelines are available [9].

Table 18.3. The intensive care management of severe head injury.

Ventilation	• $PaO_2 > 13$ kPa
	• $PaCO_2$ 4.5–5.0 kPa
	• PEEP (£10 cm H_2O) to maintain oxygenation
	• routine strategies to minimise risk of pneumonia
Cardiovascular	• MAP > 90 mmHg
	• Euvolaemia
	• vaspressors/inotropes if insufficient response to fluid
ICP and CPP targets	• CPP 50 – 70 mmHg
	• ICP < 20 mmHg
ICP and CPP management	• sedation/analgesia
	• volume expansion plus norepinephrine to maintain CPP
	• osmotic therapy (mannitol or hypertonic saline)
Resistant intracranial hypertension	• moderate hyperventilation ($PaCO_2$ 4.0–4.5kPa)
	• moderate hypothermia
	• CSF drainage
	• Barbiturates
	• decompressive craniectomy
General	• normothermia
	• normoglycaemia
	• enteral nutrition
	• thromboembolic prophylaxis
	• seizure control

18.2.4.1 *Ventilation*

Control of partial pressure of oxygen in arterial blood (PaO_2) and partial pressure of carbon dioxide in arterial blood ($PaCO_2$) is essential to maintain favourable cerebral haemodynamics and oxygenation and mechanical ventilation is a key part of management. Patients with severe TBI are at high risk of developing acute lung injury and ventilator management can be challenging [10]. The classic teaching of no or low-level positive end-expiratory pressure (PEEP) to prevent rises in ICP is inappropriate because ventilation without PEEP often fails to correct hypoxaemia. With adequate-volume resuscitation PEEP often decreases ICP because of improved cerebral oxygenation.

18.2.4.2 *Cardiovascular support*

Even short periods of hypotension (MAP <90 mmHg) are associated with adverse neurological outcome and should be avoided [11]. Higher mean pressures may be necessary to maintain an adequate CPP in the presence of intracranial hypertension. Euvolaemia is the primary resuscitative goal and crystalloids and colloids may be used to support CPP [1,2]. Glucose-containing solutions should be avoided because they are a source of free water that can worsen cerebral oedema and because anaerobic metabolism of glucose in the ischaemic brain leads to local lactate production and worsened secondary injury. A vasoactive agent, such as norepinephrine, is required if adequate blood pressure cannot be achieved with fluid resuscitation alone.

18.2.4.3 *ICP- and CPP-guided therapy*

Over the last decade there has been a shift of emphasis from primary control of ICP to a multi-faceted approach of maintenance of CPP and brain protection. Although there is debate about the optimal level for CPP, there is a consensus that it should be maintained between 50–70 mmHg [9] as higher targets are often achieved only at the expense of significant complications [12].

18.2.4.4 *Management of intracranial hypertension*

Guidelines recommend that ICP >20 mmHg should be treated [9] and simple measures, such as optimisation of sedation and elevation of the head of the bed, are often sufficient.

18.2.4.4.1 Hyperventilation

Hyperventilation was once the cornerstone of ICP control but it is now known that empirical and excessive hyperventilation is associated with adverse neurological outcome because of the risk of cerebral ischaemia secondary to reduced-$PaCO_2$-related cerebral vasoconstriction [13]. Current guidance recommends routine $PaCO_2$ targets of 4.0–4.5 kPa [9]. Although modest hyperventilation may be used to control intracranial hypertension in selected cases, cerebral oxygenation monitoring should be used to ensure that it does not worsen cerebral ischaemia.

18.2.4.4.2 Osmotic therapy

Mannitol effectively reduces elevated ICP and improves CBF in certain settings of intracranial hypertension. It is often used to 'buy time' pending definitive treatment such as evacuation of an intracranial haematoma. On the ICU, ICP-directed treatment is more beneficial than treatment directed by neurological signs or physiological indicators [14]. Repeated administration of mannitol may result in high serum osmolality (>320 mOsm/l) and associated neurological and renal complications. Hypertonic saline (HS) is an effective alternative to mannitol and its beneficial effects are related not only to its osmotic action but also to haemodynamic, vasoregulatory, immunological and neurochemical effects [15]. HS is effective in controlling ICP resistant to mannitol and is associated with fewer side effects. In particular, the large intravascular volume shifts seen with mannitol are absent and renal complications are less frequent. There are many different concentrations of HS available (1.7–29.2%) and the optimal osmolar load to lower elevated ICP has not been defined.

18.2.4.4.3 Barbiturates

Thiopental reduces ICP and, in association with other barbiturates, has protective effects in the context of focal ischaemia. However, the clinical use of thiopental for the control of refractory intracranial hypertension is contentious and any potential beneficial effects may be offset by side effects, particularly hypotension.

18.2.4.4.4 Surgical methods

Evacuation of an expanding or mass-effect-producing intracranial haematoma is the primary goal of surgical treatment. Drainage of cerebrospinal fluid (CSF) via a ventricular catheter is an effective means of reducing ICP. Another option for treating refractory intracranial hypertension is decompressive craniectomy, an operation to remove a large area of skull to increase the volume of the cranial cavity and thereby decrease its pressure [2]. Recently, a multicentre randomised trial has reported higher mortality in patients treated with craniectomy [16]. However, some have raised concerns about the heterogeneity in the craniectomy group. There is currently a randomised, controlled multicentre trial comparing thiopentone with decompressive craniectomy in patients with refractory elevation of ICP.

18.2.4.4.5 Glycaemic control

Severely head-injured patients frequently develop hyperglycaemia and this exacerbates secondary injury and worsens neurological outcome because of hyperosmolality, lactic acid production and increases in excitatory amino-acids. Glycaemic control may improve outcome after TBI and is widely employed [1,2], although the optimum systemic glucose targets remain controversial.

18.2.4.4.6 Therapeutic hypothermia

Despite benefit in animal models, the results of moderate hypothermia (33–35°C) in human trials have been disappointing. A prospective, randomised study of moderate hypothermia (33°C) in TBI was terminated early because of increased morbidity in patients over 45 years of age treated with hypothermia [17]. There was possible benefit to patients who presented already hypothermic but older patients had such high rates of medical complications that hypothermia was detrimental regardless of admission temperature. However, moderate hypothermia is an effective method of reducing raised ICP and remains a treatment option in younger patients [2]. Increased systemic and brain temperature is associated with worse outcome after TBI and core temperature should be monitored and pyrexia treated [18].

18.2.4.5 *Systemic complications*

Systemic complications are common after TBI and are independent contributors to morbidity and mortality [19]. They represent risk factors which are potentially amenable to treatment but their management can be challenging because optimum treatment for the failing systemic organ system may have potentially adverse effects on the injured brain and *vice versa* [10]. Respiratory complications are most frequent, occurring in up to 80% of patients. Ventilator-acquired pneumonia is a particular problem and occurs in 45–60% of patients. ECG changes and other cardiovascular complications also occur frequently. Head injury is often complicated by disorders of sodium and water balance secondary to central diabetes insipidus, the cerebral salt wasting syndrome and the syndrome of inappropriate antidiuretic hormone secretion [20].

18.2.4.6 *Outcome*

The mortality of severe TBI is around 23%, with over 60% of survivors having residual deficits including cognitive impairment and behavioural problems that affect functional status and quality of life. The introduction of evidence-based protocols to guide the intensive care management of patients with severe head injury is associated with a significant reduction in both ICU and hospital mortality and potentially improved outcome in survivors.

18.3 Cerebral Haemorrhage

Cerebral haemorrhage remains a major cause of death and neurological disability, and is most commonly a result trauma (see above), subarachnoid haemorrhage or an intracerebral bleed.

18.3.1 *Subarachnoid haemorrhage*

Despite improvements in outcome over the last decade, aneurysmal subarachnoid haemorrhage (SAH) remains a potentially devastating disease. The mortality rate is high and one-third of those who survive need lifelong care and a further 40% have residual impairment. Prognosis depends on three factors: (i) the severity of the initial bleed, (ii) the success of the procedure to secure the aneurysm and (iii) the occurrence and severity of sequelae, including cerebral vasospasm [21].

18.3.1.1 *Grading of SAH*

Several grading scales have been developed to describe the severity of SAH and assess prognosis [22]. That described by the World Federation of

Neurosurgeons (WFNS) is widely used and based on the GCS and presence or absence of a motor deficit.

- Grade 1 — GCS 15 and no motor deficit.
- Grade 2 — GCS 14–13 and no motor deficit.
- Grade 3 — GCS 14–13 with motor deficit.
- Grade 4 — GCS 12–7 with or without motor deficit.
- Grade 5 — GCS 6–3 with or without motor deficit.

18.3.1.2 *Management*

The ICU management is targeted at optimising cardiovascular variables, securing the ruptured aneurysm, detecting and treating intracranial complications, including the prevention and treatment of cerebral vasospasm, and managing systemic complications [23]. Hydrocephalus occurs in ~ 25% patients after SAH and temporary external ventricular drainage may be required.

18.3.1.2.1 Cardiovascular control

Prior to control of the aneurysm, systemic blood pressure should be carefully controlled in the 'high normal' range to maintain cerebral perfusion whilst minimising the risk of re-bleeding. Hypotension should be treated initially with intravenous fluids followed by vasopressors, but hypertension should only be treated if systolic blood pressure exceeds 160 mmHg in a previously normotensive patient.

18.3.1.2.2 Protection of aneurysm

Re-bleeding occurs in 7% cases and is prevented by early protection of the ruptured aneurysm. Endovascular intervention is now the treatment of choice for the majority of intracranial aneurysms, although the efficacy and risks associated with re-treatments must be determined by longer-term outcome studies [24].

18.3.1.2.3 Vasospasm

With the current emphasis on early protection of ruptured aneurysms, cerebral vasospasm and delayed ischaemic neurological deficit (DIND) is the most common cause of mortality and morbidity after SAH. Vasospasm peaks at between four and ten days and persists for several days. Although its exact cause remains obscure, the risk of vasospasm is related to blood load in the basal cisterns. Constituents of oxyhaemoglobin are likely spasmogenic factors and several mechanisms coexist, including release of endothelin and inhibition of nitric oxide [25]. Adventitial inflammation and intimal hyperplasia also occur in affected vessels.

Vasospasm is detected clinically in conscious patients by a reduction in consciousness level with or without a focal neurological deficit. Cerebral angiography is the gold standard for diagnosis of cerebral vasospasm, although TCD ultrasonography is routinely used in its bedside assessment [23].

Triple-H therapy (hypervolaemia, hypertension and haemodilution) is widely used to prevent and treat cerebral vasospasm after SAH [25]. Crystalloids and colloids should be infused (>3000 ml/24 hours) to achieve a daily positive fluid balance, and supra-normal systemic blood pressure maintained using vasopressors/inotropes. Haemodilution is the most controversial component of triple-H therapy and is not universally applied. Triple-H therapy may exacerbate the cardiopulmonary complications of SAH and cause intracranial complications such as cerebral oedema and intracranial haemorrhage. Balloon angioplasty and direct intra-arterial infusion of vasodilator agents are useful in patients with symptomatic vasospasm resistant to triple-H therapy.

18.3.1.2.4 Cerebral protection

Nimodipine, a specific antagonist of the L-type voltage-gated calcium channel, is the only pharmacological agent proven to improve outcome after SAH and is administered routinely for 21 days. Magnesium and statins are promising treatments, with small studies demonstrating reductions in the incidence of DIND and improved outcome.

18.3.1.2.5 Systemic complications

Systemic complications occur in up to 79% patients after SAH and are independently associated with higher mortality and poor outcome [26].

Electrocardogram changes, particularly T-wave and conduction abnormalities, and 'stunned' myocardium syndrome are related to endogenous catecholamine release and activation of adrenoceptors. The challenge is to differentiate between a centrally mediated effect, which is often self-limiting, and an acute coronary syndrome. Pulmonary complications occur because of pulmonary expression of a systemic inflammatory response, neurogenic pulmonary oedema and as a complication of triple-H therapy.

18.3.2 *Intracerebal haemorrhage*

Intracerebral haemorrhage (ICH) accounts for 10–30% of all strokes but is one of the major causes of stroke-related death and disability. The majority of primary ICH is associated with hypertension and secondary ICH with anticoagulation therapy.

18.3.2.1 *Management*

ICH is a medical emergency since delays in treatment are associated with worse outcome.

18.3.2.1.1 Cardiovascular control

Hypertension is common in the first six hours after ICH, even in previously normotensive patients. Treatment should balance the risks of hypertension-related haematoma expansion against excessive reduction in cerebral perfusion pressure and peri-haematoma ischaemia [26]. Blood pressure targets should be individualised but, in general terms, hypertension should not be treated unless >180/105 mmHg.

18.3.2.1.2 Control of intracranial pressure

Emergency measures to control ICP are required for comatose patients or those who develop clinical signs of brainstem herniation. Medical methods may be sufficient but in some patients surgery may be required. Surgical interventional is controversial but some sub-groups, such as younger patients with lobar haemorrhages causing significant mass effect, are likely to derive benefit from surgery. A cerebellar haematoma over 3 cm in diameter should also be evacuated because of the high risk of early deterioration.

18.3.2.1.3 Haemostatic therapy

Emergency reversal of oral anticoagulant therapy is recommended in warfarin-associated ICH. Despite promise in early studies, recombinant activated factor VII has no place in controlling intracerebral bleeding and reducing haematoma volume after ICH [28].

18.3.2.2 *Outcome*

ICH has a 30–55% six-month mortality overall, rising to 67% in patients receiving oral anticoagulant therapy. Fewer than 20% of survivors regain functional independence by six months.

18.4 Ischaemic Stroke

Ischaemic stroke is the second most common cause of death worldwide after ischaemic heart disease. It is caused by occlusion of vessels supplying brain tissue, which causes death of tissue in the immediate area supplied by those vessels. However, surrounding this area is tissue (the ischaemic penumbra) which may survive if perfusion can be restored [29]. Recognition of this has resulted in early and more aggressive treatment of stroke, often in acute stroke units which have been shown to improve outcome.

18.4.1 *Clinical features*

Acute stroke characteristically results in a sudden loss of neurological function, which is usually unilateral. Symptoms include limb weakness, dysarthria, dysphasia, hemianopia, sensory loss and neglect. Consciousness is usually maintained with anterior circulation strokes.

18.4.2 *Acute management*

If a stroke is suspected, the patient must undergo immediate CT to distinguish cerebral infarction from intracerebral haemorrhage. Emergency room care includes tracheal intubation if the GCS is less than or equal to 8, adequate fluid resuscitation and attention to blood pressure control. In patients ineligible for thrombolysis, a diastolic blood pressure of below 120 mmHg is generally acceptable; labetalol is the treatment of choice for pressures above this. For those eligible for thrombolysis, systolic blood pressure must be less than 185 mmHg and diastolic blood pressure less than 110 mmHg; again, labetalol is a suitable agent.

If an ischaemic stroke is diagnosed within 4.5 hours of the onset of symptoms, intravenous thrombolysis with recombinant tissue-type plasminogen activator (rt-PA) (alteplase) is indicated [30]. Studies including the National Institute of Neurological Disorders (NINDS) rt-PA Stroke Study have demonstrated a more favourable functional outcome in those treated with intravenous thrombolysis [31], and the earlier intravenous thrombolysis is initiated, the greater the benefit [32]. The risk of intracerebral haemorrhage is increased following intravenous thrombolysis, especially in those with severe stroke and in older patients. Intra-arterial thrombolysis (IAT), which should be safer than intravenous administration as a lower dose of thrombolytic agent is delivered directly to the thrombus, is the preserve of specialist units and the results of randomised trials are awaited. There are reports of success of treating vertebrobasilar occlusion with IAT in combination with vascular stenting.

Aspirin, started within 48 hours following ischaemic stroke and continued for two weeks, has been shown to reduce mortality and dependence at six months, probably by decreasing the risk of recurrent strokes [33]; although the benefit is small, the use of aspirin is recommended. No randomised controlled trials of the use of other antiplatelet agents, such as dipyridamole or clopidogrel, have appeared.

18.4.3 *Intensive care treatment of ischaemic stroke*

General measures for the care of stroke patients, include nursing of the patient head up, early assessment of swallowing and treatment with H_2

receptor antagonists to help prevent aspiration pneumonia, early initiation of enteral feeding, good glycaemic control and measures to prevent thromboembolism. Therapeutic hypothermia is not recommended at present. Seizures occur in 5–7% of patients and should be aggressively treated.

Large middle cerebral artery (MCA) infarcts may result in massive swelling of the cerebral hemisphere with subsequent herniation or compression of the brainstem. The so-called 'malignant MCA syndrome' typically occurs two to five days after the stroke and is characterised by a deteriorating level of consciousness and progressive deterioration of neurological function. Mortality is very high and wide decompressive craniectomy has been suggested as a treatment. Although mortality may be reduced by this manoeuvre, the results of randomised trials on functional outcome are awaited.

18.4.4 *Cerebral venous sinus thrombosis*

Occlusion of the cerebral venous sinuses or a cortical vein results in cortical venous infarction, often with haemorrhagic transformation [34]. Predisposing factors include hypercoagulable states (including pregnancy and the use of the oral contraceptive pill), dehydration and local infection (e.g. mastoiditis). Symptoms include headache, nausea and vomiting, seizures and focal neurological signs. Diagnosis requires MRI and magnetic resonance venography. Treatment consists of anticoagulation with heparin; if unsuccessful, direct infusion of thrombolytic agents into the clot has been advocated.

18.5 Management of Spinal Cord Injury

The annual incidence of spinal cord injury (SCI) in the UK is approximately 40 cases per million of the population, with road traffic accidents accounting for about 50% of cases. About 50% of cases involve people aged between 16 and 30. The commonest level of cervical spine injury is C5. Of patients with SCI, 65% have associated injuries including head, thoracic, abdominal or vascular injuries [35].

Primary injury occurs at the time of the injury and involves mechanical disruption of the spinal cord neural elements, often associated with fracture/dislocation of the spine, although in some cases there may be no radiological evidence of disruption. Secondary ischaemic injury follows as a consequence of hypotension, hypoxia, oedema and the presence of toxic inflammatory mediators [36]. The intensive care management of patients with spinal cord injury is therefore directed towards rapid resuscitation and maintenance of normal physiological variables.

Hypotension is common following SCI and may the result of hypovolaemia due to associated injuries or neurogenic (spinal) shock; the latter is characterised by the triad of hypotension, bradycardia and peripheral vasodilatation and is usually seen in SCI above the level of thoracic vertebra T6 and is due to disruption of sympathetic nervous system control. Treatment of neurogenic shock consists of fluid, inotropic therapy and anticholinergic therapy (e.g. atropine).

SCI affecting cervical C3–6 levels disrupts phrenic nerve outflow and necessitates tracheal intubation and mechanical ventilation. Patients with complete transection of the spinal cord above C3 will require permanent ventilatory support.

18.5.1 *Intensive care treatment*

Although most patients with SCI will be cared for in specialised units, they are often treated in general ICUs until a bed becomes available. Careful attention must be paid to a number of considerations.

The patient with SCI should be nursed supine initially with careful regular 'log-rolling'. Analgesic drugs should be used appropriately to allow pain-free physiotherapy. After a few days, the patient can be nursed slightly head up. Great care must be taken to prevent the development of pressure sores.

Early enteral nutrition helps reduce muscle loss due to catabolism seen following SCI. Paralytic ileus is common and results in poor absorption of feed, nausea and vomiting and constipation, which need to be treated with prokinetic agents, anti-emetic drugs and laxatives respectively. Total parenteral nutrition may be necessary.

Depending on the level of injury, long-term urinary catheterisation is usually needed in SCI and many authorities favour early suprapubic catheterisation.

18.5.2 *Surgical treatment*

Surgery may be necessary to decompress the swollen spinal cord and for fixation of unstable spinal fractures. This is usually performed early to allow safe and effective passive mobilisation of the patient; it also permits safe transport to a specialised unit.

18.5.3 *Corticosteroid therapy*

The National Acute Spinal Cord Injuries Studies (NASCIS) II and III and a Cochrane review [37,38] of these and various other studies have verified an improvement in both motor and sensory function in complete and incomplete SCI patients who were treated with high-dose methylprednisolone within eight hours of injury. However, doubts have been raised about the validity of the NASCIS study and the clinical gains seen with corticosteroid therapy [39]. As a result, many units do not recommend their routine use.

18.6 Status Epilepticus

Status epilepticus (SE) [40] is defined as continuous seizure activity lasting 30 minutes or more or intermittent seizure activity lasting 30 minutes or more during which consciousness is not regained [41]. Its incidence is approximately 50 per 100,000 of the population per annum. The definition recognises that seizures lasting more than 30 minutes are associated with physiological and biochemical changes resulting in permanent neuronal damage.

Generalised tonic–clonic (grand mal) SE is the commonest form although partial and non-convulsive SE (which manifests in altered mental state or consciousness) occurs and may be a cause of unexplained altered consciousness in the ICU [42].

Causes of SE include low antiepileptic drug (AED) levels in known epileptics, electrolyte imbalance (especially hyponatraemia), drug toxicity (especially alcohol and cocaine), cerebrovascular accidents, central nervous system infection (especially encephalitis) and traumatic brain injury (including surgery). SE in children may be precipitated by pyrexia.

Diagnosis of SE is usually obvious in the early stages but after a period of a few hours, abnormal movements may become subtle despite ongoing cerebral seizure activity; electroencephalographic studies may be necessary to confirm the diagnosis in this situation.

Systemic complications of SE include cerebral hypoxia, oedema, haemorrhage and venous thrombosis, myocardial infarction, arrhythmias, cardiac arrest, respiratory failure, aspiration pneumonia, pulmonary embolus, metabolic derangements, multiple organ dysfunction syndrome (MODS), rhabdomyolysis, renal failure and fractures [40].

First-line treatment of SE consists of rapid resuscitation ensuring adequate oxygenation and ventilation, establishing appropriate monitoring and maintaining circulatory support. Intravenous lorazepam (0.1 mg/kg to a maximum of 7 mg) is the initial drug of choice; its longer half-life confers advantages over diazepam in stopping SE and preventing recurrence [43]. It is effective in aborting up to 90% of SE. If SE persists, the second-line treatment consists of the intravenous administration of phenytoin (15–20 mg/kg) or fosphenytoin (the water-soluble prodrug of phenytoin). If, in spite of these interventions, SE continues, the stage of refractory SE is reached and requires general anaesthesia with propofol or thiopental in a specialised unit with electroencephalogram monitoring whilst optimising levels of various classes of AEDs [44].

Mortality of SE varies between 5–60%, depending on the duration, aetiology and age of the patient.

18.7 Neuromuscular Diseases in the ICU

The causes of acute generalised weakness requiring intensive care support are many but may be classified on an anatomical basis (Table 18.4) [45]; although many are rare and will tend to be confined to specialist neurological ICUs, others will be encountered on the general ICU. This account details some of the latter conditions.

18.7.1 *Guillain–Barré syndrome*

Guillain–Barré syndrome (GBS) [46] is the commonest cause of acute neuromuscular paralysis with an annual incidence of 2 per 100,000 of the

Table 18.4. Spinal cord and neuromuscular causes of respiratory failure.

Spinal cord	Acute transverse myelitis
	Cord infarction
	Acute compression
	Tetanus
Anterior horn cell disease	Motor neurone disease
	Poliomyelitis
Multiple radiculopathies	Carcinomatous meningitis
	AIDS polyradiculitis
Polyneuropathies	Guillain–Barré syndromes
	Critical illness neuropathy
	Acute porphyria
Neuromuscular junction diseases	Myasthenia gravis
	Lambert–Eaton myasthenic syndrome
	Botulism
	Organophosphate poisoning
Muscle diseases	Critical illness myopathy
	Muscular dystrophies
	Myotonic dystrophy
	Mitochondrial disease
	Periodic paralysis

population. It is characterised by an ascending limb weakness, areflexia and mild sensory symptoms; however, there is a wide clinical spectrum which includes the Fisher syndrome (ophthalmoplegia, ataxia and absent tendon reflexes) and acute motor and sensory axonal neuropathy.

A history of an antecedent upper respiratory tract infection or diarrhoeal illness is present in 70% of patients, which strongly suggests an immune basis for the condition. The most commonly identified organism is *Campylobacter jejuni*. Although the diagnosis is usually obvious, it should be confirmed by examination of the CSF (which classically shows an increase in protein without the presence of white cells) and electrophysiological studies which, in the majority, show evidence of a demyelinating neuropathy. However, axonal involvement may be evident in 10% of patients.

Acute respiratory failure, often accompanied by bulbar failure requiring tracheal intubation and mechanical ventilation, occurs in 30% of patients with GBS and may occur over a few hours in severe cases [47]. Suxamethonium for intubation must be avoided as it may cause fatal hyperkalaemia. ICU management of GBS includes early tracheostomy if ventilatory support is needed for more than ten days, treatment of arrhythmias (due to autonomic involvement), pain (which may be musculoskeletal or neuropathic) and thromboembolic prophylaxis. Psychological support is essential for patients requiring prolonged ventilation.

Specific therapy for GBS consists of plasma exchange or intravenous immunoglobulin and randomised trials of the two therapies suggest that both hasten recovery equally [48]. There appears to be no evidence of further improvement from combining the two therapies. Corticosteroids have been shown to have no role in treatment.

Mortality in those who require mechanical ventilation is approximately 7% [49] and whilst most recover sufficiently to walk independently after six months, some (especially the elderly and those with a history of a preceding diarrhoeal illness) remain permanently disabled.

18.7.2 *Critical illness neuropathy and myopathy*

Critical illness neuropathy and myopathy [50] are common acute neuromuscular disorders seen in the ICU and result in generalised weakness, often leading to failure to wean from mechanical ventilation.

Critical illness neuropathy (CIP) is an acute axonal sensory and motor neuropathy which occurs in approximately 50% of adult ICU patients; its incidence rises towards 100% of patients with sepsis, the systemic inflammatory response syndrome (SIRS) and multiple organ dysfunction syndrome (MODS). It probably represents the neurological manifestation of the latter and is thought to be due to neuronal microcirculatory changes leading to neuronal energy failure. Bacterial endotoxins and antibodies raised to neuronal gangliosides may play a role. Other associated factors include the use of corticosteroid therapy, non-depolarising neuromuscular blocking agents, total parenteral nutrition and aminoglycoside antibiotic agents, although these may merely reflect the severity of the underlying illness.

Clinical features of CIP include generalised muscle weakness and wasting and a flaccid tetraparesis (legs more often involved than arms). Reflexes are usually reduced or absent although are normal in 30%. Diagnosis requires exclusion of other causes of weakness and electrophysiological testing, which characteristically shows reduced motor and sensory compound muscle action potentials with normal conduction velocities indicating axonal damage [51].

Prevention of CIP consists of rapid treatment of SIRS and avoidance of the agents implicated in its pathogenesis. Recently, it has been suggested that tight glycaemic control may reduce its incidence. Treatment of CIP is largely supportive whilst awaiting recovery which, in the majority of cases, occurs over several weeks. Most patients, however, report long-lasting impairment in quality of life following the condition.

Critical illness myopathy (CIM) is an acute primary myopathy seen in a similar population of patients to those with CIP; indeed, the two conditions may co-exist and the term critical illness polyneuromyopathy has been suggested. The proposed mechanism for the development of CIM is bioenergetic failure due to mitochondrial dysfunction and unavailability of energy substrates. There appears to be a more robust association between the use of high-dose corticosteroids and neuromuscular blocking drugs in CIM than CIP [52]. Definitive diagnosis requires muscle biopsy as neurophysiological testing in an uncooperative patient often fails to differentiate the two conditions.

Treatment of CIM is again supportive whilst awaiting recovery.

18.7.3 *Myasthenia gravis*

Myasthenia gravis (MG) is an autoimmune condition in which immunoglobulin G antibodies are directed towards the post-synaptic acetylcholine receptors at the neuromuscular junction; the resultant decrease in receptor density produces the characteristic skeletal muscle fatigability [53]. Although the precise aetiology remains obscure, the thymus gland seems to play a central role in the pathogenesis of the disease. The annual incidence in the general population is 1 per 20,000. Diagnosis of MG relies on clinical history, response to the edrophonium (Tensilon®) test, repetitive nerve conduction testing and electromyography.

Approximately 15% of myasthenic patients will require mechanical ventilation during the course of their disease. When this occurs, it is referred to as a myasthenic crisis. It is often precipitated by infection, surgery, inadequate treatment or initiation of high-dose corticosteroid therapy. Admission to the ICU should be determined by the rate of progression of the weakness, the presence of bulbar failure and the clinical state of the patient rather than relying on measurement of the vital capacity alone [54].

ICU management of myasthenic crisis involves providing respiratory support (often via a tracheostomy) whilst awaiting recovery. Specific therapies to encourage improvement include the optimisation of anticholinesterase and corticosteroid therapy, plasma exchange to remove the autoantibodies and intravenous immunoglobulin [55]. With careful management mortality should not exceed 5%.

18.7.4 *Botulism*

Botulism [56] is a syndrome caused by neurotoxins (usually type A, B or E) produced by the Gram-positive organism *Clostridium botulinum*. It is classified according to the source of infection (i.e. foodborne, wound or infant botulism). Although rare, a form of wound botulism due to 'skin popping' black tar heroin by drug abusers seems to be increasing. Symptoms of the condition include nausea, vomiting, abdominal pain and autonomic dysfunction (blurred vision, diplopia, bradycardia, hypotension) followed by a descending flaccid paralysis. Diagnosis relies mainly on clinical suspicion while awaiting positive detection of botulinum toxin from the relevant specimen.

Patients with suspected botulism should be nursed in a high-dependency area as the development of ventilatory failure may be rapid. The toxin also blocks cholinergic synapses in the autonomic system and cardiovascular instability, gastrointestinal stasis and urinary retention are common.

ICU care is largely supportive until recovery occurs. Specific treatment with either ABE antitoxin or human botulism immunoglobulin dramatically reduces the course of the disease but requires careful co-ordination with the microbiology department. Mortality is below 10% with modern ICU management.

18.7.5 *Tetanus*

Tetanus [57] is a syndrome caused by the neurotoxin tetanospasmin produced by the Gram-positive organism *Clostridium tetani* under anaerobic conditions. Although vaccination has made tetanus rare in the UK, it causes approximately one million deaths worldwide per annum. Tetanospasmin binds to peripheral nerve terminals and then migrates through retrograde axonal transport to the spinal cord and brainstem. Eventually it spreads to presynaptic terminals where it exerts its effect. Tetanus is characterised by increased muscle tone and spasms, typically starting with trismus ('lockjaw') and then spreading to involve the neck, shoulder and back muscles and being provoked by the slightest stimulus. Respiratory muscle failure and autonomic dysfunction (labile blood pressure, arrhythmias, profuse sweating) are the most serious complications requiring ICU treatment. Diagnosis is made mainly on clinical grounds.

Treatment consists of thorough debridement of the wound, administration of penicillin (to eradicate surviving organisms) and human anti-tetanus immunoglobulin as early as possible. Muscular spasm is treated with sedation and neuromuscular-blocking drugs whilst ensuring adequate mechanical ventilation. Dantrolene and magnesium sulphate may have a role. Mortality with modern ICU facilities is less than 10%.

18.8 Clinical Case

A 25-year-old 70-kg man presented to the Accident and Emergency department complaining of shortness of breath and difficulty with swallowing. He gave a history of a diarrhoeal illness ten days previously followed by parasthesiae in his hands and feet accompanied by weakness in both legs making walking unaided impossible.

On examination he was found to be tachypnoeic and using his accessory respiratory muscles. He was tachycardic and hypertensive. Neurological examination revealed normal intellectual function. Cranial nerve examination showed bilateral facial weakness, partial ophthalmoplegia, reduced tongue movement and an absent gag reflex. Distal and proximal weakness was noted in all limbs, legs more affected than arms. Tendon reflexes were absent. Examination of the sensory system was normal. Vital capacity measured using a face mask was 950 ml. Arterial blood gas analysis showed a type 2 respiratory failure.

Although there are many causes of a motor neuropathy (including myasthenia gravis, poliomyelitis and botulism), the history and examination was highly suggestive of Guillain–Barré syndrome.

A lumbar puncture revealed the typical findings of a raised protein, normal glucose and no white cells. Electromyography revealed marked slowing of nerve conduction with increases in distal motor latencies; no axonal loss was demonstrated.

Treatment with intravenous immunoglobulin was started but over the next 12 hours his vital capacity fell further and he required tracheal intubation and mechanical ventilation. Tracheostomy was subsequently performed. Two weeks after the initiation of mechanical ventilation his vital capacity began to increase and bulbar function returned; after a further two weeks he was fully weaned from the ventilator. His tracheostomy was removed and following a period of rehabilitation he made a full recovery.

References

[1] Moppett, I. (2007). Traumatic brain injury: assessment, resuscitation and early management, *Brit J Anaesth*, **99**, 18–31.

[2] Helmy, A., Vizcaychipi, M. and Gupta, A. (2007). Traumatic brain injury: intensive care management, *Br J Anaesth*, **99**, 32–42.

[3] Tisdall, M. and Smith, M. (2007). Multimodal monitoring in traumatic brain injury: current status and future directions, *Br J Anaesth*, **99**, 61–67.

[4] Smith, M. (2008). Monitoring intracranial pressure in traumatic brain injury, *Anesth Analg*, **106**, 240–248.

[5] Nortje, J. and Gupta, A. (2006). The role of tissue oxygen monitoring in patients with acute brain injury, *Br J Anaesth*, **97**, 95–106.

[6] Tisdall, M. and Smith, M. (2006). Cerebral microdialysis: research technique or clinical tool? *Brit J Anaesth*, **97**, 18–25.

[7] Roberts, I., Schierhout, G. and Alderson P. (1998). Absence of evidence for the effectiveness of five interventions routinely used in the intensive care management of severe head injury: a systematic review, *J Neurol Neurosurg Psychiatry*, **65**, 729–733.

[8] Smith, M. (2004). Neurocritical care: has it come of age? *Br J Anaesth*, **93**, 753–755.

[9] Brain Trauma Foundation (2007). Guidelines for the management of severe traumatic brain injury, third edition, *J Neurotrauma*, **24**, (Suppl. 1), S1–S106.
[10] Lim, H. and Smith, M. (2007). Systemic complications after head injury: a clinical review, *Anaesthesia*, **62**, 474–482.
[11] Chesnut, R.M. (1997). Avoidance of hypotension: *conditio sine qua non* of successful severe head-injury management, *J Trauma*, **42**, S4–S9.
[12] Robertson, C.S., Valadka, A.B., Hannay, H.J. *et al.* (1999). Prevention of secondary ischemic insults after severe head injury, *Crit Care Med*, **27**, 2086–2095.
[13] Coles, J.P., Minhas, P.S., Fryer, T.D. *et al.* (2002). Effect of hyperventilation on cerebral blood flow in traumatic head injury: clinical relevance and monitoring correlates, *Crit Care Med*, **30**, 1950–1959.
[14] Wakai, A., Roberts, I. and Schierhout, G. (2005). Mannitol for acute traumatic brain injury, *Cochrane Database Sys Rev*, CD001049.
[15] Himmelseher, S. (2007). Hypertonic saline solutions for treatment of intracranial hypertension, *Curr Opin Anaesthesiol*, **20**, 414–426.
[16] Cooper, D.J., Rosenfeld, J.V., Murray, L. *et al.* (2011). Decompressive craniectomy in diffuse traumatic brain injury, *N Engl J Med*, **364**, 1493–1502.
[17] Clifton, G.L., Miller, E.R., Choi, S.C. *et al.* (2001). Lack of effect of induction of hypothermia after acute brain injury, *N Engl J Med*, **344**, 566–563.
[18] Polderman, K., Ely, E., Badr, A. *et al.* (2004). Induced hypothermia in traumatic brain injury: considering the conflicting results of meta-analyses and moving forward, *Crit Care Med*, **30**,1860–1864.
[19] Zygun, D. (2005). Non-neurological organ dysfunction in neurocritical care: impact on outcome and etiological considerations, *Curr Opin Crit Care*, **11**, 139–143.
[20] Tisdall, M., Crocker, M., Watkiss, J. *et al.* (2006). Disturbances of sodium in critically ill adult neurologic patients, *J Neurosurg Anesthesiol*, **18**, 57–63.
[21] Suarez, J., Tarr, R., Selman, W. *et al.* (2006). Aneurysmal subarachnoid hemorrhage, *N Engl J Med*, **354**, 387–396.
[22] Wilson, S., Hirsch, N. and Appleby, I. (2005). Management of subarachnoid haemorrhage in a non-neurosurgical centre, *Anaesthesia*, **60**, 470–485.
[23] Smith, M. (2007). Intensive care management of patients with subarachnoid haemorrhage, *Curr Opin Anesthesiol*, **20**, 400–407.
[24] Diringer, M.N. (2005). To clip or to coil acutely ruptured intracranial aneurysms: update on the debate, *Curr Opin Crit Care*, **11**, 121–125.
[25] Janjua, N. and Mayer, S.A. (2003). Cerebral vasospasm after subarachnoid hemorrhage, *Curr Opin Crit Care*, **9**, 113–119.
[26] Wartenberg, K.E. and Mayer, S.A. (2006). Medical complications after subarachnoid hemorrhage: new strategies for prevention and management, *Curr Opin Crit Care*, **12**, 78–84.

[27] Mayer, S. and Rincon F. (2005). Treatment of intracerebral haemorrhage, *Lancet Neurol*, **4**, 662–672.

[28] Mayer, S. (2007). Recombinant activated factor VII for acute intracerebral hemorrhage, *Stroke*, **38**, 763–767.

[29] Mergenthaler, P., Dirnagl, U. and Meisel, A. (2004). Pathophysiology of stroke: lessons from animal models, *Metab Brain Dis*, **19**, 151–167.

[30] Hacke, W., Kaste, M., Bluhmke, E. *et al.* (2008). Thrombolysis with alteplase 3 to 4.5 hours after ischemic stroke, *N Engl J Med*, **359**, 1393–1395.

[31] Wardlaw, J.M., del Zoppo, G., Yamaguchi, T. *et al.* (2003). Thrombolysis for acute ischaemic stroke, *Cochrane Database Syst Rev*, **3**, CD000213.

[32] Hacke, W., Donnan, G., Fieschi, C., *et al.* (2004). Association of outcome with early stroke treatment: pooled analysis of ATLANTIS, ECASS and NINDS rt-PA stroke trials, *Lancet*, **363**, 768–774.

[33] Chen, Z.M., Sandercock, P., Han, H.C. *et al.* (2000). Indications for early aspirin use in acute ischemic stroke: a combined analysis of 40 000 randomized patients from the Chinese Acute Stroke Trial and the International Stroke Trial, *Stroke*, **31**, 1240–1249.

[34] Stam, J. (2005). Thrombosis of the cerebral veins and sinuses, *N Engl J Med*, **352**, 1791–1798.

[35] McDonald, J.W. and Sadowsky, C. (2002). Spinal-cord injury, *Lancet*, **359**, 417–425.

[36] Kwon, B.K., Tetzlaff, W., Grauer, J.N. *et al.* (2004). Pathophysiology and pharmacologic treatment of acute spinal cord injury, *Spine*, **4**, 451–464.

[37] Bracken, M.B., Shepard, M.J., Collins, W.F., *et al.* (1990). A randomized, controlled trial of methylprednisolone or naloxone in the treatment of acute spinal-cord injury. Results of the Second National Acute Spinal Cord Injury Study, *N Engl J Med*, **322**, 1405–1411.

[38] Bracken, M.B., Shepard, M.J., Holford, T.R., *et al.* (1998). Methylprednisolone or tirilazad mesylate administration after acute spinal cord injury: 1-year follow up. Results of the third National Acute Spinal Cord Injury randomized controlled trial, *J Neurosurg*, **89**, 699–706.

[39] Spencer, M.T. and Bazarian, J.J. (2003). Are corticosteroids effective in traumatic spinal cord injury? *Ann Emerg Med*, **41**, 410–413.

[40] Chapman, M.G., Smith, M. and Hirsch, N.P. (2001). Status epilepticus, *Anaesthesia*, **56**, 648–659.

[41] Epilepsy Foundation of America's Working Group on Status Epilepticus (1993). Treatment of convulsive status epilepticus, Recommendations of the epilepsy foundation of America's working group on status epilepticus, *JAMA*, **270**, 854–859.

[42] Towne, A.R., Waterhouse, E.G., Boggs, J.G. *et al.* (2000). Prevalence of non-convulsive status epilepticus in comatose patients, *Neurology*, **54**, 340–345.

[43] Prasad, K., Al-Rooni, K., Krishnan, P.R. *et al.* (2005). Anticonvulsant therapy for status epilepticus, *Cochrane Database Syst Rev*, **4**, CD003723.

[44] Walker, M.C., Howard, R.S., Smith, S.J. *et al.* (1996). Diagnosis and treatment of status epilepticus on a neurological intensive care unit, *Q J Med*, **89**, 913–920.

[45] Howard, R.S., Kullmann, D.M., Hirsch, N.P. (2003). Admission to neurological intensive care: who, when and why? *J Neurol Neurosurg Psychiatry*, **74** (Suppl. III): iii2–iii9.

[46] Hughes, R.A.C. and Cornblath, D.R. (2005). Guillain–Barré syndrome, *Lancet*, **366**, 1653–1666.

[47] Lawn, N.D., Fletcher, D.D., Henderson, R.D. *et al.* (2001). Anticipating mechanical ventilation in Guillain–Barré syndrome, *Arch Neurol*, **58**, 893–898.

[48] Hughes, R.A., Swan, A.V., Raphael, J.C. *et al.* (2007). Immunotherapy for, Guillain–Barré syndrome: a systematic review, *Brain*, **130**, 2245–2257.

[49] Ng, K.K.P., Howard, R.S., Fish, D.R. *et al.* (1995). Management and outcome of severe Guillain–Barré syndrome, *Q J Med*, **88**, 243–250.

[50] Latronico, N., Peli, E., Bottero, M. *et al.* (2005). Critical illness myopathy and neuropathy, *Curr Opin Crit Care*, **11**, 126–132.

[51] Hund, E.F., Fogel, W., Krieger, D. *et al.* (1996). Critical illness polyneuropathy: clinical findings and outcomes of a frequent cause of neuromuscular weaning failure, *Crit Care Med*, **24**, 1328–1333.

[52] Bolton, C.F. (2005). Neuromuscular manifestations of critical illness, *Muscle Nerve*, **32**, 140–163.

[53] Vincent, A., Palace, J. and Hilton-Jones, D. (2001). Myasthenia gravis, *Lancet*, **357**, 2122–2128.

[54] Lacomis, D. (2005). Myasthenic crisis, *Neurocrit Care*, **03,** 189–194.

[55] O'Riordan, J.I., Miller, D.H., Mottershead, J.P. *et al.* (1998). The management and outcome of patients treated acutely in a neurological intensive care unit, *Eur J Neurol*, **5**, 137–142.

[56] Caya, J.G., Agni, R. and Miller, J.E. (2004). *Clostridium botulinum* and the clinical laboratorian, *Arch Pathol Lab Med*, **128**, 653–662.

[57] Cook, T.M., Protheroe, R.T. and Handel, J.M. (2001). Tetanus: a review of the literature, *Br J Anaesth*, **87**, 477–487.

19

Cardiopulmonary Intensive Care

Marius Gota, Allen Bashour and Michael O'Connor

19.1 Introduction

Every year more than 500,000 open heart procedures are performed in the USA [1], and all these patients are admitted post-operatively to an intensive care unit (ICU).

Cardiac surgery almost never brings an immediate improvement in the patient's well-being and functional status. On the contrary, short-term it often means added insult to an organism already compromised by the cardiac disease as well as by a host of comorbidities. Post-operative morbidity is frequent and mortality varies from 1% in low-risk patients undergoing elective, 'simple procedures' (i.e. isolated coronary artery bypass graft (CABG)) to significantly higher for higher-risk patients and/or more complex procedures [2, 3]. Occurrence of major morbidities with extended ICU length of stay affects both short- and long-term survival [4]. Counteracting these insults and the longer-term complications in the attempt to re-establish the organism's autonomy is the object of post-operative critical care.

Significant advances in surgical, perfusion and anaesthetic technique as well as in post-operative care resulted in shorter ICU length of stay and better outcomes despite this surgery being delivered to an increasingly sicker and older patient population.

19.2 The Initial Post-Operative Period

Major bleeding needing re-exploration, haemodynamic instability, arrhythmias, metabolic and respiratory disturbances can occur frequently in the immediate post-operative period. The same level of monitoring as in the operating room (OR), with the exception of transoesophageal echo (TEE), is preserved during this time. This includes two-lead electrocardiogram (ECG), pulse oximetry, invasive arterial and central venous pressures, urinary output and ventilation parameters. Outcome data favouring pulmonary-artery-catheter-derived benefits are lacking [5, 6], however, in most busy hospitals in North America, pulmonary artery catheters are routinely used as a tool to rapidly derive information incorporated in haemodynamic management protocols. While the incidence of minor complications related to pulmonary catheter placement and usage may be higher, major complications related to its use are exceedingly rare [7]. Capnography in addition to pulse oximetry reduces the need for frequent arterial blood gas (ABG) determinations in stable patients.

Routine laboratory tests are obtained to detect major abnormalities. Unless mandated by signs and symptoms or monitoring parameters, ABG is measured about 30 minutes after mechanical ventilation is instituted. A chest X-ray to confirm position of endotracheal tubes, monitoring catheters and surgical drains and to rule out mechanical complications (pneumothorax, haemothorax and mediastinal enlargement due to bleeding) as well as a 12-lead ECG are performed as soon as the transfer of care is complete.

To allow for a smooth emergence and identification of early complications the vast majority of patients are transferred from the OR to the ICU intubated, while recovering from the effect of anaesthetics. Short-acting, easily titratable sedatives are employed in most instances with the purpose of ensuring a smooth transition from the OR to the ICU, facilitating the transfer of care and assessment of the patient. Propofol and dexmedetomidine are the agents of choice for this period. While propofol has a short elimination half-life, awakening is mostly dependent on its rapid redistribution and even after prolonged ICU infusion, awakening time is short. Another important characteristic of propofol is that it does not produce reliable amnesia unless it is administered at hypnotic doses. While this may be a disadvantage in the OR setting, it is advantageous when rapid emergence and reorientation of the patient is desired, more often than not in the ICU setting. However, propofol is not an analgesic and patients awakening from propofol sedation will be in pain and possibly agitated, unless this is addressed by analgesic (i.e. opioid) medication.

In contrast, dexmedetomidine, a highly selective and potent alpha-2 agonist, has analgesic properties. Sedation by dexmedetomidine is felt by some to come close to the ideal for conscious sedation as it does not induce full hypnosis or amnesia so the patient reorients, is easily rousable and is able to follow commands comfortably. Additionally, dexmedetomidine does not depress respiration, so the drug does not need to be discontinued for extubation. Dexmedetomidine appears to significantly decrease the incidence of post-operative delirium, decreases the use of analgesics and has a variety of favourable physiological benefits with only minor side effects [8, 9].

Incomplete rewarming before separation from the heart–lung machine results in post-operative hypothermia with unwanted consequences: coagulopathy (i.e. platelet dysfunction), vasoconstriction, shivering with increased oxygen consumption and carbon dioxide production resulting in both metabolic (lactic) and respiratory acidosis. Forced air heating blankets in combination with drug adjuncts, such as small doses of meperidine (or other opioids) and muscle relaxants (if mechanical ventilation is difficult or acidosis worsening) usually result in fast rewarming. The vasoconstriction that accompanies hypothermia is soon followed by vasodilatation with increasing fluid requirements and, if the post-operative inflammatory response is intense, possible need for vasoconstrictors.

Cardiac output is an important predictor of outcome after cardiac surgery. A patient with warm extremities, fast capillary refill, stable heart rhythm and rate, blood pressure and producing adequate urine is likely to have a good cardiac output.

The haemodynamic syndrome (Table 19.1) is often the starting point in the differential diagnosis of various and potential life-threatening post-operative complications.

Low cardiac output has a variety of aetiologies. Hypovolaemia is frequently caused by overt or concealed post-operative bleeding, third spacing as a result of the systemic inflammatory response to surgery and cardiopulmonary bypass (CPB) and/or polyuria resulting from hypothermia as well as the intra-operative use of mannitol. No resuscitation fluid

Table 19.1. Haemodynamic syndrome. CI, cardiac index; PAWP, pulmonary artery wedge pressure; CVP, central venous pressure; SVR, systemic vascular resistance; N, normal.

		Haemodynamic parameter			
		CI	PAWP	CVP	SVR
Shock type	Hypovolemic	low	low	low	high
	Cardiogenic	low	high	N/high	high
	Distributive	high	N/low	N/low	low

has proven its superiority so far [10,11]. Large amounts of crystalloids have been traditionally avoided in cardiac surgery due to the fear of worsening tissue oedema and congestive heart failure. On the other hand, colloids are expensive and have side effects of their own (i.e. allergic reactions, coagulopathy, platelet and reticulo-endothelial system dysfunction etc.) which limit their use. Ultimately, the timing, aggressiveness and adequacy of resuscitation are the determinant factors in limiting the extent of end-organ dysfunction [12,13]. During active fluid resuscitation, vasoconstrictors can be temporarily employed to maintain adequate perfusion pressures to the vital organs. One should not forget that the indiscriminate use of vasopressors may mask hypovolaemia. Increasing pressor requirement, persistent low urine and cardiac output, evidence of high oxygen extraction and worsening metabolic acidosis should prompt a careful search for the cause of hypovolaemia (i.e. concealed bleeding, massive third spacing in catastrophic abdominal complications — i.e. mesenteric ischaemia, pancreatitis).

A low cardiac output or hypotension with clinical evidence of organ hypoperfusion and elevated filling pressures should point towards cardiogenic shock. Pre-existent myocardial dysfunction is one of the most important predictors of post-operative function and is often compounded by intra-operative myocardial injury or stunning. In the operating room, post cardiopulmonary bypass, all determinants of cardiac function are addressed in a systematic fashion. Adequate preloading, rate and rhythm (if necessary using epicardial pacing and/or anti-arrhythmics), contractility (using various inotropes) and afterload (using either pressors or vasodilators) are ensured before the transport of the patient to the ICU.

The patient is usually returned from the OR in stable condition and with a well characterised (using intra-operative TEE as well as invasive monitoring) heart function and haemodynamics. From this baseline, any unexpected worsening of a previously stable patient should determine a prompt search for the aetiology of the cardiogenic shock. Aetiologies that require prompt diagnosis and treatment include:

- Cardiac tamponade (pericardial effusion or resulting from tissue oedema).
- Acute ischaemia secondary to acute graft occlusion or spasm or incomplete revascularisation.
- Uncorrected or unrecognised valvular abnormalities.

Echocardiography is an invaluable tool in getting a timely diagnosis and therapy. The post-operative ICU patient, however, confronts the echocardiographer with problems stemming from presence of surgical dressings, chest tubes, mechanical ventilation, an uncooperative patient, presence of pneumothorax or pneumomediastinum, all resulting in poor transthoracic echo windows and a difficult exam. TEE proves to be of particular benefit in this setting and success rate in obtaining adequate TEE images is high (> 90%) [14].

19.2.1 *Cardiac tamponade*

Cardiac tamponade is rare but potentially life-threatening. Its incidence is reported to be between 0.5–5.8% in different studies and it most often occurs in the early post-operative period [15]. Early post-operative cardiac tamponade is usually related to surgical bleeding and post cardiopulmonary bypass coagulopathy. Leaving the anterior pericardial sac open does not appear to be protective. The classical clinical triad of hypotension, elevated venous pressure and a small quiet heart as well as pulsus paradoxus and equalisation of diastolic pressures (right atrial (RA) = right ventricular (RV) = pulmonary artery diastolic (PAD)) on pulmonary artery catheter (PAC) tracing is rare after heart surgery [16]. Localised pericardial effusions or clots with selective cardiac chamber compression are frequent and result in a blunted clinical picture [17]. Most often post-operative tamponade manifests as hypodynamic shock with organ hypoperfusion and hypotension. A sudden decrease in a previously abundant chest tube output with an enlarged mediastinum on the chest X-ray suggests tamponade. Acute left ventricular (LV) and especially RV failure can be a difficult differential diagnosis when only routine clinical, haemodynamic and radiological tools are used. The typical echocardiographic signs of right atrial late diastolic and right ventricular early diastolic collapse as well as paradoxical septal motion and transmitral and transtricuspid respirophasic flow variations are common in circumferential pericardial effusion but may be absent in the presence of a localised compression or as a consequence of elevated filling pressures from aggressive resuscitation. TEE, however, can reveal loculated effusions with selective compression in the majority of patients and provide useful elements for the differential (see Fig. 19.1) [17]. The reopening of the sternum is the treatment of choice in the early post-operative period, achieving clot evacuation and also definitive surgical haemostasis. Substernal pericardial window or, rarely, percutaneous drainage are used for late pericardial tamponade

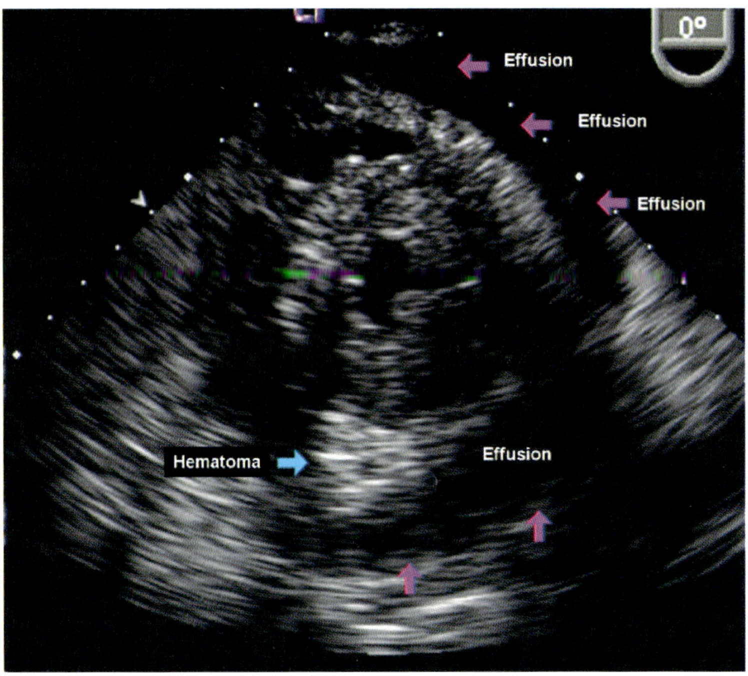

Figure 19.1. Early post-operative cardiac tamponade. (Reproduced courtesy of Dr Robert M. Savage).

19.2.2 *Peri-operative ischaemia/infarction*

Peri-operative ischaemia/infarction occurs in 5–10% of cases after CABG [18]. Causes include graft occlusion (thrombosis, spasm, kinking), wrong anastomosis, incomplete revascularisation, displaced graft and poor run-off [19]. Diagnosis is based on detection of new localised ECG changes in the setting of coronary heart failure (CHF)/shock and/or rhythm instability (especially polymorphic ventricular tachycardia (VT) or ventricular fibrillation). The surgeon's opinion is critical for such details as severity of coronary artery disease, quality of targets and conduits and completeness of revascularisation. Enzymatic diagnosis is difficult since cardiac surgery is almost always associated with an increase in the markers of myocardial necrosis [20]. New wall motion abnormalities (especially if in territories other than septum) by echocardiography support the diagnosis. A stable patient should undergo an urgent coronary angiography followed by revascularisation or medical treatment when the former is not possible. Unstable patients are taken directly to the operating room where the grafts are inspected and repaired or additional bypasses are performed. In patients without contraindication to its use, bedside placement of an intra-aortic balloon pump increases coronary perfusion pressure and unloads the left ventricle, thus limiting the extent of ischaemia until the definitive intervention is performed. Adequate pain control and oxygenation, reduction of unnecessary stresses and oxygen consumption as well as antiplatelet agents (aspirin) and, wherever the situation allows, β-blockers and anticoagulation should be employed as soon as possible.

19.2.3 *Uncorrected or unrecognised valvular abnormalities*

Uncorrected or unrecognised valvular abnormalities (dynamic left ventricular outflow tract (LVOT) obstruction and systolic anterior motion (SAM) of the mitral valve with mitral regurgitation, paravalvular leaks, patient–prosthesis mismatch) are all causes of haemodynamic compromise and can be best recognised by echocardiography and in particular by transoesophageal studies. A particularly difficult problem after heart surgery is RV failure as a cause of haemodynamic instability. Pre-existent RV dysfunction, imperfect intra-operative myocardial protection and subsequent ischaemia–reperfusion injury, air emboli lodging in the right coronary ostium, exacerbation of pulmonary hypertension after CPB and protamine reactions are involved in the pathogenesis of post-operative RV failure [21]. When the contractile reserve and the Frank–Starling compensatory mechanism of the RV reach their limits, ischaemia of the RV free wall ensues, with a precipitous decrease in cardiac output and hypotension [22].

Hypodynamic shock with elevated right-sided filling pressures and low PAWP are diagnostic of RV failure. Echocardiography can confirm this and help differentiate it from cardiac tamponade. Typical echocardiographic findings are: RV dilatation and hypokinesis, tricuspid regurgitation, flattening of the interventricular septum with paradoxical motion and dilated inferior vena cava with lack of inspiratory collapse. RV failure with pulmonary hypertension (PHTN) is secondary to LV dysfunction, chronic thromboembolic disease or pulmonary vascular disease of various aetiologies. Acute hypoxemia, acute lung injury/acute respiratory distress syndrome (ARDS) as well as acute acid-base abnormalities are important causes of PHTN in ICU. An acutely decompensated RV without pulmonary hypertension is caused by right-sided valvular disease or has an ischaemic/cardiomyopathic mechanism (RV infarction, poor protection, primary cardiomyopathies) [23]. Means to stabilise the patient include: volume resuscitation, various pressors and inotropes and pulmonary vasodilators as well as mechanical circulatory support.

A relatively stable patient can benefit from small fluid boluses. Increasing the CVP to more than 12–15 mmHg is of no benefit or can be even detrimental. If cardiac output decreases in response to a fluid challenge, diuresis or ultrafiltration can be used to reduce preload. To break the vicious circle of hypotension leading to RV ischaemia leading to more hypotension, the use of pressors is mandatory. Norepinephrine, epinephrine and dopamine have all been used successfully. Interestingly, besides ensuring perfusion pressures to the RV and vital organs, vasoconstriction is also beneficial by increasing the left ventricular end diastolic pressure and left ventricular end diastolic volume. This could restore the normal crescent shape of the interventricular septum, thus providing contractile support to the RV free wall. Once adequate perfusion pressure and preload have been established, inotropes are employed to increase the RV contractility.

Right-sided heart inotropes are isoproterenol, dobutamine and milrinone. Isoproterenol is used preponderantly in the setting of heart transplantation, where it acts also as a potent chronotrope. Dobutamine has been shown to improve haemodynamics in the setting of RV failure with pulmonary hypertension, where it does not increase pulmonary vascular resistance as well as in the case of RV ischaemia/infarction where it is considered the inotropic agent of choice. Milrinone's inodilator properties are useful in the decompensated RV. Vasopressin has been used to counteract the systemic vasodilatation produced by milrinone without producing important pulmonary vasoconstriction.

For RV failure with pulmonary hypertension, the use of pulmonary vasodilators is logical. Inhaled nitric oxide (iNO) is devoid of any systemic effects, and possibly the best choice in the acute setting. Its use is hampered, however, by the high cost. Prostacyclin and prostaglandin E1, as well as nitroglycerine and nitroprusside can produce systemic hypotension and worsen ventilation–perfusion mismatch. Oral sildenafil is an alternative agent that can be used to facilitate weaning of inhaled and intravenous pulmonary vasodilators [24, 25]. The intra-aortic balloon pump (IABP) has been used in RV failure with the goal of increasing coronary perfusion to reduce RV ischaemia. Limiting positive end-expiratory pressure (PEEP)/auto-PEEP, as well as the mean airway pressure resulting from aggressive ventilation, correction of hypercarbia and metabolic acidosis are basic therapeutic strategies to limit unwarranted increases in RV afterload. For refractory cases mechanical circulatory support by extra-corporeal membrane oxygenation (ECMO), or ventricular-assist devices, as appropriate, can bridge the patient to recovery or transplant.

19.2.4 *Vasodilatory shock*

Vasodilatory shock is estimated to occur in 5–8% of patients undergoing cardiopulmonary bypass and is higher in sicker patients [26]. Risk factors are left ventricular ejection fraction (LVEF) < 35%, insertion of left ventricular assist devices for end-stage heart failure, long cross-clamp time and cardiopulmonary bypass time as well as pre-operative use of angiotensin converting enzyme inhibitors [26, 27]. Blood contact with the foreign surface of the CPB circuit, endotoxinaemia resulting from gut hypoperfusion, heparin–protamine interaction and the surgical act itself are initiating factors of the systemic inflammatory response post open heart surgery. Treatment remains largely supportive and focussed on ensuring an adequate perfusion pressure and oxygen delivery to end organs.

Alpha-1-mediated vasoconstriction to increase perfusion pressure is achieved by the use of a variety of sympathetic agonists. Norepinephrine is ideally suited for this purpose, but clear advantage compared with dopamine or epinephrine is lacking. A relative or absolute vasopressin deficiency is common post cardiopulmonary bypass. Low-dose vasopressin can increase mean arterial pressure and decrease norepinephrine administration and side effects [26, 28]. Nitric oxide (NO), which acts through activation of soluble guanylate cyclase, has been involved in pathophysiology of post CPB-vasodilatory shock. Methylene blue, a guanylate cyclase inhibitor, was shown to be effective in reversing the vasoplegic syndrome after cardiopulmonary bypass and possibly improving the outcome of these patients [29].

Overt or concealed post-operative bleeding is frequent after cardiac surgery with both bleeding and re-exploration being independent predictors of adverse outcome. Some degree of bleeding is common but diminishes over the first ten hours after the operation. It is related to coagulopathy after cardiopulmonary bypass as well as to the mediastinal dissection. Increased age, non-elective surgery, low body surface area, CPB time longer than 150 minutes, complex surgery (combined valve–CABG or high number of bypass grafts), re-operations, as well as pre-operative use of antiplatelet agents have been associated with excessive post-operative bleeding [30]. Heparin rebound [31] (heparin released in circulation from endothelial surfaced and shorter half-life of protamine) suggested by an increased activated partial thromboplastin time (APTT) is treated with small doses of protamine [32]. One should remember that APTT is a better detector of residual heparin effect at low concentrations than activated clotting time (ACT). CPB reduces platelet count, but thrombocytopenia below 50–100 k is rare and should be treated with platelet transfusion. Rarely is platelet transfusion needed when the platelet count exceeds 100 k, however it should be born in mind that pre-operative use of antiplatelet agents (aspirin, clopidogrel), as well as prolonged CPB, induce platelet dysfunction. This is not usually explored with routine post-operative coagulation tests, and platelet transfusion is warranted when there is clinical bleeding unexplained otherwise. Factor-deficiency coagulopathy is expected in the presence of pre-operative liver dysfunction or the use of warfarin. After CPB, there is a predictable fall in coagulation factors (II, V, VII, IX, X, XIII) related to dilution (massive transfusion) and/or consumption [30]. When this is accompanied by clinical bleeding the recommended dose of fresh frozen plasma is 10 ml/kg. Cryoprecipitate, which supplies fibrinogen, factor VIII, VIII-vW, XIII and fibronectin, is usually reserved for patients with fibrinogen levels below 100 mg/dl. The role of activated factor VII in cardiac surgery is still to be established. Bleeding exceeding 500 cm^3 in the first hour, 400 ml/hour over two hours, 300 ml/hour over 3 hours, or 200 ml/hour over four hours, together with tamponade or bleeding causing haemodynamic instability are typical indications for mediastinal re-exploration. While re-exploration is an independent risk factor for septic complications (i.e. deep sternal wound infection) and prolonged ICU course, it seems that early re-operation for bleeding can decrease the number of subsequent complications [33]. Frequent sites of surgical bleeding include branches of the mammary artery or saphenous vein grafts, coronary anastomoses and sites of cannulation (aortic, cardioplegia or venous). Frequently only diffuse bleeding is noted but removal of clot and fibrinolytic byproducts may decrease further bleeding and reduce longer-term complications.

19.2.5 *Acute dysrhythmias*

Acute dysrhythmias are frequent in the post-operative period. They become important when associated with haemodynamic compromise or cardiac arrest, when they are persistent or when they are a sign of a more ominous complication. Atrial tachyarrhythmias are not uncommon in the first 24 hours after cardiac surgery. The most common is atrial fibrillation, which occurs in 20–40% of patients after CABG and is more frequent after valve surgery. Its peak incidence is on post-operative days two and three and it is self-limited, with most of the patients returning to sinus rhythm by six to eight weeks after surgery. Use of various inotropes, β-blocker withdrawal, inflammation and surgical trauma, as well as electrolyte abnormalities (hypokalemia and hypomagnesemia) are incriminated in its pathogenesis. Its occurrence is associated with increased risk of stroke and duration of hospitalisation [34]. Amiodarone reduces the incidence of post-operative atrial fibrillation [35]. When associated with haemodynamic instability direct-current cardioversion is performed urgently, however, for the stable patient a rate-control strategy (with anticoagulation started as soon as possible) has outcomes similar to rhythm control. It should be remembered that post-operative tachycardia is better tolerated than bradycardia, and any negative chronotropic drugs should be used with caution early after the operation.

19.2.6 *Blocks*

Blocks and slow escape/non-perfusing rhythms are related to pre-existent conduction abnormalities, drug effects and/or surgical trauma. Valve surgery increases the rate of blocks and bradycardias [36]. Almost routine placement of epicardial pacing wires (ventricular or atrial and ventricular) simplifies the immediate post-operative management of these patients. Most patients that recover conduction will do so within seven days, and blocks persisting beyond this interval require permanent pacing. Ventricular arrhythmias including frequent or non-sustained premature ventricular contractions or sustained VT/ventricular fibrillations can be the expression of same general factors that cause supraventricular arrhythmias or associated with peri-operative ischaemia–reperfusion or reduced ventricular function. Besides antiarrhythmic treatment or emergent cardioversion/defibrillation if needed, correction of gas exchange, electrolyte and metabolic abnormalities and aggressive attempts to rule out and or treat myocardial ischaemia should be undertaken. The long-term prognosis after complex ventricular arrhythmias is related to the degree of ventricular dysfunction [36].

While cardiac arrest in the ICU is usually the result of a protracted severe illness (severe heart failure, sepsis, etc.) a minority (0.7% in a large prospective cohort) of patients will sustain post-operative cardiac arrest during the first 24 hours after cardiac surgery [37]. The main causes are peri-operative myocardial infarction, mechanical impediments (tamponade and graft malfunction) or primary arrhythmias. Mechanical causes constitute an important proportion of these cases (28%) [37]. The conventional CPR measures, if not successful, are followed by open-chest CPR with the dual purpose of more efficient resuscitation and rapid identification and relieving of the mechanical cause. The results of open-chest resuscitation, especially if it is performed within five to ten minutes post arrest, are significant, with 22–38% of patients surviving to hospital discharge [37,38].

An increased alveolo–arterial O_2 gradient is common after heart surgery, and due to acute post cardiopulmonary bypass lung injury, compounded by atelectasis and hydrostatic factors. Severe acute hypoxaemia is uncommon, and when it occurs requires rapid diagnosis and treatment. Endobronchial intubation (right mainstem) and pneumothorax, are diagnosed by physical exam, careful attention to mechanical ventilation parameters and the post-operative chest X-ray and easily treated thereafter. Severe pulmonary oedema can be the consequence of the primary cardiac disease or results from capillary leak (i.e. 'pump lung', transfusion-related acute lung injury, ARDS). Besides the usual supportive measures muscle paralysis can be required to facilitate mechanical ventilation and avoid barotrauma. The newer lung-protective ventilation strategies (low tidal volumes, high PEEP) should be employed to limit the extent of ventilator-induced lung injury [39]. In severe cases iNO or short-term ECMO can be salutary and provide the time necessary for resolution of the process.

19.3 Neurological Complications

Post cardiac surgery stroke occurs in 1.5–5.2% of patients and carries a three-fold increase in the rate of death [40, 41]. Risk factors include: age, female sex, carotid artery disease, prior strokes, valve surgery, calcified aorta, renal failure, smoking and diabetes [42]. Focal ischaemic injury is the result of peri-operative macro emboli (aortic atheromas, atrial or ventricular thrombi, air or other debris) or intra-operative hypoperfusion (rarely). Haemorrhagic stroke is rare after cardiac surgery and results more often from transformation of an ischaemic stroke. Diagnosis is based on the clinical picture and can be suggested by failure of the patient to emerge from anaesthesia and follow commands within the first six hours after the surgery. The stroke team should be activated as soon as there is a clinical suspicion and a CT/computed tomography angiography should be performed to rule out intracranial bleeding and assess lesions amenable to mechanical interventions. Magnetic resonance imaging is more sensitive than CT and can detect subtle abnormalities but can be performed only in stable patients without medical devices and after the epicardial pacing wires are removed. Treatment is largely supportive (permissive hypertension, adequate oxygenation, glycaemic control, aggressive treatment of fever). Aspirin has been shown to improve outcome after ischaemic stroke and is routinely given after cardiac surgery [43]. Mechanical thrombolysis can be considered whenever it can be performed within eight hours of the onset of the ischaemic event.

19.3.1 *Encephalopathy*

Encephalopathy ranges from subtle neuropsychiatric abnormalities to delirium, seizures and, rarely, coma and occurs in up to 32% of patients. It also triples hospital mortality [41]. Risk factors include age, previous stroke and presence of a carotid bruit, hypertension and diabetes. When the patient emerges from anaesthesia with persistent combativeness and agitation the differentials include emergence delirium (i.e. residual sedative/anaesthetic effect) or encephalopathy. Adequate analgesia is key to avoiding emergence delirium. Dexmedetomidine is a sedative especially suited for this setting. Treatment includes agitation control using neuroleptics (haloperidol is the mainstay), pain control, reorientation, removal of other psychoactive medication (benzodiazepines, anticholinergics etc.) that can compound confusion and worsen agitation, correction of metabolic and electrolyte abnormalities, exclusion or treatment of sepsis. Extubation is frequently delayed until agitation is controlled.

19.4 Respiratory Management and Complications

Lung function impairment is inevitable after any major surgery and is frequently superimposed on significant pre-operative comorbidities. Respiratory mechanics are altered by sternotomy, thoracotomy and manipulation of the thoracic content which can cause atelectasis, pleural effusions or pneumothoraces. Mediastinal dissection and pericardial ice or cold saline used for myocardial protection can result in phrenic nerve injury. Pulmonary oedema, hydrostatic or inflammatory, increases the alveolo–arterial gradient.

It is not surprising then that respiratory complications are a leading cause of morbidity after cardiac surgery. In a large study of consecutive patients after cardiac surgery, 7.5% had respiratory complications, 21% of which resulted in death and 64.3% to prolonged hospitalisation [44]. It seems, however, that the major cause of poor pulmonary outcome after cardiac surgery remains cardiac dysfunction itself [45].

19.4.1 *Atelectasis*

Atelectasis is usually the product of supine position and anaesthesia with muscle relaxation and upper displacement of the diaphragm. In the left lung this is compounded by pleurotomy and compression for internal mammary artery takedown. After sternotomy, forced vital capacity and forced expiratory volume in one second may decrease by more than 50% from pre-operative values [46] and these decreases may persist for more than three months after the surgery. Together with post-operative pain these ventilatory changes can impair secretion clearance. Lobar atelectasis usually results from retained secretions and is less frequently associated with phrenic nerve injury. Early mobilisation and good pain control combined with aggressive chest physiotherapy and, when needed, therapeutic bronchoscopy is an effective means of preventing and treating significant atelectasis. There is no clear evidence that regional anaesthesia techniques (subarachnoid opioids or epidural analgesia) reduce the rate of post-operative complications and improve outcome.

19.4.2 *Pleural effusions*

Many patients develop pleural effusions after cardiac surgery. The radiographic incidence of pleural effusions after CABG, for example, is 40–50%, mostly left-sided and asymptomatic. Causes include: post-operative bleeding, leakage of fluid from the mediastinum, pleurotomy during mammary artery dissection, disruption of pleural lymphatic drainage and CHF. Late effusions (i.e. two to three weeks after surgery) can be caused by the post-pericardiotomy syndrome. Most effusions resolve spontaneously and require no treatment; however, when large and symptomatic, these effusions require thoracocenthesis, tube thoracostomy or pleurodhesis [47].

19.4.3 *Pneumothorax*

Pneumothorax occurs in 1.4% of patients [48], with a higher incidence after CABG with internal mammary artery takedown. It can result from direct surgical trauma to the lung, from central venous cannulation or as a result of ventilator-induced barotrauma in patients at risk (chronic interstitial lung disease, bullous emphysema, chronic obstructive pulmonary disease (COPD) or asthma). It can occur immediately after surgery or later, with discontinuation of the pleural or mediastinal chest tubes. Most resolve with tube thoracostomy, while a small percentage need surgery.

19.4.4 *Cardiogenic pulmonary oedema*

Cardiogenic pulmonary oedema is one of the most frequent causes of prolonged post-operative mechanical ventilation. Patients at risk have reduced left ventricular function. Interestingly, a low LVEF is more predictive of post-operative respiratory complications than abnormal pre-operative pulmonary function [45].

19.4.5 *Non-cardiogenic pulmonary oedema*

Non-cardiogenic pulmonary oedema is common after cardiac surgery. A mild degree of acute lung injury is reported in up to 12% of cases, and full blown ARDS develops in only about 2% of patients, with a mortality of approximately 75% [49, 50]. Risk factors for ARDS include redo and emergency surgery, re-exploration for bleeding and significant transfusion of blood products. Lung injury is generally believed to be the result of the damaging effects of systemic inflammatory reaction to cardiopulmonary bypass. Notably, however, both on-pump and off-pump CABG patients experience similar degrees of alveolar–arterial partial O_2 pressure difference increase and shunting, despite an attenuated inflammatory response in off-pump patients [51]. Post-operative management is largely supportive. 'Lung protective ventilation', employing low tidal volumes (6 ml/kg rather than 12 ml/kg in conventional ventilation), has emerged as a major strategy involved in avoiding further ventilator-induced lung injury and improving the chances of recovery [39]. Mortality and morbidity benefits in cardiac surgical population remain to be proven. Permissive hypercarbia frequently employed with this strategy has not been shown to have detrimental effects.

19.4.6 *Pulmonary thromboembolism*

An under-recognised complication after cardiac surgery is pulmonary thromboembolism. Frequently asymptomatic, it has a reported incidence of between 0.3% and 9.5% and is the cause of death in 4% of these patients [52]. Aspirin and elastic gradient compression stockings are routinely employed prophylactically in low-risk patients, while unfractionated heparin or low-molecular-weight heparin and sequential compression stockings are added in higher risk, bedridden patients. Diagnosis is based on a high index of suspicion, and treatment follows the same general scheme as for non-cardiac surgical patient.

19.4.7 *Weaning mechanical ventilation after cardiac surgery — the concept of 'fast tracking'*

Despite the high number of pulmonary and non-pulmonary complications that can occur after cardiac surgery, the time-honoured practice of routinely maintaining the patient intubated for the first 24 hours is not supported by literature and has been abandoned in most institutions. In a large multicentre European study, the median time to extubation was 12 hours [53]. The trend is to extubate most patients as soon as possible after surgery, ideally within between four and six hours [54]. This is incorporated in the broader concept of 'fast tracking' which seeks to reduce the ICU and hospital length of stay as well as the costs associated with surgery with the goals of maintaining safety and, if possible, ensuring better outcomes. While early extubation could reduce the rates of atelectasis and nosocomial pneumonias [55, 56], the benefit in reducing ICU and length of hospital stay is equivocal. Initially reserved for low-risk patients anaesthetised with lower doses of short-acting agents and subsequent post-operative stability, fast tracking is being extended to increasingly higher-risk patients (older age, more comorbidities, lower ventricular ejection fraction, needing inotropes or pressors in post-operative period). Factors associated with delayed extubation are: age and presence of pre-operative IABP [57], moderate/severe LVEF, acute coronary syndrome within 30 days of surgery, redo operations, extra cardiac arteriopathy, raised creatinine levels as well as urgent and complex surgery. The procedure for weaning in fresh post-operative cases is merely 'liberation' from mechanical ventilation of a patient fully recovered from anaesthesia, with intact neurological function, good gas exchange and ventilatory mechanics, not bleeding and stable from haemodynamic and metabolic perspectives. Specific extubation criteria vary and are defined by taking into account the patient population and staffing levels of any particular unit.

19.4.8 *Failure to wean from mechanical ventilation (difficult weaning)*

Failure to wean from mechanical ventilation (difficult weaning) occurs in approximately 5% of patients after cardiac surgery [58]. Their mortality and length of ICU and hospital stay is much higher than in the patients that wean successfully [59]. Post-operative respiratory failure requiring prolonged mechanical ventilation is generally associated with older age, current smoking, pre-operative presence of IABP, low ejection fraction, COPD, prolonged cardiopulmonary bypass time or post-operative complications such as bleeding with re-operation, sternal wound infections, endocarditis, gastrointestinal bleeding, mesenteric ischaemia, neurological complications and renal failure. Deep sternal wound infections and mediastinitis are devastating complications that frequently require multiple surgeries, impair chest wall mechanics and are a major cause of prolonged mechanical ventilation. When an apparent cause is not obvious, phrenic nerve injury should be suspected as a cause for weaning failure. An elevated hemidiaphragm on the chest radiography with paradoxical motion during spontaneous breathing at fluoroscopy or ultrasonography are diagnostic. Usually left-sided and short-lived, phrenic nerve paralysis can take months to resolve, or rarely, can be permanent.

Successful weaning is accomplished once the underlying cause resolves. This often leads to prolonged periods of rehabilitation to allow for the resolution of neuropathy and debilitation that accompany protracted critical illness. More important than a specific weaning method (daily spontaneous breathing trial, pressure support weaning or synchronised intermittent mandatory ventilation weaning) is a consistent approach towards weaning by a dedicated team of respiratory and physical therapists, nurses and physicians. Often this is performed in specialised weaning units where the patients are transferred once the acute process has resolved and a stable airway (i.e. tracheostomy) and enteral nutrition access are established. Timing of tracheostomy is still a controversial aspect. The consensus is that most of the patients that do not wean by 14 days require it, but new evidence is pointing towards better outcomes with even earlier tracheostomy [60].

19.5 Gastrointestinal Complications

Gastrointestinal complications occur with a frequency of 0.5–2% after cardiac surgery but carry a disproportionate mortality rate, ranging from 13.9%–63% [61]. Not surprisingly in this patient population, regional (focal ischaemic events caused by emboli of various materials and from various origins, or rarely thrombosis) or global hypoperfusion is a common denominator in many events. Risk factors are valve surgery, use of inotropic support, IABP, arrhythmias, renal dysfunction, pre-existing liver dysfunction, prolonged mechanical ventilation, sepsis, deep sternal wound infection [62, 63], as well as general risk factors for cardiac surgery.

19.5.1 *Mesenteric ischaemia*

Mesenteric ischaemia is a catastrophic complication, accounting for about two-thirds of the gastrointestinal complications and with mortality around 70% [61]. An early diagnosis is crucial for improving survival. The clinical picture is often incomplete, with the manifestation obscured by analgesics or sedatives (pain) or having alternate possible explanations (metabolic acidosis, hypotension, hypovolaemia, fever and leukocytosis). Since the vast majority of episodes occur in the first few hours to days after the surgery the symptom detection is facilitated by a fast-track protocol. While CT scan could be a useful diagnostic resource, early laparotomy based on clinical suspicion may result in intra-operative recognition of a correctable ischaemic event such as isolated superior mesenteric artery/ large vessel occlusion or segmental colonic necrosis and better outcome.

19.5.2 *Other gastrointestinal complications*

Other gastrointestinal complications such as bleeding, peptic ulcer disease, pancreatitis, calculous and acalculous cholecystitis, hollow viscous perforation and diverticulitis, usually occur later and carry a less ominous prognosis. Often, in the case of peptic ulcer, 'stress bleeding' and acalculous cholecystitis they are epiphenomena of prolonged and severe critical illness, and are managed with condition-specific interventions or therapies.

19.6 Acute Kidney Dysfunction

Renal dysfunction occurs in up to 30% of patients after cardiac surgery [64]. Although the need for dialysis is rare (1–5%), renal dysfunction results in increased morbidity, mortality as well as length of ICU and hospital stay [64, 65]. In a recent study using the newer Risk of renal dysfunction, Injury to the kidney, Failure of kidney function, Loss of kidney function and End-stage kidney disease (RIFLE) criteria, 19.3% of patients had renal dysfunction after cardiac surgery. Mortality at 90 days was between 32.5% for those with the most severe class of failure and 8.0% for those with risk only, and was higher than in the control group [66]. Risk factors include: age, pre-operative renal dysfunction (creatinine > 1.4 mg/dl), reduced left ventricular ejection fraction, duration of the cardiopulmonary bypass, use of an IABP, emergency operation as well as cardiac catheterisation within five days of surgery [64, 67]. Despite ability to identify patients at risk, the incidence of acute kidney injury needing renal replacement therapy (RRT) has not decreased. This reflects the failure of methods designed to 'protect' against kidney injury. Indeed various renal vasodilators (dopamine, fenoldopam), natriuretics (furosemide, atrial natriuretic peptide), or inflammation modulators (*N*-acetylcysteine) have failed to show any benefit or can be even harmful, when they induce further physiological insult [68]. The most likely pathological lesion after cardiac surgery is acute tubular necrosis resulting from multiple and successive haemodynamic and inflammatory insults during the pre-operative, intra-operative and post-operative periods. Providing careful support (satisfactory haemodynamics and oxygen-carrying capacity) and avoiding further nephrotoxins to allow time for body and kidney recovery is the only therapy available to date. In most studies mortality of the patients requiring RRT remains above 50% and is even higher when renal dysfunction occurs in the broader context of multiple organ dysfunction. The indications for and goals of RRT are the same as for any other patient in an intensive care setting.

19.7 Heart and Lung Transplantation

19.7.1 *Heart transplantation*

With one-year survival of 90% and five-year survival approaching 70%, heart transplantation is the treatment of choice for end-stage heart failure [69]. Physiological changes induced secondary to transplantation (i.e. denervated heart, preload and heart rate dependency of cardiac index) are dealt with the usual means (i.e. chronotropic agents, epicardial pacing and adequate volume loading) and the general immediate post-operative care of the heart transplant patient remains similar to that of any cardiac surgical patient. A combined immunosuppressive regimen is begun intra-operatively and continued according to well-developed institutional protocols. A steroid, calcineurin inhibitor and an antiproliferative agent are used most often, with the steroid being subsequently weaned. The most advantageous combination, however, has yet to be established [70]. Extubation and weaning from inotropic support are performed as soon as possible and the patient can be discharged to the surgical ward after jut a few days of ICU stay.

19.7.1.1 *Graft dysfunction*

Graft dysfunction, characterised by hypotension, elevated filling pressures and low cardiac output, is a major cause of morbidity and mortality after heart transplantation. Early graft dysfunction is evident intra-operatively or within days from surgery. Hyperacute (extremely rare, and with an ominous prognosis) or acute rejection, poorly controlled pulmonary hypertension, or technical surgical problems must be identified and addressed in a timely fashion. When severe graft dysfunction occurs intra-operatively and persists without any immunological or anatomic abnormalities, the diagnosis of primary graft dysfunction is made. Significant risk factors for primary graft failure are long ischaemic time (greater than four hours) and increased donor age. When specific therapy (i.e. plasmapheresis, intravenous immunoglobulin, induction immuno-suppression) maximal inotropic, vasodilator/pulmonary vasodilator and IABP support) fails to stabilise the patient, early ECMO can be salutary [71]. Notably, difficulties with the right heart are the most common problem after weaning off CPB, and its treatment follows the general principles described earlier in this chapter. Other complications in the heart transplant patient are those related to immunosuppression, which includes drug toxicities (renal failure, neurotoxicity, diabetes, bone marrow suppression and gastrointestinal upset) as well as infections. Nosocomial pneumonias, urinary tract, wound and bloodstream infections caused by *Pseudomonas*, *Staphylococcus* sp., *Enterococcus* and *Enterobacteriaceae* are significant morbidities that occur in the first month after transplantation and are one of the leading causes of early mortality [72, 73].

19.7.2 *Lung transplantation*

Lung transplantation is an established treatment for end-stage lung disease with approximately 90% one-year, 65% five-year and 40% ten-year survival expected in experienced centres. Surgical options are heart–lung, single lung, bilateral sequential or *en bloc* and lobar transplantation. Despite the technical success of these operations, lung transplantation remains a high-risk procedure with multiple complications that limit both long-term survival and quality of life. Early morbidity is, in many respects, not different than for any major cardiothoracic operation. Bleeding, haemodynamic instability and arrhythmias are monitored for and treated in the usual fashion. Ventilator management and weaning do not pose major problems in the majority of patients. PEEP is generally not used for COPD patients who are recipients of a single-lung transplant since it preferentially distends the native lung, and is maintained at low level in all other patients. Independent lung ventilation is rarely needed.

Ventilator weaning proceeds smoothly once the patient is stable and the graft function adequate. Pain control, using epidural patient-controlled analgesia whenever possible and especially when a thoracotomy approach has been employed, is important in facilitating aggressive post-operative chest physical therapy and preventing atelectasis. Phrenic nerve injury is frequent (3–9%) [74, 75] and should be considered when there is no obvious cause for weaning failure. Primary graft dysfunction (PGD) from ischaemic reperfusion injury is manifested as oxygenation failure with or without chest X-ray infiltrates in the first 72 hours post transplant. Confirmation of a negative crossmatch as well as the ABO group type virtually exclude hyperacute rejection, while transesophageal echocardiography, CT scan and invasive haemodynamic monitoring help in detecting other secondary aetiologies (hydrostatic pulmonary oedema, aspiration pneumonia, pulmonary vein thrombosis, lobar torsion). Mild forms of PGD are common, occurring in up to 60% of patients, with the rarer, most severe form (associated with PaO_2:fraction of inspired O_2 (FiO_2) < 200) being the cause of up to 50% of deaths in the first 90 days post transplantation [76].

While secondary graft dysfunction benefits from specific treatment, treatment for PGD is supportive only, with mechanical ventilation and diuresis to reduce any component of hydrostatic oedema until spontaneous recovery occurs. iNO improves oxygenation and may have anti-inflammatory properties, but has not been associated with improved outcome. Early use of veno–veno or veno–arterial ECMO ensures gas exchange, limits ventilator-induced lung injury, and has been shown to improve mortality in small case series of life-threatening PGD [77, 78]. Acute rejection accounts for only 4.9% of early deaths owing to the efficiency of modern immunosupressants [79]. Immunosuppression is started pre-operatively or intra-operatively and includes a steroid in combination with a calcineurin inhibitor and an antiproliferative agent, with or without the use of an induction cytolytic agent (antithymocyte globulin or orthoclone OKT3). Peri-operative bacterial and fungal infections are one of the leading causes of post-operative morbidity and mortality [79]. Broad-spectrum antibacterials and antifungals are administered to cover for any pathogen growing from donor or recipient's cultures. CMV prophylaxis is important in any CMV-negative recipient that receives a graft from a positive donor. The high risk for aspiration (due to intra-operative recurrent nerve injury and lung denervation with reduced cough reflex) with potential catastrophic effects on the transplanted lung mandates attention when oral intake is resumed. Attention should be paid to early removal of invasive monitoring devices (central catheters) and institution of routine deep vein thrombosis prophylaxis since deep venous thrombosis is frequent and pulmonary embolism may be dangerous due to the reduced pulmonary reserve [80].

19.8 Ventricular Assist Devices

Mechanical circulatory support is quickly developing as standard of care for temporary support when recovery of native heart function is anticipated (i.e. patients with acute myocarditis and postcardiotomy cardiogenic shock), as a 'bridge to transplantation' in severely sick heart transplants candidates with impending failing organs, and as 'destination therapy' in those patients not candidates for transplantation [81–83]. To date, the largest amount of clinical data has been generated for pulsatile devices, however smaller axial-flow devices have recently proven safe and could offer advantages compared with the former [84]. Most referral centres in North America have a paracorporeal device (Thoratec biventricular BVS) available for use on smaller patients when biventricular support is needed, as well as a pulsatile (electrically or pneumatically driven) implantable device (HeartMate left ventricular assist device (LVAD)), which is also approved for destination therapy.

The vast majority of ventricular assist devices (VADs) implanted are for left ventricular assistance. The most common complications of significance for the intensivist include bleeding, hypovolaemia and right ventricular failure. Post-operative bleeding is a known complication of device implantation, and often exacerbated by pre-existing coagulopathy owing to severe liver congestion and malnutrition from CHF, sequestration of platelets and activation of fibrinolysis by the VAD surfaces, extensive mediastinal dissection, pocket creation and redo surgery. Meticulous attention to surgical haemostasis, intra-operative use of antifibrinolytics and aggressive correction of coagulopathy are mandatory. Single-donor platelets should be used when needed, to avoid alloimmunisation. Despite these measures, re-operation has been reported in approximately 50% of cases in early series [85].

An important aspect of device management is assessing preload and adequate transfusion, since hypovolaemia is poorly tolerated. Another factor that determines both the adequacy of preload to the device and survival after LVAD implantation is the native right ventricular function. Left ventricular decompression from the device produces a decrease in the right ventricle afterload with a corresponding leftward shift of the interventricular septum. The net effect, in combination with pre-existent pulmonary hypertension, poor RV function and massive transfusion, is often right ventricular failure [86, 87]. Post-operative inotropic support with right-sided inotropes (milrinone, dobutamine) as well as use of pulmonary vasodilators (iNO, prostaglandin, prostacyclin) together with avoidance of hypoxaemia, acidosis and high mean airway pressures are routine measures in this setting. When an RVAD is needed after LVAD implantation, mortality is high. If hypovolaemia, right heart failure and tamponade are excluded as causes of low cardiac output after LVAD implantation, attention should be directed to the adequacy of implantation (i.e. surgical placement of the cannulas) and unrecognised valvular abnormalities that impact both the device function (i.e. aortic insufficiency, mitral stenosis) and the integrity of the device. Serious device malfunction events are rare.

Due to the high incidence of thromboembolic complications, most patients with VADs will require at least some form of anticoagulation, with the only notable exception being the HeartMate I device whose chamber eventually becomes covered by a neointima that requires only antiplatelet agents. Infectious complications following VAD implantation are reported to occur in about one-third of patients in the first three months after implantation [83]. They range in severity from localised driveline exit-site, pocket-site and mediastinal infections to the most severe device-related bloodstream infection. Epidemiology is dominated by Gram-positive skin bacteria (*Staphylococcus*), however *Enterococcus*, or Gram-negative bacteria (*Pseudomonas aeruginosa*, *Enterobacter* species and *Klebsiella* species) and fungi may occur and are associated with a poor outcome. There are no universally accepted criteria of diagnosis for the vast variety of device-related infections, and differentials with non-ventricular assist devices sources should be investigated. Empirical treatment is usually begun early with antibiotics covering the most likely source and tailored according to culture results. Endovascular infections are best treated with device removal, however, this is often not possible. Usually antibiotic therapy is attempted, with urgent transplantation or device change performed for refractory sepsis or embolic events. Duration of antibiotic treatment is not fully defined and should be individualised.

References

[1] DeFrances, C.J. and Hall, M.J. (2004). 2002 National Hospital Discharge Survey, *Adv Data*, **342**, 1–29.

[2] Hein, O.V., Birnbaum, J., Wernecke, K.D. *et al.* (2006). Three-year survival after four major post-cardiac operative complications, *Crit Care Med*, **34**, 2729–2737.

[3] Grover, F.L. (1999). The Society of Thoracic Surgeons National Database: current status and future directions, *Ann Thorac Surg*, **68**, 367–373.

[4] Bashour, C.A., Yared, J.P., Ryan, T.A. *et al.* (2000). Long-term survival and functional capacity in cardiac surgery patients after prolonged intensive care, *Crit Care Med*, **28**, 3847–3853.

[5] Ospina–Tascón, G.A., Cordioli, R.L. and Vincent, J.L. (2008). What type of monitoring has been shown to improve outcomes in acutely ill patients? *Intens Care Med*, **34**, 800–820.

[6] Ranucci, M. (2006). Which cardiac surgical patients can benefit from placement of a pulmonary artery catheter? *Critical Care*, **10** (Suppl. 3), S6.

[7] Wheeler, A.P., Bernard, G.R., Thompson, B.T. *et al.* (2006). Pulmonary-artery versus central venous catheter to guide treatment of acute lung injury, *N Engl J Med*, **25**, 2213–2224.

[8] Herr, D.L., Sum-Ping, S.T. and England, M. (2003). ICU sedation after coronary artery bypass graft surgery: dexmedetomidine-based versus propofol-based sedation regimens, *J Cardiothorac Vasc Anesth*, **17**, 576–584.

[9] Pandharipande, P.P., Pun, B.T., Herr, D.L. *et al.* (2007). Effect of sedation with dexmedetomidine vs lorazepam on acute brain dysfunction in mechanically ventilated patients: the MENDS randomized controlled trial, *JAMA*, **298**, 2644–2653.

[10] Roberts, I., Alderson, P., Bunn, F. *et al.* (2004). Colloids versus crystalloids for fluid resuscitation in critically ill patients, *Cochrane Database Syst Rev*, CD000567.

[11] Bunn, F., Trivedi, D. and Ashraf, S. (2008). Colloid solutions for fluid resuscitation, *Cochrane Database Syst Rev*, CD001319.

[12] Bagshaw, S.M. and Bellomo, R. (2007). The influence of volume management on outcome, *Curr Opin Crit Care*, **13**, 541–548.

[13] Rivers, E., Nguyen, B., Havstad, S. *et al.* (2001). Early goal-directed therapy in the treatment of severe sepsis and septic shock, *N Engl J Med*, **345**, 1368–1377.

[14] Reeves, S.T. (2005). 'TEE in the Critical Care Setting', in Savage, R.M. and Aronson, S. (eds), *Comprehensive Textbook of Intraoperative Transesophageal Echocardiography*, Lippincott Williams & Wilkins, Philadelphia, pp. 303–324.

[15] Russo, A.M., O'Connor, W.H. and Waxman, H.L. (1993). Atypical presentations and echocardiographic findings in patients with cardiac tamponade occurring early and late after cardiac surgery, *Chest*, **104**, 71–78.

[16] Chuttani, K., Tischler, M.D., Pandian, N.G. *et al.* (1994). Diagnosis of cardiac tamponade after cardiac surgery: relative value of clinical, echocardiographic, and hemodynamic signs, *Am Heart J*, **127**, 913–918.

[17] Sangalli, F., Colagrande, L., Manetti, B., *et al.* (2005). Hemodynamic instability after cardiac surgery: transesophageal echocardiographic diagnosis of a localized pericardial tamponade, *J Cardiothorac Vasc Anesth*, **19**, 775–776.

[18] Rasmussen, C., Thiis J.J., Clemmensen, P. *et al.* (1997). Significance and management of early graft failure after coronary artery bypass grafting: feasibility and results of acute angiography and re-re-vascularization, *Eur J Cardiothoracic Surg*, **12**, 847–852.

[19] Fabricius, A.M., Gerber, W., Hanke, M. *et al.* (2001). Early angiographic control of perioperative ischemia after coronary artery bypass grafting, *Eur J Cardiothoracic Surg*, **19**, 853–858.

[20] Holmvang, L., Jurlander, B., Rasmussen, C. *et al.* (2002). Use of biochemical markers of infarction for diagnosing perioperative myocardial infarction and early graft occlusion after coronary artery bypass surgery, *Chest*, **121**, 103–111.

[21] Haddad, F., Doyle, R., Murphy, D.J. *et al.* (2008). Right ventricular function in cardiovascular disease. Part II: pathophysiology, clinical importance, and management of right ventricular failure, *Circulation*, **117**, 1717–1731.

[22] Greyson, C.R. (2008). Pathophysiology of right ventricular failure, *Crit Care Med*, **36** (Suppl. 1), S57–S65.

[23] Piazza, G. and Goldhaver, S.Z. (2005). The acutely decompensated right ventricle: pathways for diagnosis and management, *Chest*, **128**, 1836–1852.

[24] Lepore, J.J., Maroo, A., Bigatello, L.M. *et al.* (2005). Hemodynamic effects of sildenafil in patients with congestive heart failure and pulmonary hypertension: combined administration with inhaled nitric oxide, *Chest*, **127**, 1647–1653.

[25] Trachte, A.L., Lobato, E.B., Urdaneta, F. *et al.* (2005). Oral sildenafil reduces pulmonary hypertension after cardiac surgery, *Ann Thorac Surg*, **79**, 194–197.

[26] Argenziano ,M., Chen, J.M., Choudhri, A.F. *et al.* (1998). Management of vasodilatory shock after cardiac surgery: identification of predisposing factors and use of a novel pressor agent, *J Thorac Cardiovasc Surg*, **116**, 973–980.

[27] Kristof, A.S. and Magder, S. (1999). Low systemic vascular resistance state in patients undergoing cardiopulmonary bypass, *Crit Care Med*, **27**, 1121–1127.

[28] Morales, D.L., Gregg, D., Helman, D.N. *et al.* (2000). Arginine vasopressin in the treatment of 50 patients with postcardiotomy vasodilatory shock, *Ann Thorac Surg*, **69**, 102–106.

[29] Leyh, R.G., Kofidis, T., Strüber, M. *et al.* (2003). Methylene blue: the drug of choice for catecholamine-refractory vasoplegia after cardiopulmonary bypass? *J Thorac Cardiovasc Surg*, **125**, 1426–1431.

[30] Whitlock, R., Crowther, M.A. and Ng, H.J. (2005). Bleeding in cardiac surgery: its prevention and treatment–an evidence-based review, *Crit Care Clin*, **21**, 589–610.

[31] Martin, P., Horkay, F., Gupta, N.K. *et al.* (1992). Heparin rebound phenomenon–much ado about nothing? *Blood Coagul Fibrinolysis*, **3**, 187–191.

[32] Pifarré, R, Babka, R., Sullivan, H.J. *et al.* (1981). Management of postoperative heparin rebound following cardiopulmonary bypass, *J Thorac Cardiovasc Surg*, **81**, 378–381.

[33] Karthik, S., Grayson, A.D., McCarron, E.E. *et al.* (2004). Reexploration for bleeding after coronary artery bypass surgery: risk factors, outcomes, and the effect of time delay, *Ann Thorac Surg*, **78**, 527–534.

[34] Villareal, R.P., Hariharan, R., Liu, B.C. *et al.* (2004).Postoperative atrial fibrillation and mortality after coronary artery bypass surgery, *J Am Coll Cardiol*, **43**, 742–748.

[35] Daoud, E.G., Strickberger, S.A., Man, K.C. *et al.* (1997). Preoperative amiodarone as prophylaxis against atrial fibrillation after heart surgery, *N Engl J Med*, **337**, 1785–1791.

[36] Chung, M.K. (2000). Cardiac surgery: postoperative arrhythmias, *Crit Care Med*, **28** (Suppl. 10), N136–N144.

[37] Anthi, A., Tzelepis, G.E., Alivizatos, P. *et al.* (1998). Unexpected cardiac arrest after cardiac surgery: incidence, predisposing causes, and outcome of open chest cardiopulmonary resuscitation, *Chest*, **113**, 15–19.

[38] Mackay, J.H., Powell, S.J., Osgathorp, J. *et al.* (2002). Six-year prospective audit of chest reopening after cardiac arrest, *Eur J Cardiothorac Surg*, **22**, 421–425.

[39] The Acute Respiratory Distress Syndrome Network (2000). Ventilation with lower tidal volumes as compared with traditional tidal volumes for acute lung injury and the acute respiratory distress syndrome, *N Engl J Med*, **342**, 1301–1308.

[40] McKhann, G.M., Goldsborough, M.A., Borowicz Jr, L.M. *et al.* (1997). Predictors of stroke risk in coronary artery bypass patients, *Ann Thorac Surg*, **63**, 516–521.

[41] McKhann, G.M., Grega, M.A, Borowicz Jr, L.M. *et al.* (2006). Stroke and encephalopathy after cardiac surgery: an update, *Stroke*, **37**, 562–571.

[42] Gardner, T.J., Horneffer, P.J., Manolio, T.A. *et al.* (1985). Stroke following coronary artery bypass grafting: a ten-year study, *Ann Thorac Surg*, **40**, 574–581.

[43] Coull, B.M., Williams, L.S., Goldstein, L.B. *et al.* (2002). Anticoagulants and antiplatelet agents in acute ischemic stroke: report of the Joint Stroke Guideline Development Committee of the American Academy of Neurology and the American Stroke Association, *Neurology*, **59**, 12–22.

[44] Welsby, I.J., Bennett-Guerrero, E., Atwell, D. *et al.* (2002). The association of complication type with mortality and prolonged stay after cardiac surgery with cardiopulmonary bypass, *Anesth Analg*, **94**, 1072–1078.

[45] Bando, K., Sun, K., Binford, R.S. *et al.* (1997). Determinants of longer duration of endotracheal intubation after adult cardiac operations, *Ann Thorac Surg*, **63**, 1026–1033.

[46] Matte, P., Jacquet, L., Van Dyck, M. *et al.* (2000). Effects of conventional physiotherapy, continuous positive airway pressure and non-invasive ventilatory support with bilevel positive airway pressure after coronary artery bypass grafting, *Acta Anaesthesiol Scand*, **44**, 75–81.

[47] Light, R.W., Rogers, J.T., Cheng, D. *et al.* (1999). Large pleural effusions occurring after coronary artery bypass grafting, *Ann Intern Med*, **130**, 891–896.

[48] Douglas, J.M. and Spaniol, S. (2002). Prevention of postoperative pneumothorax in patients undergoing cardiac surgery, *Am J Surg*, **183**, 551–553.

[49] Reeve, W.G., Ingram, S.M. and Smith, D.C. (1994). Respiratory function after cardiopulmonary bypass: a comparison of bubble and membrane oxygenators, *J Cardiothorac Vasc Anesth*, **8**, 502–508.

[50] Ng, C.S., Wan, S., Yim, A.P. *et al.* (2002). Pulmonary dysfunction after cardiac surgery, *Chest*, **121**, 1269–1277.

[51] Cox, C.M., Ascione, R., Cohen, A.M. *et al.* (2000). Effect of cardiopulmonary bypass on pulmonary gas exchange: a prospective randomized study, *Ann Thorac Surg*, **69**, 140–145.

[52] Zehr, K.J., Liddicoat, J.R., Salazar, J.D. *et al.* (1997). The autopsy: still important in cardiac surgery, *Ann Thorac Surg*, **64**, 380–383.

[53] Lassnigg, A., Hiesmayr, M.J., Bauer, P., *et al.* (2002). Effect of centre-, patient- and procedure-related factors on intensive care resource utilisation after cardiac surgery, *Intens Care Med*, **28**, 1453–1461.

[54] Liu, L.L. and Gropper, M.A. (2002). Respiratory and hemodynamic management after cardiac surgery, *Curr Treat Options Cardiovasc Med*, **4**, 161–169.

[55] Johnson, D., Thomson, D., Mycyk, T., *et al.* (1997). Respiratory outcomes with early extubation after coronary artery bypass surgery, *J Cardiothorac Vasc Anesth*, **11**, 474–480.

[56] London, M.J., Shroyer, A.L., Jernigan, V. *et al.* (1997). Fast-track cardiac surgery in a Department of Veterans Affairs patient population, *Ann Thorac Surg*, **64**, 134–141.

[57] London, M.J., Shroyer, A.L., Coll, J.R. *et al.* (1998). Early extubation following cardiac surgery in a veterans population, *Anesthesiology*, **88**, 1447–1458.

[58] Shroyer, A.L., Coombs, L.P., Peterson, E.D. *et al.* (2003). The Society of Thoracic Surgeons: 30-day operative mortality and morbidity risk models, *Ann Thorac Surg*, **75**, 1885–1864.

[59] Kern, H., Redlich, U., Hotz, H. *et al.* (2001). Risk factors for prolonged ventilation after cardiac surgery using APACHE II, SAPS II, and TISS: comparison of three different models, *Intens Care Med*, **27**, 407–415.

[60] De Leyn, P., Bedert, L., Delcroix, M. *et al.* (2007). Tracheotomy: clinical review and guidelines, *Eur J Cardiothorac Surg*, **32**, 412–421.

[61] Mangi, A.A., Christison-Lagay, E.R., Torchiana, D.F. *et al.* (2005). Gastrointestinal complications in patients undergoing heart operation: an analysis of 8709 consecutive cardiac surgical patients, *Ann Surg*, **241**, 901–904.

[62] Ohri, S.K., Desai, J.B., Gaer, J.A. *et al.* (1991). Intraabdominal complications after cardiopulmonary bypass, *Ann Thorac Surg*, **52**, 826–831.

[63] D'Ancona, G., Baillot, R., Poirier, B. *et al.* (2003). Determinants of gastrointestinal complications in cardiac surgery, *Tex Heart Inst J*, **30**, 280–285.
[64] Bove, T., Calabrò, M.G., Landoni, G. *et al.* (2004). The incidence and risk of acute renal failure after cardiac surgery, *J Cardiothorac Vasc Anesth*, **18**, 442–445.
[65] Chertow, G.M., Levy, E.M., Hammermeister, K.E. *et al.* (1998). Independent association between acute renal failure and mortality following cardiac surgery, *Am J Med*, **104**, 342–348.
[66] Kuitunen, A., Vento, A., Suojaranta-Ylinen, R. *et al.* (2006). Acute renal failure after cardiac surgery: evaluation of the RIFLE classification, *Ann Thorac Surg*, **81**, 542–546.
[67] Del Duca, D., Iqbal, S., Rahme, E. *et al.* (2007). Renal failure after cardiac surgery: timing of cardiac catheterization and other perioperative risk factors, *Ann Thorac Surg*, **84**, 1264–1271.
[68] Stafford-Smith, M. (2005). Evidence-based renal protection in cardiac surgery, *Semin Cardiothorac Vasc Anesth*, **9**, 65–76.
[69] Taylor, D.O., Edwards, L.B., Boucek, M.M. *et al.* (2007). Registry of the International Society for Heart and Lung Transplantation: twenty-fourth official adult heart transplant report — 2007, *J Heart Lung Transplant*, **26**, 769–781.
[70] Kobashigawa, J.A. and Patel, J.K. (2006). Immunosuppression for heart transplantation: where are we now? *Nat Clin Pract Cardiovasc Med*, **3**, 203–212.
[71] Marasco S.F., Esmore, D.S., Negri, J. *et al.* (2005). Early institution of mechanical support improves outcomes in primary cardiac allograft failure, *J Heart Lung Transplant*, **24**, 2037–2042.
[72] Miniati, D.N. and Robbins, R.C. (2002). Heart transplantation: a thirty-year perspective, *Annu Rev Med*, **53**, 189–205.
[73] Montoya, J.G., Giraldo, L.F., Efron, B. *et al.* (2001). Infectious complications among 620 consecutive heart transplant patients at Stanford University Medical Center, *Clin Infect Dis*, **33**, 629–640.
[74] Maziak, D.E., Maurer, J.R. and Kesten, S. (1996). Diaphragmatic paralysis: a complication of lung transplantation, *Ann Thorac Surg*, **61**, 170–173.
[75] Ferdinande, P., Bruyninckx, F., Van Raemdonck, D. *et al.* (2004). Phrenic nerve dysfunction after heart-lung and lung transplantation, *J Heart Lung Transplant*, **23**, 105–109.
[76] Carter, Y.M. and Davis, R.D. (2006). Primary Graft Dysfunction in Lung Transplantation, *Semin Respir Crit Care Med*, **27**, 501–507.
[77] Wigfield, C.H., Lindsey, J.D., Steffens, T.G. *et al.* (2007). Early institution of extracorporeal membrane oxygenation for primary graft dysfunction

after lung transplantation improves outcome, *J Heart Lung Transplant*, **26**, 331–338.

[78] Fischer S., Bohn, D., Rycus, P. *et al.* (2007). Extracorporeal membrane oxygenation for primary graft dysfunction after lung transplantation: analysis of the Extracorporeal Life Support Organization (ELSO) registry, *J Heart Lung Transplant*, **26**, 472–477.

[79] Studer, S.M., Levy, R.D., McNeil, K. *et al.* (2004). Lung transplant outcomes: a review of survival, graft function, physiology, health-related quality of life and cost-effectiveness, *Eur Respir J*, **24**, 674–685.

[80] Kroshus, T.J., Kshettry, V.R., Hertz, M. I. *et al.* (1995). Deep venous thrombosis and pulmonary embolism after lung transplantation, *J Thorac Cardiovasc Surg*, **110**, 540–544.

[81] Vitali, E., Colombo, T., Bruschi, G. *et al.* (2005). Different clinical scenarios for circulatory mechanical support in acute and chronic heart failure, *Am J Cardiol*, **96**, 34L–41L.

[82] Birks, E.J., Tansley, P.D., Hardy, J. *et al.* (2006). Left ventricular assist device and drug therapy for the reversal of heart failure, *N Engl J Med*, **355**, 1873–1884.

[83] Rose, E.A., Gelijns, A.C., Moskowitz, A.J. *et al.* (2001). Long-term use of a left ventricular assist device for end-stage heart failure, *N Engl J Med*, **345**, 1435–1443.

[84] Miller L.W., Pagani, F.D., Russell, S.D. *et al.* (2007). Use of a continuous-flow device in patients awaiting heart transplantation, *N Engl J Med*, **357**, 885–896.

[85] McCarthy, P.M. and Sabik, J.F. (1994). Implantable circulatory support devices as a bridge to heart transplantation, *Semin Thorac Cardiovasc Surg*, **6**, 174–180.

[86] Patel, N.D., Weiss, E.S., Schaffer, J. *et al.* (2008). Right heart dysfunction after left ventricular assist device implantation: a comparison of the pulsatile HeartMate I and axial-flow HeartMate II devices, *Ann Thorac Surg*, **86**, 832–840.

[87] Nakatani, S., Thomas, J.D., Savage, R.M. *et al.* (1996). Prediction of right ventricular dysfunction after left ventricular assist device implantation, *Circulation*, **94**, (Suppl. 9), II 216–221.

20
Respiratory Intensive Care

Sarah L. Stirling and Mark J. D. Griffiths

20.1 Acute Respiratory Failure

Acute respiratory failure is a common indication for intensive care unit (ICU) admission [1]. Patients often deteriorate rapidly and need timely endotracheal intubation for respiratory support which exposes them to the complications associated with mechanical ventilation (see Chapter 7). Here we discuss the presentation and ICU treatment of patients with acute respiratory distress syndrome (ARDS).

20.1.1 *Acute respiratory distress syndrome*

20.1.1.1 *Definition*

ARDS was defined by the North American–European Consensus Conference (NAECC) as the acute onset of refractory hypoxaemia in association with bilateral pulmonary infiltrates with evidence that this was not caused primarily by an elevated left atrial pressure (Table 20.1) [2]. The syndrome has no definitive diagnostic test, the chest radiograph criteria are subjective and the oxygenation criteria do not allow for the provision of ventilatory support. Whilst the syndrome is traditionally divided into acute lung injury (ALI) and ARDS on the basis of the oxygen gradient (Table 20.1), this practice has been questioned as the outcome between ALI and ARDS is similar [3].

Table 20.1. NAECC definitions of ALI and ARDS. $PaO_2:FiO_2$, arterial partial pressure of oxygen:inspired oxygen fraction; PAOP, pulmonary artery occlusion pressure.

	Oxygenation	Chest radiograph	Exclusion of cardiogenic pulmonary oedema
ALI	$PaO_2:FiO_2 \leq 300$ mmHg (40 kPa)	Bilateral opacities consistent with pulmonary oedema	PAOP ≤18mmHg if measured or no clinical evidence of left atrial hypertension
ARDS	$PaO_2:FiO_2 \leq 200$ mmHg (26.7 kPa)		

20.1.1.2 *Clinical features and investigations*

The initial clinical assessment aims to identify the underlying cause of ARDS as well as any failing organ systems requiring urgent support. Whilst a cardiogenic cause for pulmonary oedema can be initially excluded based on patient history, chest X-ray, electrocardiogram and echocardiography, further information obtained from pulmonary artery catheterisation may be beneficial in selected cases. Thereafter, investigations focus on detecting the complications of ARDS and critical illness such as hospital-acquired infection.

20.1.1.3 *Management*

20.1.1.3.1 General supportive care

There is no specific treatment for ARDS. Management involves aggressive treatment of the underlying cause and prevention and treatment of the complications of critical illness (Fig. 20.1). Whilst sepsis is a common cause of ARDS, ventilator-associated pneumonia (VAP) and sepsis are also common complications of the syndrome [4]. However, VAP is often extremely difficult to diagnose in patients with ARDS because of the coexistence of pulmonary infiltrates and raised inflammatory markers. It is therefore important that appropriate microbiological investigations are undertaken and prompt protocol-driven antibiotic treatment commenced with timely de-escalation guided by culture results or expert advice [5].

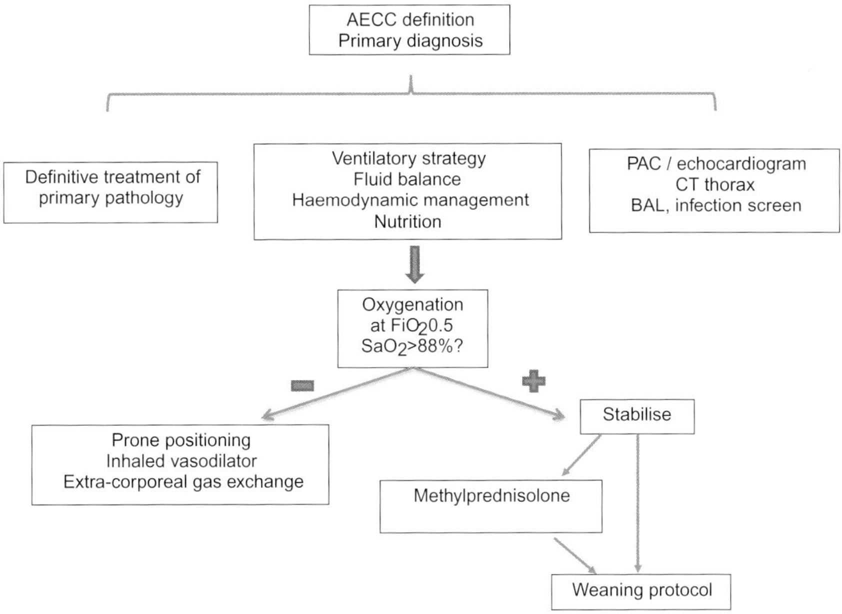

Figure 20.1. Proposed management algorithm for the ARDS. AECC, (North) American–European Consensus Conference; PAC, pulmonary artery catheter; BAL, bronchoalveolar lavage; SaO_2, oxygen saturation of arterial blood.

The pulmonary microvasculature is highly permeable in ARDS, causing both interstitial oedema and airspace fluid accumulation. Whilst removing lung water does improve respiratory function, the necessary dehydration of critically ill patients required to achieve this may decrease cardiac output and hence oxygen delivery, thereby exacerbating multiple organ failure. Available data suggest that a more conservative fluid administration policy shortens the duration of mechanical ventilation without increasing non-pulmonary-organ failures [6].

Sedation is usually necessary in the management of patients with ARDS but the available evidence shows that regular interruption of continuous sedative infusions shortens the duration of mechanical ventilation and facilitates weaning [7]. Neuromuscular blockers are also commonly required in this group but, particularly when given with corticosteroids, are associated with critical illness neuromyopathy, a major cause of morbidity in survivors (8).

20.1.1.3.2 Ventilatory management

Mechanical ventilation inevitably causes further damage to injured lung tissue and induces the release of inflammatory mediators into the systemic circulation, which is thought to contribute to multiple organ failure. Though an optimum ventilation strategy remains elusive, there are basic guidelines, which attempt to limit mediators of ventilator-induced lung injury (Table 20.2). These can be divided mechanistically into high-volume injury or volutrauma (over-distension), low-volume injury or atelectotrauma (repeated collapse and reopening of the airspace) and finally oxygen toxicity.

20.1.1.3.3 Drug treatment

Corticosteroids may modify the course of lung injury by reducing pro-inflammatory and fibrogenic mediators but are harmful when given early

Table 20.2. Ventilation guidelines in ARDS. PBW, predicted body weight.

Parameter	Aim	Comment
Tidal volume (V_t)	6 ml/kg (predicted body weight)	PBW male = 50 + 0.91(height cm −152.4) PBW female = 45.5 + 0.91(height cm −152.4)
Plateau pressure	<30 cm H_2O	If >30 cm H_2O decrease V_t if gas exchange targets still met
Respiratory rate	Up to 20/minute	> 20/minute may cause 'stacking'
pH	>7.2	Respiratory acidosis generally tolerated well Not if intracranial pressure is raised
Oxygenation	88–92%	Peripheral oxygen saturation (SpO_2) used rather than PaO_2 — major determinant of O_2 delivery
Positive end-expiratory pressure	8–15 cm H_2O	Start at high level and decrease until compliance or oxygenation deteriorate
Prone positioning	Refractory hypoxaemia improved in two-thirds of cases	No evidence of increase in survival Increased incidence of endotracheal tube displacement, pressure sores
Nitric oxide/ Inhaled vasodilators	Refractory hypoxaemia improved in two-thirds of cases	No evidence of increase in survival

in the course of the syndrome. In a recent study, methylprednisolone decreased the number of ventilator- and shock-free days with an improvement in oxygenation and compliance. However, the primary endpoint of 60-day mortality was unaltered in patients treated with methyprednisolone [9]. Though there remains some scope for investigation, it is currently unclear whether steroids have a role in the treatment of ARDS.

Deficient active surfactant in ARDS is associated with alveolar collapse, which contributes to respiratory failure. Whilst there has been success in treating neonates with respiratory distress syndrome with exogenous surfactant, multiple trials of synthetic surfactant preparations in adults with ARDS have shown no survival benefit [10]. The reasons for this failure remain unclear, though inadequate surfactant delivery to diseased lung units and poor biological activity of the synthetic preparations are possible causes.

Beta adrenergic agonists, amongst other known beneficial effects, increase fluid clearance from distal lung airspaces [11] and continuous infusion of salbutamol decreased an index of lung water in patients with ARDS [12]. Larger trials intended to determine the effect of salbutamol on mortality are underway.

20.2 Post-Operative Respiratory Failure

Patients are susceptible to respiratory failure in the peri-operative period. Understanding the pathogenesis of respiratory failure (Fig. 20.2) in this setting and implementing appropriate preventative measures can significantly improve outcomes.

20.2.1 *Pathogenesis*

Pulmonary oedema and atelectasis are the most important lung processes in this context. The metabolic response to surgery and trauma includes secretion of aldosterone and anti-diuretic hormone, both of which decrease urine output. Pulmonary venous pressure may become critically elevated and lead to oedema formation in patients with poor cardiopulmonary reserve, especially if excessive fluid is administered in response to oliguria. Similarly, patients undergoing major surgery are often exposed to risk factors for ALI which incrementally increase pulmonary vascular permeability,

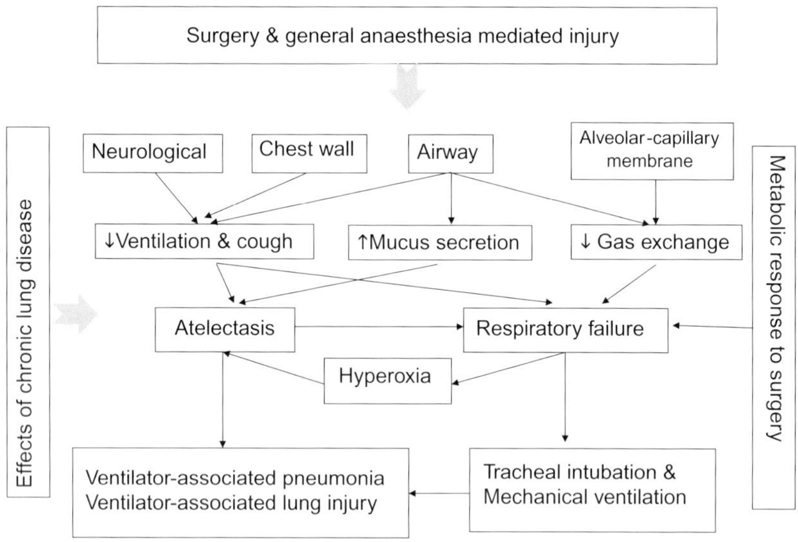

Figure 20.2. Pathogenesis of post-operative respiratory failure.

for example: sepsis, transfusion of blood products, shock, head injury and bone fractures.

Significant atelectasis occurs rapidly after the induction of anaesthesia and may be exacerbated, causing significant hypoxia in the post-operative period. In patients undergoing upper abdominal surgery, oxygenation deteriorated as the lung's functional residual capacity (FRC) fell below the closing volume, indicating collapse of the airway [13]. In healthy patients and in smokers, FRC decreases with age whilst closing volume increases. In young people, closing volume is about 10% of vital capacity but increases with age to about 40% at 65 years and can enter the FRC so that closure occurs at higher lung volumes. Similarly, FRC decreases in the supine compared with the upright position. After upper abdominal surgery, vital capacity fell within the first four hours post-operatively and was followed by a decrease in FRC which was maximal after about 24 hours [14]. This functional restrictive defect, which is due at least in part to incisional pain and to diaphragmatic dysfunction of unknown cause, decreases the ability to cough effectively to clear secretions and eventually leads to a decrease in closing volume and an increase in FRC.

Hypercarbia may result from a combination of hypoventilation related to decreased central drive (most often drug-related) and pulmonary restriction and increased carbon dioxide production associated with a post-surgical catabolic state. Anaesthetic agents and opiates not only decrease respiratory drive but also suppress coughing and may act on the airway epithelium to promote mucus plugging and decrease local defence against infection. Many anaesthetic and surgical procedures are associated with a risk of aspiration of gastric contents which, depending on the extent of airway soiling and the host response, may cause problems ranging from coughing and bronchospasm to pneumonia and ARDS. Prolonged tracheal intubation is almost inevitably associated with microaspiration of upper airway secretions that are contaminated by gut bacteria, which may lead to VAP (see Section 20.3.2).

20.2.2 *Predicting and preventing post-operative respiratory failure*

No respiratory function parameters accurately predict post-operative respiratory morbidity, although very poor results on spirometry have been proposed as predictors of complications. Apart from patient-related variables that are associated with risk (Table 20.3), prolonged anaesthesia and certain types of surgery carry a high incidence of pulmonary complications for obvious reasons; in descending order of risk are thoracic, upper abdominal, lower abdominal and superficial surgery.

Pre-operative prevention is based on measures designed to optimise respiratory and cardiac function. This will vary markedly between patients and can only be effective if pre-operative assessment identifies treatable risk factors. In some cases the risk of delaying surgery has to be weighed against the benefits of, and likely success of, measures designed to optimise function. For example, smoking cessation is commonly advised pre-operatively, however a benefit in terms of post-operative respiratory complications has only been demonstrated after abstinence of over eight weeks [15]. Otherwise, common-sense measures like treating infection and optimising the control of chronic conditions like heart failure, asthma and COPD are all advisable.

Post-operative measures aimed at preventing shock and organ failure are the essence of good critical care but again the problem is far less likely

Table 20.3. Patient-related risk factors for post-operative respiratory failure (PORF). CPAP, continuous positive airway pressure; NIV, non-invasive ventilation.

Risk factor	Mechanism	Pre-operative prevention	Post-operative prevention/ treatment	Comment
Age	Decreased FRC Increased closing volume Functional dependence carries an independent risk	Physiotherapy	Standard measures	Approximately four-fold increased risk for those aged 70–79 Take into account biological age and fitness
Post-operative confusion	Loss of cooperation with mobilisation and physio-therapy	Alcohol history	Avoid drug treatment where possible Communication aids	Small increased risk (odds ratio1.4)
Obesity, ascites	Closing volume may exceed FRC	Ascitic fluid drainage	Early mobilisation CPAP effective	Obesity not associated with increased risk of PORF Consider sleep-disordered breathing
Smoking history	Increased closing volume	Smoking cessation for > eight weeks Partial cessation or cessation for < eight weeks may increase risk	Standard measures	Small increased risk Consider COPD and ischaemic heart disease

(*Continued*)

Table 20.3. *(Continued)*

Risk factor	Mechanism	Pre-operative prevention	Post-operative prevention/ treatment	Comment
Chronic obstructive pulmonary disease (COPD)	Decreased respiratory reserve Increased sputum production Bronchopneumonia Bronchospasm	Optimise COPD treatment Treat infection Nutritional support	Physiotherapy Bronchodilation Mucolytics NIV effective	Consider sleep-disordered breathing and ischaemic heart disease
Lung cancer resection	Removal of functioning lung, damage of remaining lung Post-lung resection acute lung injury Pre-existing lung disease Post-operative pain	Optimise concurrent lung disease Consider thoracic epidural or paravertebral block for regional anaesthesia	Avoid over-hydration Early extubation and mobilisation Optimise analgesia NIV effective	Consider surgical complications Investigate for right ventricular dysfunction
American Society of Anaesthesiologists Score (ASA)	Subjective composite clinical assessment of the effects on the patient of comorbid conditions	Standard measures	Standard measures	Risk increases with increasing score — approximately four-fold increased risk in ASA >2
Heart failure	Decreased cardiac reserve — increased risk of pulmonary oedema	Optimise medical treatment Treat reversible ischaemia	Low threshold for cardiac output monitoring Inotropic support CPAP or NIV for cardiogenic pulmonary oedema	Approximately three-fold increased risk Consider renal failure

to be mitigated if it is not anticipated and the patient's risk of pulmonary complications is unrecognised or underestimated. The most difficult aspect of haemodynamic fine tuning in such patients is optimising fluid balance and perhaps the most useful tool in helping to avoid both under-perfusion associated with under-filling and pulmonary oedema is a well-performed fluid challenge (see Chapter 15). Similarly, well planned peri-operative analgesia including local techniques can help to achieve early mobilisation and secretion clearance whilst avoiding narcosis and constipation (see Chapter 15). The aims of physiotherapy in respiratory dysfunction are to improve global or regional ventilation and lung compliance, to reduce airway resistance and the work of breathing, and to clear airway secretions. Body positioning and mobilisation may improve alveolar recruitment, lung perfusion and ventilation:perfusion matching [16]. Techniques which increase inspiratory volume, expiratory flow and the effectiveness of cough in non-intubated patients are in patients with respiratory muscle weakness. Continuous positive airway pressure (CPAP) increases FRC and alveolar recruitment. Its use in patients recovering from abdominal surgery decreased respiratory complications, atelectasis and hospital-acquired pneumonia (HAP) [17]. Similarly, non-invasive ventilation (NIV) may help selected patients with respiratory pump failure to avoid reintubation. However, in a trial of over 200 unselected patients with post-operative respiratory failure the use of NIV to prevent re-intubation was no more effective than standard therapy, and delays in reintubation after the development of acute respiratory failure actually correlated with worsened survival rates [18].

When post-operative respiratory failure has occurred, adequate oxygenation has to be maintained with the caveats that hypercarbia and reabsorption atelectasis may be exacerbated in susceptible patients. VAP should be treated promptly and aggressively with antibiotics modified by microbiological results according to local guidelines. The identification of pulmonary oedema should always institute an assessment of the cardiac status of the patient. The timing of reinstitution of invasive mechanical ventilation and the need for tracheostomy has to be made on an individual-patient basis determined by the likelihood of their respiratory function improving rapidly using non-invasive methods.

20.3 Pneumonia

20.3.1 *Community-acquired pneumonia (CAP)*

CAP is a common illness with an estimated incidence of 5–11 cases per 1,000 of the population every year [19]. Between 20–30% of cases require hospital admission and up to 10% of these are admitted to ICU [20]. In this most severely affected group there is almost always associated multiple organ dysfunction, and the mortality can exceed 50% [21]. It is therefore essential that these particularly high-risk patients are quickly identified and treated (Table 20.4) with the aim of preventing further deterioration.

20.3.1.1 *Aetiology*

Worldwide patterns of infection differ considerably, but in the UK the commonest causative organism requiring admission to the ICU remains *Streptococcus pneumoniae* (12–38%). Other organisms commonly isolated are *Legionella* (0–30%), *Staphylococcus aureus* (1–18%) and Gram-negative bacilli (2–34%). However, in up to a third of cases, no organism is isolated.

20.3.1.2 *Treatment*

Antimicrobial treatment for CAP is dependent upon local resistance patterns and individual hospital policy (Table 20.5). Antibiotic resistance is an

Table 20.4. The British Thoracic Society (BTS) guidelines define severe pneumonia as the presence of two or more of the following features on hospital admission [22].

Parameter	Measurement
Respiratory rate	≥30/min
Diastolic blood pressure	≤60 mmHg
Urea	>7 mmol/l
Altered mental status*	Abbreviated Mental Test <8/10
Hypoxaemia*	PaO_2 <8 kPa / SpO_2 <90% (regardless of FiO_2)
Extent of infection*	Bilateral or more than two lobes affected on chest X-ray

*Confers 50% mortality in elderly patients [23].

Table 20.5. Recommended therapy of microbiologically documented pneumonia [15]. (See also Chapter 10.) MRSA = methicillin-resistant *Staphylococcus aureus.*

Pathogen	Preferred	Alternative
Streptococcus pneumoniae	Amoxicillin 500 mg — 1 g three times daily orally or benzylpenicillin 1.2 g four times daily intravenously	Erythromycin 500 mg four times daily orally or clarithromycin 500 mg twice daily orally or cefuroxime 0.75–1.5 g three times daily intravenously or cefotaxime 1–2 g three times daily intravenously or ceftriaxone 2 g once daily intravenously
Mycoplasma pneumoniae *Chlamydia pneumoniae*	Erythromycin 500 mg four times daily orally/intravenously or clarithromycin 500 mg twice daily orally/intravenously	Tetracycline 250–500 mg four times daily orally or fluoroquinolone orally/ intravenously
Chlamydia psittaci *Chlamydia burnetii*	Tetracycline 250 mg–500 mg four times daily orally or 500 mg twice daily intravenously	Erythromycin 500 mg four times daily orally or clarithromycin 500 mg twice daily intravenously
Legionella spp	Clarithromycin 500 mg twice daily orally/intravenously ± rifampicin 600 mg once or twice daily orally/intravenously	Fluoroquinolone orally/ intravenously
Haemophilus influenzae	Non-β-lactamase-producing: amoxicillin 500 mg three times daily orally or ampicillin 500 mg four times daily orally intravenously β-lactamase-producing: co-amoxiclav 625 mg three times daily orally or 1.2g three times daily intravenously	Cefuroxime 750 mg –1.5 g three times daily intravenously or cefotaxime 1–2 g three times daily intravenously or ceftriaxone 2 g once daily intravenously or fluoroquinolone orally/ intravenously
Gram-negative bacilli	Cefuroxime 1.5 g three times daily or cefotaxime 1–2 g three times daily intravenously or ceftriaxone 2 g once daily intravenously	Fluoroquinolone intravenously or imipenem 500 mg four times daily intravenously or meropenem 0.5–1.0 g three times daily intravenously

(*Continued*)

Table 20.5. (*Continued*)

Pathogen	Preferred	Alternative
Pseudomonas aeruginosa	Ceftazidime 2 g three times daily intravenously plus gentamicin or tobramycin (dose monitoring)	Ciprofloxacin 400 mg twice daily intravenously or piperacillin 4 g three times daily intravenously plus gentamicin or tobramycin (dose monitoring)
Staphylococcus aureus	Non-MRSA: Flucloxacillin 1–2 g four times daily intravenously ± rifampicin 600 mg once or twice daily orally/intravenously MRSA: Vancomycin 1 g twice daily intravenously (monitoring)	Teicoplanin 400 mg twice daily intravenously ± rifampicin 600 mg once or twice daily orally/intravenously linezolid 600 mg twice daily intravenously or orally

increasing problem with a number of reports of penicillin-resistant *Streptococcus pneumoniae.*

The majority of patients with severe CAP require mechanical ventilation and some develop ALI/ARDS. In this high-mortality group, most deaths are caused by multiple organ failure [24]. Renal replacement therapy and advanced cardiovascular support are commonly required and those who do survive tend to have protracted ICU admissions. Overall, the management is targeted at prevention of complications, support of failing organ systems and septic source control.

Lack of clinical response at 48 to 72 hours is widely accepted as an indication of treatment failure. The diagnosis should be reviewed and other diagnoses such as cardiac failure or pulmonary embolism considered. Microbiological culture results should also be available by this stage and may indicate that a change in antibiotics is necessary. The complications of severe infection, such as lung empyema or abscess, endocarditis, meningitis and nosocomial infection, should be sought. Fibreoptic bronchoscopy should be reconsidered to obtain further microbiological and pathological samples [25]. Unusual organisms for the UK [26] should be excluded by taking a careful foreign travel history and details of occupation, pets and hobbies: the possibility of immunosuppression should be probed.

20.3.2 *Hospital-acquired pneumonia*

Nosocomial or hospital-acquired pneumonia (HAP) is defined as pneumonia beginning at least 48 hours after hospital admission. Its incidence ranges from 5–15 per 1,000 hospital admissions and increases with age [27]. VAP accounts for over 80% of ICU nosocomial infections with a resulting mortality rate of 70% in some series. More recently, VAP has been divided into early-onset (less than five days after hospital admission) and late-onset (more than five days after hospital admission). This distinction has proved important as early VAP is more likely to be caused by aspiration of endogenous organisms [28] whereas late-onset pneumonia usually follows aspiration of secretions containing potentially drug-resistant nosocomial pathogens and is associated with a higher mortality [29].

20.3.2.1 *Pathogenesis*

For HAP to manifest there must be colonisation then overt infection of the lower respiratory tract by pathogenic organisms. During mechanical ventilation, this is thought to occur mainly via microaspiration of endogenous pathogenic bacteria around the endotracheal tube (ETT) cuff. Other recognised causes are aspiration of gastric contents, inhalation of organisms colonising the ETT, inhaled aerosolised material and direct haematogenous spread. The main risk factor for HAP is mechanical ventilation for longer than 48 hours, which increases the incidence by up to 20-fold. Other risk factors include the duration of ICU or hospital stay, severity of underlying illness and presence of comorbidities [30]. Measures that reduce the incidence of VAP/HAP are listed in Table 20.6.

20.3.2.2 *Diagnosis*

It is notoriously difficult to make the definitive diagnosis of VAP as many patients with other diseases also fit the clinical picture and laboratory investigations, as mentioned above, are at best inconsistent in their ability to confirm the diagnosis. Therefore a pragmatic clinical approach is widely adopted and all patients with new (or progressive) radiographic infiltrates, purulent sputum, raised white cell count (WCC), pyrexia or worsening oxygenation should be considered to have VAP until proven otherwise.

Table 20.6. Bedside care interventions reducing VAP and HAP. MV = mechanical ventilation.

Care aspect	Intervention
Ventilator circuit change	Change as clinically indicated — not regularly
Patient position	Semi-recumbent — 30° head up
Mechanical ventilation	Avoid MV — NIV if possible
Hand hygiene	Hand washing between interventions
Oral care	Regular with chlorhexidine 1% gel four times per day
Ventilator circuit type	Closed

Chest radiography, microbiological cultures (wherever possible before the first dose of antibiotic) and serology are the standard diagnostic tests. Wherever possible, quantitative respiratory samples should be obtained either from blind endotracheal aspirates or from fibreoptic bronchoscopy.

20.3.2.3 *Treatment*

The immediate and appropriate administration of antimicrobial treatment is associated with better outcomes [31] and inappropriate treatment is associated with an increased risk of death. Empirical treatment should be guided by time of onset as well as local microbiological resistance patterns and pathogenic organisms (Table 20.7). There is no evidence to support a specific duration of antibiotic treatment and assessment of efficacy of treatment depends on clinical improvement and falling inflammatory markers.

20.3.3 *Pneumonia in the immunocompromised host*

Regardless of the cause of immunocompromise, pneumonia carries a high mortality rate in these patients [33]. The starting point of care, as with any other cause of sepsis, is using an airway, breathing, circulation, disability, exposure (ABCDE) approach but it is imperative that the cause of immunocompromise is diagnosed. This guides the clinician to the likely microbiological culprits and therefore to the appropriate method of treatment (Table 20.8).

Table 20.7. Recommendations for empiric antimicrobial treatment of VAP. Based on the American Thoracic Society (ATS) guidelines [32].

Onset	Pathogen	Antibiotic
Early	*Streptococcus pneumoniae* *Haemophilus influenza* Methicillin-sensitive *Staphylococcus aureus* Gram-negative bacilli	Ceftriaxone or levofloxacin, moxifloxacin or ciprofloxacin or Ampicillin/sulbactam or Ertapenem
Late	All of above plus *Pseudomonas aeruginosa* *Klebsiella pneumoniae* (extended spectrum beta-lactamase^{+}) Acinetobacter species MRSA *Legionella pneumophila*	Antipseudomonal cephalosporin or antipseudomonal carbepenem or β-lactamase inhibitor plus antipseudomonal fluoroquinolone or aminoglycoside plus linezolid or vancomycin

Table 20.8. Causes of immunocompromise and likely organisms causing pneumonia [31].

Cause	Likely organisms
Human immunodeficiency virus (HIV)	*Pneumocystis jiroveci* *Streptococcus pneumoniae* *Mycobacterium avium* complex (MAC) Tuberculosis Cryptococcal pneumonia Cytomegaloviral pneumonitis
Primary immunodeficiencies	
Humoral	Recurrent bacterial
Cell-mediated	Viral
Combined	Particularly viral
Transplantation	Bacterial Tuberculosis Fungal Pneumocystis pneumonia Viral
Malignancy	Recurrent bacterial infection
Autoimmune	Bacterial
Pregnancy	*Haemophilus influenzae* *Streptococcus pneumonia*
Asplenic patients	Encapsulated organisms

Empirical antimicrobial and supportive treatment should be commenced without delay, as in immunocompetent patients, whilst a definitive diagnosis is sought. It should be remembered that chest X-ray may be normal, most notably in patients with pneumocystis pneumonia. Bronchoscopy has become a cornerstone in the evaluation of the immunocompromised patient [34]. It can provide a spectrum of samples (Table 20.9) though the procedure is often repeated, particularly for microbiological testing. The additional risks of each test, perhaps most notably the risk of pneumothorax [35] with transbronchial biopsy, must be weighed against the benefits of refining the diagnosis for each case.

20.3.3.1 *Human immunodeficiency virus*

Since human immunodeficiency virus (HIV) was discovered in 1981, there have been dramatic changes in treatment and prognosis. Even in the mid-1990s, admission to ICU in the context of acquired immune deficiency syndrome (AIDS) and pneumonia was rare and the mortality figures reached almost 100% in some series. Largely due to advances in anti-retroviral chemotherapy, this patient population has a much improved outlook and therefore, HIV and ICU physicians need to continue to collaborate closely to deliver optimal care.

20.3.3.2 *Severe acute respiratory syndrome*

Severe acute respiratory syndrome (SARS) is a viral illness that can progress to respiratory failure and death. The outbreak in China, Toronto and

Table 20.9. Bronchoscopy procedure in mechanically ventilated patients — practical considerations.

Factor	Action
Oxygenation	Set FiO_2 to 1.0
Access for fibreoptic bronchoscopy (FOB)	Use modified catheter-mount with airtight seal
Obstruction to ventilation by FOB	Minimum 8 mm ET tube
Awareness/coughing	Adequate sedation +/− paralysis
Hypercarbia	Intermittently withdraw bronchoscope Monitoring of end-tidal CO_2

Singapore in 2002–2003 carried a significant mortality rate of 9.6% [36]. There is no diagnostic test, and therefore the diagnosis of SARS is based on the presence of risk factors, symptoms and signs. The incubation period of SARS is reported to be two to seven days and the mean duration of symptoms to time of admission to hospital is three to five days [37]. Transmission is thought to occur by droplet spread leading to the main spread prevention measures centring on barrier methods. Up to 25% of SARS patients deteriorate further, requiring ICU admission [38,39], usually because of respiratory failure, and 10–15% of patients will require mechanical ventilation. The clinical picture appears similar to ARDS, and ICU management should generally follow the same principles applied to ARDS (Section 20.1.1). Other treatment focuses on two main issues; pharmacological therapy and prevention of further spread. As the diagnosis is often in doubt, empirical therapy for community-acquired pneumonia should be started, including a fluoroquinolone or macrolide. The antiviral ribavirin has been used in the majority of patients in past outbreaks but there is no evidence of benefit. Other unproven treatments include corticosteroids, interferon 1β and plasmapheresis.

As droplet spread is thought to be the method of infective spread, general ICU care is fraught with potential contamination of both healthcare providers and other patients. The SARS virus may remain viable for up to 24 hours on a dry surface [40] and, despite the use of strict infection control precautions, 18% of the infected population in the Toronto epidemic were healthcare workers. Comprehensive recommendations for ICU staff have been published (Table 20.10) [41]. Though considerable knowledge of SARS was gained in the 2002–2003 outbreaks, it remains a global threat and a model of the expected influenza epidemics: many questions remain as to how healthcare systems would cope with further epidemics of viral pneumonia.

20.4 Specific Lung Diseases

20.4.1 *Asthma*

While worldwide prevalence of asthma continues to increase, overall mortality and outcome figures are improving. Nevertheless, asthma accounts for over 1,500 deaths per year in the UK, a proportion of which occur despite

Table 20.10. Essential critical care precaution strategies in SARS [41].

Area	Action
Staff education	High risk procedures — alternatives Precautions Minimise time in room, efficiency Avoid contamination during dress precautions SARS virus infection and natural history
Dress precautions	N-95 mask wearing mandatory Eye protection Personal items — not permitted in room Powered Air Purification Hoods — use during high-risk procedures
Equipment	Negative pressure rooms and ante rooms — door closure mandatory Alcohol based disinfectants — frequent cleaning Disposable protective equipment/disposal unit Remote monitoring equipment (video) Equipment — single patient use
Transporting patients	Avoid if at all possible Intubated patients — high level filter patient side of expiratory outlet Inform infection control

the individual receiving hospital and ICU care [42]. There are well established risk factors for the development of near-fatal asthma (Table 20.11).

20.4.1.1 *Pathogenesis*

Several mechanisms have been suggested for the most severe forms of asthma, including mucous plugging and pure bronchoconstriction. Post-mortem examination has shown widespread airway plugging by dense mucous and inflammatory cells, mucosal oedema and extensive eosinophilic infiltrates. There may also be a distinct subtype of asthma in which intense bronchoconstriction alone causes respiratory failure to develop over one to three hours [43].

20.4.1.2 *Management*

The first step should be severity assessment (Table 20.12) whilst implementing first-line treatment (see Table 20.13). If initial resuscitation is

Table 20.11. Risk factors for near-fatal asthma [35].

Features of chronic brittle asthma	Previous ventilation Previous admission for asthma (especially in last year) Treatment with more than three classes of asthma medication Heavy β2 agonist use Repeated accident and emergency attendance (especially in last year)
Prior medical care/ history	Non-compliance/self-discharge Failure to attend clinic appointments Concurrent psychiatric history Drug/alcohol misuse
Social history	Employment or income problems Social isolation Childhood abuse Severe domestic, marital or legal stress

Table 20.12. Features of life-threatening asthma [35].

Features	Silent chest Poor respiratory effort Decreased respiratory rate Drowsiness/confusion Bradycardia Hypotension Pulsus paradoxus
Blood gas parameters	Normal or raised partial pressure of carbon dioxide (PCO_2) Partial pressure of oxygen (PO_2) <8 kPa/SpO_2 <92% irrespective of FiO_2 low pH
PEFR (if measurable)	<33% best normal

Table 20.13. BTS guidelines on treatment of acute asthma.

Oxygen FiO_2 0.4–0.6 via face mask
Salbutamol 5 mg via an oxygen-driven nebuliser
Prednisolone tablets 30–60 mg or intravenous hydrocortisone 200 mg
Add ipratroprium bromide 0.5 mg
Aminophylline 250 mg intravenous infusion over 20 minutes (caution if already on theophyllines)
Magnesium sulphate 1.2–2 g over 20 minutes

unsuccessful, or the patient arrives *in extremis*, mechanical ventilation is likely to be required. Signs of this are deteriorating peak expiratory flow rate (PEFR), worsening or persisting hypoxia, hypercapnia, exhaustion, poor respiratory effort, confusion, coma or respiratory arrest. The patient should be promptly transferred to a critical care setting and preparations made for intubation and mechanical ventilation. It is essential to have an understanding of the difficulties that can arise during this phase and, where possible, minimise the associated complications.

Prevention of hyperinflation is one of the primary goals of mechanical ventilation in asthmatic patients. Usually, a slow respiratory rate and prolonged expiratory time are used to achieve this, reducing gas trapping and the risk of pneumothorax. A degree of hypercapnia may ensue but this is normally well tolerated [44].

Mucous plugging and areas of collapse are common in asthmatic patients. Mucolytics, ventilation circuit humidification and chest physiotherapy should be used to aid expectoration. NIV may have a limited role in improving gas exchange, but its use should not delay moving a patient with life-threatening asthma to ICU or initiation of invasive mechanical ventilation when it is absolutely indicated [45].

Inhalational anaesthetic agents (sevoflurane and isoflurane most recently) may help to reverse bronchoconstriction. However, many ICU ventilators are unable to deliver anaesthetic agents and likewise many anaesthetic (or theatre) ventilators are unable to ventilate patients with severely elevated airway pressures. There is also the serious concern of anaesthetic gas scavenging as well as cost implications, but in recent years one system has been introduced that may allow use of volatile anaesthetic agent to be used with ITU ventilators [46]. Ketamine and adrenaline infusions have been used with some success in intractable bronchoconstriction. However, the side effect profile of both drugs, particularly the sympathomimetic properties has led to caution in their use.

Nitric oxide causes pulmonary vasodilation and has a weak bronchodilator effect and heliox causes a fall in airway pressures in ventilated patients. However neither of these treatments has been shown to improve outcome [44] and, perhaps because of the complexities involved in their delivery on ICU, are rarely used. Successful use of extracorporeal membrane oxygenation as well as a pumpless arteriovenous carbon dioxide removal system have been reported, though evidence of a positive effect on mortality is, as yet, lacking.

20.4.2 *Chronic obstructive pulmonary disease*

COPD is characterised by progressive, only partially reversible airflow obstruction with intermittent episodes of acute deterioration. It now accounts for a significant and increasing proportion of ICU referrals. In the past a poor outcome was often predicted, limiting access to ICU care, but more recent experience suggests that short-term mortality may be much lower than previously thought [48,49]. Long-term survival is poorer but figures are similar to those for left ventricular dysfunction after acute myocardial infarction [50]. In one recent study the mortality rates at six months and one, three and five years were 39.0%, 42.7%, 61.2% and 75.9%, respectively, following admission to the ICU and the median survival time for all patients was 26 months [51]. Prognosis is undoubtedly affected by the patient's premorbid condition [50] both in terms of the severity of respiratory disease as well as comorbidities (Table 20.14). Common causes of deterioration are bacterial pneumonia, disease exacerbation and heart failure [48].

20.4.2.1 *Treatment*

Patients tend to fall into three main groups — those requiring pharmacotherapy alone (Table 20.15), those needing NIV and the highest-risk group

Table 20.14. Adverse prognostic factors in COPD outcome in critical care.

Long-term oxygen therapy (LTOT)
Severity of airflow limitation
Poor exercise tolerance (<100 yards)
Presence of pulmonary hypertension
Presence of other comorbidities
Older age
Poor nutritional status

Table 20.15. Pharmacotherapy in COPD.

Drug	Setting
Antibiotics	Infection is a common cause of worsening symptoms If pyrexial, WCC or C-reactive protein is elevated, purulent sputum Choice guided by local policy
Corticosteroids	Consider for all exacerbations Oral prednisolone 30–40 mg No evidence intravenous gives a better outcome than oral but there are practical issues with ability to remove O_2 mask/distress to take oral
β2 agonists	Often little reversibility in chronic phase Can reduce bronchoconstriction acutely Routinely nebulised
Aminophylline	No clear evidence of benefit Need to consider side effects (agitation, tachycardia, seizures, diuresis)
Doxapram	Poor side effect profile (tachycardia, severe agitation, acidosis, further precipitation of fatigue) Can be used if respiratory rate low despite clinical picture Largely replaced by NIV now Can be used in addition to NIV

who require MV. As always, the decision to intubate and mechanically ventilate should be made by the most experienced clinician available. When making decisions regarding escalation of treatment based on quality of life, it is the patient who determines their quality of life not the doctor. As much background information as possible should be obtained from the patient, relatives and medical notes.

NIV (see Chapter 8) should be considered in all patients with respiratory acidosis (pH <7.3) resistant to pharmacotherapy, in the absence of contraindications (impaired consciousness, intolerance, vomiting, cardiovascular compromise). The mortality rates of COPD patients treated with NIV have been consistently better when compared with MV [52] and current recommendations are that it should be the first-line therapy when pharmacotherapy alone has failed. NIV can be used in either the ward or critical care setting, with the most important factors in its successful use being the presence of equipment, monitoring and appropriately trained staff.

Once the decision has been made to proceed to mechanical ventilation, the patient should be moved to the ICU (if not already there) and preparations made for intubation. As with severe asthmatics, this group of patients are prone to cardiovascular collapse during induction of anaesthesia. It is therefore of paramount importance that this procedure is carried out by expert clinicians. The aims of MV are to control respiratory acidosis whilst avoiding further lung hyperinflation (Section 20.4.1.2). Weaning failure occurs in up to a quarter of COPD patients requiring MV. Thought should be given to the timing of placement of a tracheostomy and referral to a specialist weaning centre. In the small number of patients who are irreversibly ventilator-dependant, the clinical team, relatives and patient will need to consider withholding escalating treatment when further deterioration occurs.

20.4.3 *Haemoptysis*

Whilst there is no widely agreed volume which constitutes a 'massive' haemoptysis, there is no doubt that the expectoration of large volumes of blood carries a high mortality [53]. The causes of massive haemoptysis are varied (Table 20.16). Whatever the cause, massive haemoptysis is a medical emergency and demands prompt, aggressive treatment in the critical care or theatre environment. The source of bleeding is the pulmonary circulation in around 5% of cases and the bronchial circulation (systemic pressure) in over 90% of cases [54]. Fibreoptic bronchoscopy may confirm the diagnosis and localise the source of bleeding, as may contrast-enhanced computed tomography or computed tomography angiography.

20.4.3.1 *Management*

Initial steps should be via an airway, breathing, circulation (ABC) approach, often including intubation to protect the upper airway and achieve effective gas exchange in the face of significant alveolar soiling, and volume resuscitation because of high intravascular losses. Large-bore intravenous access and blood transfusion are likely to be necessary. If the site of bleeding can be identified, positioning of the patient with the bleeding side down may help prevent soiling of the upper lung. A double-lumen

Table 20.16. Causes of massive haemoptysis.

Infections	Mycobacteria (mainly tuberculosis) Fungal infections (Mycetoma) Lung abscess Necrotising pneumonia e.g. *Klebsiella, Staphylococcus*
Neoplasms	Bronchogenic carcinoma Bronchial adenoma Pulmonary metastases Sarcoma
Vascular	Pulmonary embolism Arterio-bronchial fistula Arteriovenous malformations Telangiectasia
Vasculitis	Behcet's disease Wegener's granulomatosis
Inflammatory/Infective	Bronchiectasis Chronic bronchitis
Coagulopathy	Von Willibrand's disease Haemophilia Anticoagulant therapy Thrombocytopaenia/platelet dysfunction Disseminated intravascular coagulation
Trauma	Blunt/penetrating injury Suction ulcers Tracheoarterial fistula
Iatrogenic	Pulmonary artery catheter insertion/balloon inflation Bronchoscopy Transbronchial biopsy

endotracheal tube can be inserted to isolate the bleeding lung. This procedure should only be carried out by an expert as incorrect tube placement is associated with increased mortality [55]. Fibreoptic or rigid bronchoscopy can be used to identify as well as to treat life-threatening haemoptysis, for example with topical epinephrine (1:20000 solution). When available, rigid bronchoscopy can be used to guide a balloon catheter to isolate a bleeding segment or lobe.

Bronchial artery embolisation is widely accepted as the treatment of choice and is being used with increasing success in the management of life-threatening haemoptysis [56]. The immediate success rates for control of massive haemoptysis are high, though recurrence of bleeding is reported in up to half of those treated [57]. Complications are reported in up to 15% of patients, including vessel perforation, chest pain, pyrexia, haemoptysis and systemic embolisation causing neurological and vascular injury. Emergency surgery for massive haemoptysis carries a high mortality risk and is usually reserved for cases in which embolisation is unavailable or unlikely to be successful or in the presence of bleeding from chest trauma, aortic aneurysm rupture and bleeding from a mycetoma resistant to other therapy.

20.4.4 *Pulmonary thrombo-embolism*

Despite extensive, protocol-driven use of low-molecular-weight heparin in hospital patients, the in-hospital mortality rates for pulmonary thrombo-embolism (PTE) remain stubbornly high at around 15% [58]. Risk factors for PTE are summarised in Table 20.17 [59]. The presentation of PTE is variable with many symptoms and signs such as chest pain, tachycardia, haemoptysis or arrhythmia applicable to other disease processes. Acute massive PTE, where at least half of the pulmonary circulation is occluded, tends to present with cardiovascular effects ranging from sudden death to central chest pain (Fig. 20.3).

Echocardiography is the diagnostic test of choice for acute massive PTE because it can be performed at the bedside. It is unusual to directly visualise the clot, rather the effects on the right ventricle, including dilatation and regional wall motion abnormalities, are more often seen; it can therefore be used to guide therapy and have prognostic significance. Pulmonary angiography used to be the gold standard investigation but this is no longer the case with the advent of computed tomography pulmonary angiography (CTPA) scanning. Also, isotope lung or VQ scanning was extensively used in the past but low specificity has meant it has been largely discontinued as a diagnostic tool in PTE. The practicalities of transferring patients with respiratory or cardiovascular compromise for investigations have to be weighed against the possible benefits.

Table 20.17. Risk factors for the development of PTE.

Major risk factors	
Surgery	Major abdominal/pelvic surgery Lower limb surgery Post-operative intensive care admission
Obstetrics	Late pregnancy Caesarean section Puerperium
Lower limb problems	Fracture Varicose veins
Malignancy	Abdominal/pelvic Advanced/metastatic
Reduced mobility	Hospitalisation Institutionalised care Previous PTE
Procoagulant states	Protein C/S deficiency Factor V Leiden deficiency
Minor risk factors	
Cardiovascular	Congenital heart disease Congestive cardiac failure Hypertension Superficial venous thrombosis Indwelling central venous catheter
Oestrogens	Oral contraceptive Hormone replacement
Miscellaneous	COPD Neurological disability Occult malignancy Thrombotic disorders Long distance travel Obesity

20.4.4.1 *Management*

Patients requiring admission to ICU with PTE often presented with cardiovascular collapse and have a high mortality despite treatment. After initial resuscitation, the aim is to remove or disperse the pulmonary

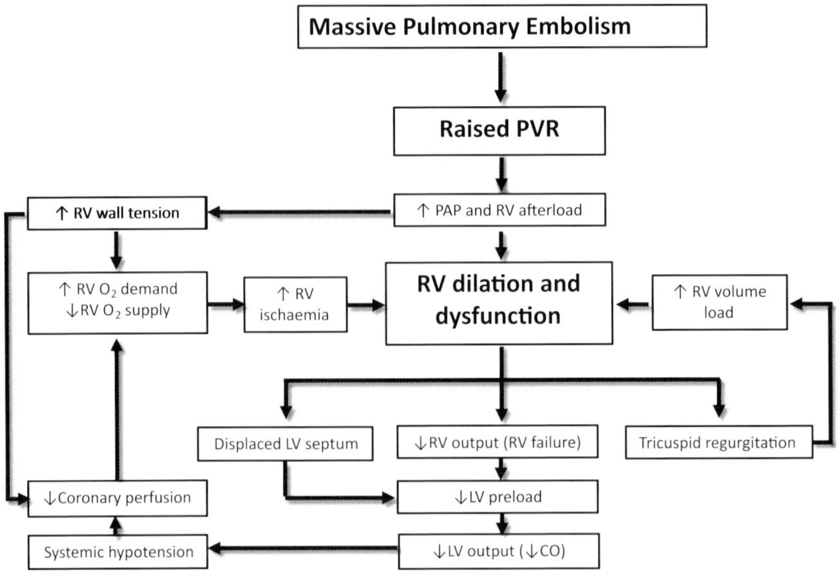

Figure 20.3. Mechanisms of cardiovascular collapse following a massive pulmonary embolism. RV, right ventricular; LV, left ventricular; PAP, pulmonary artery pressure; CO, cardiac output.

arterial clot as soon as possible. As the incidence of major haemorrhage is doubled when using thrombolysis [60] compared with heparin, most clinicians reserve this treatment for those with clinically massive PTE. The current BTS recommendation is that thrombolysis should be given via a peripheral cannula as this is as effective as when given centrally. Where thrombolysis has failed or there are absolute contraindications to its use, a right heart catheter can be inserted in an attempt to mechanically disrupt the clot. Surgical embolectomy in a cardiothoracic centre is the option of last resort as the associated mortality of emergency surgery is very high.

Right heart dysfunction is a prominent feature in cardiovascularly significant PTE. In the initial stages of resuscitation large volumes of fluid are required to support cardiac output. This intravenous filling may well need to be aided by inotropic and vasopressor support if left heart dysfunction ensues as a result of right ventricular dilatation and decreased preload (Fig 20.3). The role of inhaled pulmonary vasodilators is uncertain.

Low-molecular-weight heparin is as efficacious as unfractionated heparin for the treatment of PTE [61], and is the standard of care for thrombo-prophylaxis with graded compression stockings and pneumatic sequential compression boots for all patients in ICU (see Chapter 14).

20.4.5 *Interstitial lung disease*

Despite the conditions that are grouped together as interstitial lung disease (ILD) having different characteristics (Table 20.18), difficulty in making a swift diagnosis has meant that the initial approach to this patient group is similar. ILD patients requiring ICU admission usually fall into two groups: those with an established diagnosis who have an acute deterioration and those who present with acute respiratory failure of unknown cause. Both groups require prompt investigation and treatment, and most will need ventilatory support.

Table 20.18. Classification and pathological findings in ILD.

Condition	Computed tomography/ Pathological findings	Treatment
Non-specific interstitial pneumonia (NSIP)	Preserved architecture Variable fibrosis/cellularity	Immunosupression
Idiopathic pulmonary fibrosis (IPF)	Lesions of varying ages Multiple fibroblastic foci Dense fibrosis/honeycombing	Lung transplantation Drugs appear ineffective
Desquamative interstitial pneumonia (DIP)	Diffuse pattern of fibrosis Preservation of lung architecture	Smoking cessation Immunosupression
Respiratory bronchiolitis–interstitial lung disease (RB–ILD)	Patchy bronchiolocentric inflammation	Smoking cessation Immunosupression
Hypersensitivity pneumonitis (HP)	Peribronchiolar mixed inflammatory infiltrate	Avoidance of trigger Corticosteroids
Cryptogenic organising pneumonia (COP)	Uniform fibrosing process of small bronchioles	Immunosupression
Lymphoid interstitial pneumonia (LIP)	Interstitial imflammatory cell infiltrate	Immunosupression

Unfortunately, serological tests and chest X-ray changes are usually non-specific in ILD and most critically ill patients are unable to perform lung-function tests [62]. High-resolution computed tomography has a key role in establishing the diagnosis and identifies the suitable sites for surgical lung biopsy. BAL, and in selected cases transbronchial lung biopsy, is advocated to rule out an infective cause for respiratory failure as the mainstay of treatment for ILD is immunosupression. Surgical lung biopsy has been advocated in patients where the importance of diagnostic accuracy on treatment and outcome can justify the increased incidence of perioperative complications [63].

20.4.5.1 *Management*

As mentioned above, immunosupression forms the backbone of treatment for ILD although in severe resistant cases referral for lung transplantation is necessary. Intravenous corticosteroid therapy is the initial treatment of choice and intravenous cyclophosphamide is usually administered in patients not responding to corticosteroids [64]. Mechanical ventilation is widely regarded as a strong relative contraindication to lung transplantation, in view of the risk of pneumonia, muscular de-conditioning due to immobility and other complications. However, the evidence is conflicting regarding outcome and transplantation should be considered in appropriate circumstances.

The inflammatory nature of ILD means that, theoretically, this group are at high risk of ventilator-associated lung injury and a 'protective' lung strategy has been advocated [64]. However, in the case of known IPF, the latest BTS guideline [62], suggests that, given the poor prognosis and lack of proven treatment, mechanical ventilation is unlikely to be helpful in the short- or long-term.

20.5 Investigations

Identification of the causes of respiratory failure and their complications is crucial as many diseases have specific treatments and in the critically ill time is of the essence if further deterioration is to be prevented. For example, in one recent case series of 376 patients with a clinical diagnosis of

ARDS, 169 died and 64 had post-mortem data for analysis. Post-mortem examination revealed the classical histopathological appearance of ARDS, diffuse alveolar damage in 32 patients (50%), pneumonia without diffuse alveolar damage in 16 patients (25%) and invasive pulmonary aspergillosis in eight patients (12.5%). Major unexpected findings were found in 15 patients (23%) [65]. Despite the obvious weakness of the study, these data demonstrate the difficulty of making accurate diagnoses in critically ill patients and highlight the causes of diffuse chest radiographic abnormality with respiratory failure, many of which have specific treatments (Table 20.19).

There is considerable overlap between conditions that cause ARDS and those that are also associated with a distinct pathology that may have a specific treatment.

Table 20.19. Conditions that mimic and cause ALI and ARDS but have distinct pathology.

Condition			Specific treatment
Pneumonia	Bacterial	Miliary tuberculosis	R
	Viral	Cytomegalovirus	R
		Herpes simplex	R
		Hantavirus	
	Fungal	Pneumocystis jiroveci	R
		Invasive aspergillosis	
	Others	Strongyloidiasis	R
Cryptogenic		Acute interstitial pneumonia	R
		Cryptogenic organising pneumonia	R
		Acute eosinophilic pneumonia	R
Malignancy		Bronchoalveolar cell carcinoma	
		Lymphangitis carcinomatosa	
		Acute leukaemia	R
		Lymphoma	R
Pulmonary vascular disease		Diffuse alveolar haemorrhage	R
		Sickle lung	R

20.5.1 *Bronchoscopy*

The BTS recommends that fibreoptic bronchoscopy (FOB) is available for use in all ICUs [66]. It can be used to collect samples to aid diagnosis in patients failing to respond to first-line antimicrobial therapy. Other common uses include the relief of endobronchial obstruction (e.g. by secretions), to aid ETT or percutaneous tracheostomy placement and the localisation of a bleeding source (see Section 20.4). FOB should be carefully planned as the procedure is not without serious side effects, including hypoxia, inadvertent extubation, hypercarbia or gas trapping and pneumothorax. Basic requirements are listed in Table 20.20. Although FOB may have a high false negative rate in cases of CAP, a negative BAL culture in suspected VAP virtually excludes the diagnosis (see Section 20.3).

Trans-bronchial biopsy in mechanically ventilated patients carries a substantial risk (8–14%) of pneumothorax [67]. It is therefore generally reserved for patients who have had lung transplantation, where the sensitivity and specificity are high and the potential risks are considered to be justified.

20.5.2 *Surgical lung biopsy*

This carries a significant risk of causing persistent air leaks in ventilated patients but has a high diagnostic yield [63]. Current recommendations are that at least five pieces of tissue are taken to make specific diagnoses, perhaps explaining the complication risk. There is conflicting evidence as

Table 20.20. Bronchoscopy procedure in mechanically ventilated patients — practical considerations.

Factor	Action
Oxygenation	Set FiO_2 to 1.0
Access for FOB	Use modified catheter-mount with airtight seal
Obstruction to ventilation by FOB	Minimum 8 mm ETT
Awareness/coughing	Adequate sedation with or without paralysis
Hypercarbia	Intermittently withdraw bronchoscope Monitoring of end-tidal CO_2

to the effect on mortality therefore this procedure is only carried out when the risks of failing to diagnose the patient's condition are deemed to outweigh the possible complications.

20.5.3 *Radiology*

20.5.3.1 *Chest X-ray*

Daily chest X-rays are recommended by the American College of Radiology [68] in mechanically ventilated patients. This is based on case series that reported a significant incidence (15–18%) of findings which directly led to changes in management [69]. The advent of digital imaging techniques has meant that lower radiation doses are used and allowed image manipulation to facilitate visualisation of intravenous lines and nasogastric tubes (NGTs). Chest X-rays should routinely be performed after all ETT placements and NGT, central venous catheter and pleural drain insertion.

20.5.3.2 *Thoracic ultrasound*

Fluid in the pleural space is known to affect ventilation–perfusion matching and its removal improves oxygenation and pulmonary compliance [70]. Real time ultrasound-guided drainage using small-bore drains (12 French size) inserted using the Seldinger technique is the standard of care in many units. Ultrasound has an expanding role in diagnosing thoracic pathology in critically ill patients [71].

20.5.3.3 *Thoracic computed tomography*

The transfer and monitoring of a critically ill patient for computed tomography (CT) scanning involves co-ordinating the efforts of medical, nursing and technical support staff and this should only be considered if the risks of moving a specific patient have been weighed against the well-described hazards [72]. There are standards for transporting critically ill patients which include a period of stabilisation on the transport ventilator prior to movement [72].

The indications for CT scanning in critically ill patients are manifold but the use of bedside ultrasound is increasing owing to better training of intensivists. For example, ARDS can be complicated by small, loculated pneumothoraces, empyema or abscess which may not be apparent on a plain chest X-ray [73]. In this setting, CT can be diagnostic and also guide percutaneous drainage. CT scanning of victims of serious trauma has now become routine, as clinical examination and plain radiography can miss potentially life-threatening conditions such as pneumo/haemothorax, pulmonary contusion or mediastinal injury.

20.5.4 *Lung function tests*

Though these basic tests are carried out routinely in the outpatient or general ward setting, they are often dismissed as impractical in the ICU. However, measuring respiratory muscle strength and basic spirometry may be invaluable in selected cases of weaning failure. An airtight connection between the ETT and a hand-held spirometer can give accurate, reproducible results [74]. If respiratory muscle weakness is suspected, measurements should be performed sitting and supine as a reduction of 25% or more whilst supine indicates diagphragmatic weakness. It is widely accepted that a vital capacity of 10 ml/kg is required to sustain unsupported ventilation.

20.6 Conclusions

Patients with respiratory failure on ICU are frequently unstable from either a haemodynamic or a respiratory point of view. In attempting to make a diagnosis, clinicians must carefully weigh the need for rapid diagnosis and prompt commencement of treatment against the potential harm caused by the investigative techniques. Where the decision is taken to transfer a patient to another area to carry out such investigations, strict safety guidelines must be followed and the effect of occupying a significant number of critical care personnel weighed against the benefit to each patient.

20.7 Clinical Case

A 47-year-old American man was admitted to the ICU following transfer from a local district general hospital ICU for further management of severe ARDS following Panton–Valentine leukocidin (PVL)-positive community-acquired methicillin-resistant staphylococcus aureus (MRSA) pneumonia. The medical history included mild asthma, migraine, hyperlipidaemia, hypertension and lumbar disc prolapse.

He presented to the accident and emergency department following arrival on a flight from the USA with haemoptysis and a history of several days of shortness of breath, cough and fever. An emergency CTPA excluded pulmonary embolism, but demonstrated bilateral lower lobe consolidation. He was admitted to intensive care and managed with broad-spectrum antibiotics, activated protein C, vasopressor and renal support, but he deteriorated, requiring invasive mechanical ventilation within 24 hours. During the subsequent week PVL-toxin-positive MRSA was cultured from a sputum sample; consequently Linezolid and Rifampicin were added to the antibiotic regimen. A right pneumothorax and a large left-sided pleural effusion detected on a CT thorax were drained (Fig. 20.4). However, the lung compliance worsened and blood gases on FiO_2 0.5 with a respiratory rate of 24 breaths/minute, peak pressure of 35 cm H_2O and positive end-expiratory pressure 10 cm H_2O of PO_2 8.1 kPa, PCO_2 10.9 kPa, pH 7.13, bicarbonate 21.9 mmol/l preceded a request for transfer to a cardiothoracic centre.

Prior to transfer, the retrieval team instituted invasive lung assist (iLA: Novalung) through a 15 French gauge right femoral arterial cannula and a 17 French gauge right femoral venous cannula inserted under ultrasound control. Following initiation of Novalung support, after 20 minutes on the transport ventilator the PCO_2 was 9 kPa with a PO_2 of 18 on FiO_2 of 0.8. Subsequently, with an oxygen flow of 10 l/minute through the Novalung it was possible to reduce the tidal volume and peak inspiratory pressure to 250 ml and 30 cm H_2O. A further left pleural effusion was drained. A transthoracic echocardiogram showed a moderate pericardial effusion with no evidence of haemodynamic significance, good LV function and no valvular abnormalities. A negative fluid balance was achieved on haemofiltration, a new Klebsiella nosocomial pneumonia was treated and parenteral feeding converted to enteral.

After two weeks of relative stability, it was decided that corticosteroid therapy would be used. Methylprednisolone 500 mg for three days followed by 2 mg/kg was administered for a month in total. Gradual

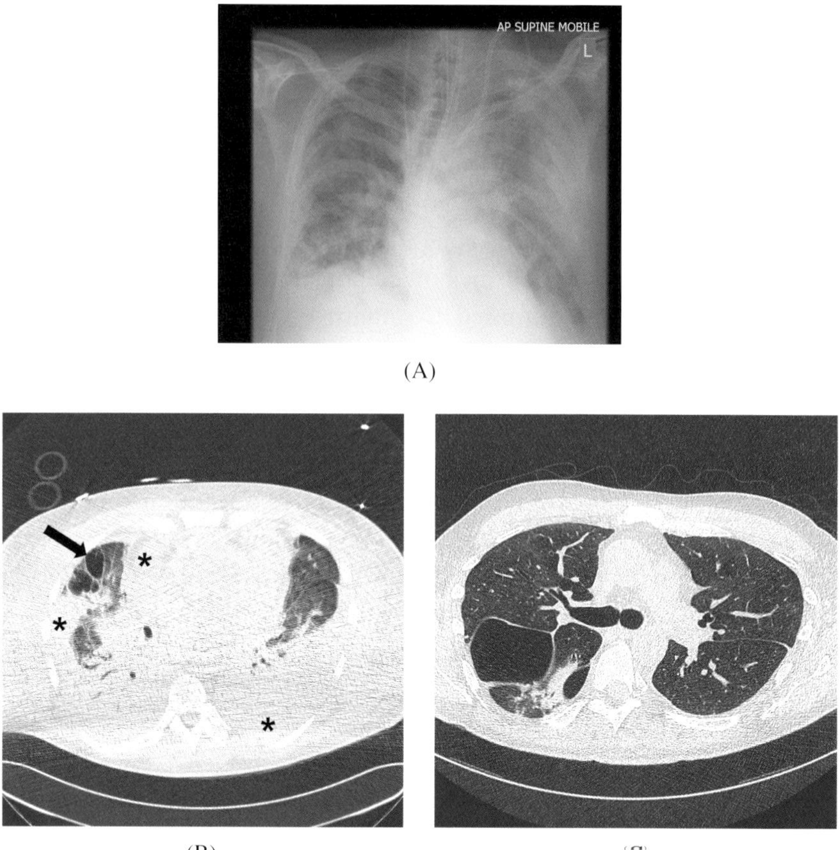

Figure 20.4 (A) Chest radiograph of illustrative case — ARDS complicating PVL toxin + MRSA pneumonia. (B) Contemporaneous CT scan of thorax showing characteristic dense bilateral consolidation, bilateral pleural and a pericardial effusion (asterix) and anterior pneumatoceles (arrow). (C) CT thorax in the recovery period showing a right-sided pneumothorax and evidence of scarring from the previous lung injury.

improvement in the patient's overall condition with recovery of gut and renal function, decreased requirement for cardiovascular support was punctuated by episodes of ventilator-associated pneumonia. Gas exchange improved such that it was possible to establish a spontaneous mechanical ventilation mode, remove the Novalung and slowly lighten sedation. On removing the arterial cannula, the femoral artery was torn requiring open surgical repair. In the recovery phase around the time of tracheal decannulation, the predominant issues were weakness, anxiety and depression.

After several weeks in hospital, the patient was keen to be repatriated. A further CT scan of the thorax was performed which demonstrated a complex persistent right-sided pneumothorax and multiple subpleural pneumatoceles anteriorly.

20.7.1 *Learning points*

(i) PVL-MRSA can cause necrotising pneumonia with a relatively high incidence of pleural complications and acute respiratory failure. Linezolid is probably the first choice antimicrobial agent for this infection; it inhibits production of the exotoxin.

(ii) iLA (Novalung) may be useful in facilitating patient transfer but its primary indication in ARDS is to facilitate a very-low-tidal-volume ventilation strategy. The major complications of its use are vascular, associated with the arterial cannula.

(iii) The role of corticosteroids in patients recovering from ARDS remains controversial.

(iv) The commonest causes of morbidity in survivors of ARDS affect muscle strength, mobility and mood.

(v) Pneumothoraces and other air leaks complicate ARDS in up to 66% of cases. After they have recovered, these patients should be reassessed for their fitness to fly.

References

[1] Garber, B.G., Hébert, P.C., Yelle, J.-D. *et al.* (1996). Adult respiratory distress syndrome: a systemic overview of incidence and risk factors, *Crit Care Med*, **24**, 687–695.

[2] Bernard, G.R., Artigas, A., Brigham, K.L. *et al.* (1994). The American–European Consensus Conference on ARDS. Definitions, mechanisms, relevant outcomes, and clinical trial coordination, *Am J Respir Crit Care Med*, **149**, 818–824.

[3] Wheeler, A.P. and Bernard, G.R. (2007). Acute lung injury and the acute respiratory distress syndrome: a clinical review, *Lancet*, **369**, 1553–1564.

[4] Griffiths, M.J.D. and Evans, TW. (2003). 'Acute respiratory distress syndrome', in Gibson, G.J., Geddes, D.M., Costabel, U., *et al.* (eds), *Respiratory Medicine*, third edition, Saunders, London, pp. 736–763.

[5] Chastre, J. (2005). Antibiotic prescribing for ventilator-associated pneumonia: get it right from the beginning but be able to rapidly deescalate, *Intens Care Med*, **31**, 1463–1465.

[6] Wiedemann, H.P. Wheeler, A., Bernard, G.R. *et al.* (2006). Comparison of two fluid-management strategies in acute lung injury, *N Engl J Med*, **354**, 2564–2575.

[7] Kress, J.P., Pohlman A.S., O'Connor, M.F. *et al.* (2000). Daily interruption of sedative infusions in critically ill patients undergoing mechanical ventilation, *N Engl J Med*, **342**, 1471–1477.

[8] Fletcher, S.N., Kennedy, D.D., Ghosh, I.R. *et al.* (2003). Persistent neuromuscular and neurophysiologic abnormalities in long-term survivors of prolonged critical illness, *Crit Care Med*, **31**, 1012–1016.

[9] Steinberg, K.P., Hudson L.D., Goodman, R.B. *et al.* (2006). Efficacy and safety of corticosteroids for persistent acute respiratory distress syndrome, *N Engl J Med*, **354**, 1671–1684.

[10] Baudouin, S.V. (2004). Exogenous surfactant replacement in ARDS — one day, someday, or never? *N Engl J Med*, **351**, 853–855.

[11] Sakuma, T., Okaniwa, G., Nakada, T. *et al.* (1994). Alveolar fluid clearance in the resected human lung, Alveolar fluid clearance in the resected human lung, *Am J Respir Crit Care Med*, **150**, 305–310.

[12] Perkins, G.D., McAuley, D.F., Thickett, D.R. *et al.* (2006). The β-agonist lung injury trial (BALTI); a randomized placebo-controlled clinical trial, *Am J Respir Crit Care Med*, **173**, 281–287.

[13] Alexander, J.I., Horton, P.W., Millar, W.T. *et al.* (1972). The effect of upper abdominal surgery on the relationship of airway closing point to end tidal position, *Clin Sci*, **43**, 137–141.

[14] Ali, J., Weisel, R.D., Layug, A.B. *et al.* (1974). Consequences of postoperative alterations in respiratory mechanics, *Am J Surg*, **128**, 376–382.

[15] Warner, M.A., Divertie, M.B. and Tinker, J.H. (1984). Preoperative cessation of smoking and pulmonary complications in coronary artery bypass patients, *Anesthesiology*, **60**, 380–383.

[16] Gosselink, R., Bott, J., Johnson, M. *et al.* (2008). Physiotherapy for adult patients with critical illness: recommendations of the European Respiratory Society and European Society of Intensive Care Medicine Task Force on Physiotherapy for critically ill patients, *Intens Care Med*, **34**, 1188–1199.

[17] Ferreyra, G.P., Baussano, I., Squadrone, V. *et al.* (2008). Continuous positive airway pressure for treatment of respiratory complications after abdominal surgery: a systematic review and meta-analysis, *Ann Surg*, **247**, 617–626.
[18] Esteban, A., Frutos-Vivar, F., Ferguson, N.D. *et al.* (2004). Noninvasive positive-pressure ventilation for respiratory failure after extubation, *N Engl J Med*, **350**, 2452–2460.
[19] Ewig, S. and Torres, A. (1999). Severe community-acquired pneumonia, *Clin Chest Med*, **20**, 575–587.
[20] Angus, D.C., Marrie, T.J., Obrosky, D.S. *et al.* (2002). Severe community-acquired pneumonia use of intensive care services and evaluation of American and British Thoracic Society diagnostic criteria, *Am J Respir Crit Care Med*, **166**, 717–723.
[21] Fine, M.J., Smith, M.A., Carson, C.A. *et al.* (1996). Prognosis and outcomes of patients with community-acquired pneumonia, a meta-analysis, *JAMA*, **275**, 134–141.
[22] The British Thoracic Society (2001). Guidelines for the management of community-acquired pneumonia in adults admitted to hospital, *Thorax*, **56** (Suppl. IV), 1–64.
[23] Garcia-Ordonez, M.A., García-Jiménez, J.M., Páez, F. *et al.* (2001). Clinical aspects and prognostic factors in elderly patients hospitalised for community-acquired pneumonia, *Eur J Clin Microbiol Infect Dis*, **20**, 14–19.
[24] The British Thoracic Society Research Committee and the Public Health Laboratory Service (1992). The aetiology, management and outcome of severe community-acquired pneumonia on the intensive care unit, *Respir Med*, **86**, 7–13.
[25] Fagon, J.Y., Chastre, J., Wolff, M. *et al.* (2000). Invasive and noninvasive strategies for management of suspected ventilator-associated pneumonia, A randomized trial, *Ann Intern Med*, **132**, 621–630.
[26] Tan, Y.K., Khoo, K.L., Chin, S.P. *et al.* (1998). Aetiology and outcome of severe community-acquired pneumonia in Singapore, *Eur Respir J*, **12**, 113–115.
[27] Rello J., Quintana, E., Ausina, V. *et al.* (1991). Incidence, etiology, and outcome of nosocomial pneumonia in mechanically ventilated patients, *Chest*, **100**, 439–444.
[28] Ewig, S., Torres, A., El-Ebiary, M. *et al* (1999). Bacterial colonization patterns in mechanically ventilated patients with traumatic and medical head injury, Incidence, risk factors, and association with ventilator-associated pneumonia, *Am J Respir Crit Care Med*, **159**, 188–198.
[29] Kollef, M.H., Silver, P., Murphy, D.M. *et al.* (1995). The effect of late-onset pneumonia in determining patient mortality, *Chest*, **108**,1655–1662.

[30] Lynch, J.P. (2001). Hospital-acquired pneumonia — risk factors, microbiology, and treatment, Chest, **119**, 373s–384s.

[31] American Thoracic Society (1996). Hospital-acquired pneumonia in adults; diagnosis, assessment, initial severity, and prevention. A consensus statement, *Am J Respir Crit Care Med*, **153**, 1711–1725.

[32] American Thoracic Society (1996). Hospital-acquired pneumonia in adults; diagnosis, assessment, initial severity, and prevention, a consensus statement, November 1995, *Am J Respir Crit Care Med*, **153**, 1711–1725.

[33] Rañó, A., Agustí, C., Sibila, O. *et al.* (2005). Pulmonary infections in non-HIV-immunocompromised patients, *Curr Opin Pulm Med*, **11**, 213–217.

[34] Baughman, R.P. (1994). Use of bronchoscopy in the diagnosis of infection in the immunocompromised host, *Thorax*, **49**, 3–7.

[35] Broaddus, C., Drake, M.D., Stulbarg, M.S. *et al.* (1985). Bronchoalveolar lavage and transbronchial biopsy for the diagnosis of pulmonary infections in the acquired immunodeficiency syndrome, *Ann Intern Med*, **102**, 747–752.

[36] Centers for Disease Control and Prevention (CDC) (2003). Update: severe acute respiratory syndrome–United States, *MMWR Morb Mortal Wkly Rep*, **52**, 570.

[37] Donnelly, C.A., Ghani, A.C., Leung, G.M. *et al.* (2003). Epidemiological determinants of spread of causal agent of severe acute respiratory syndrome in Hong Kong, *Lancet*, **361**, 1761–1766.

[38] Lew, T.W., Kwek, T.K., Tai, D. *et al.* (2003). Acute respiratory distress syndrome in critically ill patients with severe acute respiratory syndrome, *JAMA*, **290**, 374–380.

[39] Fowler R.A., Lapinsky S.E., Hallett D. *et al.* (2003). Critically ill patients with severe acute respiratory syndrome, *JAMA*, **290**, 367–373.

[40] Centers for Disease Control and Prevention (CDC). (2003). Cluster of severe acute respiratory syndrome cases among protected health-care workers–Toronto, Canada, *MMWR Morb Mortal Wkly Rep*, **52**, 433–436.

[41] Lapinsky, S.E. and Hawryluck, L. (2003). ICU management of severe acute respiratory syndrome, *Intens Care Med*, **29**, 870–875.

[42] Shugg, A.W., Kerr, S. and Butt, W.W. (1990). Mechanical ventilation of paediatric patients with asthma: short and long term outcome, *J Paediatr Child Health*, **26**, 343–346.

[43] Reid, L.M. (1987). The presence or absence of bronchial mucus in fatal asthma, *J Allergy Clin Immunol*, **80**, 415–416.

[44] Mansel, J.K., Stogner, S.W., Petrini, M.F. *et al*, (1990). Mechanical ventilation in patients with acute severe asthma, *Am J Med*, **89**, 42–48.

[45] Meduri, G.U., Turner, R.E., Abou-Shala, N. *et al.* (1996). Noninvasive positive pressure ventilation via face mask. First-line intervention in patients with acute hypercapnic and hypoxemic respiratory failure, *Chest*, **109**, 179–193.
[46] Berton, J., Sargentini, C., Nguyen, J.L. *et al.* (2007). AnaConDa reflection filter: bench and patient evaluation of safety and volatile anesthetic conservation, *Anesth Analg*, **104**, 130–134.
[47] British Thoracic Society and Scottish Intercollegiate Guidelines Network (2008). British Guideline on the Management of Asthma, *Thorax*, **63** (Suppl. 4), iv1–iv121.
[48] Nevins, M.L. and Epstein, S. K. (2001). Predictors of outcome for patients with COPD requiring invasive mechanical ventilation, *Chest*, **119**, 1840–1849.
[49] Seneff. M.G., Wagner D.P., Wagner, R.P. *et al.* (1995). Hospital and 1-year survival of patients admitted to intensive care units with acute exacerbations of chronic obstructive disease, *JAMA*, **274**, 1852–1857.
[50] Ai-Ping, C., Lee, K.H. and Lim, T.K. (2005). In-hospital and 5-year mortality of patients treated in the ICU for acute exacerbation of COPD, *Chest*, **128**, 518–524.
[51] Wildman, M.J., Sanderson, C.F., Groves, J. *et al.* (2009). Survival and quality of life for patients with COPD or asthma admitted to intensive care in a UK multicentre cohort: the COPD and Asthma Outcome Study (CAOS), *Thorax*, **64**, 128–132.
[52] Lightowler, J.V., Wedzicha, J.A., Elliott, M.W. *et al.* (2003). Non-invasive positive pressure ventilation to treat respiratory failure resulting from exacerbations of chronic obstructive pulmonary disease: Cochrane systematic review and meta-analysis, *BMJ*, **326**, 185–187.
[53] Håkanson, E., Konstantinov, I.E., Fransson, S.-G. *et al.* (2002). Management of life-threatening haemoptysis, *Br J Anaesth*, **88**, 291–295.
[54] Jean-Baptiste, E. (2000). Clinical assessment and management of massive hemoptysis, *Crit Care Med*, **28**, 1642–1647.
[55] Klein, U., Karzai, W., Bloos, F. *et al.* (1998). Role of fiberoptic bronchoscopy in conjunction with the use of double-lumen tubes for thoracic anesthesia: a prospective study, *Anesthesiology*, **88**, 346–350.
[56] Hayakawa, K., Tanaka, F., Torizuka, T. *et al.* (1992). Bronchial artery embolisation for haemoptysis: immediate and long-term results, *Cardiovasc Intervent Radiol*, **15**, 154–159.
[57] Lee. S., Chan, J.W., Chan, S.C. *et al.* (2008). Bronchial artery embolisation can be equally safe and effective in the management of chronic recurrent haemoptysis, *Hong Kong Med J*, **14**, 14–20.

[58] Aylin, P., Bottle, A., Kirkwood, G. *et al.* (2008). Trends in hospital admissions for pulmonary embolism in England: 1996/7 to 2005/6, *Clin Med*, **8**, 388–392.

[59] British Thoracic Society Standards of Care Committee Pulmonary Embolism Guideline Development Group (2003). British Thoracic Society guidelines for the management of suspected acute pulmonary embolism, *Thorax*, **48**, 470–484.

[60] Konstantinides, S., Geibel, A., Heusel, G. *et al.* (2002). Heparin plus alteplase compared with heparin alone in patients with submassive pulmonary embolism, *N Engl J Med*, **347**, 1143–1150.

[61] Hirsh, J., Warkentin, T.E., Shaughnessy, S.G. *et al.* (2001). Heparin and low-molecular-weight heparin mechanisms of action, pharmacokinetics, dosing, monitoring, efficacy, and safety, *Chest*, **119** (Suppl. 1), 64S–94S.

[62] Bradley. B., Branley, H.M., Egan, J.J. *et al.* (2008). Interstitial lung disease guideline: the British Thoracic Society in collaboration with the Thoracic Society of Australia and New Zealand and the Irish Thoracic Society, *Thorax*, **63** (Suppl. 5), v1–v58.

[63] Flabouris, A. and Myburgh J. (1999). The utility of open lung biopsy in patients requiring mechanical ventilation, *Chest*, **115**, 811–817.

[64] Baydur A. (2008). Mechanical ventilation in interstitial lung disease which patients are likely to benefit? *Chest*, **133**, 1062–1063.

[65] de Hemptinne, Q., Remmelink, M., Brimioulle, S. *et al.* (2009). ARDS: a clinicopathological confrontation, *Chest*, **135**, 944–949.

[66] British Thoracic Society (2001). British Thoracic Society Guidelines on Diagnostic Flexible Bronchoscopy, *Thorax*, **56** (Suppl. 1), 1–22.

[67] Papin, T.A., Grum, C. M. and Weg, J.G. (1986). Transbronchial biopsy during mechanical ventilation, *Chest*, **89**, 168–170.

[68] Tocino, I., Westcott, J., Davis, S.D. *et al.* (2000). Routine daily portable X-ray. American College of Radiology. ACR Appropriateness Criteria, *Radiology*, **215** (Suppl.), 621–626.

[69] Strain, D.S., Kinasewitz, G.T., Vereen, L.E. *et al.* (1985). Value of routine daily chest x-rays in the medical intensive care unit, *Critical Care Medicine*, **13**, 534–536.

[70] Agusti, A.G., Cardús, J., Roca, J. *et al.* (1997). Ventilation-perfusion mismatch in patients with pleural effusion: effects of thoracentesis, *Am J Respir Crit Care Med*, **156**, 1205–1209.

[71] Schmidt G.A. (2009). ICU ultrasound. The coming boom, *Chest*, **135**, 1407–1408.

[72] Intensive Care Society (2002). *Guidelines for the Transport of the Critically Ill Adult*, Intensive Care Society, London.
[73] Snow, N., Bergin, K.T. and Horrigan, T.P. (1990). Thoracic CT scanning in critically ill patients, Information obtained frequently alters management, *Chest*, **97**, 1467–1470.
[74] Dakin, J. and Griffiths, M. (2002). The pulmonary physician in critical care 1, pulmonary investigations for acute respiratory failure, *Thorax*, **57**, 79–85.

21

Vascular Intensive Care

Susan Jain and Carlos M. H. Gómez

21.1 Introduction

The typical vascular patient poses a challenge both to the surgeon and the intensivist. In some places, post-operative management still takes place on a general surgical ward where monitoring is not as thorough and picking up problems can be delayed through lack of experience of junior medical staff or simply because of lack of manpower.

The presence of multiple comorbidities and certain characteristics in vascular patients makes them a target group for appropriate pre-operative work up:

(i) Advanced age.
(ii) Often lifelong heavy smokers.
(iii) Cardiovascular disease — silent or otherwise.
(iv) Renal disease.
(v) Chronic obstructive pulmonary disease (COPD) coupled with general lack of fitness due to intermittent claudication.
(vi) Diabetes.

Cardiovascular complications remain the leading cause of mortality post vascular surgery. This is true for both abdominal aortic aneurysm (AAA) repair [1,2] and lower limb revascularisation. Indeed, symptomatic coronary artery disease (CAD) can have an incidence of 40–45% both in AAA and in elective lower limb revascularisation [3]. Furthermore, severe CAD was noted in 44% of patients with clinical evidence and in 15% with no clinical evidence of disease [3]. Atherosclerosis, if present in the lower limbs, will be prevalent elsewhere in the body — besides CAD, these patients may also have carotid artery disease and an AAA.

Assessment of cardiac risk pre-operatively can be beneficial in that it allows the anaesthetist to be better prepared and to further tailor the anaesthetic for the individual. The American College of Cardiology (ACC) and the American Heart Association (AHA) published guidelines in 2007 [4] to aid peri-operative evaluation for non-cardiac surgery. By using this, high-risk patients can be highlighted and further investigated (Table 21.1).

As a guideline, those in the minor risk category require no further cardiac evaluation while those in the major risk category definitely do. The intermediate risk category should be taken on an individual basis, for example one factor together with favourable clinical and functional status does not necessarily warrant further investigation while a couple of factors with questionable functional status will probably need to be looked at in more detail.

If patients have:

(i) had coronary revascularisation in the last five years, or
(ii) had a favourable coronary evaluation in the last two years, and there are no symptoms or changes to report, then there should be no cardiac testing required [5].

If this is not so, the patient must be assessed using the following criteria:

- The presence of comorbidities.
- Cardiac risk factors (as per the ACC/AHA guidelines).
- Functional status which can be evaluated using metabolic equivalents (METS).
- The risk of the proposed surgery.

Table 21.1. Clinical predictors of increased peri-operative cardiovascular risk (myocardial infarction (MI), heart failure, death).

Major
Unstable coronary syndromes
Acute or recent MI with evidence of important ischemic risk by clinical symptoms or non-invasive study
Unstable or severe angina (Canadian class III or IV)
Decompensated heart failure
Significant arrhythmias
High-grade atrioventricular block
Symptomatic ventricular arrhythmias in the presence of underlying heart disease
Supraventricular arrhythmias with uncontrolled ventricular rate
Severe valvular disease
Intermediate
Mild angina pectoris (Canadian class I or II)
Previous MI by history or pathologic Q waves
Compensated or prior heart failure
Diabetes mellitus (particularly insulin-dependent)
Renal insufficiency
Minor
Advanced age
Abnormal electrocardiogram (left ventricular hypertrophy, left bundle-branch block, ST-T abnormalities)
Rhythm other than sinus (e.g. atrial fibrillation)
Low functional capacity (e.g. inability to climb one flight of stairs with a bag of groceries)
History of stroke
Uncontrolled systemic hypertension

The use of exercise/stress testing, thallium scanning, dobutamine stress echocardiography and coronary angiography will be at the discretion of the assessing teams, which will usually include cardiologists if high-risk patients are identified.

Finally, the use of β-blockers pre-operatively has remained an unresolved issue. In 1996, 200 high-risk patients were given atenolol, commencing two days pre-operatively and continuing for seven days post-operatively: the results showed a reduced incidence of peri- and post-op MI by approximately 30% [6].

In 1999 a randomised controlled multicentre trial explored the pre-operative use of β-blockers in high-risk patients for vascular surgery [7]. Cardiac death or non-fatal MI in the bisoprolol group was 3.4% versus 34% in standard care group.

These are but two examples of the many studies undertaken in order to prove the efficacy of β-blockade in reducing mortality from cardiac causes. The most recent to add fuel to the fire was the Peri-operative Ischemic Evaluation Study (POISE) [8], which concluded that β-blockers should be continued in those already taking them, but for the rest of the population (including high-cardiac-risk patients) no clear benefit could be demonstrated and in fact there might even be a higher risk of precipitating a cerebrovascular event. The theoretical advantage of β-blockade may be clear — reduction of myocardial oxygen demand, anti-arrhythmic and even anti-inflammatory effects [9] — but for now the evidence does not seem to point in one clear direction.

With regard to renal insufficiency, COPD and diabetes mellitus, each must be assessed with regard to its:

- Severity, e.g. biochemical markers, glucose control, lung function tests.
- Effects on clinical/functional status.
- Requirement for pharmacotherapy if appropriate.

All of these factors contribute to post-operative mortality, hence the need for thorough assessment and avoidance of worsening the condition.

21.2 Physiological Impact of Major Vascular Surgery and Post-Operative Complications

Surgery and indeed trauma evoke a stress response, which can be thought of as neuroendocrine and inflammatory. The systemic inflammatory response syndrome (SIRS) is a part of this and will be discussed with reference to specific points in the vascular setting.

The value of the stress response is to enable survival after the insult. Early on, pain and hypovolaemia cause a rise in catecholamines which produces the familiar signs of tachycardia and hypertension. What is important is that there is an overall increase in myocardial oxygen consumption and hence demand so this is the first evidence of stress imposed on the body. Cortisol levels swiftly rise and can be as much as five times higher than normal. This hormone is responsible for:

- Increasing cardiac output and reducing systemic vascular resistance.
- Increasing salt and water retention via the renin–angiotensin–aldosterone axis.
- Inhibiting insulin.
- Acting as an immunosuppressant.

Other hormones released include growth hormone, glucagon, antidiuretic hormone and prolactin. The overall result is one of catabolism whereby fatty acids are mobilised, proteins are broken down to useable amino acids and hyperglycaemia ensues. This lasts on average for five days.

At the same time, the inflammatory response is characterised by the release of cytokines, primarily interleukin-1 (IL-1), IL-6 and tumour necrosis factor-α (TNF-α). These cytokines are produced by activated macrophages in damaged tissue and are then responsible for a host of effects including activation of neutrophils, production of acute-phase proteins, activation of the complement cascade and upregulation of adhesion molecules. The overall effect is one of pro-inflammation.

Part of this acute inflammatory response is SIRS which is diagnosed when two or more of the following criteria exist:

(i) White cell count < 4000 or > 12000 cells/mm^3.
(ii) Temperature < 36°C or > 38°C.
(iii) Respiratory rate > 20 breaths per minute or partial pressure of carbon dioxide (pCO_2) < 4.3 kPa.
(iv) Heart rate > 90 beats per minute.

Sepsis is present if there is SIRS with a documented infection. Persistent SIRS causes organ dysfunction (Table 21.2) whereby the involvement of two or more systems represents multiple organ failure (MOF).

Table 21.2. Possible effects of SIRS on specific organ system [10].

Organ/system	Clinical syndrome
Respiratory	Acute lung injury
Cardiovascular	Hyperdynamic hypotension
Genitourinary	Acute tubular necrosis
Gastrointestinal	Gastroparesis and intestinal ileus
Central nervous	Metabolic encephalopathy
Peripheral nervous	Critical illness polyneuropathy
Liver	Acute inflammatory hepatitis
Coagulation	Disseminated intravascular coagulation
Adrenal glands	Acute adrenal insufficiency
Skeletal muscle	Rhabdomyolysis

It is important to remember that SIRS is a spectrum and is initially a response by the body to prevent further damage [11–13].

A high incidence of SIRS after AAA repair has been demonstrated. In one series this was seen to be 89% after elective surgery, 92% after urgent surgery and 100% after emergency surgery. Those that went onto develop MOF had a significantly higher mortality than those that did not (69% versus 0%) [14].

21.2.1 *Stress specific to vascular surgery*

- Cross-clamping — prolonged ischaemia followed by reperfusion injury releases free radicals into the circulation where they act as a stimulus for cytokine production [15]. Haemorrhage and massive blood transfusion cause activation of the complement cascade.
- Endotoxaemia — occurs in vascular surgery especially as a result of intestinal hypoperfusion [16,17]. Endotoxins in turn act as stimuli for pro-inflammatory cytokines.
- Complement activation via the production of C3a and C5a has been shown to occur in major vascular surgery [18,19].

21.3 Peri-Operative and Post-Operative Complications

Although morbidity and mortality have been reduced over time by a better understanding of the pre-morbid condition of the patient, the complication rate remains rather high and thus it is wise to have a good understanding of what can occur, as well as how best to avoid or manage these problems.

The following are relevant to both aortic aneurysm repair and lower limb revascularisation, however there will be some specific complications associated with the latter described in Section 21.3.8.

It is worth noting that studies have shown a significantly lower rate of gastrointestinal complications but failed to demonstrate a significantly lower mortality with the retroperitoneal approach as opposed to the transperitoneal approach [20,21].

21.3.1 *Cardiovascular system*

This remains the most common complication, contributing to both mortality and morbidity. The cause can be thought of as due to increased oxygen demand and reduced oxygen supply (Table 21.3).

Any factor that causes tachycardia and hypertension will lead to increased myocardial oxygen demand.

In a study to analyse the risk factors for cardiac complications, four points were identified:

- Stress of surgery.
- Increased blood loss.
- Poor pre-operative cardiac status i.e. coronary heart failure, known CAD and low ejection fraction.
- Pre-operative history of coronary artery bypass graft.

A prior coronary artery bypass graft or percutaneous transluminal coronary angioplasty was only protective of mortality after a peri-operative MI had occurred but did not reduce the actual incidence of it [22,23].

Table 21.3. Factors affecting O_2 supply and demand.

Factors increasing demand	Factors reducing supply
Stress of surgery	Hypotension, e.g. hypovolaemia, SIRS
Pain	Hypoxia
Use of inotropes	Coronary plaque rupture/thrombosis
Aortic cross-clamping	Haemorrhage causing anaemia

The period of greatest risk is from within the first 24 hours up to 72 hours post-op [8,25,26] and indeed this risk is further increased if there are any prolonged (>30 minutes) episodes of myocardial ischaemia, as evidenced by ST depression, either peri-operatively or immediately post-operatively [24–28].

Cardiac monitoring post-operatively is essential and measures should be taken to avoid any further stress, for example adequate analgesia.

Care must be taken to continue pre-existing cardiac medication if appropriate, especially β-blockers as there is strong evidence to show that discontinuation is detrimental (POISE) [9].

If there are any suspicions of a cardiac event, a 12-lead electrocardiogram should be carefully examined, blood sent for the measurement of myocardial troponins and non-invasive imaging carried out with invasive imaging kept under serious consideration.

21.3.2 *Renal*

There have been a few well structured studies to show that renal dysfunction will contribute to operative mortality both after open aneurysm repair [29–31] and following endovascular aneurysm repair (EVAR) [32].

A spectrum of renal dysfunction exists, ranging from mild dysfunction with normal urine output through oliguric renal failure and culminating in anuria with significant acidosis requiring dialysis. The occurrence can be anywhere between 8% for elective AAA repair [33] to 50% for thoracoabdominal aortic aneurysm (TAAA) [34] taking into account the degrees of dysfunction.

Whilst a background of massive haemorrhage, sepsis, diabetes, hypertension, cardiac disease, peripheral vascular disease, chronic renal impairment and age all contribute [35,36], the aetiology can be conveniently divided into pre-renal (the majority in this setting), intrinsic renal and post-renal.

Two main mechanisms are responsible for the effects:

(i) Reduced renal blood flow leading to reduced ultrafiltration and tubular hypoxia.
(ii) Reduced renal perfusion pressure, which is due to an acute drop in blood pressure such that autoregulation can no longer be maintained.

Once acute renal failure is established, a cycle ensues consisting of further release of cytokines that is likely to cause dysfunction of other organ systems.

Intra-operative situations that contribute to the above factors, especially the former, are:

- Hypovolaemia — absolute and relative.
- Suprarenal cross-clamping, which can reduce renal blood flow by 80% [10] as opposed to around 38% in infrarenal cross-clamping [37]. Renal vascular resistance rises and blood flow is redistribute from the cortex.
- Ischaemia–reperfusion injury is paramount in the development of acute renal failure (ARF). Initially ischaemia causes vasoconstriction, tubular damage and release of endothelial factors. Once reperfusion is allowed, activated neutrophils release damaging free radicals, recruit polymorphs and activate the arachidonic acid cascade [38]. In an ideal world, a one-hour limit to cross-clamping would greatly reduce the incidence of problems associated with it, however, in reality, this is not always possible.
- Coronary hypoperfusion and depression of myocardial contractility occur as a result of onset (increased left ventricular afterload) and release of the cross-clamp (sudden reduction in aortic pressure).

As expected, emergency procedures have a much higher incidence of renal failure largely due to the long period of pre-operative hypotension, length of operation, increased blood loss and the likely positioning of the cross-clamp above the origin of the renal arteries.

Despite many attempts in the past to maintain renal perfusion with dopamine and mannitol, there is no evidence to show that these agents have significantly reduced renal injury.

The rules to preventing renal dysfunction apply both peri-operatively and post-operatively:

- Maintain good cardiac output.
- Maintain a blood pressure appropriate to the patient.
- Provide adequate intravascular volume at all times.

- Monitor haemodynamic variables and be prepared to manipulate them in order to achieve the above factors.

21.3.3 *Pulmonary*

Respiratory failure can occur in up to 8% of elective AAA repairs [39] and in as many as 47% of ruptured AAA repairs [40]. As well as pre-existing lung diseases such as COPD (specifically a forced expiratory volume in one second or forced vital capacity of less than 70% predicted [41]), many other factors predict post-operative pulmonary complications [42–44].

- Inadequate post-operative analgesia — the use of epidurals can improve pain relief considerably and help to reduce atelectasis after AAA surgery [45].
- Continued cigarette smoking — this needs to stop at least eight weeks prior to surgery to allow improvement in ciliary action.
- Age > 70.
- Obesity.
- Operation time > five hours.
- American Society of Anaesthesiologists (ASA) class IV.

The common complications tend to be pneumonia, atelectasis, bronchospasm and respiratory failure leading to a longer time on the ventilator [43]. Acute lung injury can occur as a result of vascular surgical factors such as hypovolaemia, cross-clamping, blood transfusion, prolonged SIRS and endotoxaemia [46] all of which initiate the process of free radical and cytokine formation, in turn activating the large pool of neutrophils in the lungs. There then follows a cascade of responses, which will ultimately cause tissue damage.

Unfortunately there is little that can be done to avoid these complications. EVAR avoids the need for cross-clamping and also potentially requires less use of blood products.

Adequate pre-operative assessment, good analgesia and early physiotherapy remain the mainstay of minimising complications. Once established, any lower respiratory tract infections should be treated aggressively and advice sought early from the microbiologists.

21.3.4 *Gastrointestinal*

During the operation, there is considerable manipulation of the bowel so it follows that some of the problems encountered in this setting are similar to those seen after major gastrointestinal surgery. Aneurysm surgery has been shown to increase intestinal permeability [47] — the result is a period of endotoxaemia.

Commonly, paralytic ileus ensues and indeed function seems to resume more quickly following a retroperitoneal approach [20]. Another factor deemed to be beneficial is the use of epidurals [48–50].

In one series, other complications that occurred in very small numbers were upper gastrointestinal bleeding, acute cholecystitis, *Clostridium difficile* enterocolitis, mechanical obstruction, ascites and ischaemic colitis [51].

Although uncommon, ischaemic colitis is a serious problem and should be diagnosed as soon as possible. It has an approximate incidence of 1–7% in elective open AAA repair [52] with a few predictive factors:

- A ligated inferior mesenteric artery at operation — hence risk can be reduced by ensuring reimplantation of the inferior mesenteric artery in the aortic graft or bypass grafting [53–55].
- Prolonged operation.
- Absence of mesenteric Doppler signals post-operatively.
- Elderly patients with multiple comorbidities.

Ruptured AAA repairs pose the greatest risk and up to 60% can develop colonic ischaemia [56].

The disease process can manifest as early as 24 hours and as late as two weeks post-operatively.

Signs and symptoms of ischaemic colitis:

- Excessive fluid requirements.
- Abdominal pain.
- Fever.
- Diarrhoea/bloody stools.
- Raised white cell count (WCC).
- Lactic acidosis.

Flexible sigmoidoscopy and multiplanar computed tomography (CT) imaging should be considered in patients exhibiting signs. Once a diagnosis is made, the main method of treatment is supportive — that is, maintain adequate cardiac output and mean arterial pressure, preferably avoiding vasopressors as they may worsen the ischaemia. If the situation is advanced, then further surgery is necessary either to attempt revascularisation or to resect dead bowel.

The abdominal compartment syndrome, which is defined as an intra-abdominal pressure of greater than 20 mmHg in the presence of organ dysfunction, can occur in patients having AAA repair, particularly ruptured cases. Once established, it can have detrimental effects on the other systems such as cardiovascular, respiratory, renal and central nervous, thus early recognition and decompression are essential.

21.3.5 *Haematological*

Usually a physiological balance is present which allows coagulation and thrombolysis to exist in the same environment without any major changes. However, vascular surgery lays open the door to a number of different settings which generally disrupt normality:

- Relative hypothermia.
- Acidosis.
- Large volume shifts.
- Massive blood transfusion.
- Drugs to alter coagulation.

A situation called heparin rebound may arise in which heparin is initially bound to non-specific plasma proteins only to be released back into the circulation up to six hours later [57].

Clotting should be monitored carefully:

- Platelets should be kept above 50×10^9 per litre.
- Activated partial thromboplastin time (APTT) (intrinsic clotting system) is prolonged by heparin and thus can be corrected if required.
- Prothrombin time (PT) and international normalised ratio (extrinsic clotting) can be corrected with fresh frozen plasma (FFP) with or without

vitamin K; usually 1.5 is the upper limit that is pre-operatively desirable.
- Fibrinogen levels can fall due to consumption or dilution.
- Thromboelastography (measures the interaction of platelets with the coagulation cascade and looks at clot strength) [58].

Disseminated intravascular coagulation will prolong APTT and PT as well as reduce platelet count and fibrinogen.

Maintenance of haemostasis is a combination of replacement of factors where possible once surgical bleeding has been ruled out or controlled (or indeed as an adjunct to this). The use of recombinant factor VIIa remains at the discretion of the intensivist who must weigh up patient suitability against the risks of thrombogenesis, which has more serious implications for the vascular patient.

21.3.6 *Graft infection*

Although a relatively rare occurrence, this must be considered in those who have unexplained fever, raised WCC and general malaise. It can present any time post-operatively with the risk being greater if the graft extends to the femoral arteries.

The source is usually skin flora but can come from the gastrointestinal system (Gram-negative organisms) or bacteria within the atherosclerotic plaque. The majority of infections will be due to *Staphylococcus aureus*, *Staphylococcus epidermidis* and *Escherichia coli*.

As well as prophylactic antibiotics at induction of anaesthesia, any post-operative infection must be treated adequately and if necessary, the graft should be replaced.

21.3.7 *Aortoenteric fistula (AEF)*

Primary AEF is when the AAA invades the duodenum, usually secondary to an infection or simply a rather inflammatory aneurysm [59].

Secondary AEF refers to the occurrence after AAA repair and can be at any time. In this case the causes are mechanical (pseudoaneurysm formation) or non-mechanical (infection).

Presentation is characterised by fever and anaemia due to hidden gastrointestinal bleeding.

21.3.8 *Complications of lower limb revascularisation*

As discussed earlier in the chapter, this cohort of patients share the same the comorbidities as those who have vascular insufficiency higher up the arterial tree.

Common complications after infrainguinal surgery are:

(i) Myocardial ischaemia.
(ii) Graft failure of either the biological or prosthetic graft. Higher incidence in end-stage renal disease and diabetes with peripheral vascular disease [60,61].
(iii) Graft infection.
(iv) Haemorrhage.
(v) Anastomotic pseudoaneurysms — most often at the femoral anastomosis.
(vi) Amputation.

21.4 Endovascular Repair

Endovascular aneurysm repair (EVAR) is the procedure by which flow within the aneurysm is excluded from the main circulation by means of an endograft, which itself is introduced via a remote-access vessel and positioned by radiological guidance.

Following its introduction in 1991 [62] this method has increased in popularity owing to its non-invasive nature and relative technical ease as well as potentially reduced complications.

At the outset, there were greater limitations on patient suitability for EVAR but with time, experience and the development of newer stent-graft devices, this has expanded [63]. Current devices are now in their third generation and on the whole tend to be of the modular bifurcated type. This type of graft can use the internal iliac artery for fixation at a distal point, thus keeping the iliac artery patent while also avoiding a femoral–femoral cross over graft [10].

Relative contraindications include:

- The involvement of critical branched vessels within the aneurysm — this can sometimes be remedied by using branched or fenestrated endografts, which allow critical perfusion during fixation [64], however, the procedure is made more lengthy and open to further complication.
- Thrombus or calcification at the site of implantation may reduce the chances of success.

Pre-operative preparation should be the same as for an open repair, that is, as detailed in its cardiovascular and respiratory work up, since conversion to open remains a possibility.

Post-operative follow up requires regular attendance for CT scans, usually at 1, 3, 6 and 12 months and sometimes this may be important when choosing suitable patients who will be compliant.

21.4.1 *Open versus endovascular repair — what can we expect?*

Unsurprisingly, since the advent of EVAR, there have been many retrospective reviews and some prospective clinical trials which overall seem to have been in favour of EVAR when looking at the peri-operative and immediate post-operative periods [63,65].

However, more recently, two large randomised controlled trials have added important information and provided medium-term follow-up data previously unavailable. Participants were chosen according to suitability for open or endovascular repair taking into account their aneurysm anatomy and their comorbidities.

The Dutch Randomized Endovascular Management (DREAM-) trial enrolled 345 patients [66] and the EVAR-1 trial enrolled 1,082 patients [67]. Both trials showed the following:

- Lower peri-operative mortality with EVAR as opposed to open, e.g. 1.2% versus 4.6% in DREAM.
- Less blood loss, shorter operative times, less time on the ventilator and shorter hospital stays.

- All-cause mortality at mid-term (two years for DREAM and 4 years for EVAR-1) was similar in both the endovascular and open groups, however there was still a lower incidence of aneurysm-related deaths in the endovascular group, e.g. 4% versus 7% in EVAR-1 [68,69].
- A higher rate of reintervention over time if the repair was endovascular as opposed to open, e.g. 20% versus 6% in EVAR-1.

Separate findings included from EVAR-1 noted a higher rate of secondary interventions at 30 days in the endovascular group (9.8% versus 5.8%).

There are yet to be results of the long-term follow up from both these trials but results so far are useful in determining patient suitability for each type of repair.

21.4.2 *Possible complications of endovascular aneurysm repair (EVAR)*

As with any surgery, the patient's pre-operative condition has been shown to be a guide to post-operative morbidity and mortality [70]. The same complications with regard to the cardiovascular, respiratory and renal systems exist in EVAR as they do in open surgery although early on, the EVAR groups seem to do better. This could be due to:

(i) Less intra-operative blood loss.
(ii) Shorter operative times.
(iii) Avoidance of aortic cross-clamp.
(iv) Anaesthetic considerations such as the use of regional techniques, thus avoiding general anaesthesia.

For example, in one randomised study, myocardial ischaemia occurred more frequently in open repair (56% versus 26%) however there was no difference in mortality due to a cardiac cause [65].

The complications that differ are:

(i) Endoleak — which is the persistence of blood flow outside the graft but within the aneurysmal sac. Four types exist and can be early (<30 days) or late (>30 days)

Type I — Proximal or distal seal problem of the attachment sites of the graft. Will need either another endovascular repair or open approach
Type II — Collateral flow from the inferior or mesenteric arteries usually. Can usually be dealt with endovascularly.
Type III — A seal problem between modular components, e.g. tears.
Type IV — Continued blood flow through the intact fabric of the graft, which usually thromboses with time [10].

(ii) Migration of the stent graft which itself may cause endoleak or arterial occlusion.
(iii) Conversion to open repair either at the time of surgery or later on. Reasons for the latter may include endoleak and migration.
(iv) Secondary intervention to manage graft infection, thrombosis and local wound problems.
(v) Paraplegia is still a possibility with EVAR thought to be due to microembolisation [71].
(vi) Large blood loss — although usually 400 ml would be the acceptable average compared to 800 ml for open.

One study looked at 96 EVAR procedures to see if they could determine risk factors of complications [72]. Unsurprisingly, pre-operative renal dysfunction and poor coronary and respiratory status were significant in contributing to both early and mid-term (around 27 months) mortality. Type II endoleaks were also seen to be the most frequent type of endoleak, as previously noted [73,74]. This may have been the case due to the use of magnetic resonance imaging to diagnose the problem — it is more sensitive than helical CT imaging [75].

EVAR is also used for ruptured cases, and this was done for the first time in 1994 [76,77]. Unfortunately, there have not been any randomised controlled trials looking at a comparison between open and endovascular outcomes in the ruptured setting. Meta-analysis has suggested that poorer clinical outcomes are expected with open surgery based on the patients' haemodynamic condition. However, this only extends to short-term follow-up data taken from observational and non-randomised studies [78,79]. More work needs to be done in order to establish the true role of EVAR for ruptured aneurysms.

21.5 Spinal Cord Protection

As already mentioned earlier, paraplegia is an unfortunate complication of surgical repair of thoracic and thoracoabdominal aneurysms.

The general risk of spinal cord ischaemia can vary from 0.3–25%. The factors which have been associated with a higher incidence are:

(i) The type of TAAA — type II repairs pose the highest risk by virtue of the extent of the aorta involved.
(ii) Surgical circumstances — emergency surgery can increase the risk by ten times in certain instances and may be due to the level of cross-clamping established during the procedure.
(iii) The practice of spinal cord protection by various methods which will be discussed.
(iv) Age of the patient .
(v) Pre-operative renal function.
(vi) Previous aortic surgery.
(vii) Dissection as the cause [80,81].

Before discussing the pathophysiology of spinal cord ischaemia, it is important to delineate the anatomy of the spinal cord in order to explain why the cord is so vulnerable to ischaemia in the first place.

The anterior spinal artery, which provides two-thirds of the blood supply, arises from each of the vertebral arteries at the foramen magnum and supplies the whole of the cord anteriorly. It is thus responsible for the corticospinal (motor) and spinothalamic (pain and temperature) tracts.

Two posterior spinal arteries, which provide one-third of the blood supply, originate from the posterior inferior cerebellar arteries at the foramen magnum and lie anterior and posterior to the dorsal nerve roots. They supply the dorsal columns (vibration and proprioception).

Radicular arteries enter via the intervertebral foramina and link up with the spinal arteries thus adding to perfusion. The largest of these is the arteria radicularis magna (ARM) or the Artery of Adamkiewicz, which can originate anywhere from thoracic vertebra T5 to lumbar vertebra L3 but most commonly from T9 to T12 on the left.

The anterior spinal artery relies heavily on the radicular arteries and also the intercostals, especially in its lower thoracic and lumbar regions, hence the susceptibility to ischaemia. Since the number and origin of the radicular arteries varies from person to person, so too will the extra perfusion to the anterior spinal artery.

It has been demonstrated that there exists a significant collateral network of blood vessels, which is contributed to not only by the segmental vessels but also the subclavian and hypogastric arteries. As is often the case in degenerative disease of the aorta, the intercostals and lumbar arteries are blocked and this is where the collateral network assumes an even greater importance [82].

The main causes of paraplegia in TAAA repairs are:

(i) Unavoidable cord ischaemia during cross-clamping of the aorta. If we imagine spinal cord perfusion to be dependent on the difference between mean arterial pressure (MAP) and cerebrospinal fluid pressure (CSFP), then during the cross-clamp, distal aortic pressure and hence MAP decreases markedly at the same time as an increase in central venous pressure and hence CSFP. These two factors lead to a decrease in spinal cord perfusion [10].
(ii) Reperfusion injury after the release of the cross-clamp is due to substances produced during the ischaemic period, e.g. lactate and potassium, which directly contribute to cord injury. In addition, the actual process of restoration of blood results in a cord hyperaemia which causes spinal cord oedema [83].
(iii) Vascular injury during surgery may lead to thrombosis, embolisation and trauma, especially the intercostal arteries [81].
(iv) Poor perfusion of the spinal cord post-operatively may be due to general factors or SIRS causing low MAP.

There are various practices which have been developed over the past few years which are aimed at trying to reduce spinal cord injury and hence paraplegia.

21.5.1 *Cerebrospinal fluid drainage*

Drainage of cerebrospinal fluid (CSF) is a method that was first trialled in 1960 by Miyamoto *et al.* [84] with Cooley and Blaisdell following shortly after to prove that CSF drainage in canines did indeed reduce the incidence of paraplegia [84,85]. This paved the way for further studies, the most significant ones being done over the last 15 years — overall the trend has been to show that this method can reduce paraplegia but it is also important the remember the multifactorial aetiology of this complication [80,86,87].

Before the operation, an intrathecal catheter is introduced at the L3/4 or L4/5 interspace and advanced to an estimated position of T12 — L1. It is secured in place and is then used to drain CSF to a specified pressure — usually maintained around 10 mmHg.

The drain is usually left *in situ* for 72 hours.

21.5.2 *Distal aortic perfusion*

This can be performed via left-heart bypass or femoro–femoral cannulation. The left heart can be accessed via the pulmonary vein. With this method, MAP can be maintained at a level of at least 60 mmHg depending on the characteristics of the patient, for example known to be hypertensive. High flow rates are utilised (3–3.5 litres per minute) and lower-body blood pressure is monitored [86,88,89].

21.5.3 *Passive hypothermia*

Allowing the core body temperature to drift down to 32°C has been found to be beneficial and safe from a cardiac complication standpoint [90,91]. Some places are even practicing profound hypothermia together with cardiopulmonary bypass, which allows for greater tolerance of cord ischaemia.

21.5.4 *Pre-operative imaging of spinal vasculature*

Angiographic imaging via magnetic resonance or computed tomography enables the surgical team to visualise the ARM and its collateral circulation to a certain extent [92]. This information can be used alone or in conjunction with the monitoring of motor evoked potentials intra-operatively.

21.5.5 *Measuring motor evoked potentials (MEPs)*

This can be done to assess spinal cord integrity intra-operatively and provides real-time information for the surgeon, and hence, if applied correctly, it can prevent significant paraplegia as a result of unrecognised spinal cord ischaemia.

Usually the brain is stimulated via electroencephalographic electrodes and a train of five stimuli of 500 V/1 Amp applied. The resulting MEPs are picked up from the abductor pollicis brevis and anterior tibial muscles bilaterally — these can be recorded every 5 to 10 minutes before aortic cross-clamping and every minute during. Most studies using this method have found that only reductions of MEPs greater than 50% were significant, since there can be fluctuations of up to 50% without any intervention occurring [93]. Ideally, the aorta should be sequentially cross-clamped in order to adequately assess the MEPs [94]. Additionally, as the MEPs are seen to disappear, implantation of the lumbar with or without the intercostal arteries can be performed to minimise ischaemia [95] and if this is not possible, collateral supply has been identified by performing endarterectomy of the aortic wall to reveal back-bleeding segmental vessels.

There are currently no strong prospective studies to show that monitoring MEPs alone reduces the incidence of spinal cord injury. However, there is a consensus that it provides a sensitive and quick method of detecting ischaemia during the procedure and when used in conjunction with other methods (distal aortic perfusion, CSF drainage and hypothermia) does reduce the incidence of paraplegia [94,96,97].

21.5.6 *Pharmacological protection*

The aim of using drugs is to increase the tolerance of the spinal cord to ischaemia — examples of such drugs include methylprednisolone, mannitol, naloxone, allopurinol, activated protein C, adenosine, prostaglandin and insulin-like growth factor-1 [86,98].

Spinal cord injury has multiple aetiologies and so complete prevention currently seems unachievable.

Post-operative vigilance is imperative and maintenance of MAP and haematocrit feature as part of spinal cord protection as much as to prevent other complications. In addition, monitoring of motor, bowel and bladder function should be routine, allowing any changes to be brought up early.

21.6 Monitoring Limb Ischaemia

This is potential problem of both AAA repairs and lower limb revascularisation and as such must be prevented wherever possible.

Post-operatively it is the joint responsibility of the surgeon, intensivist and nursing staff to clinically examine the patient and use any tools available to check for viable circulation.

There is spectrum of the process that ranges from acute to chronic, but severity must also be considered and this is usually described in terms of limb viability.

Often there will be a portable Doppler machine available on the ICU or vascular ward which can be used to check for the main pulses — this should be done at least once a day and documented in the patients' notes so that any change can be quickly and accurately picked up by the next person who happens to be on shift.

Of course, if the patient is awake, they will be able to give you discriminatory answers and will be the best judge of how and indeed if things have changed in the post-operative course compared with pre-operatively.

A few mechanisms are responsible for limb ischaemia:

- Distal embolisation of the intraluminal plaque.
    - Macroembolisation affecting the larger arteries such as the femorals.
    - Microembolisation which is responsible for trash foot syndrome (cyanosis of toes and feet leading to gangrene) and the appearance of livedo reticularis.
    - Can also be air emboli.
- Graft failure — early (within 30 days post-operatively), which is often caused by thrombosis, and late (after 30 days), which is often due to ongoing atherosclerosis.

Management depends on severity and the acute nature of the situation but can be thought of as:

(i) Medical — antiplatelet, anticoagulant or thrombolytic therapy.
(ii) Surgical — embolectomy, graft replacement, alternative route bypass or amputation.

Amputation is the unfortunate result of a failure to revascularise and expectedly occurs more commonly in those with pre-existing renal failure and diabetes, which may be the reason for its unexpectedly high mortality rate [99].

References

[1] Diehl, J.T., Cali, R.F., Hertzer, N.R. *et al.* (1983). Complications of abdominal aortic reconstruction. An analysis of perioperative risk factors in 557 patients, *Ann Surg*, **197**, 49–56.

[2] Crawford, E.S., Saleh, S.A., Babb 3rd, J.W. *et al.* (1981). Infrarenal abdominal aortic aneurysm: factors influencing survival after operation performed over a 25-year period, *Ann Surg*, **193**, 699–709.

[3] Hertzer, N.R., Beven, E.G., Young, J.R. *et al.* (1984). Coronary artery disease in peripheral vascular patients. A classification of 1000 coronary angiograms and results of surgical management, *Ann Surg*, **199**, 223–233.

[4] Fleisher, L.A., Beckman, J.A., Brown, K.A. *et al.* (2007). ACC/AHA 2007 guidelines on perioperative cardiovascular evaluation and care for non-cardiac surgery: a report of the American College of Cardiology/American Heart Association, Task Force on Practice, Guidelines (Writing, Committee to Revise the 2002 Guidelines on Perioperative Cardiovascular Evaluation for Noncardiac, Surgery): developed in collaboration with the American Society of, Echocardiography, American Society of Nuclear Cardiology, Heart, Rhythm, Society, Society of, Cardiovascular Anesthesiologists, Society for, Cardiovascular, Angiography and Interventions, Society for Vascular, Medicine and Biology and Society for Vascular Surgery, *Circulation*, **116**, e418–e499.

[5] Venkataraman, R. (2006). Vascular surgery critical care: perioperative cardiac optimization to improve survival, *Crit Care Med*, **34** (Suppl. 9), S200–S207.

[6] Mangano, D.T., Layug, E.L., Wallace, A. *et al.* (1996). Effect of atenolol on mortality and cardiovascular morbidity after noncardiac surgery. Multicenter Study of Perioperative Ischemia Research Group, *N Engl J Med*, **335**, 1713–1720.

[7] Poldermans, D., Boersma, E., Bax, J.J. *et al.* (1999). The effect of bisoprolol on perioperative mortality and myocardial infarction in high-risk patients undergoing vascular surgery. Dutch Echocardiographic Cardiac Risk Evaluation Applying Stress Echocardiography Study Group, *N Engl J Med*, **341**, 1789–1794.

[8] Devereaux, P.J., Yang, H., Yusuf, S. *et al.* (2008). Effects of extended-release metoprolol succinate in patients undergoing non-cardiac surgery (POISE trial): a randomised controlled trial, *Lancet*, **371**, 1839–1847.

[9] London, M.J., Zaugg, M., Schaub, M.C. *et al.* (2004). Perioperative β-adrenergic receptor blockade: physiologic foundations and clinical controversies, *Anesthesiology*, **100**, 170–175.

[10] Ghansah, J.N. and Murphy, J.T. (2004). Complications of major aortic and lower extremity vascular surgery, *Semin Cardiothorac Vasc Anesth*, **8**, 335–361.

[11] Bone, R.C., Balk, R.A., Cerra, F.B. *et al.* (1992). Definitions for sepsis and organ failure and guidelines for the use of innovative therapies in sepsis. The ACCP/SCCM Consensus Conference Committee, American College of Chest Physicians/Society of Critical Care Medicine, *Chest*, **101**, 1644–1655.

[12] Bone, R.C. (1996). Toward a theory regarding the pathogenesis of the systemic inflammatory response syndrome: what we do and do not know about cytokine regulation, *Crit Care Med*, **24**, 163–172.

[13] Davies, M.G. and Hagen, P.O. (1997). Systemic inflammatory response syndrome, *Br J Surg*, **84**, 920–935.

[14] Bown, M.J., Nicholson, M.L., Bell, P.R. *et al.* (2003). The systemic inflammatory response syndrome, organ failure, and mortality after abdominal aortic aneurysm repair, *J Vasc Surg*, **37**, 600–606.

[15] Grace, P.A. (1994). Ischaemia-reperfusion injury, *Br J Surg*, **81**, 637–647.

[16] Welch, M., Douglas, J.T., Smyth, J.V. *et al.* (1995). Systemic endotoxaemia and fibrinolysis during aortic surgery, *Eur J Vasc Endovasc Surg*, **9**, 228–232.

[17] Soong, C.V., Blair, P.H., Halliday, M.I. *et al.* (1993). Endotoxaemia, the generation of the cytokines and their relationship to intramucosal acidosis of the sigmoid colon in elective abdominal aortic aneurysm repair, *Eur J Vasc Surg*, **7**, 534–539.

[18] Bengtson, A. and Heideman, M. (1986). Altered anaphylatoxin activity during induced hypoperfusion in acute and elective abdominal aortic surgery, *J Trauma*, **26**, 631–637.

[19] Fosse, E., Mollnes, T.E. and Ingvaldsen, B. (1987). Complement activation during major operations with or without cardiopulmonary bypass, *J Thorac Cardiovasc Surg*, **93**, 860–866.

[20] Sicard, G.A., Reilly, J.M., Rubin, B.G. *et al.* (1995). Transabdominal versus retroperitoneal incision for abdominal aortic surgery: report of a prospective randomized trial, *J Vasc Surg*, **21**, 174–181. Discussion 181–183.

[21] Lacroix, H. (1997). *The Optimal Surgical Approach for the Elective Reconstruction of the Infra and Juxtarenal Abdominal Aorta: A Randomized Prospective Study* (*Acta Biomedica Lovaniensia vol. 157*), Leuven University Press, Leuven.

[22] Sprung, J., Abdelmalak, B., Gottlieb, A. *et al.* (2000). Analysis of risk factors for myocardial infarction and cardiac mortality after major vascular surgery, *Anesthesiology*, **93**, 129–140.

[23] Mangano, D.T. and Goldman, L. (1995). Preoperative assessment of patients with known or suspected coronary disease, *N Engl J Med*, **333**, 1750–1756.

[24] Badner, N.H., Knill, R.L., Brown, J.E. *et al.* (1998). Myocardial infarction after noncardiac surgery, *Anesthesiology*, **88**, 572–578.

[25] Mangano, D.T. (1990). Perioperative cardiac morbidity, *Anesthesiology*, **72**, 153–184.

[26] Landesberg, G., Luria, M.H., Cotev, S. *et al.* (1993). Importance of long-duration postoperative, S.T-segment depression in cardiac morbidity after vascular surgery, *Lancet*, **341**, 715–719.

[27] Fleisher, L.A. (2001). Risk indices: what is their value to the clinician and patient? *Anesthesiology*, **94**, 191–193.

[28] Rapp, H.J., Rabethge, S., Luiz, T. *et al.* (1999). Perioperative ST-segment depression and troponin T release. Identification of patients with highest risk for myocardial damage, *Acta Anaesthesiol Scand*, **43**, 124–129.

[29] Hertzer, N.R., Mascha, E.J., Karafa, M.T. *et al.* (2002). Open infrarenal abdominal aortic aneurysm repair: the Cleveland Clinic experience from 1989 to 1998, *J Vasc Surg*, **35**, 1145–1154.

[30] Steyerberg, E.W., Kievit, J., de Mol Van Otterloo, J.C. *et al.* (1995). Perioperative mortality of elective abdominal aortic aneurysm surgery. A clinical prediction rule based on literature and individual patient data, *Arch Intern Med*, **155**, 1998–2004.

[31] Menard, M.T., Chew, D.K., Chan, R.K. *et al.* (2003). Outcome in patients at high risk after open surgical repair of abdominal aortic aneurysm, *J Vasc Surg*, **37**, 285–292.

[32] van, Eps, R.G., Leurs, L.J., Hobo, R. *et al.* (2007). Impact of renal dysfunction on operative mortality following endovascular abdominal aortic aneurysm surgery, *Br J Surg*, **94**, 174–178.

[33] Castronuovo, J.J. and Flanigan, D.P. (1985). 'Renal failure complicating vascular surgery', in Bernhard, V.M., Towne, J.B. (eds), *Complications in Vascular Surgery*, Grune & Stratton, Orlando, pp. 258–274.

[34] Bertolissi, M. (1999). Prevention of acute renal failure in major vascular surgery, *Minerva Anestesiol*, **65**, 867–877.

[35] Hoste, E.A., Lameire, N.H., Vanholder, R.C. *et al.* (2003). Acute renal failure in patients with sepsis in a surgical ICU: predictive factors, incidence, comorbidity, and outcome, *J Am Soc Nephrol*, **14**, 1022–1030.

[36] Shusterman, N., Strom, B.L., Murray, T.G. *et al.* (1987). Risk factors and outcome of hospital-acquired acute renal failure. Clinical epidemiologic study, *Am J Med*, **83**, 65–71.

[37] Gamulin, Z., Forster, A., Morel, D. *et al.* (1984). Effects of infrarenal aortic cross-clamping on renal hemodynamics in humans, *Anesthesiology*, **61**, 394–399.

[38] Kerrigan, C.L. and Stotland, M.A. (1993). Ischemia reperfusion injury: a review, *Microsurgery*, **14**, 165–175.

[39] Cordingley, J. and Palazzo, M. (1996). 'Renal rescue: management of impending renal failure', in Vincent, J.L. (ed.), *Yearbook of Intensive Care and Emergency Medicine*, Springer, Berlin, pp. 675–689.

[40] Prough, D.S. and Bauman, L.A. (1991). 'Protecting the kidneys during vascular surgery', in Kaplan, J.A. (ed.), *Vascular Anesthesia*, Churchill Livingstone, New York, pp. 521–547.

[41] Roizen, M.F. (1990). 'Anesthesia goals for surgery to relieve or prevent visceral ischemia', in Roizen, M.F. (ed.), *Anesthesia for Vascular Surgery*, Churchill Livingstone, New York, pp. 171–196.

[42] Gracey, D.R., Divertie, M.B. and Didier, E.P. (1979). Preoperative pulmonary preparation of patients with chronic obstructive pulmonary disease: a prospective study, *Chest*, **76**, 123–129.

[43] Calligaro, K.D., Azurin, D.J., Dougherty, M.J. *et al.* (1993). Pulmonary risk factors of elective abdominal aortic surgery, *J Vasc Surg*, **18**, 914–920. Discussion 920–921.

[44] Smetana, G.W. (1999). Preoperative pulmonary evaluation, *N Engl J Med*, **340**, 937–944.

[45] Major Jr, C.P., Greer, M.S., Russell, W.L. *et al.* (1996). Postoperative pulmonary complications and morbidity after abdominal aneurysmectomy: a comparison of postoperative epidural versus parenteral opioid analgesia, *Am Surg*, **62**, 45–51.

[46] Pararajasingam, R., Nicholson, M.L., Bell, P.R. *et al.* (1999). Non-cardiogenic pulmonary oedema in vascular surgery, *Eur J Vasc Endovasc Surg*, **17**, 93–105.

[47] Roumen, R.M., van der Vliet, J.A., Wevers, R.A. *et al.* (1993). Intestinal permeability is increased after major vascular surgery, *J Vasc Surg*, **17**, 734–737.

[48] Scheinin, B., Asantila, R. and Orko, R. (1987). The effect of bupivacaine and morphine on pain and bowel function after colonic surgery, *Acta Anaesthesiol Scand*, **31**, 161–164.

[49] Liu, S.S., Carpenter, R.L., Mackey, D.C. *et al.* (1995). Effects of perioperative analgesic technique on rate of recovery after colon surgery, *Anesthesiology*, **83**, 757–765.

[50] Carli, F., Trudel, J.L. and Belliveau, P. (2001). The effect of intraoperative thoracic epidural anesthesia and postoperative analgesia on bowel function after colorectal surgery: a prospective, randomized trial, *Dis Colon Rectum*, **44**, 1083–1089.

[51] Valentine, R.J., Hagino, R.T., Jackson, M.R. *et al.* (1998). Gastrointestinal complications after aortic surgery, *J Vasc Surg*, **28**, 404–411. Discussion 411–412.

[52] Bjorck, M., Bergqvist, D. and Troeng, T. (1996). Incidence and clinical presentation of bowel ischaemia after aortoiliac surgery –2930 operations from a population-based registry in Sweden, *Eur J Vasc Endovasc Surg*, **12**, 139–144.

[53] Bjorck, M., Troeng, T. and Bergqvist, D. (1997). Risk factors for intestinal ischaemia after aortoiliac surgery: a combined cohort and case-control study of 2824 operations, *Eur J Vasc Endovasc Surg*, **13**, 531–539.

[54] Schneider, D.B., Nelken, N.A., Messina, L.M. *et al.* (1999). Isolated inferior mesenteric artery revascularization for chronic visceral ischemia, *J Vasc Surg*, **30**, 51–58.

[55] Rapp, J.H., Reilly, L.M., Qvarfordt, P.G. *et al.* (1986). Durability of endarterectomy and antegrade grafts in the treatment of chronic visceral ischemia, *J Vasc Surg*, **3**, 799–806.

[56] Redaelli, C.A., Schilling, M.K. and Carrel, T.P. (1998). Intraoperative assessment of intestinal viability by laser, Doppler flowmetry for surgery of ruptured abdominal aortic aneurysms, *World J Surg*, **22**, 283–289.

[57] Teoh, K.H., Young, E., Blackall, M.H. *et al.* (2004). Can extra protamine eliminate heparin rebound following cardiopulmonary bypass surgery? *J Thorac Cardiovas Surg*, **128**, 211–219.

[58] Untch, B.R., Turek, J.W., Manson, R.J. *et al.* (2007). Management of hemostasis in vascular surgery, *Surgery*, **142**, S26–S33.

[59] Trout 3rd, H.H., Kozloff, L. and Giordano, J.M. (1984). Priority of revascularization in patients with graft eteric fistulas, infected arteries, or infected arterial prostheses, *Ann Surg*, **199**, 669–683.

[60] Jaar, B.G., Astor, B.C., Berns, J.S. *et al.* (2004). Predictors of amputation and survival following lower extremity revascularization in hemodialysis patients, *Kidney Int*, **65**, 613–620.

[61] Abou-Zamzam Jr., A.M., Teruya, T.H., Killeen, J.D. *et al.* (2003). Major lower extremity amputation in an academic vascular center, *Ann Vasc Surg*, **17**, 86–90.

[62] Parodi, J.C., Palmaz, J.C. and Barone, H.D. (1991). Transfemoral intraluminal graft implantation for abdominal aortic aneurysms, *Ann Vasc Surg*, **5**, 491–499.

[63] Baril, D.T., Jacobs, T.S. and Marin, M.L. (2007). Surgery insight: advances in endovascular repair of abdominal aortic aneurysms, *Nat Clin Pract Cardiovasc Med*, **4**, 206–213.

[64] Franks, S., Lloyd, G., Fishwick, G. *et al.* (2006). Endovascular treatment of ruptured and symptomatic abdominal aortic aneurysms, *Eur J Vasc Endovasc Surg*, **31**, 345–350.

[65] Cuypers, P.W., Gardien, M., Buth, J. *et al.* (2001).Randomized study comparing cardiac response in endovascular and open abdominal aortic aneurysm repair, *Br J Surg*, **88**, 1059–1065.

[66] Prinssen, M., Verhoeven, E.L., Buth, J. *et al.* (2004). A randomized trial comparing conventional and endovascular repair of abdominal aortic aneurysms, *N Engl J Med*, **351**, 1607–1618.

[67] Greenhalgh, R.M., Brown, L.C., Kwong, G.P. *et al.* (2004). Comparison of endovascular aneurysm repair with open repair in patients with abdominal aortic aneurysm (EVAR trial 1), 30–day operative mortality results: randomised controlled trial, *Lancet*, **364**, 843–848.

[68] Blankensteijn, J.D., de Jong, S.E., Prinssen, M. *et al.* (2005). Two-year outcomes after conventional or endovascular repair of abdominal aortic aneurysms, *N Engl J Med*, **352**, 2398–2405.

[69] Evar trial participants (2005). Endovascular aneurysm repair versus open repair in patients with abdominal aortic aneurysm (EVAR trial 1): randomised controlled trial, *Lancet*, **365**, 2179–2186.

[70] Buth, J., and Laheij, R.J. (2000). Early complications and endoleaks after endovascular abdominal aortic aneurysm repair: report of a multicenter study, *J Vasc Surg*, **31**, 134–146.

[71] Berg, P., Kaufmann, D., van Marrewijk, C.J. *et al.* (2001). Spinal cord ischaemia after stent-graft treatment for infra-renal abdominal aortic aneurysms., Analysis of the Eurostar database, *Eur J Vasc Endovasc Surg*, **22**, 342–347.

[72] Haulon, S., Devos, P., Willoteaux, S. *et al.* (2003). Risk factors of early and late complications in patients undergoing endovascular aneurysm repair, *Eur J Vasc Endovasc Surg*, **25**, 118–124.

[73] Cuypers, P., Buth, J., Harris, P.L. *et al.* (1999). Realistic expectations for patients with stent-graft treatment of abdominal aortic aneurysms. Results of a European multicentre registry, *Eur J Vasc Endovasc Surg*, **17**, 507–516.

[74] Haulon, S., Willoteaux, S., Koussa, M. *et al.* (2001). Diagnosis and treatment of type II endoleak after stent placement for exclusion of an abdominal aortic aneurysm, *Ann Vasc Surg*, **15**, 148–154.

[75] Engellau, L., Larsson, E.M., Albrechtsson, U. *et al.* (1998). Magnetic resonance imaging and MR angiography of endoluminally treated abdominal aortic aneurysms, *Eur J Vasc Endovasc Surg*, **15**, 212–219.
[76] Marin, M.L., Veith, F.J., Cynamon, J. *et al.* (1995). Initial experience with transluminally placed endovascular grafts for the treatment of complex vascular lesions, *Ann Surg*, **222**, 449–465. Discussion 465–469.
[77] Yusuf, S.W., Whitaker, S.C., Chuter, T.A. *et al.* (1994). Emergency endovascular repair of leaking aortic aneurysm, *Lancet*, **344**, 1645.
[78] Mastracci, T.M., Garrido-Olivares, L., Cina, C.S. *et al.* (2008). Endovascular repair of ruptured abdominal aortic aneurysms: a systematic review and meta-analysis, *J Vasc Surg*, **47**, 214–221.
[79] Visser, J.J., van Sambeek, M.R., Hamza, T.H. *et al.* (2007). Ruptured abdominal aortic aneurysms: endovascular repair versus open surgery — systematic review, *Radiology*, **245**, 122–129.
[80] Safi, H.J., Hess, K.R., Randel, M. *et al.* (1996). Cerebrospinal fluid drainage and distal aortic perfusion: reducing neurologic complications in repair of thoracoabdominal aortic aneurysm types I and II, *J Vasc Surg*, **23**, 223–228. Discussion 229.
[81] Murray, M.J., Bower, T.C., Oliver Jr, W.C. *et al.* (1993). Effects of cerebrospinal fluid drainage in patients undergoing thoracic and thoracoabdominal aortic surgery, *J Cardiothorac Vasc Anesth*, **7**, 266–272.
[82] Jacobs, M.J. de, Mol, B.A., Elenbaas, T. *et al.* (2002). Spinal cord blood supply in patients with thoracoabdominal aortic aneurysms, *J Vasc Surg*, **35**, 30–37.
[83] Barone, G.W., Joob, A.W., Flanagan, T.L. *et al.* (1988). The effect of hyperemia on spinal cord function after temporary thoracic aortic occlusion, *J Vasc Surg*, **8**, 535–540.
[84] Miyamoto, K., Ueno, A., Wada, T. *et al.* (1960). A new and simple method of preventing spinal cord damage following temporary occlusion of the thoracic aorta by draining the cerebrospinal fluid, *J Cardiovasc Surg (Torino)*, **1**, 188–197.
[85] Blaisdell, F.W. and Cooley, D.A. (1962). The mechanism of paraplegia after temporary thoracic aortic occlusion and its relationship to spinal fluid pressure, *Surgery*, **51**, 351–355.
[86] Griepp, R.B. and Griepp, E.B. (2007). Spinal cord perfusion and protection during descending thoracic and thoracoabdominal aortic surgery: the collateral network concept, *Ann Thorac Surg*, **83**, S865–S869. Discussion, S890–S892.
[87] Cina, C.S., Abouzahr, L., Arena, G.O. *et al.* (2004). Cerebrospinal fluid drainage to prevent paraplegia during thoracic and thoracoabdominal aortic

aneurysm surgery: a systematic review and meta-analysis, *J Vasc Surg*, **40**, 36–44.

[88] Safi, H.J., Campbell, M.P., Miller 3rd, C.C. *et al.* (1997). Cerebral spinal fluid drainage and distal aortic perfusion decrease the incidence of neurological deficit: the results of 343 descending and thoracoabdominal aortic aneurysm repairs, *Eur J Vasc Endovasc Surg*, **14**, 118–124.

[89] Coselli, J.S. and LeMaire, S.A. (1999). Left heart bypass reduces paraplegia rates after thoracoabdominal aortic aneurysm repair, *Ann Thorac Surg*, **67**, 1931–1934. Discussion 1953–1958.

[90] Kouchoukos, N.T., Masetti, P. and Murphy, S.F. (2003). Hypothermic cardiopulmonary bypass and circulatory arrest in the management of extensive thoracic and thoracoabdominal aortic aneurysms, *Semin Thorac Cardiovasc Surg*, **15**, 333–339.

[91] Svensson, L.G., Khitin, L., Nadolny, E.M. *et al.* (2003). Systemic temperature and paralysis after thoracoabdominal and descending aortic operations, *Arch Surg*, **138**, 175–179. Discussion 180.

[92] Nijenhuis, R.J., Gerretsen, S., Leiner, T. *et al.* (2005). Comparison of 0.5–M Gd-DTPA with 1.0–M gadobutrol for magnetic resonance angiography of the supplying arteries of the spinal cord in thoracoabdominal aortic aneurysm patients, *J Magn Reson Imaging*, **22**, 136–144.

[93] Schurink, G.W., Nijenhuis, R.J., Backes, W.H. *et al.* (2007). Assessment of spinal cord circulation and function in endovascular treatment of thoracic aortic aneurysms, *Ann Thorac Surg*, **83**, S890–892. Discussion, S877–S881.

[94] Jacobs, M.J., Mommertz, G., Koeppel, T.A. *et al.* (2007). Surgical repair of thoracoabdominal aortic aneurysms, *J Cardiovasc Surg (Torino)*, **48**, 49–58.

[95] Svensson, L.G., Hess, K.R., Coselli, J.S. *et al.* (1994). Influence of segmental arteries, extent, and atriofemoral bypass on postoperative paraplegia after thoracoabdominal aortic operations, *J Vasc Surg*, **20**, 255–262.

[96] Etz, C.D., Halstead, J.C., Spielvogel, D., *et al.*, (2006). Thoracic and thoracoabdominal aneurysm repair: is reimplantation of spinal cord arteries a waste of time? *Ann Thorac Surg*, **82**, 1670–1677.

[97] Jacobs, M.J., Mess, W., Mochtar, B. *et al.* (2006). The value of motor evoked potentials in reducing paraplegia during thoracoabdominal aneurysm repair, *J Vasc Surg*, **43**, 239–246.

[98] Acher, C.W. and Wynn, M.M. (1999). Thoracoabdominal aortic aneurysm. How we do it, *Cardiovasc Surg*, **7**, 593–596.

[99] Calle-Pascual, A.L., Duran, A., Diaz, A. *et al.* (2001). Comparison of peripheral arterial reconstruction in diabetic and non-diabetic patients: a prospective clinic-based study, *Diabetes Res Clin Pract*, **53**, 129–136.

22
Liver Intensive Care

Julia Wendon and Patrick Ward

22.1 Definition and Introduction

The incidence of cirrhosis amongst the general population is steadily rising by virtue of increasing viral disease (predominantly hepatitis C), alcohol-related cirrhosis and non-alcoholic fatty liver disease (as a component of the metabolic syndrome) [1].

The cirrhotic patient, by definition, has a chronic disease process with scarring of the liver and development of portal hypertension [2]. Patients may present with either a complication of their liver disease (variceal bleed, encephalopathy, renal failure) or with decompensation of their liver disease in association with another process (alcoholic hepatitis, elective surgery, sepsis).

Acute liver failure (ALF), by contrast, defines a patient without previous liver disease. ALF requires the presence of coagulaopthy and hepatic encephalopathy. Acute liver dysfunction is defined as acute hepatic injury without the presence of encephalopathy [3,4].

22.2 Acute Liver Failure

ALF has a heterogeneous group of aetiologies that display variability in terms of incidence, clinical presentation, time course and prognosis [3,4]. In the developing world the leading cause of ALF is predominated by the viral hepatitides, particularly hepatitis B, with hepatitis E being particularly prevalent in the Indian sub-continent [5]. In the USA and a large proportion of Europe the main aetiologies are paracetamol (acetominophen) ingestion, idiosyncratic drug reactions and sero-negative hepatitis [6–9]. Ischaemic hepatitis (hypoxic hepatitis) is also increasing in incidence, and is seen most commonly in patients with underlying cardiorespiratory disease resulting in a congested and primed liver [10,11]. In both paracetamol and ischaemic hepatitis the levels of transaminases are often in excess of 6,000–10,000 and bilirubin is only marginally elevated as compared with other aetiologies. Aetiological factors are delineated in Table 22.1.

The prognosis of ALF depends on age, aetiology and the time course over which the disease evolves. Hyperacute aetiologies, with a very short time course of less than seven days, have the highest incidence of complications (cardiovascular, renal failure and grade III/IV encephalopathy (Table 22.2) with significant risk of cerebral oedema and intracranial hypertension).

Table 22.1. Classifications of ALF (time from jaundice to onset of encephalopathy).

Definition	Time (days)	Commonest aetiologies
Hyperacute	<7 days	Paracetamol overdose, hepatitis A and B
Fulminant	<2 weeks	—
Acute	8–28 days	Paracetamol overdose, hepatitis A, B and E
Subacute	29 days–12 weeks	Idiosyncratic drug reactions, seronegative hepatitis
Subfulminant	>2 weeks <24 weeks	—

Table 22.2. Aetiology of acute liver failure.

Cause	Agent responsible
Viral hepatitis	Hepatitis A, B, D E, cytomegalovirus, herpes simplex virus, seronegative hepatitis (14–25% of cases in UK)
Drug related	Dose related (e.g. paracetamol) and idiosyncratic reactions (e.g. Anti-tuberculous drugs, statins, Recreational drugs, anticonvulsants, non-steroidal anti-inflammatory agents, cyproterone and many others)
Toxins	Carbon tetrachloride, *Amanita phalloides*
Vascular events	Ischaemic hepatitis, veno-occlusive disease, Budd–Chiari heatstroke
Other	Pregnancy related liver diseases, Wilson disease, lymphoma, carcinoma, trauma

Interestingly, these carry the greatest chance of spontaneous recovery, whilst those with a subacute course (4–24 weeks) have a low risk of intracranial hypertension and cardiovascular failure but a very high mortality following the development of poor prognostic signs [9,12].

The chance of survival of ALF without transplantation, even in those with the most severe disease, has improved to between 40% and 90% [13–15]. This is related both to improved critical care management and better prognostic assessment.

The management of ALF is focussed on the support of all organ systems and the prevention and treatment of complications, in particular sepsis. Liver necrosis acts as a focus of inflammation, driving vasoplegia and leading to cardiovascular collapse which in turn exacerbates dysfunction of other vital organs, particularly the kidney and brain. The identification and treatment of the cause of the underlying liver injury should be the primary goal, whilst maintaining a focus on the optimisation of circulation in order to promote hepatocellular regeneration and to prevent further damage from ischaemic injury.

Liver transplantation with excision of the necrotic liver mass offers the best chance of survival for those with poor prognostic criteria and this can be achieved with various surgical options. The standard operation would be that of full orthotopic transplantation, although increasingly living-related transplantation is offered, especially in those countries where orthotopic transplantation may not be readily available. In a sub-group of patients the decision may be to undertake auxiliary transplantation — this allows the patients to be supported by the transplanted liver but over time the remaining native liver will regenerate and then immunosuppressive drugs may be slowly withdrawn and the transplanted liver will undergo fibrosis [16–20].

The decision to prioritise for transplantation requires a multidisciplinary team approach incorporating specialist liver transplant surgeons, hepatologists and intensivists who can utilise established prognostic criteria along with the daily assessment of the levels of organ support in order to best determine which patients are likely to benefit from being priority listed and indeed proceeding to orthotopic transplantation if levels of organ support permit. Various criteria for transplantation have been described (King's, Clichy, Model for End-Stage Liver Disease (MELD), bilirubin–lactate–etiology (BiLE) scores). Recently, criteria have also been described for patients in India [21–25].

It is important to recognise patients with ALF and enter into discussion with transplant centres in order to ascertain whether transfer or local management is appropriate. Early discussion is always advisable, even if the patient does not require transfer. Potential indicators for discussion are listed in Table 22.3.

Basic management should include fluid resuscitation and high index of suspicion for infection. The use of *N*-acetyl cysteine has a role in both paracetamol and non-paracetamol aetiologies and is usually given for a period of one to five days [26–31]. The development of encephalopathy is a poor prognostic sign and deep levels of coma may be associated with cerebral oedema and intracranial hypertension. The development of grade III/IV coma requires intubation and ventilation with sedation, normally utilising a mix of propofol and an opiate. The development of

Table 22.3. Guidance for referral/discussion with transplant centre.

Paracetamol and other hyperacute causes
Metabolic acidosis
Oliguria or evidence of acute kidney injury
Hypoglycaemia
Coagulaopthy
Encephalopathy
Non-paracetamol and acute and subacute aetiologies
Coagulopathy
Encephalopathy
Metabolic acidosis
Oliguria or evidence of acute kidney injury
Hypoglycaemia
Shrinking liver volume
Hyponatraemia
Bilirubin >250 μmol/l
In children any coagulopathy should be referred
In Budd–Chairi or pregnancy-related aetiologies all such cases should be discussed

grade III/IV coma would normally necessitate transfer to a transplant centre. Management of the risk of cerebral oedema/intracranial hypertension is essential. Avoidance of fever is beneficial, as is maintenance of serum sodium at the top end of the normal range. Close neurological observations should be undertaken. The presence of dilated pupils with sluggish response to light should be treated as an emergency with bolus infusion of 20% mannitol (150 ml) or hypertonic saline. Serum osmolarity should be maintained at <320 mOsm/l. Hypoglycaemia should be avoided. Renal failure is frequent and may be associated with hyperammonaemia, systemic inflammatory response syndrome (SIRS) and increased risk of developing hepatic encephalopathy [32–34].

22.3 Critically Ill Cirrhotic (CIC)

Critical care support for patients with cirrhosis has traditionally been viewed with a degree of scepticism and as having inevitably poor prognosis. It should be recognised, however, that management of varices and renal dysfunction have improved significantly and there is a greater understanding of the options of treatment available for alcoholic hepatitis. Furthermore, liver transplantation has radically changed the outcome of cirrhotics and, although this is rarely undertaken from the critical care unit, survivors of an episode of critical illness or decompensation should be referred to a liver transplant centre for assessment [32,35–37].

22.3.1 *Ventilation*

Hypoxemia may be multifactorial and axial imaging (computed tomography (CT)) should be considered, as should echocardiography, incorporating contrast, to exclude either hepatopulmonary syndrome or patent foramen ovale with shunting as a cause of decreased arterial oxygenation levels. Intra-abdominal hypertension may also contribute to hypoxemia.

Hydrothoraces are not uncommon and may contribute to hypoxia and can normally be drained indirectly by paracentesis of ascites.

The evidence for early tracheostomy is lacking although in some instances it may be applicable in this cohort of patients whose management may be facilitated by ensuring control of airway and avoidance of sedation in the encephalopathic patient. Percutaneous tracheostomy can be undertaken without increased risk [38].

22.3.2 *Cardiovascular status*

In the setting of cirrhosis with an acute deterioration in organ function similar aims should be considered as per any patients with acute deterioration in clinical status. Although as a group they will frequently exhibit ascites and peripheral oedema they are centrally volume-deplete, despite an increase in total blood volume.

They will nearly all exhibit a hyperdynamic circulation regardless of volume status and as such central venous oxygen saturation ($ScvO_2$) is not an accurate reflection of volume requirements. Equally, as in critically ill patients generally, pressure measures are unlikely to reflect volume status, and this is compounded in the cirrhotic with ascites where intra-abdominal pressures will affect measured cardiac filling pressures. Indeed a recent meta-analysis by Marik *et al.* showed that central venous pressure measurements were not predictive of volume responsiveness [39]. Delta lactate may well be of benefit, albeit accepting that initial elevations of lactate may reflect volume status and tissue perfusion whilst persistent elevations are more likely to represent accelerated aerobic glycolysis as opposed to tissue hypoperfusion [40]. The use of straight-leg raising [41] has not been fully assessed in cirrhotics but it may not be useful given the frequent presence of elevated intra-abdominal pressures and compression of the inferior vena cava. Volume responsiveness is most likely to be reflected in dynamic measures such as stroke volume or pulse pressure variation. Echocardiography should be undertaken both to assess volume status but also to assess ventricular function. Cardiomyopathy related to disease aetiology (alcohol and haemachromatosis) is relatively rare, but detailed cardiac examination should include assessment of right heart function and pulmonary artery pressures to exclude porto-pulmonary syndrome. This may be seen in up to 20% of patients with cirrhosis and elevated pulmonary pressure and pulmonary vascular resistance is often amenable to treatment with similar agents to those utilised in primary pulmonary hypertension [42]. CIC may also frequently demonstrate a cirrhotic cardiomyopathy with decreased response to stress, autonomic dysfunction and diastolic dysfunction [43–45].

High venous pressure may be detrimental to liver function with development of venous congestion, as is seen in right heart failure and associated ascites and oedema. Given that the data supports the view that excessive use of fluid is associated with increased mortality in the cirrhotic population, early use of pressors, such as terlipressin, in the precritical care environment should be considered when the patient is no longer volume responsive [46–49].

Regardless of the fluid used it should be administered in a manner compatible with a fluid challenge and dynamic variables (stroke volume) assessed pre- and post-fluid loading. The role of albumin remains controversial but remains the favoured solution for hepatologists in managing cirrhotic patients. Data in patients with cirrhosis and bacterial peritonitis in a ward environment showed benefit in the albumin-treated group, and albumin (20%) was found by Fernandez *et al.* [51] to have improved vasoactive and neurohumeral effects when compared with a starch solution. However, albumin has not been examined in the context of the critically ill cirrhotic population [50,51].

When undertaking large-volume paracentesis (>6 l), there is evidence of neurohumeral dysfunction and central-volume depletion, which may be countered by the infusion of 20% albumin [52–54]. There is a little evidence that terlipressin may also be effective [55,56].

The choice of vasopressor in the hypotensive patient with cirrhosis should be guided by the general critical care literature, with norepinephrine as the first agent of choice and vasopressin being added as a second agent. There is one randomised controlled study [57] of the use of hydrocortisone in patients with cirrhosis requiring vasopressors. The result of this study was similar to that seen in the general literature with decreased time to be free of vasopressors but without evidence of mortality benefit. In patients with liver disease the decision to use steroids should always be preceded by considering the possibility of hepatitis B. The use of steroids in this setting may result in immune activation of the disease process with development of ALF, which has a high mortality. Patients should be screened for hepatitis B and if there is evidence of carriage, treatment with steroids should be covered with concurrent antiviral therapy (usually lamivudine or tenofovir).

22.3.3 *Renal failure*

Aetiology of renal dysfunction in patients with cirrhosis frequently gets labelled as hepatorenal failure, with an associated poor prognosis. However, there has recently been a trend to reflect the type of kidney dysfunction as it is defined in the critical care and renal literatures, where the distinction is made between acute (type 1) and chronic (type 2) hepatorenal failure. Equally powerful is data demonstrating that prognosis for renal failure in patients with cirrhosis is greatly dependent upon the aetiology of the renal insult. Renal failure may be related to associated disease states (diabetes, hypertension), to the underlying liver disease (glomerulonephritis, Immunoglobulin A nephropathy) or concurrent events (hypovolaemia, interstitial nephritis) and/or hepatorenal failure [58,59].

Outcome may be improved by earlier treatment with terlipressin and albumin therapy. Equally, the negative effect of intra-abdominal pressure (IAP) on renal perfusion pressure should not be disregarded. In this context, use of vasopressors may improve renal perfusion and thereby function; equally effective may be small-volume paracentesis to decrease IAP and improve renal perfusion pressure. The data of Dünser and Varpula [60,61] suggest no apparent benefit in targeting a mean arterial pressure of greater than 65 mmHg over the first 48 hours. Similarly the work of Bourgoin *et al.* [62] showed no improvement in renal function when comparing a mean arterial pressure of 68 versus 85 mmHg.

Renal failure that progresses despite treatment to renal replacement therapy (RRT) should not be viewed as carrying an inevitably poor prognosis. When associated with ventilatory and cardiovascular failure prognosis is indeed poor. However, in isolated renal failure RRT should be offered. Timing of initiation of RRT can be difficult. Urea will frequently not increase as in other patients (given that the urea cycle is dependent upon liver function) and creatinine similarly is a poor representation of renal function due to decreased creatine production and decreased creatinine in association with decreased muscle mass. Early consideration of RRT may be worthwhile in those with hepatic encephalopathy since ammonia clearance is markedly impaired in renal dysfunction.

22.3.4 *Nutrition and gastrointestinal status*

Nutritional support, addressing vitamin and trace metal supplement action, is essential in the management of the CIC. Gut function may be significantly impaired in those with recurrent bacterial peritonitis where a fibrosing peritonitis develops with a cocoon forming around the small bowel and resulting in a picture of subacute obstruction.

Delivery of normal protein and calorie load to a functioning gastrointestinal tract does not delay recovery of encephalopathy, as demonstrated in the work of Córdoba *et al.* [63], and indeed appeared to mitigate against catabolism and protein breakdown. The role of ammonia-lowering agents in the management of CIC has not been subjected to formal study although molecular adsorbent recirculating system (MARS) therapy was shown to decrease time taken to improve degree of encephalopathy [64,65].

The presence of spontaneous bacterial peritonitis (SBP) should always be considered in the sick cirrhotic patient. A sterile aspirate of fluid should be sent for both culture and white blood cell count alongside protein and albumin. A polymorphonuclear leukocyte count of $>250\,\text{mm/cm}^3$ is compatible with a diagnosis of SBP. A low protein count is associated with greater risk of subsequent development of bacterial peritonitis ($<1\,\text{g/dl}$) whilst the finding of an exudate should raise suspicion of venous outflow obstruction, cardiac failure, constrictive pericarditis or malignancy.

The discovery of blood within the ascites should raise the suspicion of an ectopic variceal bleed or puncture of a cutaneous varix during needling/drainage of ascites. Haemoperitoneum is also a frequent presentation of a ruptured hepatocellular carcinoma, usually in association with significant drop in haemoglobin and cardiovascular compromise. Diagnosis may be confirmed by CT angiography and control of bleeding can normally be achieved with selective arterial embolisation.

22.4 Variceal Bleeding

Elective intubation and ventilation of patients with active variceal haemorrhage or in those with encephalopathy who require endoscopic therapy is an accepted essential component of optimal care, although it has never been examined in a trial setting. Providing airway control allows the endoscopist an optimal environment to achieve haemostasis and prevents the substantial risk of micro-/macro-aspiration and subsequent chest sepsis. Antibiotics are indicated in the management of acute variceal bleeding. A large proportion of patients will have positive cultures prior to the onset of a bleed, and as such antibiotic therapy can be viewed as pre-emptive as opposed to prophylactic. There is also evidence demonstrating decreased risk of re-bleeding and decreased mortality in those who receive antibiotic therapy [66–68]. Changes in thromboelastography can be demonstrated in those cirrhotic with active infection, perhaps further explaining the relationship between sepsis and bleeding [69].

Optimal endoscopic control is achieved with banding therapy for oesophageal varices and glue for gastric varices. The combination of vasocontrictor therapy, such as terlipressin, along with endoscopic therapy in comparison to terlipressin alone decreases risk of re-bleeding but does not affect survival [70,71]. Identification of patients who are likely to fail endoscopic therapy needs to be considered early in their clinical course, with recourse to other therapeutic options such as transjugular intrahepatic porto system shunting (TIPS). Portal pressure measurements of >20 mmHg have significantly improved prognosis if offered TIPS as compared with ongoing endoscopic therapy. Those with portal pressure less than 20 mmHg had a greater than 80% 12-month survival with endoscopic therapy whilst those with pressure greater than 20 mmHg had a survival of greater 70% if they proceeded to TIPS compared with only 40% in those managed endoscopically [72–74]. Many centres do not have the option to measure portal pressure within 24 to 48 hours of admission and recent data suggests that this high-risk group can be equally identified by Child Pugh score, with 80% of Child Pugh C patients having a portal pressure over 20 mmHg. Risk of re-bleed can also be predicted by active bleeding at the time of endoscopy and a blood transfusion of more than four units in the first 24 hours [75–78].

In gastric varices Procaccini *et al.* [79] reported TIPS versus cyanoacrylate glue injection. In this single-centre study of 105 patients there was no difference in survival comparing the two treatment options. A recent study [80] compared early TIPS shunt (offered to Child Pugh C score 10–13, or active bleeding at endoscopy if Child Pugh was 7–9) to drug therapy and endoscopic band ligation and demonstrated significantly improved 24-month survival in the TIPS group (over 80% versus 60%).

In some patients endoscopic control cannot be achieved, or a patient may be bleeding profusely and has such haemodynamic instability that endoscopic therapy cannot be achieved in a timely manner. In these settings balloon tamponade can be life-saving. Control of bleeding can nearly always be achieved by inflation of the gastric balloon only. Smooth traction should be achieved against the gastro-oesophageal junction, undertaken by taping the tube to the patient's cheek or to a helmet; this prevents variable traction, as would occur if a bag of fluid is attached to the Sengstaken–Blakemore or Minnesota tube. Although potentially life-saving, balloon tamponade is associated with significant morbidity and potential mortality. Complications may relate to aspiration, ulceration and potentially oesophageal rupture if the oesophageal balloon is inflated in an incorrect position.

Admission of patients with acute variceal haemorrhage to a critical care environment facilitates resuscitation, safe endoscopic management and decision making in regard of TIPS shunting.

22.5 Hepatic Encephalopathy

Hepatic encephalopathy (HE) (Table 22.4) can be challenging to manage in a ward environment, and its presence is associated with a worse outcome when compared with patients who do not develop this complication.

Hepatic encephalopathy may also result in impaired outcome due to poor compliance with therapy secondary to agitation and confusion. In addition, patients with HE are at increased risk of sepsis, particularly respiratory due to microaspiration.

Hepatic encephalopathy can resolve with remarkable speed or can persist for prolonged periods. Admission to a critical care environment allows close monitoring and intubation, should it be required to protect airway competence or control agitation in those patients that become a danger to themselves and are unable to comply with treatment. The aetiology of encephalopathy is almost certainly multifactorial with regard to putative mediators; at present, however, the most likely mediator is thought to be ammonia.

Table 22.4. Grading of hepatic encephalopathy. Modified parsons-smith scale of hepatic encephalopathy [82,83].

Grade	Clinical features	Neurological signs	Glasgow Coma scale
0	Normal	Only seen on neuropsychometric testing	15
I	Trivial lack of awareness, shortened attention span	Tremor, apraxia, incoordination	15
II	Lethargy, disorientation, personality change	Asterixis, ataxia, dysarthria	11–15
III	Confusion, somnolence to semi-stupor, responsive to stimuli	Asterixis, ataxia	8–11
IV	Coma	Decerebration	<8

In a recent study [81] of patients with grade III and IV HE, inflammatory response rather than arterial ammonia level separated survivors from non-survivors. Differences were also observed for SIRS, Sequential Organ Failure Assessment (SOFA), MELD and Acute Physiology and Chronic Health Evaluation (APACHE) II scores.

Ammonia may have other significant effects, however, and recent data suggests that increased ammonia concentrations impair neutrophil function, and hence may predispose to infection and sepsis [84].

Use of the MARS extracorporeal support system has been shown to decrease time to improvement in level of encephalopathy in a randomised control trial in chronic liver disease [64,65].

Ammonia-lowering therapies, such as L-ornithine and L-arginine, have not been assessed in critically ill cirrhotics but may potentially have a role. More important, however, is the need to address and treat possible aetiological factors; sepsis, dehydration, variceal bleed or administration of neuroactive drugs being the commonest precipitants to consider.

22.6 Alcoholic Hepatitis

Acute Alcoholic Hepatitis (AAH) has been almost entirely examined in a ward-based environment. The scoring systems that have developed over the years have allowed delineation of those patients who are most likely to respond to steroid therapy [85,86]. A multicentre study in France [87] has demonstrated benefit from *N*-acetylcysteine in AAH at one month but not at three months. Similarly the use of pentoxyfylline has been shown to improve outcome in a single-centre study of AAH, with the main benefit being to decrease risk of developing acute kidney injury [88]. The Glasgow Hepatitis Score (based upon white blood cells, bilirubin, age, coagulation and urea) can separate survivors from non-survivors [89]. In addition it identifies those who are most likely to benefit from steroids. French investigators have also described the Lille criteria, incorporating a delta fall in bilirubin over the first week of treatment with steroids, in addition to age, renal function, international normalised ratio (INR), baseline bilirubin and albumin as being highly predictive of outcome [90]. Utilising this prognostic model the French group identified a highly selected group of alcoholic hepatitis patients who had not responded to therapy with a predicted mortality of 80%; liver transplantation was offered to this selected group with excellent outcome and low recidivism rates. It is noteworthy that there was a high incidence of aspergillosis in those patients who died following liver transplantation.

22.7 Elective Surgery

Patients with cirrhosis are increasingly being admitted to critical care areas following elective surgical procedures, either as a planned admission or following decompensation. Mortality at 30 and 90 days can be predicted from baseline MELD score [91]. In those undergoing cardiac surgery, mortality is similarly related to severity of underlying disease, with reasonable survivals being recorded in those with Child Pugh A patients.

22.8 Prognostication

One of the main challenges in the management of the CIC is prognostication (Table 22.5) and ensuring appropriate utilisation of resources in this ever-growing patient group. Recent data would suggest that prognosis is better than ten years ago, and this is seen especially in patients whose initial presentation is variceal bleeding. Recent data suggests that SOFA score may be adapted and haematological scores excluded, resulting in improved sensitivity

Table 22.5. Prognostic models.

King's College Hospital Criteria for non-paracetamol-induced liver failure [95]

- Prothombin time >100 seconds (INR >6.5)

  Or any three of the following:

- Age <10 years
- Age >40 years
- Seronegative hepatitis (non A,B,C,E,F), Hep C, Halothane or other drug reaction
- Duration of jaundice >7 days before encephalopathy
- Prothrombin time >50 seconds (INR >3.5)
- Bilirubin >300 mol/l

King's College Hospital Criteria in paracetamol-induced fulminant hepatic failure [95]

- pH <7.3 (following fluid resuscitation)

  Or the coexistence of:

- Prothrombin time >100 (INR >6.5), creatinine >300 mol/l and grade III or worse encephalopathy.

The Clichy Criteria in viral FHF [96]

- Coma or confusion (grade III/IV)

  and / or

- Factor V <20% if patient under 30 years old
- Factor V <30% if patient over 30 years old

MELD score (97) >30

BiLe score [98]

Bilirubin (μmol/l)/100 + lactate (mmol/l)

+4 (in the case of indeterminate ALF, Budd–Chiari or phenprocoumon toxicity)-

2 (in case of acetaminophen toxicity)

0 (in case of any other aetiology)

and specificity and optimal prognostic value being seen at day three post-admission. Similar data has been reported by the Royal Free Group, where mean score over two days appears optimal in prognostication [92–94].

The prognosis of a cirrhotic population, requiring RRT and intensive care was examined by Fang *et al.* [99]. They developed and validated an MBRS score (mean arterial blood pressure <80 mmHg, Bilirubin >80 μmol/l, respiratory failure and sepsis; allocating 1 point for each factor). Scores of 0 and 1 were associated with survival of 62% and 58%, respectively, while survival fell to 10% for a score of 3. A score of 4 was associated with a mortality of 100%.

It is noteworthy that scores encompassing severity of organ dysfunction appear to be best at elucidating outcome as opposed to liver-based scores (MELD [97] and Child–Pugh [100,101]). Further improvements in prognosis may be achieved by earlier admission to critical care areas and identification of those patients who have an acute and hence reversible precipitant in liver function, as opposed to those who present with inexorable and inevitable deterioration in liver function and subsequent development of extra-hepatic organ failure.

22.9 Liver Transplantation

Increasingly, patients who have received liver transplants will present to critical care with a variety of illnesses related or unrelated to their liver condition.

Immunosupression (steroids, calciurin inhibitors and or mycofenylate) result in an increased risk of post-transplant lymphoma, proliferative disease, malignancy, cardiovascular disease, diabetes, hyperlipidaemia, renal dysfunction and sepsis.

With regard to immunosuppression, in the first instance it should be continued, calciurin inhibitors being well absorbed orally. Clearance is based on hepatic function but increased levels are associated with increased renal toxicity and potentially neurotoxicity.

Liver function tests should be undertaken and ultrasound should integrate abdominal organs, with particular attention being addressed to patency of the hepatic and portal veins and arteries as well as of the biliary tree. It is important to contact the transplant centre that has been undertaking follow-up to ascertain the patients transplant procedure, normal immunosuppression levels and liver function tests.

In addition to standard investigations and samples for infectious agents, consideration should be given to viral infections and cytomegalovirus, and herpes simplex virus polymerase chain reactions should be undertaken looking for active viral infection. Fungal infection may also be seen, and there should be a low threshold to undertake axial imaging of head, chest and abdomen as clinically indicated.

References

[1] Sweeting, M.J., De Angelis, D., Brant, L.J. *et al.* (2007). The burden of hepatitis C in England, *J Viral Hepat,* **14**, 570–576.

[2] Sohrabpour, A.A., Mohamadnejad, M. and Malekzadeh, R. (2012). Review article: the reversibility of cirrhosis, *Aliment Pharmacol Ther*, **36**, 824–832.

[3] Wlodzimirow, K.A., Eslami, S., Abu-Hanna, A. *et al.* (2012). Systematic review: acute liver failure — one disease, more than 40 definitions, *Aliment Pharmacol Ther*, **35**, 1245–1256.

[4] Lee, W.M.R. (2012). Recent developments in acute liver failure, *Best Pract Res Clin Gastroenterol*, **26**, 3–16.

[5] Abraham, P. (2012). Viral hepatitis in India, *Clin Lab Med*, **32**, 159–174.

[6] Averhoff, F.M., Glass, N. and Holtzman, D. (2012). Global burden of hepatitis C: considerations for healthcare providers in the United States, *Clin Infect Dis*, **55** (Suppl. 1), S10–S15.

[7] Franco, E., Meleleo, C., Serino, L. *et al.* (2012). Hepatitis A: epidemiology and prevention in developing countries, *World J Hepatol*, **4**, 68–73.

[8] Abbas Z. and Siddiqui, A.R. (2011). Management of hepatitis B in developing countries, *World J Hepatol*, **3**, 292–299.

[9] Lee, W.M.E. (2008). Etiologies of acute liver failure, *Semin Liver Dis*, **28**, 142–152.

[10] Seeto, R.K.F, Fenn, B. and Rockey, D.C. (2000). Ischemic hepatitis: clinical presentation and pathogenesis, *Am J Med*, **109**, 109–113.

[11] Taylor, R.M., Tujios, S., Jinjuvadia, K. *et al.* (2012). Short and long-term outcomes in patients with acute liver failure due to ischemic hepatitis, *Dig Dis Sci*, **57**, 777–785

[12] Williams, R. (1996). Classification, etiology, and considerations of outcome in acute liver failure, *Semin Liver Dis*, **16**, 343–348.

[13] Larson, A.M. (2010). Diagnosis and management of acute liver failure, *Curr Opin Gastroenterol*, **26**, 214–221.

[14] Marudanayagam, R.S., Shanmugam, V., Gunson, B. *et al.* (2009). Aetiology and outcome of acute liver failure, *HPB (Oxford)*, **11**, 429–434.

[15] Mindikoglu, A.L., Magder, L.S.R. and Regev, A., A. (2009). Outcome of liver transplantation for drug-induced acute liver failure in the United States: analysis of the United Network for Organ Sharing database, *Liver Transpl*, **15**, 719–729.

[16] Zuckerman, M., M. and Loveland, J. (2012). Selection and work-up for liver transplantation, S Afr Med J,**102**, 876–878.

[17] Nandhakumar, A., McCluskey, S.A.S, Srinivas, C. *et al.* (2012). Liver transplantation: advances and perioperative care, *Indian J Anaesth*, **56**, 326–335.
[18] Gómez Cabeza de Vaca, V., Bernal Bellido, C., Alamo Martínez, J.N. *et al.* (2012). Liver transplantation due to fulminant hepatic failure, *Transplant Proc*, **44**, 2076–2077.
[19] Muñoz, L.E., Nañez, H., Rositas, F. *et al.* (2010). Long-term complications and survival of patients after orthotopic liver transplantation, *Transplant Proc*, **42**, 2381–2382.
[20] Belghiti, J.S., Sommacale, D., Dondéro, F. *et al.* (2004). Auxiliary liver transplantation for acute liver failure, *HPB (Oxford)*, **6**, 83–87.
[21] Varma, V., Mehta, N., Kumaran, V. *et al.* (2011). Indications and contraindications for liver transplantation, *Int J Hepatol*, 121862.
[22] Sibal, A.R, Rajasekar, R.S. and Sooin, A.S. (1999). Liver transplantation in the developing world, *Indian J Pediatr*, **66** (Suppl. 1), S120–S123.
[23] Dutkowski, P., Oberkofler, C.E., Slankamenac, K. *et al.* (2011). Are there better guidelines for allocation in liver transplantation? A novel score targeting justice and utility in the model for end-stage liver disease era, *Ann S Surg*, **254**, 745–753; discussion 753.
[24] Biselli, M., Gitto, S., Gramenzi, A. *et al.* (2010). Six score systems to evaluate candidates with advanced cirrhosis for orthotopic liver transplant: Which is the winner? *Liver Transpl*, **16**, 964–973.
[25] Perkins, J.D. (2009). Another formula to determine the prognosis of patients with acute liver failure, *Liver Trranspl*, **15**, 986–991.
[26] Filik, L.N. (2010). *N*-Acetylcysteine in non-acetaminophen-induced acute liver failure, *Hepatol Int*, **4**, 535.
[27] Koch, A., and Trautwein, C.N. (2010). *N*-Aacetylcysteine on its way to a broader application in patients with acute liver failure, *Hepatology*, **51**, 338–340.
[28] Mumtaz, K., Azam, Z., Hamid, S. *et al.* (2009). Role of *N*-acetylcysteine in adults with non-acetaminophen-induced acute liver failure in a center without the facility of liver transplantation, *Hepatol Int*, **3**, 563–570.
[29] Trotter, J.F. (2009). Practical management of acute liver failure in the Intensive Care Unit, *Curr Opin Crit Care*, **15**, 163–167.
[30] Chun, L.J.T., Toong, M.J., Busuttil, R.W. *et al.* (2009). Acetaminophen hepatotoxicity and acute liver failure, *J Clin Gastroenterol*, **43**, 342–349.
[31] Betten, D.P., Cantrell, F.L., Thomas, S.C. *et al.* (2007). A prospective evaluation of shortened course oral, *N*-acetylcysteine for the treatment of acute acetaminophen poisoning, *Ann E Emerg Med*, **50**, 272–279.

[32] Poddar, B., Saigal, S., Kumar, A. *et al.* (2012). Factors associated with outcome in acute liver failure in an intensive care unit, *Indian J Gastroenterol*, epub.

[33] Garg, H., Kumar, A., Garg, V. *et al.* (2012). Clinical profile and predictors of mortality in patients of acute-on-chronic liver failure. *Dig Liver Dis*, **44**, 166–171.

[34] Guevara, M., Baccaro, M.E., Ríos, J. *et al.* (2010). Risk factors for hepatic encephalopathy in patients with cirrhosis and refractory ascites: relevance of serum sodium concentration, *Liver Int*, **30**, 1137–1142.

[35] Dasher, K. and Trotter, J.F. (2012). Intensive care unit management of liver-related coagulation disorders, *Crit Care Clln*, **28**, 389–398, vi.

[36] Figueiredo, A.R., Romero-Bermejo, F., Peerdigoto, R. *et al.* (2012). The end-organ impairment in liver cirrhosis: appointments for critical care, *Crit Care Res Pract*, 539412.

[37] Olson, J.C., Wendon, J.A., Kramer, D.J. *et al.* (2011). Intensive care of the patient with cirrhosis, Hepatology, **54**, 1864–1872.

[38] Auzinger, G., O'Callaghan, G.P., Bernal, W. *et al.* (2007). Percutaneous tracheostomy in patients with severe liver disease and a high incidence of refractory coagulopathy: a prospective trial, *Crit Care*, **11**, R110.

[39] Marik, P.E., Baram, M., Vahid, B. (2008). Does central venous pressure predict fluid responsiveness? A systematic review of the literature and the tale of seven mares, *Chest*, **134**, 172–178.

[40] De Backer, D. (2003). Lactic acidosis, *Minerva Anestesiol*, **69**, 281–284.

[41] De Backer, D. (2006). Can passive leg raising be used to guide fluid administration? *Crit Care*, **10**, 170.

[42] Nayak, R.P., Li, D. and Matuschak, G.M. (2009). Portopulmonary hypertension, *Curr Gastroenterol Rep*, **11**, 56–63.

[43] Alexopoulou, A., Papatheodoridis, G., Pouriki, S. *et al.* (2012). Diastolic myocardial dysfunction does not affect survival in patients with cirrhosis., *Transpl Int*, **25**, 1174–1181.

[44] Timoh, T., Protano, M.A., Wagman, G. *et al.* (2011). A perspective on cirrhotic cardiomyopathy, *Transplant Proc*, **43**, 1649–1653.

[45] Zardi, E.M., Abbate, A., Zardi, D.M. *et al.* (2010). Cirrhotic cardiomyopathy, *J Am Coll Cardiol*, **56**, 539–549.

[46] Moore, K.P. and Aithal, G.P. (2006). Guidelines on the management of ascites in cirrhosis, *Gut*, **55** (Suppl. 6), vi1–12.

[47] Martin, P.Y. and Schrier, R.W. (1997). Pathogenesis of water and sodium retention in cirrhosis, *Kidney Int Suppl*, **59**, S43–S49.

[48] Fimiani, B., Guardia, D.D., Puoti, C. *et al.* (2011). The use of terlipressin in cirrhotic patients with refractory ascites and normal renal function: a multicentric study, *Eur J Intern Med*, **22**, 587–590.
[49] Biecker, E. (2011). Diagnosis and therapy of ascites in liver cirrhosis, *World J Gastroenterol*, **17**, 1237–1248.
[50] Chen, T.A., Tsao Y.C., Chen, A. *et al.* (2009). Effect of intravenous albumin on endotoxin removal, cytokines, and nitric oxide production in patients with cirrhosis and spontaneous bacterial peritonitis, *Scand J Gastroenterol*, **44**, 619–625.
[51] Fernández, J., Monteagudo, J., Bargallo, X. *et al.* (2005). A randomized unblinded pilot study comparing albumin versus hydroxyethyl starch in spontaneous bacterial peritonitis, *Hepatology*, **42**, 627–634.
[52] Alessandria, C., Elia, C., Mezzabotta, L. *et al.* (2011). Prevention of paracentesis-induced circulatory dysfunction in cirrhosis: standard vs half albumin doses. A prospective, randomized, unblinded pilot study, *Dig Liver Dis*, **43**, 881–886.
[53] Nasr, G., Hassan, A., Ahmed, S. *et al.* (2010). Predictors of large volume paracantesis induced circulatory dysfunction in patients with massive hepatic ascites, *J Cardiovasc Dis Res*, **1**, 136–144.
[54] Polli, F. and Gattinoni, L. (2010). Balancing volume resuscitation and ascites management in cirrhosis, *Curr Opin Anaesthesiol*, **23**, 151–158.
[55] Singh, V., Kumar, R., Nain, C.K. *et al.* (2006). Terlipressin versus albumin in paracentesis-induced circulatory dysfunction in cirrhosis: a randomized study, *J Gastroenterol Hepato*l, **21**, 303–307.
[56] Moreau, R., Asselah, T., Condat, B. *et al.* (2002). Comparison of the effect of terlipressin and albumin on arterial blood volume in patients with cirrhosis and tense ascites treated by paracentesis: a randomised pilot study, *Gut*, **50**, 90–94.
[57] Arabi, Y.M., Aljumah, A., Dabbagh, O, *et al.* (2010). Low-dose hydrocortisone in patients with cirrhosis and septic shock: a randomized controlled trial, *CMAJ*, **182**, 1971–1977.
[58] Angeli, P., Sanyal, A., Moller, S. *et al.* (2013). Current limits and future challenges in the management of renal dysfunction in patients with cirrhosis: report from the International Club of Ascites, *Liver Int*, **33**, 16–23.
[59] Muciño-Bermejo, J., Carrillo-Esper, R., Uribe, M. *et al.* (2012). Acute kidney injury in critically ill cirrhotic patients: a review, *Ann Hepatol*, **11**, 301–310.
[60] Dünser, M.W., Ruokonen, E., Pettilä, V. *et al.* (2009). Association of arterial blood pressure and vasopressor load with septic shock mortality: a post hoc analysis of a multicenter trial, *Crit Care*, **13**, R181.

[61] Varpula, M., Tallgren, M., Saukkonen, K. *et al.* (2005). Hemodynamic variables related to outcome in septic shock, *Intens Care Med*, **31**, 1066–1071.

[62] Bourgoin, A., Leone, M., Delmas, A. *et al.* (2005). Increasing mean arterial pressure in patients with septic shock: effects on oxygen variables and renal function, *Crit Care Med*, **33**, 780–786.

[63] Córdoba, J., Mínguez, B. and Vergara, M. (2005). Treatment of hepatic encephalopathy, *Lancet*, **365**, 1384–1385.

[64] Kobashi-Margáin, R.A., Gavilanes-Espinar, J.G., Gutiérrez-Grobe, Y. *et al.* (2011). Albumin dialysis with molecular adsorbent recirculating system (MARS) for the treatment of hepatic encephalopathy in liver failure, *Ann Hepatol*, **10** (Suppl. 2), S70–S76.

[65] Butterworth, R.F. (2003). Role of circulating neurotoxins in the pathogenesis of hepatic encephalopathy: potential for improvement following their removal by liver assist devices, *Liver Int*, **23** (Suppl. 3), 5–9.

[66] Brown, M.R., Jones, G., Nash, K.L. *et al.* (2010). Antibiotic prophylaxis in variceal hemorrhage: timing, effectiveness and *Clostridium difficile* rates, *World J Gastroenterol*, **16**, 5317–5323.

[67] Pohl, J., Pollmann, K., Sauer, P. *et al.* (2004). Antibiotic prophylaxis after variceal hemorrhage reduces incidence of early rebleeding, *Hepatogastroenterology*, **51**, 541–546.

[68] Hou, M.C., Lin, H.C., Liu, T.T. *et al.* (2004). Antibiotic prophylaxis after endoscopic therapy prevents rebleeding in acute variceal hemorrhage: a randomized trial, *Hepatology*, **39**, 746–753.

[69] Chau, T.N., Chan, Y.W., Patch, D. *et al.* (1998). Thrombelastographic changes and early rebleeding in cirrhotic patients with variceal bleeding, *Gut*, **43**, 267–271.

[70] Bendtsen, F., Krag, A. and Møller, S. (2008). Treatment of acute variceal bleeding, *Dig Liver Dis*, **40**, 328–336.

[71] Ioannou, G., Doust, J. and Rockey D.C. (2003). Terlipressin for acute esophageal variceal haemorrhage, *Cochrane Database Syst Rev*, CD002147.

[72] Addley, J., Tham, T.C. and Cash, W.J. (2012). Use of portal pressure studies in the management of variceal haemorrhage, *World J Gastrointest Endosc*, **4**, 281–289.

[73] Monescillo, A., Martínez-Lagares, F., Ruiz-del-Arbol, L. *et al.* (2004). Influence of portal hypertension and its early decompression by TIPS placement on the outcome of variceal bleeding, *Hepatology*, **40**, 793–801.

[74] Lopera, J.E. (2005). Role of emergency transjugular intrahepatic portosystemic shunts, *Semin Intervent Radiol*, **22**, 253–265.

[75] Xu, L., Ji, F., Xu, Q.W. *et al.* (2011). Risk factors for predicting early variceal rebleeding after endoscopic variceal ligation, *World J Gastroenterol*, **17**, 3347–3352.
[76] Lee, S.W., Lee, T.Y. and Chang, C.S. (2009). Independent factors associated with recurrent bleeding in cirrhotic patients with esophageal variceal haemorrhage, *Dig Dis Sci*, **54**, 1128–1134.
[77] Wang, M.T., Liu, T., Ma, X.Q. *et al.* (2011). Prognostic factors associated with rebleeding in cirrhotic inpatients complicated with esophageal variceal bleeding, *Chin Med J (Engl)*, **124**, 1493–1497.
[78] Krige, J.E., Kotze U.K., Distiller, G. *et al.* (2009).Predictive factors for rebleeding and death in alcoholic cirrhotic patients with acute variceal bleeding: a multivariate analysis, *World J Surg*, **33**, 127–135.
[79] Procaccini, N.J., Al-Osaimi, A.M., Northup, P. *et al.* (2009). Endoscopic cyanoacrylate versus transjugular intrahepatic portosystemic shunt for gastric variceal bleeding: a single-center US analysis, *Gastrointest Endosc*, **70**, 881–887.
[80] García-Pagán, J.C., Caca, K., Bureau, C. *et al.* (2010). Early use of TIPS in patients with cirrhosis and variceal bleeding, *N Engl J Med*, **362**, 2370–2379.
[81] Shawcross, D.L., Sharifi, Y., Canavan, J.B. *et al.* (2011). Infection and systemic inflammation, not ammonia, are associated with Grade 3/4 hepatic encephalopathy, but not mortality in cirrhosis, *J Hepatol*, **54**, 640–649.
[82] Parsons-Smith, B.G., Summerskill, W.H., Dawson, A.M. *et al.* (1957). The electroencephalograph in liver disease, *Lancet*, **273**, 867–871.
[83] Ferenci, P., Lockwood, A., Mullen, K. *et al.* (2002). Hepatic encephalopathy-definition, nomenclature, diagnosis, and quantificaton: final report of the working party at the 11th World Congress of Gastroenterology, Vienna, 1998, *Hepatology*, **35**, 716–721.
[84] Shawcross, D.L., Shabbir, S.S., Taylor, N.J. *et al.* (2010). Ammonia and the neutrophil in the pathogenesis of hepatic encephalopathy in cirrhosis, *Hepatology*, **51**, 1062–1069.
[85] Carey, W.D. (1992). Steroids in alcoholic hepatitis: another salvo of data, *Am J Gastroenterol*, **87**, 1219–1220.
[86] Daures, J.P., Peray, P., Bories, P. *et al.* (1991). Corticoid therapy in the treatment of acute alcoholic hepatitis. Results of a meta-analysis, *Gastroenterol Clin Biol*, **15**, 223–228.
[87] Nguyen-Khac, E., Thevenot, T., Piquet, M.A. *et al.* (2011). Glucocorticoids plus *N*-acetylcysteine in severe alcoholic hepatitis, *N Engl J Med*, **365**, 1781–1789.
[88] Akriviadis, E., Botla, R., Briggs, W. *et al.* (2000). Pentoxifylline improves short-term survival in severe acute alcoholic hepatitis: a double-blind, placebo-controlled trial, *Gastroenterology*, **119**, 1637–1648.

[89] Forrest, E.H., Evans, C.D. and Stewart, S. (2005). Analysis of factors predictive of mortality in alcoholic hepatitis and derivation and validation of the Glasgow alcoholic hepatitis score, *Gut*, **54**, 1174–1179.

[90] Louvet, A., Naveau, S. and Abdelnour, M. (2007). The Lille model, a new tool for therapeutic strategy in patients with severe alcoholic hepatitis treated with steroids, *Hepatology*, **45**, 1348–1354.

[91] Neeff, H., Mariaskin, D., Spangenberg, H.C. *et al.* (2011). Perioperative mortality after nonhepatic general surgery in patients with liver cirrhosis, an analysis of 138 operations in the 2000s using Child and MELD scores, *J Gastrointest Surg*, **15**, 1–11.

[92] Tu, K.H., Jenq, C.C., Tsai, M.H. *et al.* (2011). Outcome scoring systems for short-term prognosis in critically ill cirrhotic patients, *Shock*, **36**, 445–450.

[93] Cholongitas, E., Senzolo, M., Patch, D. *et al.* (2006). Review article, scoring systems for assessing prognosis in critically ill adult cirrhotics, *Aliment Pharmacol Ther*, **24**, 453–464.

[94] Cholongitas, E., Senzolo, M., Patch, D. *et al.* (2006). Risk factors, sequential organ failure assessment and model for end-stage liver disease scores for predicting short term mortality in cirrhotic patients admitted to intensive care unit, *Aliment Pharmacol Ther*, **23**, 883–893.

[95] O'Grady, J.G., Alexander, G.J., Hayllar, K.M. *et al.* (1989). Early indicators of prognosis in fulminant hepatic failure, *Gastroenterology*, **97**, 439–445.

[96] Bernuau, J., Goudeau, A., Poynard, T. *et al.* (1986). Multivariate analysis of prognostic factors in fulminant hepatitis B, *Hepatology*, **6**, 648–651.

[97] Kamath, P.S. and Kim, W.R. (2007). The model for end-stage liver disease (MELD), *Hepatology*, **45**, 797–805.

[98] Hadem, J., Stiefel, P., Bahr, M.J *et al.* (1989). Prognostic implications of lactate, bilirubin, and etiology in German patients with acute liver failure, *Gastroenterology*, **97**, 439–445.

[99] Fang, J.T., Tsai, M.H., Tian Y.C. *et al.* (2008). Outcome predictors and new score of critically ill cirrhotic patients with acute renal failure, *Nephrol Dial Transplant*, **23**, 1961–1969.

[100] Child, C.G. and Turcotte, J.G. (1964). 'Surgery and portal hypertension', in, Child C.G. (ed.), *The Liver and Portal Hypertension*, Saunders, Philadelphia, pp. 50–64.

[101] Pugh, R.N., Murray-Lyon, I.M., Dawson, J.L. *et al.* (1973). Transection of the oesophagus for bleeding oesophageal varices, *Br J Surg*, **60**, 646–649.

23

Acute Kidney Injury in Intensive Care

Shaikh A. Nurmohamed, Marc G. Vervloet and A. B. Johan Groeneveld

23.1 Defining Acute Renal Failure (ARF)

Acute renal failure in the intensive care unit (ICU) is common and carries a high mortality. The reported incidence of acute renal failure in the critically ill varies from 1–25% with a hospital mortality of 28–90% [1–5]. The reason for these wide ranges is the lack of consensus definition for acute kidney injury (AKI). A uniform definition and classification system is necessary for standardising entry criteria and endpoints in clinical trials. The Acute Dialysis Quality Initiative Group developed the Risk of renal dysfunction, Injury to the kidney, Failure of kidney function, Loss of kidney function and End-stage kidney disease (RIFLE) classification system through broad consensus by experts (Fig. 23.1) [6,7]. The RIFLE criteria have been validated in several studies and appeared useful in predicting hospital outcome [8,9]. RIFLE is an acronym for three levels of severity: risk, injury and failure, and two outcomes: persistent acute renal failure for more than four weeks, termed loss, and renal function loss for more than three months, termed end-stage renal disease (ESRD).

Whilst this definition was developed, several studies showed the clinical importance of renal dysfunction even before reaching the stage of failure. Mild loss of renal function seems to be associated with adverse outcomes [8,10]. These new insights have led the Acute Kidney Injury Network to propose some small modifications to the RIFLE criteria (Table 23.1) [11].

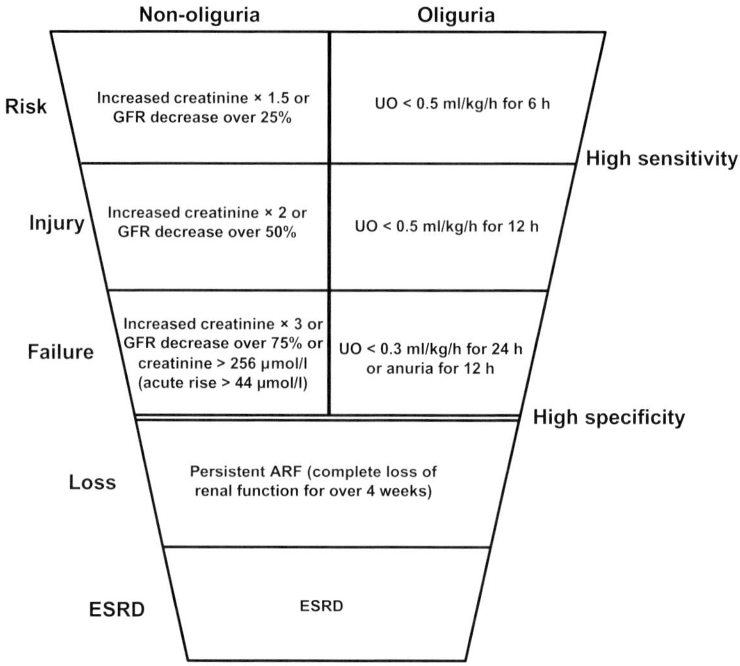

Figure 23.1. RIFLE criteria for the classification of acute renal failure. GFR, glomerular filtration rate; UO, urine output; ARF, acute renal failure; ESRD, end-stage renal disease [6]. (Reproduced with permission.)

Table 23.1. Classification/staging system for acute kidney injury [11].

Classification/staging system for kidney injury*

Stage	Serum creatinine criteria	Urine output criteria
1	Increase in serum creatinine of more than or equal to 26.4 μmol/l (≥0.3 mg/dl) or increase to more than or equal to 150% to 200% (1.5–2-fold) from baseline	Less than 0.5 ml/kg per hour for more than 6 hours
2	Increase in serum creatinine to more than 200% (> two-fold to three-fold) from baseline	Less than 0.5 ml/kg per hour for more than 12 hours
3†	Increase in serum creatinine to more than 300% (> three-fold) from baseline (or serum creatinine of more than or equal to 354 μmol/l (≥4.0 mg/dl) with an increase of at least 44 μmol/l (0.5 mg/dl)	Less than 0.3 ml/kg per hour for 24 hours or anuria for 12 hours

*Modified from RIFLE criteria. Only one criterion (creatinine or urine output) has to be fulfilled to qualify for a stage.

†Individuals receiving renal replacement therapy (RRT) are considered to have met the criteria for stage 3 irrespective of the stage they are in at the time of RRT.

The diagnostic criteria for AKI were broadened: an abrupt (within 48 hours) reduction in kidney function defined by an absolute increase in serum creatinine of more than or equal to 26.4 μmol/l, a percentage increase in serum creatinine of more than or equal to 50%, or a reduction in urinary output (documented oliguria of less than 0.5 ml/kg/h for more than six hours). Also, the staging system was altered. The 'risk' category has the same criteria for the diagnosis of stage 1 AKI. The 'injury' and 'failure' categories are now stages 2 and 3 of AKI. Patients receiving renal replacement therapy are categorised as stage 3. The new system is yet to be validated.

23.2 Pathogenesis and Prevention of Acute Renal Failure

The causes of acute renal failure can be classified into three broad categories: prerenal, postrenal and intrinsic renal. The pathogenesis of acute renal failure depends on its aetiology, varying from immune- or infection-mediated-glomerular damage to drug-induced tubulo-interstitial nephritis (Fig. 23.2).

23.2.1 *Pathogenesis*

In the ICU the prerenal form is by far the most common cause of acute renal failure, associated with diminished renal perfusion but the absence of tissue damage. There are several conditions that can cause a decreased

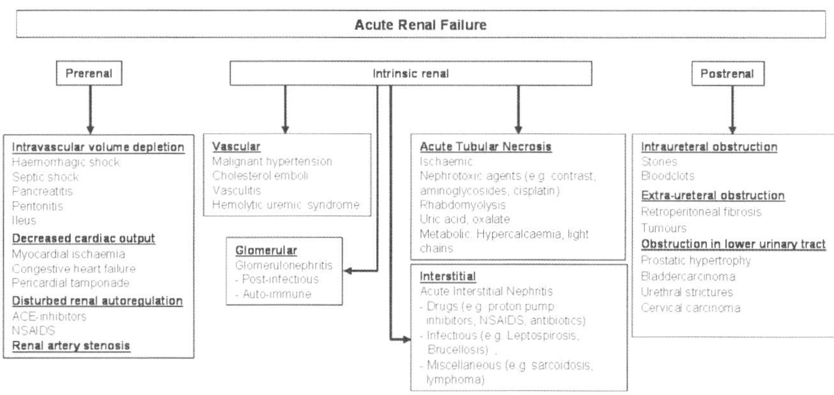

Figure 23.2. Classification of acute renal failure. ACE = angiotensin converting enzyme; NSAIDs = non-steroidal anti inflammatory drugs.

renal perfusion, such as reduced cardiac output and any cause of shock or intravascular volume depletion. These conditions will typically result in oliguric acute renal failure. If renal hypoperfusion is prolonged, tissue injury will eventually occur, resulting in acute tubular damage (resulting in apoptosis or necrosis and AKI). The mechanisms of acute intrinsic renal failure involve both vascular and tubular factors. In view of medullary hypoxia, the proximal tubule and the thick ascending limb of the loop of Henle appear to be particularly susceptible to ischaemia [12]. The tubular ischaemia results in apoptosis with rapid loss of cytoskeletal integrity and cell polarity. Some cells manifest ischemic necrosis. The cells are desquamated and normal ion transport is disturbed. Sodium chloride is pumped back into the tubular lumen and ultrafiltrate diffuses back into the interstitium, causing interstitial oedema [13]. The tubuloglomerular feedback causes constriction of afferent arterioles due to high distal sodium chloride delivery, with subsequent decrease in glomerular filtration rate and urinary output. Tubular obstruction will occur as the damaged and necrotic cells and cellular debris form casts. Renal ischaemia also induces an inflammatory response in which endothelial and epithelial cells, leucocytes and T-lymphocytes are involved. The inflammatory cells are recruited during reperfusion and release several chemokines and cytokines that further fuel the inflammatory cascade [14,15].

23.2.2 *Prevention*

The most important measure in preventing acute renal failure, especially acute tubular necrosis, is optimisation of intravascular volume and cardiac output. Furthermore, nephrotoxic agents such as radiocontrast and aminoglycosides should be avoided as much as possible. These measures are especially important in those patients in whom renal function and blood flow are already compromised. Drugs that interfere with renal autoregulation (angiotensin converting enzyme inhibitors, non-steroidal anti-inflammatory drugs, angiotensin-II receptor blockers) should be used with caution. There is much debate concerning the type of fluid to be used to restore intravascular volume. Resuscitation with crystalloids is not associated with an improved survival compared with colloids [16]. The use of starch-containing volume expanders should be avoided, especially in sepsis, since it may be associated with irreversible kidney injury [17,18]. Especially in case of oliguria or anuria, caution is warranted with excessive volume expansion, which may cause pulmonary oedema. If hypotension persists in spite of adequate volume expansion, vasopressors should be considered in order to preserve renal perfusion. In patients with septic shock, norepinephrine is preferable to dopamine [19].

In the past, several pharmacological agents had been assigned renoprotective capacities, but it still remains unclear whether or not these agents are of benefit to the kidney. The use of 'renal dose' dopamine was an accepted strategy to prevent or even treat renal dysfunction, by increasing renal blood flow and resulting in short-term increases of glomerular filtration rate with an increased urinary output. Prospective trials and meta-analyses, however, have shown that the use of dopamine is not associated with reduced mortality and is ineffective in preventing or treating renal dysfunction [20]. Fenoldopam, a selective dopamine-1-receptor agonist, has been shown to increase renal blood flow and glomerular filtration rate [21]. There are some promising reports that this agent might be useful in preventing AKI from causes other than contrast exposure and in reducing mortality [22,23]. However, data concerning this issue are conflicting [24]. Future studies will hopefully give some clarifications, although hypotension as a side effect remains a major drawback. Loop diuretics have the potential to alter an oliguric state to a non-oliguric state. Several trials and meta-analyses, however, did not reveal any beneficial effects of these agents in acute renal failure [20]. Loop diuretics are not associated with diminished need for renal replacement therapy or decreased mortality, but there is an association with a shorter duration of renal replacement therapy and increased urinary output [25]. There are conflicting data regarding whether the use of diuretics in acute renal failure is associated with increased mortality [26,27]. Moreover, high-dose furosemide may cause serious adverse events such as tinnitus and deafness. Hence, caution is warranted when administering loop diuretics in the critically ill with acute renal failure. Mannitol has only proven to be beneficial in preventing acute renal failure when administered just before clamp release during cadaveric renal transplant surgery [28]. Though never formally investigated, the preventive use of mannitol together with forced alkaline diuresis is generally accepted as a preventive measure for acute renal failure in rhabdomyolysis [29]. Animal studies have demonstrated that erythroprotein, by virtue of its ability to inhibit apoptosis and enhance tubular epithelial regeneration, seems to be a promising agent with which to protect the kidney against ischaemia/reperfusion injury [30–32]. The effectiveness of this agent in acute renal failure in humans, however, is yet to be proven.

23.3 Contrast-Induced Nephropathy

A type of acute renal failure that deserves separate discussion in the context of critical illness is contrast-induced nephropathy (CIN). Indeed, critically ill patients frequently undergo diagnostic and interventional radiographic procedures in which iodinated radiocontrast media are used. Administration may result in a usually reversible form of acute renal failure. Contrast-induced acute renal failure accounts for a significant number of cases of hospital-acquired AKI [33]. CIN is the third most common cause of AKI in hospitalised patients, accounting for 11% of cases. The European Society of Urogenital Radiology precisely defined CIN as an absolute increase of serum creatinine level of ≥44 μmol/l (= 0.5 mg/dl) or a 25% increase from baseline within 72 hours after contrast administration [34]. The definition of AKI as proposed by The Acute Kidney Injury Network is a rise in serum creatinine of 26.4 μmol/l (= 0.3 mg/dl) with oliguria (Table 23.1). So, a rise in creatinine of 26.4 μmol/l (AKI stage 1) after contrast exposure in the ICU theoretically fulfills the criterion for CIN; this, of course, is debatable.

23.3.1 *Pathophysiology*

The pathogenesis of CIN is unclear. Altered renal haemodyamics and direct tubular toxicity are potential contributory factors, as outlined in Fig. 23.3. After injection of contrast agent there is an acute and transient increase in renal plasma flow, diuresis and natriuresis. These effects activate the tubuloglomerular feedback, which is responsible for renal vasoconstriction. These processes increase the renal demand for oxygen; in case of sepsis or hypovolaemia the contrast-induced increased oxygen demand may cause medullary ischaemia. If the release of protective endogenous vasodilators (such as nitric oxide and prostaglandins) is inhibited (for example by non-steroidal

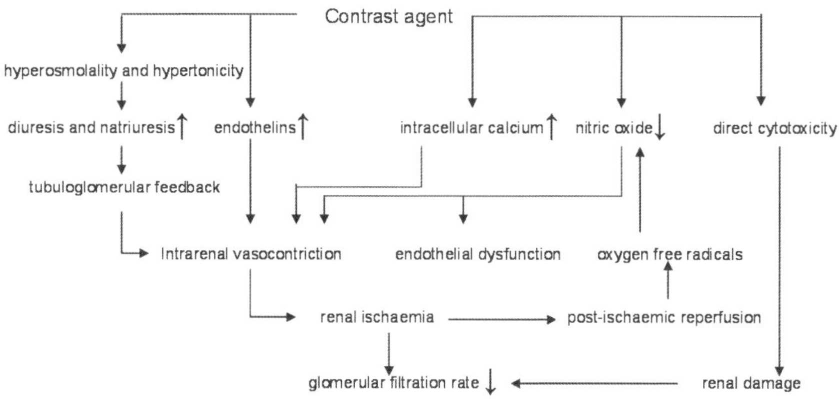

Figure 23.3. Possible mechanisms of contrast-induced nephropathy. Adapted from Meschi *et al.* [35]. (Reproduced with permission.)

anti-inflammatory drugs), medullary ischaemia and tubular necrosis may develop. In animal studies, contrast agents may have a direct tubular toxic effect due to the release of oxygen free radicals. Medullary ischaemia may also result in the formation of reactive oxygen species leading to injury.

23.3.2 *Epidemiology and risk factors*

The reported incidence of CIN greatly varies in the literature and ranges from 0–50%, depending on study population, definition of CIN, the amount and type of contrast-agent used, and the radiological procedure. Even though the mortality rate is about 14% [36], several studies reported attributable mortality in patients developing CIN [37–39]. After adjusting for co-morbidity, patients developing CIN had a more than five-fold-increased risk of death compared with those without [40]. Furthermore, the development of CIN is associated with an increased risk of adverse cardiovascular outcome and a prolonged hospital stay [41–44].

Patients developing CIN have more co-morbidity than patients exposed to contrast who do not develop CIN. Pre-existing renal impairment is associated with the highest risk for developing CIN [45]. The higher the baseline creatinine level the higher the risk: 2% in patients with a serum creatinine of < 132 μmol/l and 20% in patients with a serum creatinine level of > 220 μmol/l [46]. Historically, diabetes was known to be associated with an increased risk. However, the risk of developing CIN in diabetic patients without renal impairment is similar to healthy individuals [47]. Many elderly patients develop CIN, but they also have extensive co-morbidity such as atherosclerosis and renal impairment. Multiple myeloma is often regarded as a specific risk factor, although in the absence of hypovolaemia this has been questioned. All conditions leading to hypovolaemia or hypotension, such as heart failure, cirrhosis and sepsis are considered to be risk factors for CIN. The conditions result in a compromised renal perfusion rendering the kidneys susceptible to contrast-induced injury. Others conditions and drugs inhibiting protective renal vasodilators can also contribute to CIN.

Iodinated contrast agents are either ionic or non-ionic, also having variable osmolality. A general rule is that the higher the osmolality of the agent the greater its nephrotoxic effects [48]. The non-ionic low-osmolality contrast agents still have an osmolality of 500–850 mOsm/l/kg (iohexol, iopamidol, iopromide), which is significantly higher than plasma. The iso-osmolar contrast agents (290 mmol/kg) such as iodixanol, seem to be the least nephrotoxic, as demonstrated in a pooled analysis of 16 trials in which the compound was compared with low-osmolality contrast agents [49]. This advantage of iso-osmolar contrast may only pertain to high risk patients. In a trial in which iso-osmolar contrast was compared with a low-osmolar agent in low-risk patients, the rates of CIN were similar to those reported previously [50,51]. However, a randomised double-blind trial, comparing low-osmolar with iso-osmolar contrast agents in patients with diabetes and chronic kidney disease at risk for CIN, suggested that the incidence of CIN was similar in both groups [52]. Although there is a relationship between volume of contrast agent and incidence of CIN [53], even small volumes of contrast agent can be nephrotoxic in the high-risk patient.

23.3.3 *Clinical characteristics*

CIN typically develops within 24 hours of exposure. The AKI is usually non-oliguric and recovery may occur within three to five days. In high-risk patients the decline in renal function may temporarily require renal replacement therapy. Occasionally, renal failure is persistent, especially in patients with pre-existent, severe chronic kidney disease and extensive co-morbidity (for example diabetic nephropathy or heart failure). The diagnosis of CIN is usually made in the absence of any other causes of AKI. There are no diagnostic tests to confirm the diagnosis. After percutaneous arterial interventions, AKI can also be caused by atheromatous, cholesterol emboli or by haemorrhagic shock.

23.3.4 *Preventive strategy*

There are few modifiable risk factors that can be used to lower the risk of CIN. In high-risk patients it is preferable to use small volumes of low- or iso-osmolar contrast agents. Furthermore, dehydration and hypovolaemia should be pretreated. Isotonic saline seems more effective than half normal saline [54]. In small trials, isotonic bicarbonate seems superior to isotonic saline in preventing CIN [55,56]. However, sodium bicarbonate was associated with an increased incidence of CIN in a retrospective study [57]. There is no consensus concerning the optimal rate and duration of infusion. In elective procedures, it is recommended to administer isotonic saline from 12 hours before until 12 hours after exposure to contrast at a rate of 1 ml/kg/h [56,58]. In urgent situations, isotonic saline can be administrated at a rate of 3 ml/kg/h, starting one hour prior to the procedure and 1 ml/kg/h for six hours afterwards [56]. If rehydration prior to the procedure is not possible, it is recommended to administer isotonic saline after the procedure for several hours. Clearly, there is a need for randomised trials addressing issues like rate, duration and composition of volume expansion.

Several pharmacological agents have been tried to prevent CIN. Vasodilators such as dopamine, fenoldopam, calcium channel blockers and theophylline proved ineffective. N-acetylcysteine (600–1200 mg orally twice a day before and on the day of the procedure) has gained wide popularity because of its anti-oxidative effects and negligible side effects. Data and numerous meta-analyses concerning its effectiveness are conflicting, however. Other agents, such as statins, ascorbic acid and atrial natriuretic peptide have been tried to prevent CIN, all without success [59–61]. The concept of removing the toxic contrast agent with dialysis or filtration is charming, but there are no convincing data to show a decrease in the incidence of CIN [62].

23.4 Renal Replacement Therapy

23.4.1 *Historical background*

Renal replacement therapy became feasible when Kolff developed the artificial kidney in the mid-1940s. In the 1950s haemodialysis was not widely used yet and still considered as an emergency treatment in near-hopeless situations. In the 1960s several chronic dialysis programmes were initiated in developed countries, but availability was still limited. The increasing application of renal replacement caused mortality from acute renal failure to drop from 90% to 30%. At the end of the 1960s well structured ICUs were introduced in hospitals worldwide. Haemodialysis was the dominant form of renal replacement in the 1970s. Major drawbacks of this technique, however, were acute hypotension and difficulties in fluid management; also the rapid electrolyte shifts were considered undesirable. Because of these shortcomings, in 1977 Kramer developed a system called continuous arteriovenous haemofiltration (CAVH) [63]. The major advantages, as he described, are low stress on the cardiovascular system, high effective fluid withdrawal, absence of danger of air embolism and no need for electricity, for highly specialised staff and for high investments. The disadvantages are, however, limited urea clearance due to low filtration rate and lack of its applicability in patients with atherosclerosis [64]. The introduction of continuous arteriovenous haemodialysis (CAVHD) and continuous arteriovenous haemodiafiltration (CAVHDF) increased azotemic control. With continuous venovenous haemofiltration (CVVH), continuous venovenous haemodialysis (CVVHD) and continuous venovenous haemodiafiltration (CVVHDF) the urea clearance was guaranteed, because the extracorporeal blood flow no longer depended on the arterial pressure. With the venovenous technique, however, renal replacement therapy became more complicated as compared with the arteriovenous technique, because of the introduction of a pump and a balancing system.

Renal replacement therapy modalities are categorised by intermittent versus continuous techniques and by mechanisms of solute and fluid removal. There is as yet no clarity on which renal replacement mode is best considering patient-centred outcomes, so that the choice is mainly dictated by availability, expertise, haemodynamics, vascular access and reasons for starting renal replacement therapy.

23.4.2 *Diffusion versus convection*

Ultrafiltration is the term used to describe fluid removal in renal replacement therapy, a process by which plasma water and ultrasoluble solutes are removed from whole blood across a semi-permeable membrane driven by pressure. The two primary principles of solute removal are diffusion and convection. Diffusion concerns solute transport across a semi-permeable membrane generated by a concentration gradient; molecules move from the compartment with a high concentration to the compartment with a low concentration (Fig. 23.4A). In general, solutes move from the blood compartment to the dialysate compartment. In haemodialysis, solutes are removed by diffusive clearance. The dialysate fluid, generally containing sodium, chloride, bicarbonate, calcium and magnesium, runs countercurrent to the blood flow, thereby maximising the concentration gradient. Factors affecting the rate of solute removal are the solute molecular weight, concentration gradient across the membrane, dialysis duration, blood and dialysate flow rates, and surface

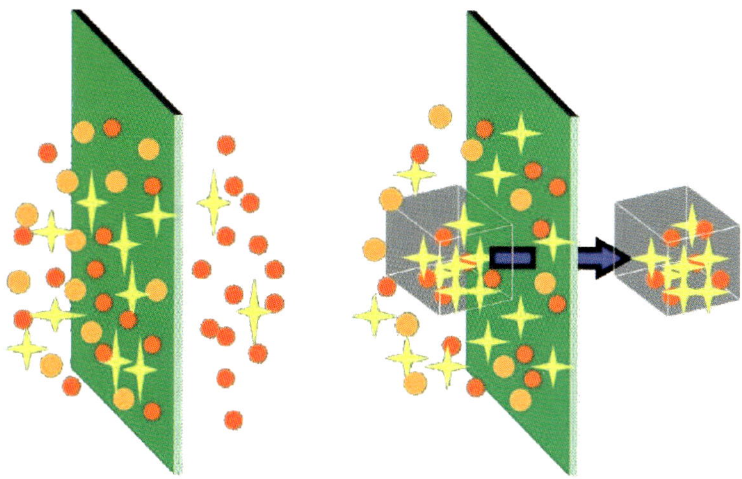

(A) Diffusion (B) Convection

Figure 23.4. Principles of solute removal. (A) Diffusion: removal of solutes across a semi-permeable membrane by a concentration gradient. (B) Convection: removal of solutes across a semi-permeable membrane by filtration (solvent drag); solutes together with the solvent are dragged from a high hydrostatic pressure compartment to a low pressure compartment.

area and permeability of the haemofilter. Low-molecular-weight solutes (<500 Da), such as blood urea nitrogen, potassium creatinine and some drugs such as lithium, are most effectively cleared by haemodialysis.

Convection concerns solute transport across a semi-permeable membrane generated by a hydrostatic pressure gradient; molecules move from the compartment with a higher pressure to the compartment with a lower pressure together with the solvent (solvent drag) (Fig. 23.4B). During haemofiltration, solutes are removed by convective clearance. Solute removal is primarily dependent on the ultrafiltration rate, the concentration in plasma water, and the surface area and permeability of the haemofilter. Apart from the low-molecular-weight solutes, medium-molecular-weight molecules are also removed by haemofiltration. It requires the use of a replacement solution to prevent acidosis, electrolyte disturbances and excessive fluid removal. The replacement solution generally contains sodium, chloride, magnesium, calcium, glucose and bicarbonate/lactate and some potassium. Hence, the concentration of solutes in plasma is gradually decreased during haemofiltration and the concentrations of electrolytes gradually move towards the concentration in the replacement solution. The replacement solution can be delivered prefilter (predilution) or postfilter (postdilution). The prefilter administration decreases the plasma solute concentration and thereby solute clearance. However, diluting the plasma with replacement solution may increase the filter life, which has a favourable effect on uraemic control. Conversely, postdilution continuous renal replacement therapy may be associated with a reduced filter life without any beneficial effects on metabolic control, as compared with predilution continuous renal replacement therapy [64]. Worldwide, both predilution and postdilution continuous renal replacement therapy remain widely practiced. In haemodiafiltration, diffusive and convective clearances are combined, allowing improved clearance of both small and large molecular weight substances.

23.4.3 *Renal replacement therapy modalities*

There are several options for renal replacement therapies. The three primary modalities are intermittent haemodialysis (IHD), sustained low extended dialysis (SLED) and the continuous forms of renal replacement therapy (CRRT). Peritoneal dialysis, which is a commonly used modality in chronic renal failure is generally not used in the critically ill. In IHD, solutes are removed by diffusion and fluid by ultrafiltration. In AKI, IHD is generally prescribed for three to six hours per session, three to four times a week. The major advantages of IHD include rapid solute or fluid removal, relatively low costs and complexity and less anticoagulation requirements. The major disadvantages are the risk for haemodynamic instability and the disequilibrium syndrome. SLED is a form of IHD where treatment time is prolonged to between 8 and 12 hours per session. In SLED, the blood flow is lowered and the fluid and solute removal is correspondingly slower. CRRT is performed continuously through arteriovenous or venovenous access. The blood flow rate used in CRRT is much lower than in IHD.

The most commonly applied submodalities of CRRT are CVVH, CVVHD and CVVHDF (Fig. 23.5) and their characteristics are described in Table 23.2. The arteriovenous techniques are no longer applied, because of the high rates of access complication and the development of external circuit pumps. CRRT provides slower solute clearance per unit of time

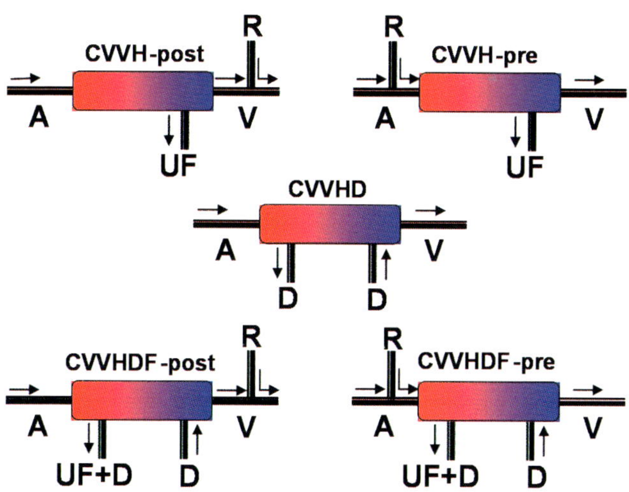

Figure 23.5. Different types of CRRT. CVVH-post: postdilution CVVH; CVVH-pre: predilution CVVH; CVVHDF-post: postdilution CVVHDF; CVVHDF-pre: predilution CVVHDF; A, blood in; V, blood out; R, replacement solution; UF, ultrafiltration; D, dialysate.

Table 23.2. Different modes and characteristics of continuous venovenous renal replacement techniques.

	Solute transport	Blood flow	Dialysate flow	Replacement solution	Ultrafiltration flow
Continuous venovenous haemofiltration (CVVH)	Convection	100–200	None	Yes	Equal to replacement solution flow. More ultrafiltration results in volume loss.
Continuous v enovenous haemodialysis (CVVHD)	Diffusion	100–200	1–2 l/h	No	No ultrafiltration. Ultrafiltration results in volume loss.
Continuous venovenous haemodiafiltration (CVVHDF)	Convection and diffusion	100–200	1–2 l/h	Yes	Equal to replacement solution flow. More ultrafiltration results in volume loss.

compared with IHD, but the 24-hour clearance may exceed that provided by intermittent techniques. Fluid is also removed more slowly as compared with IHD. A major drawback of continuous techniques is the use of continuous anticoagulation to prevent clotting of the filter; this, of course, carries an increased bleeding risk.

23.4.4 *Indication, timing, modality and dialysis dose*

The way renal replacement therapy is practiced around the world varies greatly, particularly with respect to indications, timing, modality and dialysis doses.

23.4.4.1 *Indication and timing*

There is no doubt that volume overload, uraemic complications, severe electrolyte disturbances and overt metabolic acidosis due to renal failure are clear reasons to start renal replacement therapy. Moreover, renal replacement therapy has to be initiated before these complications arise. The exact timing of renal replacement therapy, however, is unclear and randomised trials addressing this issue are scarce. In one trial, the effects of the initiation time of CVVH were studied in critically ill patients, developing early oliguric acute renal failure [67]. A group of 35 patients were treated with early high-volume haemofiltration (72–96 l per 24 hours) and 35 patients received late and low-volume haemofiltration (24–36 l per 24 hours). Early was defined as a start within 12 hours after a six-hour period of oliguria (<30 ml per hours). Survival at 28 days and recovery of renal function did not differ between the groups. Data from an observational study nevertheless suggest that mortality of patients starting renal replacement therapy with a urea less than 27 mmol/l is lower than in patients with urea of more than 27 mmol/l. It cannot be excluded that the results were confounded by severity of illness, however [67]. One major concern in starting renal replacement therapy early is that spontaneous recovery of renal function, which occurs in about 10% of patients, is not allowed to develop [66].

23.4.4.2 *Modality*

As outlined before, there are different modalities of renal replacement therapy. The continuous techniques have beneficial effects over IHD regarding haemodynamic stability, solute clearance and ultrafiltration capacity. These advantages are, however, limited when compared with slow haemodialysis. There are not many randomised trials comparing IHD with CRRT. In one study, the 28-day mortality rate was lower in IHD as compared with CRRT (42% versus 60%) [68]. Unfortunately, randomisation appeared unbalanced; patients in the CRRT group had higher disease severities and prevalence of liver failure. There are few randomised trials showing no differences in outcome between CRRT and IHD [69,70]. One large prospective randomised multicentre study has been performed comparing CVVHDF with IHD for acute renal failure in patients with multiple organ dysfunction syndrome: the rate of survival at 60 days was similar [71]. In the multicentre observational study on AKI, CRRT seemed associated with an increased mortality as compared with IHD. Several meta-analyses could not demonstrate convincing benefits of CRRT over IHD with regard to mortality and/or recovery of renal function [72–74]. Taken together, there are no data proving benefits of CRRT as compared with IHD in the critically ill.

23.4.4.3 *Dose*

The issue of dosage is controversial. The dosage is defined as the amount of blood purification achieved by renal replacement therapy techniques per unit of time. Uniformly, in chronic dialysis urea clearance is used as a marker of small solute removal. In patients with ESRD the correlation between dialysis intensity and mortality has been extensively studied and there is consensus that intensity really matters up to a certain level [75]. In chronic dialysis, the dose is expressed as Kt/V urea (K is the dialyser urea clearance, t represents time on dialysis and V is the volume of distribution for urea). It is advised to deliver an equilibrated Kt/V of at least 1.2 per session to chronic IHD patients. However, the Kt/V as an expression of dose is not applicable in critically ill patients with AKI, as the volume of distribution of urea is dynamic and more difficult to establish. Also, the generation of urea varies and is not in a steady state, and some residual renal function may be present. Furthermore, the delivery of dose in AKI is difficult to predict because it depends on technical issues such as malfunctioning catheters, variable blood flows and off time due to filter clotting or transport of patients (for radiology or surgery). Therefore, treatment dose in CRRT is expressed as effluent rate per kg of body weight per hour, with postfilter replacement. In a landmark study in 2000, Ronco *et al.* demonstrated an association between CRRT dose and mortality [76]. Survival in a group assigned to an ultrafiltration rate of 20 ml/kg/h was lower (41%) than in groups assigned to 35 ml/kg/h (57%) and 45 ml/kg/h (58%). The recommendation was to prescribe ultrafiltration dose according to patient's body weight, i.e. 35 ml/kg/h at minimum and many ICU's have changed their policies accordingly. Because of several drawbacks of the study, the controversies concerning CRRT dose remain, with persistent variations in prescribed doses of CRRT worldwide, as demonstrated in Fig. 23.6 [77].

Indeed, Bouman *et al.* did not observe a difference in mortality between high (48.2 ml/kg/h) and low (20.1 ml/kg/h) ultrafiltration rates in a

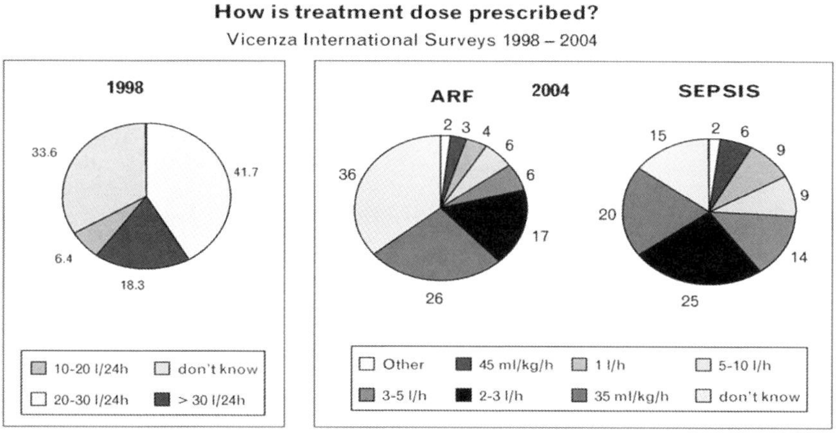

Figure 23.6. Results from the Vicenza International Surveys on CRRT carried out in 1998 and 2004. Adopted from Ronco *et al.* [77]. (Reproduced with permission).

randomised trial [66]. Saudan *et al.* showed that increasing the renal replacement dose by adding a dialysis dose to CVVH improved survival [78]. However, in a recent comparison between high- (35 ml/kg/h) and standard-dosage (20 ml/kg/h) CVVHDF, no difference in survival was found [79]. The Acute Renal Failure Trial Network also gave answers on the dosage issue [80]. In this large multicentre randomised trial, a comparison was made between intensive renal replacement therapy (IHD or SLED six times per week or CVVHDF with an ultrafiltration of 35 ml/kg/h) and less intensive renal replacement therapy (IHD or SLED on alternate days or CVVHDF with ultrafiltration rate of 20 ml/kg/h). The intensive treatment strategy did not decrease mortality, accelerate renal function recovery or change the rate of non-renal organ failure, as compared with the less-intensive strategy. The main conclusion of the authors is that other treatment strategies will be necessary to decrease mortality in the critically ill with AKI. These results were corroborated by the Randomized Evaluation of Normal versus Augmented Level of renal replacement therapy (RENAL) trial. In this large multicentre randomised trial involving over 1,400 intensive care patients throughout Australia and New Zealand, the higher intensity continuous renal replacement of 40 ml/kg/h did not reduce mortality at 90 days when compared with the 'normal' renal replacement dose of 25 ml/kg/h [81].

23.5 Non-Renal Indications for Continuous Renal Replacement Therapy

The renal indications for CRRT are based on the capability of convective and diffusive techniques to remove substances from plasma, which normally should have been removed by the kidneys. By these extracorporeal treatments it is also possible to remove substances that even normal kidneys would not remove. This feature forms the cornerstone of the so called non-renal indications for CRRT. These indications are less well established as compared with the classic ones. Non-renal indications are based on the removal of pro-inflammatory mediators in sepsis or sepsis-like syndromes, the removal of fluid in chronic heart failure, the removal of endogenous toxins or the removal of drugs in intoxications.

23.5.1 *Removal of inflammatory mediators*

Infection, tissue injury and ischaemia evoke a systemic inflammatory response as part of the body's defence mechanism. The production by macrophages, monocytes, lymphocytes and neutrophils of pro-inflammatory cytokines such as tumour necrosis factor-α (TNF-α), interleukin 1β (IL-1β) and IL-6 initiate an inflammatory cascade involving the complement, coagulation and fibrinolytic systems. The pro-inflammatory response is normally counterbalanced by inhibitors of inflammation: the compensatory anti-inflammatory response syndrome. Anti-inflammatory mediators, such as IL-10 and soluble cytokine receptors, are produced. Several decades ago, it was proposed that CRRT could play a role in attenuating the inflammatory response by extracorporeal removal of harmful cytokines and other mediators [82]. Most of the immune mediators are water soluble with a middle molecular weight; theoretically these mediators can be removed by convection as in haemofiltration. Filters utilised in standard CRRT usually have a molecular weight exclusion limit of 50,000 Da. Considering their molecular weight, thromboxane A2, leukotrienes, prostaglandins, histamine, serotonin and platelet-activated factor (all <1000 Da) are likely to be removed. Also complement (C) 3a (10,000 Da), C5a (11,200 Da), IL-1β (16,800 Da) and IL-6 (22,000 Da) can theoretically be removed if there are no interactions with the filter. One should bear in mind, however, that removal of these substances is highly variable because of interaction with proteins and cells. Based upon this rationale, several workers have investigated the effects of CRRT in animal models of sepsis and demonstrated beneficial effects [83–85]. Studies have demonstrated that inflammatory mediators can be removed during CRRT, a little by convection, but mainly by membrane adsorption [86]. Optimal mediator removal may thus be obtained by frequent filter changes, which is both expensive and impractical. To date, however, it is still controversial as to whether it makes sense and does no harm to non-specifically remove inflammatory mediators from the blood. In a trial performed in 2002, patients with sepsis were randomised to receive CVVH at 2 l/h or no CVVH [87]. In this trial, CVVH failed to reduce the circulating concentrations of several cytokines and anaphylatoxins associated with septic shock, or to attenuate the organ dysfunction that followed severe sepsis. Earlier, Cole *et al.* showed a beneficial effect of high-volume haemofiltration (HVHF) (6 l/h) compared with standard CVVH (1 l/h) regarding vasopressor requirements. Also, HVHF was associated with greater removal of C3a and C5a, mostly due to absorption rather than filtration [88].

An alternative approach to increase cytokine removal is to increase the porosity of the haemofilter with a cut-off point varying between 50 and 100 kDa. Treatment using high-cut-off filters has beneficial effects on immune cell function and increases survival in animal models of sepsis. Preliminary clinical studies show that these filters decrease plasma cytokine levels and the need for vasopressor therapy. Firm data considering clinical course and outcome are, however, still lacking [89]. A drawback of this technique is the loss of several proteins such as albumin, protein C and antithrombin, which all have a molecular weight of approximately 66 kDa. Another rather new technique is coupled plasma filtration and adsorption. In this system plasma filtration and adsorption, using a sorbent cartridge, is combined with standard renal replacement therapy (Fig. 23.7). The isolated plasma is redirected through a synthetic sorbent in which inflammatory mediators are non-selectively removed; after adsorption the endogenous plasma is returned to the blood and because of coupling with a haemofilter, further renal replacement therapy can be provided. Animal studies have already shown the efficacy of this technique regarding removal of inflammatory mediators, modulation of the immune system and survival [90]. Human studies are scarce but promising [91,92].

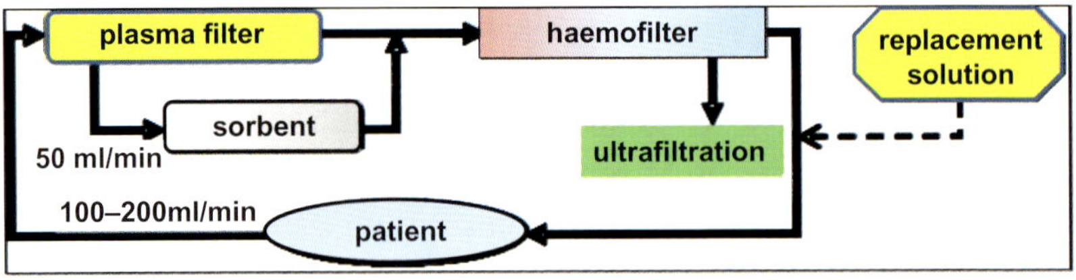

Figure 23.7. Coupled plasma filtration and adsorption. After isolation in the plasma filter, the endogenous plasma is directed to the sorbent, in which inflammatory mediators are adsorbed, the plasma then reunites with blood. Because of coupling with a haemofilter, standard renal replacement therapy can be provided [93]. (Reproduced with permission.)

In 2004, Ronco *et al.* developed the "peak concentration hypothesis" [94]. During systemic pro- and anti-inflammatory responses, systemic mediator overflow may result in immunodysregulation. There are two theories: in the sequential theory, peaks of pro-inflammatory mediators are followed by peaks of anti-inflammatory mediators; in the parallel theory, a mixture of pro- an anti-inflammatory mediators coexist. In both theories the hypothesis is that by non-selectively removing the excess of pro- and anti-inflammatory mediators (peak concentration) a situation of immunohomeostasis is restored (Fig. 23.8).

With CRRT, it is possible to remove excess pro- and anti-inflammatory mediators, but HVHF and frequent filter changes are mandatory. There are, however, some major technical requirements of HVHF: high blood flow and tight ultrafiltration control, necessitating large amounts of costly replacement fluids. These requirements combined with the crucial frequent filter change render HVHF labour-intensive. Moreover, there are increased losses of beneficial substances such as electrolytes, vitamins, trace elements and amino acids during HVHF. To reduce costs and workload several, non-controlled small trials were performed with pulse-HVHF: for example an ultrafiltration rate of 85 ml/kg/h for six hours per day followed by standard CVVH. Several of the studies concerning HVHF or pulse-HVHF showed promising results [95–97]. To date, however, the evidence is too little to propagate haemofiltration as an adjunctive therapy in critically ill patients with sepsis [98]. The use of HVHF in sepsis with or without AKI must be considered experimental and large-scale randomised studies are urgently needed. The IVOIRE (high volume in intensive care) study will perhaps give some answers as regards this issue.

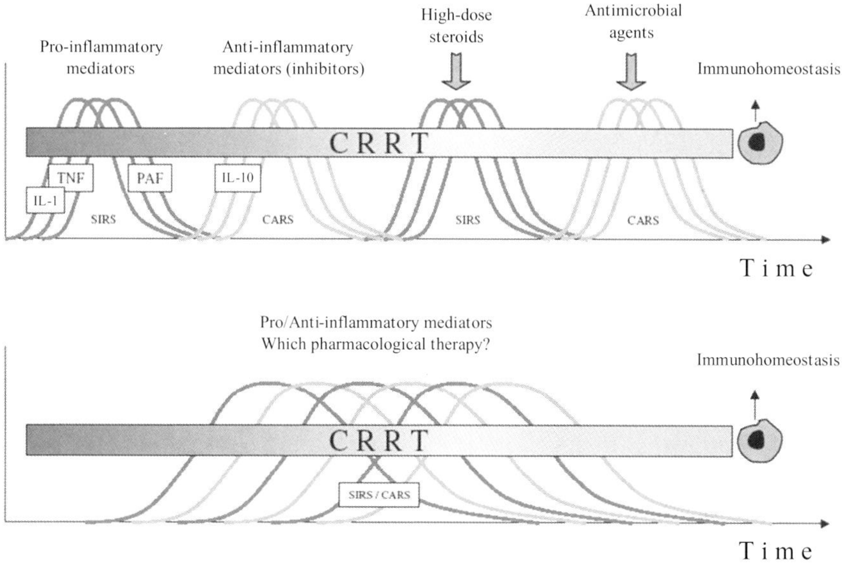

Figure 23.8. The peak concentration hypothesis. In the sequential as well as in the parallel theory the hypothesis suggests that by non-selective removal by CRRT, excess of pro- and anti-inflammatory mediators a situation of immunohomeostasis is restored. SIRS, systemic inflammatory response syndrome; CARS, compensatory anti-inflammatory response syndrome. (Adopted from Ronco *et al.* [94]. (Reproduced with permission.)

23.5.2 *Removal of fluid*

Patients on the ICU with compromised cardiac function and renal failure are best treated by CRRT. In patients with heart failure resistant to diuretics, CRRT is the best technique to restore dry body weight and improve diuresis and heart function. In congestive heart failure, the decreased effective circulating volume results in the activation of several neurohumoral systems such as the sympathetic system and the renin–angiotensin–aldosterone system and in the release of vasopressin. In case of refractory congestive heart failure, ultrafiltration by CRRT can decrease neurohumoral activation by removal of fluid and sodium [99].

23.5.3 *Removal of uric acid and phosphate*

Patients treated for malignancies may develop tumour lysis syndrome, which may result in AKI due to tubular obstruction by uric acid crystals or hyperphosphataemia with deposition of calcium phosphate crystals in renal interstitium and tubuli. Hyperhydration, and allopurinol or rasburicase may help to prevent AKI. If, however, AKI still develops, renal function recovery depends on normalisation of phosphate and uric acid levels. Both phosphate and uric acid are small molecules and are easily removed by diffusive clearance; in this setting conventional haemodialysis seems more effective than haemofiltration [100,101]. The major advantage of CRRT is the absence of a rebound hyperphosphataemia, which is often seen after intermittent haemodialysis. CRRT can also be used to prevent AKI due to tumour lysis syndrome [102].

23.5.4 *Removal of drugs in intoxications*

In the intoxicated patient, IHD has several advantages over CRRT. Especially the relatively slower clearance rate in CRRT is a major drawback in patients intoxicated with a dialysable substance. In haemodynamically unstable patients, however, CRRT is a more attractive renal replacement modality. There are no randomised controlled trials addressing this issue, however. Hence, the optimal method of extracorporeal blood purification is frequently a matter of debate. In each situation, a clinical judgement has to be made, to see if extracorporeal blood purification is beneficial and, if so, which modality is best. One has to keep in mind that in the case of an intoxication, rapid blood purification may be beneficial [103,104].

23.6 Practical Issues

23.6.1 *Vascular access*

For arteriovenous circuits (CAVH, CAVHD, CAVHDF), where the blood pressure is the driving force for blood flow, large-bore, small-length catheters are inserted, usually in the femoral artery and vein. With use of arteriovenous circuits, they carry a high risk for arterial thrombosis. In pumped systems (CVVH, CVVHD, CVVHDF, IHD) double-lumen catheters are usually used. The size depends on the location of insertion: the subclavian, jugular or femoral vein. If possible, insertion in the subclavian vein should be avoided because of a high incidence of subsequent stenosis [105]. Use of short catheters in the femoral vein may result in significant blood flow recirculation but this can be avoided by using longer catheters (19–15 cm) [106].

23.6.2 *Haemofilter*

Adequacy of renal replacement therapy also concerns the choice of the haemofilter. Haemofilters used for IHD and CRRT are characterised in terms of flux (the permeability to water and solutes) and biocompatibility (degree to which complement is activated by exposing the membrane to blood). Despite the fact that there is no evidence of superiority compared with low-flux filters, high-flux (high permeable) filters are generally recommended for CRRT, since increased permeability to water facilitates haemofiltration. The solute-removal capacity of a filter (KoA = mass transfer area coefficient) is of minor importance in CRRT, since solute clearance is largely determined by ultrafiltration/dialysate flow rate. In IHD, where therapy is given over a relatively short period, the KoA is important. Blood–filter contact may cause several undesirable effects; there are data suggesting that the use of bio-incompatible cellulose (cuprophane) haemofilters with IHD is associated with delayed recovery of renal failure and decreased survival in the critically ill compared with the use of more biocompatible filters [107].

23.6.3 *Replacement/dialysate solutions*

Dialysate for haemodialysis is produced by the dialysis machine from a combination of ultra-pure water and several electrolytes. The ultra-pure water, which does not have to be sterile, is purified by treatment with reverse osmosis, deionisation and the use of charcoal filters. Replacement solutions used for haemofiltration are in fact administered directly to the blood compartment and have to be sterile. The replacement solutions consist of balanced electrolyte solutions that closely resemble the composition of the ultrafiltrate minus the waste products that accumulate in renal failure. They contain sodium, chloride, magnesium, calcium, glucose and some potassium. These solutions also contain a buffer to correct for the metabolic acidosis. The buffer can be bicarbonate, acetate, lactate or citrate. Acetate, lactate and citrate are converted to bicarbonate; in multiple organ failure the conversion can be limited. Trials comparing lactate with acetate and lactate with bicarbonate did not demonstrate any difference in the risk of death [108,109]. It is, however, clear that lactate or bicarbonate solutions offer a better control of acid–base balance and improved cardiovascular stability compared with acetate-buffered solution [110]. The composition of the replacement solution can vary extensively in order to achieve specific metabolic goals; by varying specific electrolytes for example, imbalances can be corrected.

23.6.4 *Anticoagulation*

During renal replacement therapy, the patient's blood is in the extracorporeal circuit and in contact with artificial tubing and haemofilters. The passage of blood through the extracorporeal circuit results in activation of platelets, coagulation proteins, complement and white blood cells, resulting in microthrombus formation with subsequent platelet and fibrin deposition on the surface of the dialyser membrane [111,112]. To maintain dialyser efficacy and circuit longevity, adequate anticoagulation is important. Inadequate anticoagulation results in deterioration of filter performance, the filter may eventually clot, contributing to blood loss. Excessive anticoagulation, however, may result in bleeding complications, which is reported to occur in 5–26% of treatments [113,114]. Ideally, the anticoagulation is delivered regionally, which means that only the extracorporeal circuit is anticoagulated.

As with IHD, many anticoagulation strategies have been pursued for CRRT, including low-dose heparin, low-molecular-weight heparin, prostanoids, mesylates and regional citrate anticoagulation [115–117]. Heparin continues to be the most commonly used anticoagulant for CRRT. It is relatively easy to use and to monitor its effect. It provides adequate extracorporeal anticoagulation. However, there is a high risk of bleeding and the development of heparin-induced thrombocytopoenia and thrombosis [118]. Low-molecular-weight heparin is infrequently used due to the need to monitor factor Xa levels; and if bleeding occurs it is difficult to reverse its effects.

Citrate offers an anticoagulant effect through its ability to chelate calcium. Calcium has an essential role in activation of several clotting factors

(II, V, VII, VIII, IX, X, XIII) and in the conversion of fibrinogen to fibrin. Citrate acts regionally when administered pre-filter and thus reduces the risk of bleeding. The anticoagulant effect is overwhelmed and neutralised when citrated blood from the extracorporeal circuit returns and mixes with central venous blood containing sufficient amounts of calcium. Citrate is cleared by the tricarboxycyclic acid pathway in the liver, skeletal muscles and renal cortex, producing bicarbonate. Thus, citrate can be used to anticoagulate an extracorporeal circuit, without systemic anticoagulation, resulting in regional anticoagulation. The method carries the risk of hypocalcaemia when insufficiently counteracted by calcium infusion after passage of blood through the filter. Also, metabolic alkalosis may develop when too much citrate enters the blood. Citrate has been widely used for conventional IHD and has been successfully adapted for use in CAVHD/F and CVVH(DF) [119]. Two methods of regional citrate anticoagulation are being used effectively. The first and most frequently used method employs concentrated trisodium citrate together with the use of hypotonic alkali-free replacement solution as reported by Mehta *et al.* and Kutsogiannis *et al.* [120,121]. The second method employs trisodium-citrate-containing replacement solution that is isotonic and has an adjusted concentration of citrate, so that the amount of bicarbonate equivalent is similar to that employed when lactate or bicarbonate-buffered solutions are used [122,123]. Citrate CRRT carries the potential risk of citrate accumulation. Accumulation can occur as free citrate or as calcium citrate complexes. The main dangers are those of hypocalcaemia [124]. When free citrate accumulates, there is a rise in the anion gap. Accumulation of calcium citrate complexes will increase the total to ionised calcium ratio [125]. There is accumulating evidence that citrate anticoagulation is at least equivalent or even superior to heparin in CRRT concerning filter life and/or transfusion rate [126–128]. However, whether regional anticoagulation with citrate is associated with a lower mortality compared with heparin has not been proven yet. The advantages of citrate must be balanced against its increased complexity and its potential for metabolic complications.

In the absence of a citrate protocol, thrombin inhibitors such as argatroban or hirudin are good alternatives to heparin, especially in case of heparin-induced thrombocytopoenia [129,130]. Currently, none of the anticoagulants is ideal and the choice is frequently influenced by patient factors. The experiences of the ICU staff with the different anticoagulants are major determinants of the success of any anticoagulation regimen.

23.6.5 *Complications*

Renal replacement therapy is not free from risks. Timing and indications of CRRT can be controversial and the adverse effects of renal replacement therapy must be considered. These are the potential complications of catheter insertion (bleeding, pneumothorax, air embolism, thrombosis and infection), the hazards of continuous anticoagulation and the risk of significant blood loss associated with filter clotting. In addition, after initiation of CRRT drug dosing becomes generally more difficult.

23.7 Future Trends: Renal Cell Therapy and the Bioartificial Kidney

In chronic renal failure, transplantation is the best form of renal replacement, if possible, because normal kidney function is closely mimicked. A simplified comparison is that haemofiltration mimics the glomerulus and haemodialysis mimics the diffusive transport in the tubules. However, the tubules do have more functions than solely passive diffusive exchange of solutes, such as active bicarbonate and glucose transport, glutathione degradation, ammonia production and activation of vitamin D. A lesser known feature of the kidney is its immunological function. The renal proximal tubules possess antigen-presenting capacities and produce several inflammatory mediators [131–133]. Proximal tubular cells have a pivotal role in the metabolic, endocrine and immune functions of the kidney. In ESRD as well as in AKI these functions are compromised and simply cannot be replaced by an artificial, synthetic haemofilter. ESRD is associated with a state of chronic inflammation. It is also suggested that the propensity of patients with AKI to develop sepsis suggests that renal function, specifically renal tubule cell function secondary to acute tubular necrosis, plays a critical immunomodulating role in stress [134]. Humes *et al.* developed a method to isolate and culture renal proximal tubule cells and used these to create the renal tubule cell assist device (RAD) [135]. The RAD is in fact a haemofilter containing over 10^9 human renal tubule cells grown as confluent monolayers along the inner surface of the hollow fibres. These cells remain immunoprotected from the patient's blood by a semi-permeable membrane. By coupling the RAD to a conventional CVVH system, a bio-artificial kidney was created as outlined in Fig. 23.9. Blood pumped out of the patient first passes through the haemofilter, where ultrafiltrate is formed; this process mimics the glomerular function. This ultrafiltrate then passes through the hollow fibres of the RAD, where it is in close contact with the renal tubule cells. The filtered blood coming from the haemofilter enters the RAD through the extracapillary port. The process in the RAD mimics tubular function. The blood coming from the RAD returns to the patient and the processed ultrafiltrate is a waste product just like urine. Preclinical and animal studies have demonstrated that the tubule

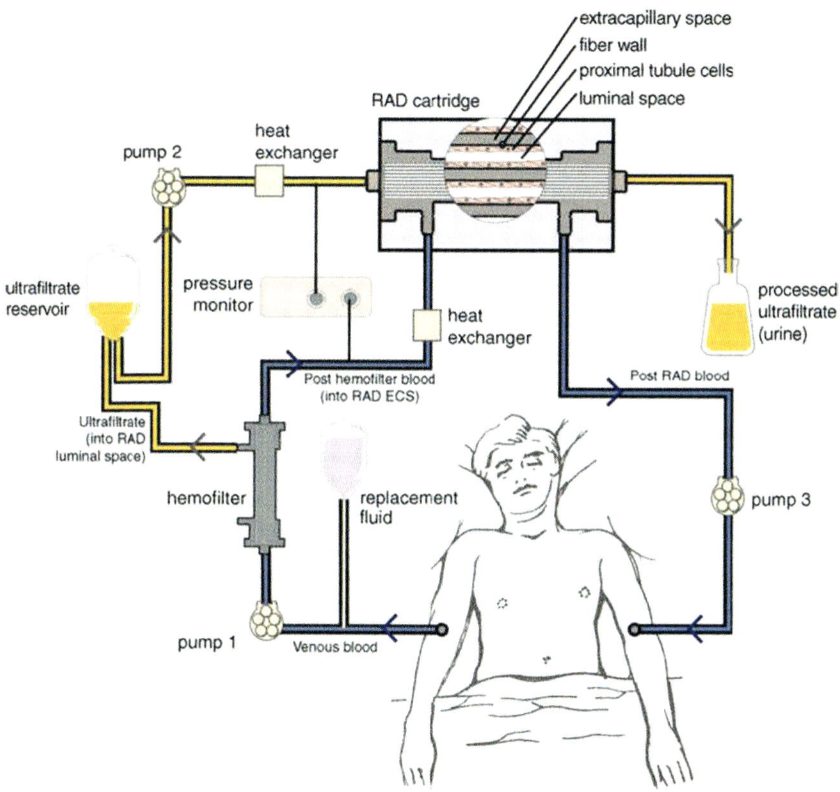

Figure. 23.9. Scheme of the extracorporeal circuit for the bioartificial kidney consisting of a haemofilter and a renal assist device (RAD) cartridge [138]. (Reproduced with permission.)

cells maintain their transport, endocrine as well as metabolic activities [135,136]. A phase II, multicentre, randomised controlled open-label trial comparing CVVH + RAD with CRRT revealed a reduced mortality rate in the first treatment group. RAD therapy was also associated with more rapid recovery of renal function. The treatment was well tolerated [137].

23.8 Prognosis

Patients with AKI are amongst the most severely ill in the ICU. The mortality of patients admitted to the ICU with AKI being treated by renal replacement therapy is approximately 60% [139]. After an initial decline in mortality during recent decades, the mortality from acute renal failure has climbed considerably despite increasing clinical experience and knowledge. The explanation for this phenomenon is that the population in the ICU's has changed with time. More patients are surviving trauma, acute coronary and vascular events and serious infections. Also, surgeons can perform more complicated surgical procedures in older patients with a considerable risk of developing acute renal failure. Many of these patients who previously might have died nowadays survive but develop acute renal failure [140]. As a consequence more patients overall develop renal failure. Conversely, the observed mortality in patients with AKI is significantly higher than predicted from the underlying disease. Therefore, AKI is an independent risk factor for mortality [5]. Even minor deterioration of renal function is associated with an increased mortality rate in ICU and non-ICU patients [8,10,40]. The majority of patients surviving the ICU and hospital stay regain normal or near-normal renal function. The long-term effects of AKI are still unclear, because of the paucity of long-term follow-up studies. The long-term mortality, however, in those patients who survived AKI is higher when compared with critically ill patients without AKI. This could be explained by the fact that a great number of survivors of AKI, varying between 19% and 31%, will eventually develop chronic kidney disease [141]. As a result of the increased risk of mortality and development of chronic kidney disease, patients with partial recovery of renal function should be monitored closely in the outpatient clinic [142,143]. Approximately 13% of patients will remain on renal replacement therapy because of the development of ESRD [139].

23.9 Clinical Case

A 29-year-old woman presented at the emergency department because of shortness of breath. Four weeks earlier she had given birth to a healthy son. Because of some neck pain she used ibuprofen daily for several days. For about two weeks she had complained of nausea and vomiting. Two days prior to her presentation she developed shortness of breath. There was no fever or coughing. On physical examination she was a pale young woman with a blood pressure of 144/95 mmHg, a heart rate of 88 beats per minute and a respiratory rate of 30 breaths per minute. She had no fever. Examination of the thorax, abdomen and extremities was normal. Laboratory analysis revealed the following abnormalities: haemoglobin: 3.6 mmol/l; white blood cell count: 13.7×10^9/l; reticulocytes: 184‰; potassium: 7.8 mmol/l; creatinine: 1851 μmol/l; blood urea nitrogen: 35.6 mmol/l; phosphorus: 3.17 mmol/l; lactate dehydrogenase: 1786 U/l. The arterial blood gas measurements showed: pH: 7.23; partial pressure of oxygen: 73 mmHg; partial pressure of carbon dioxide: 20 mmHg; base excess: −17.4 mmol/l. The blood smear demonstrated schizocytes. The chest X-ray showed bilateral pulmonary oedema. The electrocardiogram demonstrated peaked T-waves. Because of anuria there was no urinary analysis. The diagnosis was a postpartum haemolytic uraemic syndrome. Because of respiratory failure she was intubated for mechanical ventilation and sedation. Renal replacement was initiated; in order to lower the potassium and to remove the excess of fluid rapidly, the first choice of modality was haemodialysis. After haemodialysis, daily plasma exchange therapy was started combined with IHD. Recovery to spontaneous ventilation was rapid and smooth. Unfortunately, the renal failure persisted and the patient remained dependent on IHD.

References

[1] Chertow, G.M., Levy, E.M., Hammermeister, K.E. *et al.* (1998). Independent association between acute renal failure and mortality following cardiac surgery, *Am J Med*, **104**, 343–382.

[2] de Mendonça, A., Vincent, J.L., Suter, P.M. *et al.* (2000). Acute renal failure in the ICU: risk factors and outcome evaluated by the SOFA score, *Intens Care Med*, **26**, 915–921.

[3] Metnitz, P.G., Krenn, C.G., Steltzer, H. *et al.* (2002). Effect of acute renal failure requiring renal replacement therapy on outcome in critically ill patients, *Crit Care Med*, **30**, 2051–2058.

[4] Cosentino, F., Chaff, C. and Piedmonte, M. (1994). Risk factors influencing survival in ICU acute renal failure, *Nephrol Dial Transplant*, **9** (Suppl. 4), 179–182.

[5] Hoste, E.A. and Kellum, J.A. (2007). Incidence, classification and outcome of acute kidney injury, *Contrib Nephrol*, **156**, 32–38.

[6] Bellomo, R., Ronco, C., Kellum, J.A. *et al.* (2004). Acute renal failure; definition, outcome measures, animal models, fluid therapy and information technology needs: The Second International Consensus Conference of the Acute Dialysis Quality Initiative (ADQI) Group, *Crit Care*, **8**, R204–R212.

[7] Abosaif, N.Y., Tolba, Y.A., Heap, M. *et al.* (2005). The outcome of acute renal failure in the intensive care unit according to RIFLE: model application, sensitivity and predictability, *Am J Kidney Dis*, **46**, 1038–1048.

[8] Uchino, S., Bellomo, R., Goldsmith, D. *et al.* (2006). An assessment of the RIFLE criteria for acute renal failure in hospitalized patients, *Crit Care Med*, **34**, 1913–1917.

[9] Jenq, C.C., Tsai, M.H., Tian, Y.C. *et al.* (2007). RIFLE classification can predict short-term prognosis in critically ill cirrhotic patients, *Intens Care Med*, **33**, 1921–1930.

[10] Chertow, G.M., Burdick, E., Honour, M. *et al.* (2005). Acute kidney injury, mortality, length of stay, and costs in hospitalized patients, *J Am Soc Nephrol*, 16, 3365–3370.

[11] Mehta, R.L., Kellum, J.A., Shah, S.V. *et al.* (2007). Acute Kidney Injury Network: report of an initiative to improve outcomes in acute kidney injury, *Crit Care*, **11**, R31.

[12] Brezis, M. and Rosen, S. (1995). Hypoxia of the renal medulla — its implications for disease, *N Engl J Med*, **332**, 647–655.

[13] Burke, T.J., Cronin, R.E., Duchin, K.L. *et al.* (1980). Ischemia and tubule obstruction during acute renal failure in dogs: mannitol in protection, *Am J Physiol*, **238**, F305–F314.

[14] Bonventre, J.V. and Zuk, A. (2004). Ischemic acute renal failure: an inflammatory disease? *Kidney Int*, **66**, 480–485.

[15] Ysebaert, D.K., De Greef, K.E., De Beuf, A. *et al.* (2004). T cells as mediators in renal ischemia/reperfusion injury, *Kidney Int*, **66**, 491–496.

[16] Roberts, I., Alderson, P. and Bunn, F. (2004). Colloids versus crystalloids for fluid resuscitation in critically ill patients, *Cochrane Database Syst Rev*, CD000567.

[17] Dickenmann, M., Oettl, T. and Mihatsch, M.J. (2008). Osmotic nephrosis: acute kidney injury with accumulation of proximal tubular lysosomes due to administration of exogenous solutes, *Am J Kidney Dis*, **51**, 491–503.

[18] Wiedermann, C.J. (2008). Systematic review of randomized clinical trials on the use of hydroxyethyl starch for fluid management in sepsis, *BMC Emerg Med*, **8**, 1.

[19] Martin, C., Viviand, X., Leone, M. *et al.* (2000). Effect of norepinephrine on the outcome of septic shock, *Crit Care Med*, **28**, 2758–2765.

[20] Kellum, J.A. and M. Decker, J. (2001). Use of dopamine in acute renal failure: a meta-analysis, *Crit Care Med*, **29**, 1526–1531.

[21] Halpenny, M., Markos, F., Snow, H.M. *et al.* (2000). The effects of fenoldopam on renal blood flow and tubular function during aortic cross-clamping in anaesthetized dogs, *Eur J Anaesthesiol*, **17**, 491–498.

[22] Landoni, G., Biondi-Zoccai, G.G., Tumlin, J.A. *et al.* (2007). Beneficial impact of fenoldopam in critically ill patients with or at risk for acute renal failure: a meta-analysis of randomized clinical trials, *Am J Kidney Dis*, **49**, 56–68.

[23] Landoni, G., Biondi-Zoccai, G.G., Marino, G. *et al.* (2008). Fenoldopam reduces the need for renal replacement therapy and in-hospital death in cardiovascular surgery: a meta-analysis, *J Cardiothorac Vasc Anesth*, **22**, 27–33.

[24] Tumlin, J.A., Finkel, K.W., Murray, P.T. *et al.* (2005). Fenoldopam mesylate in early acute tubular necrosis: a randomized, double-blind, placebo-controlled clinical trial, *Am J Kidney Dis*, **46**, 26–34.

[25] Bagshaw, S.M., Delaney, A., Haase, M. *et al.* (2007). Loop diuretics in the management of acute renal failure: a systematic review and meta-analysis, *Crit Care Resusc*, **9**, 60–68.

[26] Mehta, R.L., Pascual, M.T., Soroko, S. *et al.* (2002). Diuretics, mortality, and nonrecovery of renal function in acute renal failure, *JAMA*, **288**, 2547–2553.

[27] Uchino, S., Doig, G.S., Bellomo, R. *et al.* (2004). Diuretics and mortality in acute renal failure, *Crit Care Med*, **32**, 1669–1677.

[28] Van Valenberg, P.L., Hoitsma, A.J., Tiggeler, R.G. *et al.* (1987). Mannitol as an indispensable constituent of an intraoperative hydration protocol for the prevention of acute renal failure after renal cadaveric transplantation, *Transplantation*, **44**, 784–788.

[29] Vanholder, R., Sever, M.S., Erek, E. *et al.* (2000). Rhabdomyolysis, *J Am Soc Nephrol*, **11**, 1553–1561.

[30] Patel, N.S., Sharples, E.J., Cuzzocrea, S. *et al.* (2004). Pretreatment with, EPO reduces the injury and dysfunction caused by ischemia/reperfusion in the mouse kidney in vivo, *Kidney Int*, **66**, 983–989.

[31] Sharples, E.J., Patel, N., Brown, P. *et al.* (2004). Erythropoietin protects the kidney against the injury and dysfunction caused by ischemia-reperfusion, *J Am Soc Nephrol*, **15**, 2115–2124.
[32] Johnson, D.W., Pat, B., Vesey, D.A. *et al.* (2006). Delayed administration of darbepoetin or erythropoietin protects against ischemic acute renal injury and failure, *Kidney Int*, **69**, 1806–1813.
[33] McCullough, P.A. and Soman, S.S. (2005). Contrast-induced nephropathy, *Crit Care Clin*, **21**, 261–280.
[34] Thomsen, H.S. (2003). Guidelines for contrast media from the European Society of Urogenital Radiology, *AJR Am J Roentgenol*, **181**, 1463–1471.
[35] Meschi, M., Detrenis, S. and Musini, S. (2006). Facts and fallacies concerning the prevention of contrast medium-induced nephroptahy, *Crit Care Med*, **34**, 2060–2068.
[36] Nash, K., Hafeez, A. and Hou, S. (2002). Hospital-acquired renal insufficiency, *Am J Kidney Dis*, **39**, 930–936.
[37] McCullough, P.A., Wolyn, R., Rocher, L.L. *et al.* (1997). Acute renal failure after coronary intervention: incidence, risk factors, and relationship to mortality, *Am J Med*, **103**, 368–375.
[38] Rihal, C.S., Textor, S.C., Grill, D.E. *et al.* (2002). Incidence and prognostic importance of acute renal failure after percutaneous coronary intervention, *Circulation*, **105**, 2259–2264.
[39] Gruberg, L., Mintz, G.S., Mehran, R. *et al.* (2000). The prognostic implications of further renal function deterioration within 48 h of interventional coronary procedures in patients with pre-existent chronic renal insufficiency, *J Am Coll Cardiol*, **36**, 1542–1548.
[40] Levy, E.M., Viscoli, C.M. and Horwitz, R.I. (1996). The effect of acute renal failure on mortality: A cohort analysis, *JAMA*, **275**, 1489–1494.
[41] Marenzi, G., Lauri, G., Assanelli, E. *et al.* (2004). Contrast-induced nephropathy in patients undergoing primary angioplasty for acute myocardial infarction, *J Am Coll Cardiol*, **44**, 1780–1785.
[42] Lindsay, J., Apple, S., Pinnow, E.E. *et al.* (2003). Percutaneous coronary intervention-associated nephropathy foreshadows increased risk of late adverse events in patients with normal baseline serum creatinine, *Catheter Cardiovasc Interv*, **59**, 338–343.
[43] Dangas, G., Iakovou, I., Nikolsky, E. *et al.* (2005). Contrast-induced nephropathy after percutaneous coronary interventions in relation to chronic kidney disease and hemodynamic variables, *Am J Cardiol*, **95**, 13–19.
[44] Lindsay, J., Canos, D.A., Apple, S. *et al.* (2004). Causes of acute renal dysfunction after percutaneous coronary intervention and comparison of late

mortality rates with postprocedure rise of creatine kinase-MB versus rise of serum creatinine, *Am J Cardiol*, **94**, 786–789.
[45] Parfrey, P. (2005). The clinical epidemiology of contrast induced nephropathy, *Cardiovasc Intervent Radiol*, **28** (Suppl. 2), S3–S11.
[46] Moore, R.D., Steinberg, E.P., Powe, N.R. *et al.* (1992). Nephrotoxicity of high-osmolality versus low-osmolality contrast media: Randomized clinical trial, *Radiology*, **182**, 649–655.
[47] Parfrey, P.S., Griffiths, S.M., Barrett, B.J. *et al.* (1989). Contrast material-induced renal failure in patients with diabetes mellitus, renal insufficiency, or both: A prospective controlled study, *N Engl J Med*, **320**, 143–149.
[48] Barret, B.J. and Carlisle, E.J. (1993). Metaanalysis of the relative nephrotoxicity of high- and low-osmolality iodinated contrast media, *Radiology*, **188**, 171–178.
[49] McCullough, P.A., Bertrand, M.E., Brinker, J.A. *et al.* (2006). A meta-analysis of the renal safety of isoosmolar iodixanol compared with low-osmolar contrast-media, *J Am Coll, Cardiol*, **48**, 692–699.
[50] Barrett, B.J., Katzberg, R.W., Thomsen, H.S. *et al.* (2006). Contrast-induced nephropathy in patients with chronic kidney disease undergoing computed tomography: a double-blind comparison of iodixanol and iopamidol, *Invest Radiol*, **41**, 815–821.
[51] Solomon, R.J., Natarajan, M.K., Doucet, S. *et al.* (2007). Cardiac Angiography in Renally Impaired Patients (CARE) study: a randomized double-blind trial of contrast-induced nephropathy in patients with chronic kidney disease, *Circulation*, **115**, 3189–3196.
[52] Kuhn, M.J., Chen, N., Sahani, D.V. *et al.* (2008). The PREDICT study: A randomized double-blind comparison of contrast-induced nephropathy after low- or isoosmolar contrast agent exposure, *AJR Am J Roentgenol*, **191**, 151–157.
[53] Barrett, B.J. and Parfrey, P.S. (2006). Clinical practice. Preventing nephropathy induced by contrast medium, *N Engl J Med*, **354**, 379–386.
[54] Mueller, C., Buerkle, G., Buettner, H.J. *et al.* (2002). Prevention of contrast media-associated nephropathy: randomized comparison of 2 hydration regimens in 1620 patients undergoing coronoary angioplasty, *Arch Intern Med*, **162**, 329–336.
[55] Briguori, C., Airoldi, F., D'Andrea, D. *et al.* (2007). Renal insufficiency Following Contrast Media Administration Trial (REMEDIAL): a randomized comparison of 3 preventive strategies, *Circulation*, **115**, 1211–1217.
[56] Merten, G.J., Burgess, W.P., Gray, L.V. *et al.* (2004). Prevention of contrast-induced nephropathy with sodium bicarbonate: a randomized controlled trial, *JAMA*, **291**, 2328–2334.

[57] From, A.M., Bartholmai, B.J., Williams, A.W. *et al.* (2008). Sodium bicarbonate is associated with an increased incidence of contrast nephropathy: A retrospective cohort, study of 7977, patients at Mayo Clinic, *Clin J Am Soc Nephrol*, **3**, 10–18.
[58] Solomon, R., Werner, C., Mann, D. *et al.* (1994). Effects of saline, mannitol, and furosemide to prevent acute decreases in renal function induced by radiocontrast agents, *N Engl J Med*, **331**, 1416–1420.
[59] Jo, S.H., Koo, B.K., Park, J.S. *et al.* (2008). Prevention of radiocontrast medium-induced nephropathy using short-term high-dose simvastatin in patients with renal insufficiency undergoing coronary angiography (PROMISS) trial — a randomized controlled study, *Am Heart*, **155**, 499e1–e8.
[60] Boscheri, A., Weinbrenner, C., Botzek, B. *et al.* (2007). Failure of ascorbic acid to prevent contrast-media induced nephropathy in patients with renal dysfunction, *Clin Nephrol*, **68**, 279–286.
[61] Stacul, F., Adam, A., Becker, C.R., *et al.* (2006). Strategies to reduce the risk of contrast-induced nephropathy, *Am J Cardiol*, **98**, 59K–77K.
[62] Cruz, D.N., Perazella, M.A., Bellomo, R. *et al.* (2006). Extracorporeal blood purification therapies for prevention of radiocontrast-induced nephropathy: a systematic review, *Am J Kidney Dis*, **48**, 361–371.
[63] Kramer, P., Wigger, W., Rieger, J. *et al.* (1977). Arteriovenous haemofiltration: a new and simple method for treatment of over-hydrated patients resistant to diuretics, *Klin Wochenschr*, **55**, 1121–1122.
[64] Kramer, P., Schrader, J., Bohnsack, W. *et al.* (1981). Continuous arteriovenous haemofiltration. A. new kidney replacement therapy, *Proc Eur Dial Transplant Assoc*, **18**, 743–749.
[65] Uchino, S., Fealy, N., Baldwin, I. *et al.* (2003). Pre-dilution vs. post-dilution during continuous veno-venous hemofiltration: impact on filter life and azotemic control, *Nephron Clin Pract*, **94**, c94–c98.
[66] Bouman, C.S.C., Oudemans-Van Straaten, H.M., Tijssen, J.G.P. *et al.* (2002). Effects of early high-volume continuous venovenous hemofiltration on survival and recovery of renal function in intensive care patients with acute renal failure: a prospective, randomized trial, *Crit Care Med*, **30**, 2205–2211.
[67] Liu, K.D., Himmelfarb, J., Paganini, E. *et al.* (2006). Timing of initiation of dialysis in critically ill patients with acute kidney injury, *Clin J Am Soc Nephrol*, **1**, 915–919.
[68] Mehta, R.L., McDonald, B., Gabbai, F.B. *et al.* (2001). A randomized clinical trial of continuous versus intermittent dialysis for acute renal failure, *Kidney Int*, **60**, 1154–1163.

[69] Uehlinger, D.E., Jakob, S.M., Ferrari, P. *et al.* (2005). Comparison of continuous and intermittent renal replacement therapy for acute renal failure, *Nephrol Dial Transplant*, **20**, 1630–1637.
[70] Augustine, J.J., Sandy, D., Seifert, T.H. *et al.* (2004). A randomized controlled trial comparing intermittent with continuous dialysis in patients with ARF, *Am J Kidney Dis*, **44**, 1000–1007.
[71] Vinsonneau, C., Camus, C., Combes, A. *et al.* (2006). Continuous venovenous haemodiafiltration versus intermittent haemodialysis for acute renal failure in patients with multiple-organ dysfunction syndrome: a multicentre randomised trial, *Lancet*, **368**, 379–385.
[72] Kellum, J.A., Angus, D.C., Johnson, J.P. *et al.* (2002). Continuous versus intermittent renal replacement therapy: a meta-analysis, *Intens Care Med*, **28**, 29–37.
[73] Tonelli, M., Manns, B. and Feller-Kopman, D. (2002). Acute renal failure in the intensive care unit: a systematic review of the impact of dialytic modality on mortality and renal recovery, *Am J Kidney Dis*, **40**, 875–885.
[74] Bagshaw, S.M., Berthiaume, L.R., Delaney, A. *et al.* (2008). Continuous versus intermittent renal replacement therapy for critically ill patients with acute kidney injury: a meta-analysis, *Crit Care Med*, **36**, 610–617.
[75] Eknoyan, G., Beck, G.J., Cheung, A.K. *et al.* (2002). Effect of dialysis dose and membrane flux in maintenance hemodialysis, *N Engl J Med*, **347**, 2010–2019.
[76] Ronco, C., Bellomo, R., Homel, P. *et al.* (2000). Effects of different doses in continuous veno-venous haemofiltration on outcomes of acute renal failure: a prospective randomised trial, *Lancet*, **356**, 26–30.
[77] Ronco, C., Ricci, Z. and Bellomo, R. (2006). Current worldwide practice of dialysis dose prescription in acute renal failure, *Curr Opin Crit Care*, **12**, 551–556.
[78] Saudan, P., Niederberger, M., De, Seigneux, S. *et al.* (2006). Adding a dialysis dose to continuous hemofiltration increases survival in patients with acute renal failure, *Kidney Int*, **70**, 1312–1317.
[79] Tolwani, A.J., Campbell, R.C., Stofan, B.S. *et al.* (2008). Standard versus high-dose, CVVHDF for ICU-related acute renal failure, *J Am Soc Nephrol*, **19**, 1233–1238.
[80] The VA/NIH Acute Renal Failure Trial Network (2008). Intensity of renal support in critically ill patients with acute kidney injury, *N Eng J Med*, **359**, 7–20.
[81] Renal Replacement Therapy Study Investigators (2009). Intensity of continuous renal-replacement therapy in critically ill patients, *N Engl J Med*, **361**, 1627–38.

[82] Gotloib, L., Barzilay, E., Shustak, A. *et al.* (1986). Hemofiltration in septic, ARDS. The artificial kidney as an artificial endocrine lung, *Resuscitation*, **13**, 123–132.

[83] Grootendorst, A.F., Van Bommel, E.F.H., Van der Hoven, B. *et al.* (1992). High volume hemofiltration improves right ventricular function in endotoxin-induced shock in pig, *Intens Care Med*, **18**, 235–240.

[84] Yekebas, E.F., Eisenberger, C.F., Ohnesorge, H. *et al.* (2001). Attenuation of sepsis-related immunoparalysis by continuous veno-venous hemofiltration in experimental porcine pancreatitis, *Crit Care Med*, **29**, 1423–1430.

[85] Gomez, A., Wang, R., Unruh, H. *et al.* (1990). Hemofiltration reverses left ventricular dysfunction during sepsis in dogs, *Anesthesiology*, **73**, 671–685.

[86] De Vriese, A.S., Vanholder, R.C., Pascual, M. *et al.* (1999). Can inflammatory cytokines be removed efficiently by continuous renal replacement therapies, *Intens Care Med*, **25**, 903–910.

[87] Cole, L., Bellomo, R., Hart, G. *et al.* (2002). A phase II randomized, controlled trial of continuous hemofiltration in sepsis, *Crit Care Med*, **30**, 100–106.

[88] Cole, L., Bellomo, R., Journois, D. *et al.* (2001).High-volume haemofiltration in human septic shock, *Intens Care Med*, **27**, 978–986.

[89] Haase, M., Bellomo, R., Morgera, S. *et al.* (2007). High cut-off point membranes in septic acute renal failure: a systematic review, *Int J Artif Organs*, **30**, 1031–1041.

[90] Tetta, C., Gianotti, L., Cavaillon, J.M. *et al.* (2000). Coupled plasma filtration-adsorption in a rabbit model of endotoxic shock, *Crit Care Med*, **28**, 1526–1533.

[91] Ronco, C., Brendolan, A., Lonnemann, G. *et al.* (2002). A pilot study of coupled plasma filtration with adsorption in septic shock, *Crit Care Med*, **30**, 1250–1255.

[92] Formica, M., Olivieri, C., Livigni, S. *et al.* (2003). Hemodynamic response to coupled plasmafiltration-adsorption in human septic shock, *Intens Care Med*, **29**, 703–708.

[93] Tetta, C., Bellomo, R., Brendolan, A. *et al.* (1999). Use of adsorptive mechanisms in continuous renal replacement therapies in the critically ill, *Kidney Int Suppl*, **72**, S15–S19.

[94] Ronco, C., Bonello, M., Bordoni, V. *et al.* (2004). Extracorporeal therapies in non-renal disease: treatment of sepsis and the peak concentration hypothesis, *Blood Purif*, **22**, 164–174.

[95] Ratanarat, R., Brendolan, A., Piccinni, P. *et al.* (2005). Pulse high-volume haemofiltration for treatment of severe sepsis: effects on hemodynamics and survival, *Crit Care*, **9**, R294–R302.

[96] Ratanarat, R., Brendolan, A., Ricci, Z. *et al.* (2006). Pulse high-volume hemofiltration in critically ill patients: a new approach for patients with septic shock, *Semin Dial*, **19**, 69–74.
[97] Oudemans-van Straaten, H.M., Bosman, R.J. van der Spoel, J.I. *et al.* (1999). Outcome of critically ill patients treated with intermittent high-volume haemofiltration: a prospective cohort analysis, *Intens Care Med*, **25**, 814–821.
[98] Bouman, C.S., Oudemans-van Straaten, H.M., Schultz, M.J. *et al.* (2007). Hemofiltration in sepsis and systemic inflammatory response syndrome: the role of dosing and timing. *J Crit Care*, **22**, 1–12.
[99] Cipolla, C.M., Grazi, S., Rimondini, A. *et al.* (1990). Changes in circulating norepinephrine with hemofiltration in advanced congestive heart failure, *Am J Cardiol*, **66**, 987–994.
[100] Pichette, V., Leblanc, M., Bonnardeaux, A. *et al.* (1994). High dialysate flow rate continuous arteriovenous hemodialysis: a new approach for the treatment of acute renal failure and tumor lysis syndrome, *Am J Kidney Dis*, **23**, 591–596.
[101] Sakarcan, A. and Quigley, R. (1994). Hyperphosphatemia in tumor lysis syndrome: the role of hemodialysis and continuous veno-venous hemofiltration, *Pediatr Nephrol*, **8**, 351–353.
[102] Saccente, S.L., Kohaut, E.C. and Berkow, R.L. (1995). Prevention of tumor lysis syndrome using continuous veno-venous hemofiltration, *Pediatr Nephrol*, **9**, 569–573.
[103] Feinfeld, D.A., Rosenberg, J.W. and Winchester, J.F. (2006). Three controversial issues in extracorporeal toxin removal, *Semin Dial*, **19**, 358–362.
[104] Goodman, J.W. and Goldfarb, D.S. (2006). The role of continuous renal replacement therapy in the treatment of poisoning, *Semin Dial*, **19**, 402–407.
[105] Bambauer, R., Inniger, R., Pirrung, K.J. *et al.* (1994). Complications and side effects associated with large-bore catheters in the subclavian and internal jugular veins, *Artif Organs*, **18**, 318–321.
[106] Kelber, J., Delmez, J.A. and Windus, D.W. (1993). Factors affecting delivery of high-efficiency dialysis using temporary vascular access, *Am J Kidney Dis*, **22**, 24–29.
[107] Jörres, A., Gahl, G.M., Dobis, C. *et al.* (1999). Haemodialysis-membrane biocompatibility and mortality of patients with dialysis-dependent acute renal failure: a prospective randomised multicentre trial, International Multicentre Study Group, *Lancet*, **354**, 1337–1341.
[108] Morgera, S., Heering, P., Szentandrasi, T. *et al.* (1997). Comparison of a lactate-versus acetate-based hemofiltration replacement fluid in patients with acute renal failure, *Ren Fail*, **19**, 155–164.

[109] Barenbrock, M., Hausberg, M., Matzkies, F. *et al.* (2000). Effects of bicarbonate- and lactate-buffered replacement fluids on cardiovascular outcome in CVVH patients, *Kidney Int*, **58**, 1751–1757.

[110] Heering, P., Ivens, K., Thümer, O. *et al.* (1999). The use of different buffers during continuous hemofiltration in critically ill patients with acute renal failure, *Intens Care Med*, **25**, 1244–1251.

[111] Davenport, A. (1997).The coagulation system in the critically ill patient with acute renal failure and the effect of an extracorporeal circuit, *Am J Kidney Dis*, **30** (5, Suppl. 4), S20–S27.

[112] Webb, A.R., Mythen, M.G., Jacobsen, D. *et al.* (1995). Maintaining blood flow in the extracorporeal circuit: haemostasis and anticoagulation, *Intens Care Med*, **21**, 84–93.

[113] Martin, P.Y., Chevrolet, J.C., Suter, P. *et al.* (1994). Anticoagulation in patients treated by continuous venovenous hemofiltration: a retrospective study, *Am J Kidney Dis*, **24**, 806–812.

[114] Ward, D.M. and Mehta, R.L. (1993). Extracorporeal management of acute renal failure patients at high risk of bleeding, *Kidney Int*, **41**, S237–S244.

[115] Metha, R.L. (1998). 'Continuous renal replacement therapy', in Ronco, C. and Bellomo, R. (eds), *Critical Care Nephrology*, Kluwer Academic Publishers, Dordrecht, pp. 1161–1335.

[116] Abramson, S., Niles, J.L. (1999). Anticoagulation in continuous renal replacement therapy, *Curr Opin Nephrol Hypertens*, **8**, 701–707.

[117] Mehta, R.L., Dobos, G.J. and Ward, D.M. (1992). Anticoagulation in continuous renal replacement procedures, *Semin Dial*, **5**, 61–68.

[118] Lamme, S.J. de Rooij, P.D., Huijgens, P.C. *et al.* (1994). The HITT syndrome: heparin-induced thrombocytopenia and thrombosis as a cause of paradoxically occurring thromboembolisms, *Ned Tijdschr Geneeskd*, **138**, 189–193.

[119] Vervloet, M.G. and Nurmohamed, S.A. (2007). How do I use citrate-based CVVH in predilution, *Neth J Crit Care*, **11**, 8–12.

[120] Mehta, R.L., McDonald, B.R., Aguilar, M.M. *et al.* (1990). Regional citrate anticoagulation for continuous arteriovenous hemodialysis in critically ill patients, *Kidney Int*, **38**, 976–981.

[121] Kutsogiannis, D.J., Mayers, I., Chin, W.D.N. *et al.* (2000). Regional citrate anticoagulation in continuous venovenous hemodiafiltration, *Am J Kidney Dis*, **35**, 802–811.

[122] Palsson, R. and Niles, J.L. (1999). Regional citrate anticoagulation in continuous venovenous hemofiltration in critically ill patients with a high risk of bleeding, *Kidney Int*, **55**, 1991–1997.

[123] Nurmohamed, S.A., Vervloet, M.G., Girbes, A.R. *et al.* (2007). Continuous venovenous hemofiltration with or without predilution regional citrate anticoagulation: a prospective study, *Blood Purif*, **25**, 316–323.

[124] Meier-Kriesche, H.U., Finkel, K.W., Gitomer, J.J. *et al.* (1999). Unexpected severe hypocalcemia during continuous venovenous hemodialysis with regional citrate anticoagulation, *Am J Kidney Dis*, **33**, e8.

[125] Meier-Kriesche, H.U., Gitomer, J., Finkel, K. *et al.* (2001). Increased total to ionized calcium ratio during continuous venovenous hemodialysis with regional citrate anticoagulation, *Crit Care Med*, **29**, 748–752.

[126] Monchi, M., Berghmans, D., Ledoux, D. *et al.* (2004). Citrate vs heparin for anticoagulation in continuous venovenous hemofiltration: a prospective randomized study, *Intens Care Med*, **30**, 260–265.

[127] Betjes, M.G., van Oosterom, D., van Agteren, M. *et al.* (2007). Regional citrate versus heparin anticoagulation during venovenous hemofiltration in patients at low risk for bleeding: similar hemofilter survival but significantly less bleeding, *J Nephrol*, **20**, 602–608.

[128] Fealy, N., Baldwin, I., Johnstone, M. *et al.* (2007). A pilot randomized controlled crossover study comparing regional heparinization to regional citrate anticoagulation for continuous venovenous hemofiltration, *Int J Artif Organs*, **30**, 301–307.

[129] Tang, I.Y., Cox, D.S., Patel, K. *et al.* (2005). Argatroban and renal replacement therapy in patients with heparin-induced thrombocytopenia, *Ann Pharmacother*, **39**, 231–236.

[130] Hein, O.V. von Heymann, C., Diehl, T. *et al.* (2004). Intermittent hirudin versus continuous heparin for anticoagulation in continuous renal replacement therapy, *Ren Fail*, **26**, 297–303.

[131] Bishop, G.A., Waugh, J.A. and Hall, B.M. (1988). Expression of, HLA antigens on renal tubular cells in culture II. Effect of increased HLA antigen expression on tubular cell stimulation of lymphocyte activation and on their vulnerability to cell-mediated lysis, *Transplantation*, **46**, 303–310.

[132] Leonard, M., Ryan, M.P., Watson, A.J. *et al.* (1999). Role of, MAP kinase pathways in mediating IL-6 production in human primary mesangial and proximal tubular cells, *Kidney Int*, **56**, 1366–1377.

[133] Yard, B.A., Daha, M.R., Kooymans-Couthino, M. *et al.* (1992). IL-1α stimulated, TNFα production by cultured human proximal tubular epithelial cells, *Kidney Int*, **42**, 383–389.

[134] Humes, H.D., Weitzel, W.F. and Fissell, W.H. (2004). Renal cell therapy in the treatment of patients with acute and chronic renal failure, *Blood Purif*, **22**, 60–72.

[135] Humes, H.D., MacKay, S.M., Funke, A.J. *et al.* (1999). Tissue engineering of a bioartificial renal tubule assist device: *In vitro* transport and metabolic characteristics, *Kidney Int*, **55**, 2502–2514.
[136] Fissell, W.H., Lou, L., Abrishami, S. *et al.* (2003). Bioartificial kidney ameliorates Gram-negative bacteria-induced septic shock in uremic animals, *J Am Soc Nephrol*, **14**, 454–461.
[137] Tumlin, J., Wali, R., Williams, W. *et al.* (2008). Efficacy and safety of renal tubule cell therapy for acute renal failure, *J Am Soc Nephrol*, **19**, 1034–1040.
[138] Trianathanagul, K., Eiam-Ong, S. and Humes, H.D. (2005). The future of renal support: high-flux dialysis to bioartificial kidneys, *Crit Care Clin*, **21**, 379–394.
[139] Uchino, S., Kellum, J.A., Bellomo, R. *et al.* (2005). Acute renal failure in critically ill patients: a multinational, multicenter study, *JAMA*, **294**, 813–818.
[140] Bellomo, R. (2006). The epidemiology of acute renal failure: 1975 versus 2005, *Curr Opin Crit Care*, **12**, 557–560.
[141] Goldberg, R. and Dennen, P. (2008). Long-term outcomes of acute kidney injury, *Adv Chronic Kidney Dis*, **15**, 297–307.
[142] Schiffl, H. and Fischer, R. (2008). Five-year outcomes of severe acute kidney injury requiring renal replacement therapy, *Nephrol Dial Transplant*, **23**, 2235–2241.
[143] Ponte, B., Felipe, C. Muriel, A. *et al.* (2008). Long-term functional evolution after an acute kidney injury: a 10–year study, *Nephrol Dial Transplant*, **23**, 3859–3866.

24

Obstetrics Problems in Intensive Care

Surbi Malhotra

24.1 Introduction

Critically ill obstetric patients present many challenges for intensive care clinicians. Treatment and management requires consideration of two lives: mother and baby. Furthermore, the multiple physiological changes that occur in pregnancy may reduce the normal reserve of organ systems and alter their response to pathological events. Additionally, certain medical conditions are specific to pregnancy and therefore infrequently seen in general critical care settings.

Admission rates to the intensive care are quoted at 0.2–9 per 1,000 deliveries [1,2] with most admissions lasting between three and four days. Mortality data is difficult to ascertain as the usual objective predictability tests are obscured by standard scoring systems (e.g. Acute Physiology and Chronic Health Evaluation (APACHE)) and do not allow for obstetric factors. Despite this, mortality rates in the UK are frequently quoted at approximately 3–4%.

24.2 Physiological Changes of Pregnancy

The management of critically ill obstetric patients requires an understanding of the basic physiological changes that occur during pregnancy. These physiological changes are a result of hormonal factors and the mechanical factors of a gravid uterus.

24.2.1 *Hormonal changes*

Following fertilisation, corpus luteum secretes progesterone, oestrogen and relaxin. After six to eight weeks these hormones are then produced by the placenta.

Progesterone is responsible for most of the hormone-related physiological changes, including:

- Smooth muscle relaxation.
- Vasodilatation.
- Bronchodilation.
- Slowing of the gastrointestinal tract.
- Increase in maternal basal temperature.

24.2.2 *Mechanical changes*

As pregnancy progresses, the uterus enlarges and displaces the diaphragm upwards, compressing the rib cage.

24.2.3 *Cardiovascular changes*

During pregnancy, cardiac output increases by 40–50% [3]. In the first two trimesters, this is a result of an increase in stroke volume, while in the third trimester the increase in cardiac output is mainly due to an increase in heart rate. This is of relevance in pregnant patients with fixed cardiac output states (e.g. severe mitral stenosis) as these patients may not be able to be increase their cardiac output in comparison with normal pregnant patients. During labour, cardiac output increases by another 25–30% as a result of sympathetic nervous system activity. Epidural analgesia attenuates the sympathetic nervous system and may be beneficial in patients with cardiac disease by decreasing pain (and thus stress) on the myocardium.

At 15 to 20 minutes after delivery of the foetus and placenta, a substantial increase in cardiac output occurs as blood is no longer diverted to the uteroplacental vascular bed. Approximately 500 ml of blood is redirected to the maternal circulation due to the 'auto-transfusion' effect of pregnancy. This effect can cause cardiac output to increase by 60–80%. Elevated cardiac output persists for approximately two days postpartum and returns to normal between two weeks and three months.

The release of progesterone during pregnancy results in a decrease in systemic vascular resistance (SVR) and pulmonary vascular resistance (PVR). This is an important consideration for critically ill pregnant patients with sepsis, in which SVR may be decreased secondary to endotoxin. Furthermore, the decrease in PVR may increase shunting in patients with cardiac septal defects.

The heart is dramatically remodelled during pregnancy leading to an enlargement of all four chambers, particularly the left atrium. This may predispose to supraventricular and atrial arrhythmias. The enlarging gravid uterus elevates the diaphragm, causing rotation of the heart upward and to the left. Thus, left axis deviation is seen on the electrocardiogram and cardiomegaly on the chest radiograph.

24.2.4 *Respiratory changes*

Progesterone stimulates the respiratory centre, leading to an increased tidal volume and minute volume. Consequently, arterial partial pressure of CO_2 is lowered to a normal pregnancy level of approximately 4 kPa. Compensation for this primary respiratory alkalosis occurs through excretion of bicarbonate via the kidney.

Functional residual capacity falls to 80% of pre-pregnancy values due to an increased intra-abdominal pressure and upward displacement of the diaphragm by the gravid uterus. Residual volume and expiratory reserve volume both decrease. Total lung capacity is also minimally decreased.

Oxygen consumption increases due to increased metabolic needs of the mother and foetus. A combination of the decreased functional residual capacity and the increased oxygen consumption decreases the total oxygen reserve of the mother. Thus, if apnoea occurs, the onset of hypoxia occurs more rapidly in the pregnant state.

24.2.5 *Haematological changes*

Dilutional anaemia occurs secondary to the increase in plasma volume relative to red blood cell volume [4].

There may be a relative leucocytosis, which may lead to an inappropriate diagnosis of infection.

All procoagulants are increased, including fibrinogen, which increases by 50%. Combined with a reduction in fibrinolysis, these changes contribute to the hypercoagulable state of pregnancy.

The platelet count is unchanged, although a benign condition known as gestational thrombocytopenia may occur in 5–7% of patients.

24.2.6 *Urinary system*

Renal plasma flow and glomerular filtration rate both increase. The increase in glomerular filtration rate approaches 50%, which reduces the upper limit of normal for serum creatinine.

A decrease in both the colloid osmotic pressure and the pulmonary occlusion pressure occurs. This may make pregnant patients more susceptible to fluid overload and pulmonary oedema, especially in the presence of severe preeclampsia.

24.2.7 *Gastrointestinal system*

Progesterone relaxes the lower oesophageal sphincter.

Intragastric pressure rises due to the mechanical effects of the enlarging uterus.

Consequently a decrease in the gastro-oesophageal barrier occurs with an increased risk of regurgitation and aspiration.

Gastric volume is increased and remains so for up to 48 hours after delivery

Gastric emptying is not delayed in pregnancy or in labour. However, if opioids are administered during labour, gastric emptying is reduced.

24.3 Major Obstetric Haemorrhage

Haemorrhage accounts for 30% of maternal mortality worldwide [5] and is the leading cause of maternal death. In the UK, maternal haemorrhage is also a major cause of maternal morbidity, with many deaths resulting from substandard care and failure to recognise women at risk of bleeding [6]. Maternal haemorrhage has been identified as one of the main reasons for admission to the intensive care unit [1].

Several definitions of maternal haemorrhage exist in the literature and it must be remembered that obstetric bleeding is often under-estimated (blood loss is often hidden: blood may be mixed with amniotic fluid, hidden in the vagina or between the legs, or it may be occult, as in placental abruption).

Major obstetric haemorrhage (MOH) should be considered if one or more of the following criteria are fulfilled [7]:

- An estimated blood loss of 2500 ml or more.
- Transfusion of five or more units of blood.
- Coagulopathy which requires treatment.

Obstetric haemorrhage may be antepartum or postpartum. The main antepartum causes are placental abruption or placenta praevia. Uterine atony, retained products and genital tract trauma all cause postpartum haemorrhage and account for over half of all cases of major haemorrhage.

Resuscitation of the patient is the first priority and should involve all members of the labour ward team. A system now exists in many UK hospitals where a 'MOH call' is placed via the main switchboard. This alerts key team members including senior midwife, obstetric registrar and consultant, anaesthetic registrar and consultant, haematologists, blood transfusion laboratory and duty porter.

Recognition of the deteriorating clinical condition is vital for the treatment of any patient with MOH. As these women are often young and healthy, significant physiological compensation occurs. Consequently, the presence of hypotension and peripheral vasoconstriction indicates that significant blood loss has occurred. Blood and blood products should be replaced according to the clinical status of the patient and not based on blood results.

Hypothermia must also be treated aggressively to avoid its detrimental effect on coagulation. All fluids should be warmed and the patient kept warm with active warming devices or warmed blankets.

Diagnosis of the cause of bleeding should be done concomitantly with active continued resuscitation. If a surgical procedure is required, existing hypovolaemia and the presence of a possible coagulopathy may preclude regional anaesthesia and general anaesthesia may be required.

Further control of bleeding may be achieved by pharmacological or surgical methods. Pharmacological measures aid uterine contraction and include:

- Oxytocin, which is the drug of choice [8] for the prevention and treatment of an atonic uterus. Following an initial intravenous bolus of 5–10 units, an infusion of 10 units per hour may be administered.
- Ergometrine is the second-line agent to be used at a dose of 0.5 mg intravenously or intramuscularly. However, it is associated with severe nausea and vomiting and is contraindicated in patients with hypertensive disorders as it significantly elevates blood pressure.
- Hemabate (250 mg intramuscularly, repeated three or four times) is a prostaglandin and a potent smooth muscle constrictor. It has been associated with life-threatening bronchospasm [9] and should be used cautiously.
- Misoprostol is also a prostaglandin and may be administered orally, sublingually or rectally in a dose of 800–1000 μg.

When pharmacological methods fail to control bleeding, surgery must be considered early. Surgical options include aortic compression, uterine or iliac artery ligation or hysterectomy. Embolisation of the uterine arteries under radiological control has been successfully reported with 90% success rates [10] and is recommended for use both in elective placenta praevia/accreta cases [11] and in emergency situations [12]. However, its use must be tempered by the implications of the transferring of a potentially unstable patient to a possibly isolated radiology suite.

Although the use of the blood cell saver is well established in other clinical areas, concerns regarding rhesus immunisation and amniotic fluid embolism initially limited its use in the obstetric population [13]. Amniotic fluid embolism is now thought to be an immunological process rather than an embolic event and there have been no reports of its occurrence whilst using cell salvage. Rhesus immunisation may be avoided by appropriate Kleihauer testing and anti-D treatment.

Recombinant factor VII has been successfully used for intractable haemorrhage [14,15], although it is not currently licensed for use in obstetrics. No standard of practice exists with regards to dose and timing of administration, and it is not a substitute for adequate resuscitation and correction of coagulopathy. Furthermore, the value of its benefit has been questioned by recent case reports of non-responders and its association with thromboembolic complications [16].

Recently, the use of methotrexate in aiding involution of the placenta has been advocated, in circumstances where repeated attempts to remove a very adherent placenta have resulted in catastrophic haemorrhage [17]. However, the use of methotrexate for this purpose is controversial, as bleeding and infection are associated complications.

24.4 Cardiac Disease in Pregnancy

The incidence of cardiac disease in pregnant women is approximately 0.5–1%. Many of these conditions present acutely in women with no known pre-existing disease. In the UK, maternal mortality due to cardiac disease over the last 30 years has more than doubled [18]. There are a number of possible reasons for this, such as the potential that more women with cardiac disease are giving birth, females with congenital heart disease are now surviving to childbearing age [19,20], women with pre-existing disease may be encouraged by advances in medical care to embark on pregnancy, and more women are having children later in life [21–23]. These factors combined with a higher incidence of other cardiac risk factors amongst young women such as smoking and obesity [21–23] may account for the increase in the incidence of ischaemic heart disease and other related cardiac conditions. Identification of risk factors for cardiac disease in women of childbearing age and recognition of acute symptoms during pregnancy and the puerperium may help improve chances of survival in these women.

24.4.1 *Ischaemic heart disease*

Acute myocardial infarction in pregnancy is an uncommon event, and is estimated to have occurred in 6.2 of every 100,000 deliveries in the USA between 2000 and 2002 [24]. Maternal mortality due to acute coronary syndromes (ACS) and ischaemic heart disease (IHD) in the UK has risen four-fold in the last decade. This increase is one of the main reasons why cardiac disease remains the single largest cause of maternal death in the UK.

Management of ACS in pregnancy and the puerperium should be the same as that for non-pregnant patients. In any pregnant woman, who presents with chest pain, a high index of suspicion is necessary. ACS is a condition where the mother should be treated first, whatever the gestational age, as the risk of delivery to the mother with an untreated ACS is high. Close liaison with a cardiologist is mandatory.

The data available on the use of thrombolysis for myocardial infarction in pregnancy is limited, but as the complication rate for thrombolysis for pulmonary embolism in pregnancy is only 1%, thrombolysis should not be withheld from pregnant women, especially if percutaneous stenting is unavailable. Coronary artery bypass grafting in pregnancy is associated with significant maternal mortality (13%) and a high risk of miscarriage (30%).

In a pregnant patient who has been diagnosed with AMI antenatally, no consensus exists with regards to the optimal mode of delivery. Vaginal delivery avoids the stress of surgery and the need for anaesthesia. However, caesarean section may allow time for invasive monitoring to be established and cardiothoracic surgical support to be organised. The benefits of caesarean section need to be considered against the increased risk of bleeding and thromboembolism which occurs with an operative delivery. If vaginal delivery is chosen then epidural analgesia using low-dose local anaesthetic solutions combined with opioids is beneficial as it reduces the cardiovascular stress of labour pain while maintaining haemodynamic stability.

Both regional and general anaesthesia have been used successfully for caesarean section. The main concern with general anaesthesia is the risk of uncontrolled hypertension on intubation and the risk of precipitating arrhythmias. With regional anaesthesia, hypotension induced by a sympathetic blockade may be poorly tolerated in a patient with cardiac disease. Thus, single-shot spinals are avoided. The choice of regional technique would be a low-dose combined spinal-epidural, where the epidural component may be used to incrementally extend the sensory block as necessary. Some clinicians have also reported the use of continuous spinal anaesthesia in these circumstances.

The ideal tocolytic management of the third stage in cardiac patients is a slow infusion of oxytocin. Ergometrine is contraindicated as it results in severe acute hypertension and large boluses of oxytocin may result in hypotension.

Fluid shifts that are associated with the contracting uterus may also contribute to cardiovascular instability in the postpartum period and so the mother should be managed in a high-dependency environment for 48 to 72 hours with invasive monitoring.

24.4.2 *Aortic dissection*

The overall incidence of thoracic aortic aneurysm is estimated to be around 6 per 100,000 patients [25]. There are several heritable disorders that affect the thoracic aorta, predisposing patients to both aneurysm formation and aortic dissection, including Marfan syndrome, bicuspid aortic valve, Ehlers–Danlos syndrome and familial forms of aortic dissection [26]. Although women with such inherited conditions are at higher risk of aortic dissection, normal pregnant women may also suffer from aortic dissection. The physiological changes which result in an elevated cardiac output in pregnancy also increase the susceptibility of pregnant women to aortic dissection. In women who are known to have an enlarged aortic root diameter the risks of pregnancy should be discussed before conception. Counselling is important in all these patients with known aortic pathology and complete clinical evaluation should be performed (including imaging of the entire aorta) if possible, prior to pregnancy [27].

During pregnancy serial echocardiography should be done every six to eight weeks in patients with known aortic pathology. If dilatation of the aorta is diagnosed during pregnancy and prior to 30 weeks gestation then aortic repair before delivery is recommended, as there is no extra risk to the mother compared with the non-pregnant state [27]. After 30 weeks of gestation, caesarean section followed directly by cardiac surgery is the preferred option to save the lives of both the mother and the foetus [28].

If the aortic root is less than 4.5 cm, vaginal delivery may be considered but a prolonged second stage should be avoided [28]. Caesarean section is the optimal method of delivery in women with an aortic root diameter of over 4.5 cm. The use of regional analgesia and anaesthesia, for labour and operative delivery respectively, avoids blood pressure peaks. Concomitant invasive arterial monitoring should also be instituted.

In the acute situation, aortic dissection most frequently occurs in the last trimester of pregnancy or the early postpartum period. The presence of interscapular or chest pain should never be dismissed, as this may be indicative of aortic dissection, especially in the presence of systolic hypertension. Transthoracic echocardiography may show dissection, but more appropriate imaging includes either urgent computed tomography or magnetic resonance imaging [28].

If aortic dissection is diagnosed, then this is a surgical emergency; senior cardiothoracic, cardiology, obstetric and anaesthetic consultants must act rapidly to deliver the foetus (if viable) by caesarean section and proceed directly to repair the dissection. The risk of obstetric bleeding due to anticoagulation during cardiopulmonary bypass must be weighed against the risk of delaying repair of the dissection for a few hours post-delivery.

24.4.3 *Congenital heart disease*

Eighty percent of patients with congenital heart disease now survive to adulthood although mortality is still high, with patients with cyanotic heart disease having a higher mortality than those with non-cyanotic lesions [28].

Identification of patients with congenital heart disease (CHD) is mandatory in early pregnancy. These patients require appropriate antenatal counselling, investigations and a management plan for labour and delivery.

Women with corrected disorders are usually asymptomatic but some may have mild residual pulmonary hypertension.

The clinical condition of patients with cyanotic disorders may worsen during pregnancy due to a combination of increased oxygen requirements and shunting, the latter as a consequence of reduced systemic vascular resistance. Thus, fulminant heart failure may occur as pregnancy progresses.

Management of pregnancy in women with CHD requires a multidisciplinary approach.

Planned caesarean section is not necessary unless there is clinical deterioration in the mother's condition or there are specific obstetric indications. Anaesthesia for caesarean section may be provided by general or regional anaesthesia. For all patients, invasive arterial monitoring should be instituted, except in those with mild conditions.

Anticoagulation and prophylactic antibiotic cover is mandatory for all of these patients.

24.4.4 *Valvular disease*

24.4.4.1 *Mitral stenosis*

In pregnant women, mitral stenosis (MS) is usually secondary to rheumatic heart disease and often presents for the first time during pregnancy when the woman becomes symptomatic. In the UK, there was a decline in the incidence of rheumatic fever in the early 1950s, but the increasing immigrant population has resulted in a recent resurgence of MS. Many mothers who present with MS have communication difficulties and consequently, have poor access to healthcare facilities. These factors, combined with the inexperience of medical staff in diagnosing and managing MS, may lead to failure of diagnosis and a poor outcome. The major risk factors for maternal morbidity and mortality are severe MS and a pre-pregnancy cardiac event. The risk to the foetus (e.g. intrauterine growth restriction, prematurity) depends on the severity of the defect.

MS is poorly tolerated in pregnancy. The increased heart rate and stroke volume of pregnancy, and the poor flow through a stenotic valve results in a high left atrial pressure with an impaired cardiac output [28]. Superimposed atrial fibrillation may exacerbate symptoms and lead to fulminate pulmonary oedema. Pulmonary hypertension and right ventricular failure may occur.

Symptoms of MS may only become apparent as pregnancy progresses. Exertional dyspnoea with a poor exercise tolerance occurs usually in the second trimester. Other symptoms include orthopnoea, dyspnoea and a dry cough.

A chest X-ray may show signs of pulmonary congestion with a dilated left atrium. Transthoracic echocardiogram will allow assessment of the severity of the stenosis, and also reveal any other associated lesions. Valve area is more reliable in identifying the severity of MS than pressure gradient [28].

Treatment involves mainly controlling the heart rate and this is achieved by beta-blockade, a diuretic and bed rest.

If clinical deterioration occurs, then management is dependent on the gestational age of the foetus. The optimal time to make decisions with regards to treatment is usually 26 to 30 weeks gestation [28].

If the foetus is viable then delivery should be expedited followed by definitive management of the MS. If the foetus is not yet mature then balloon mitral valvotomy may be attempted, as this relieves symptoms and allows pregnancy to continue. Vaginal delivery is the preferred mode of delivery.

24.4.4.2 *Aortic stenosis*

In the UK, aortic stenosis (AS) is not a common condition in pregnancy and is usually secondary to a bicuspid aortic valve. Other conditions such as coarctation of the aorta may exist and should be considered in women with AS [28].

AS is well tolerated in pregnancy if mild to moderate disease exists. However, in severe disease an increasing cardiac output through a narrowed valve may present with symptoms of angina, dyspnoea, syncope, pulmonary oedema and even sudden death [28].

In patients with severe AS, termination of pregnancy must be discussed. Medical management is aimed at reducing the heart rate and is best achieved with beta-blockade and bed rest.

If clinical deterioration occurs, management is dependent on the gestational age of the foetus. Treatment options include balloon valvotomy, surgical valvotomy or valve replacement. Balloon valvotomy is usually performed in order to relieve symptoms and to allow the pregnancy to proceed until the foetus is viable. If surgery is necessary then aortic valve replacement is likely to be required. Cardiopulmonary bypass is associated with a high risk of maternal and foetal mortality [29,30] for a number of reasons: maternal tissues are more friable than in the non-pregnant state due to pregnancy-related hormonal changes; placental perfusion is reduced during bypass and there is a risk of placental bleeding as a result of anticoagulation.

In patients not requiring intervention vaginal delivery is the preferred mode of delivery. Invasive arterial monitoring should be established and fluid balance carefully monitored. Antibiotic prophylaxis is mandatory.

24.4.5 *Peripartum cardiomyopathy*

Peripartum cardiomyopathy (PPCM) was first recognised in 1937 by Gouley *et al.* [31] and is still considered to be a cardiomyopathy of unknown aetiology. Associations with a viral myocarditis, an immune-mediated reaction, drugs, familial or nutritional causes have all been suggested [32,34]. The quoted prevalence of PPCM ranges from 1 in 4,000 to 1 in 15,000 [34]. This variation in incidence is due to geographic differences and also disparities in case-reporting. Mortality is significant (9–56%) [35–37] with the majority of deaths occurring in the first three months of the postpartum period. Risk factors for PPCM include advanced maternal age, multiparity, multiple pregnancy, African–American race, preeclampsia and tocolytic therapy [37].

The definition and diagnosis of PPCM is based on the presence of four essential criteria : (i) development of cardiac failure in the last month of pregnancy or within five months after delivery (ii) absence of a demonstrable cause for the cardiac failure, (iii) absence of demonstrable heart disease before the last month of pregnancy and (iv) documented systolic dysfunction [37].

Presentation of PPCM is similar to that of other dilated cardiomyopathies. Dysponoea, orthopnoea, weight gain, fluid retention and fatigue are common features. These symptoms overlap with those of normal late pregnancy. Therefore, it is important that a high index of suspicion be maintained to identify the rare cases of PPCM.

Cardiac investigations are directed at excluding cardiomyopathy secondary to other causes. Transthoracic echocardiogram is crucial. Patients with PPCM exhibit left-ventricular systolic dysfunction, including decreased fractional shortening and a low ejection fraction.

Treatment is the same as for acute and chronic heart failure, with the aim being to optimise preload and decrease afterload. Drugs with teratogenic effects must be avoided when possible if presentation is prior to delivery, and in the postpartum period the presence of drug metabolites in breast milk should be considered.

Treatment involves oxygen, the use of positive inotropes, diuretics and vasodilators. Angiotensin converting enzyme inhibitors may be used in the postpartum period but are contraindicated antenatally due to the risk of renal agenesis in the foetus. The combination of diuretics and vasodilators may cause excessive dehydration leading to placental hypoperfusion, particularly in the already vasodilated pregnant woman. Calcium channel blockers have negative inotropic effects with the exception of amlodipine. Amlodipine has been shown to be beneficial in patients with non-ischaemic cardiomyopathy. If maximum medical therapy is not effective, heart or both heart and lung transplant may be required.

Anticoagulation should be considered for all patients diagnosed with PPCM. A combination of the hypercoagulable state of pregnancy, reduced ejection fraction, stasis and turbulent flow in the dilated heart make the risk of embolic events high in this population.

Early delivery is not necessary if medical management is effective. However, if presentation is antenatal and the mother is decompensating, then delivery must be expedited following stabilisation of the clinical state. Caesarean section may be necessary unless conditions are favourable for induction of labour.

Prognosis of patients with PPCM is dependent on recovery of systolic function. If symptoms persist longer than six months, myocardial damage is probably irreversible and the prognosis consequently poor. Currently there is no consensus with regards to future pregnancies. Patients with residual ventricular dysfunction should be advised that subsequent pregnancies are contraindicated. If after one year there is residual systolic dysfunction then the risk of mortality is 20% in the next pregnancy.

24.4.6 *Pulmonary arterial hypertension*

Pulmonary arterial hypertension (PAH) is the term given to a spectrum of life-threatening conditions characterised by a mean pulmonary artery pressure greater than 25 mmHg at rest or 30 mmHg during exercise.

PAH may be divided into primary and secondary. Eisenmenger's syndrome is the main cause of primary PAH in women of childbearing age, while idiopathic primary PAH is thought to occur more commonly in these women. Secondary PAH is a result of other vascular arterial pulmonary diseases, for example chronic thromboembolic disease, connective tissue diseases, such as scleroderma, and side effects from certain drugs, such as anorectic agents.

Maternal mortality rates due to PAH are high (30–50%) [38,39]. Pregnant patients with PAH have a fixed pulmonary vascular resistance, and so have a limited ability to compensate for the cardiovascular changes of pregnancy. The highest risk of death is usually immediately after delivery, in the first 72 hours postpartum.

Antenatal advice is given to women with existing PAH to avoid pregnancy, but this is often ignored. If a women with PAH becomes pregnant then termination should be offered, although this itself is associated with significant maternal mortality [40].

Pregnant patients with PAH should be managed by a multidisciplinary team throughout pregnancy. Follow-up on a monthly basis at a specialist clinic is necessary with serial transthoracic echocardiogram measurements. Hospital admission is often advised during the second trimester because of the increased risk of preterm labour and possible maternal decompensation as pregnancy progresses.

Treatment is similar to that of the non-pregnant patient. Diuretics are usually avoided during pregnancy, but some patients who develop right heart failure may require diuretics and these can be prescribed under close supervision.

Anticoagulation is mandatory and low-molecular-weight heparin (LMWH) is usually preferred.

The use of pulmonary vasoactive drugs has been described in non-pregnant patients but in the pregnant patient there are particular risks. Endothelin receptor antagonists are teratogenic and so are contraindicated in pregnancy. Although the use of sildenafil has been described in pregnancy without complications, there is limited literature available supporting its use [41]. Prostacyclin is a potent vasodilator of both the pulmonary and systemic circulations. However, the oral preparation is contraindicated in pregnancy and so, if considered to be necessary for treatment, continuous intravenous epoprostenol (prostacyclin) is used. Although nebulised prostacyclin is available, the frequency of treatment leads often to poor compliance.

There are several case reports [42,43] describing the successful use of nitric oxide in the puerpurium. However there is limited data and no randomised controlled trials of the use of nitric oxide in pregnancy. Limitations of the use of nitric oxide include poor tolerance of administration by face mask, platelet inhibition, methemoglobinaemia, and possible formation of toxic nitrite metabolites, as well as the high cost associated with its use.

Other treatment options for PAH include atrial septostomy, pulmonary thromboendarterectomy or lung transplantation. Patients with pulmonary hypertension secondary to known cardiac and respiratory disorders may benefit from therapy specifically targeted at their primary disease, such as treatment of heart failure, biventricular pacing or conventional cardiac surgery. Other therapeutic agents in the future may include lipid-lowering drugs, anti-inflammatory agents, monoclonal antibodies and antiplatelet agents.

24.4.7 *Venous thromboembolic disease*

In the UK, venous thromboembolism (VTE) is the leading cause of maternal mortality and accounts for one-third of all maternal deaths [6]. Many of these deaths are due to either delayed diagnosis and treatment or inadequate treatment [6].

As pregnancy is a hypercoaguable state, the risk of arterial (cerebrovascular accidents and heart disease) and venous thromboses (deep venous thrombosis, pulmonary embolism) is increased by between three-fold and five-fold relative to the non-pregnant population. This hypercoagulable state results from a combination of physical, hormonal and haematological changes. An increase in venous distensibility and capacity secondary to progesterone results in increased venous stasis, which combined with higher level of circulating clotting factors accounts for the increased incidence of VTE in the pregnant state.

Risk factors for VTE include increased maternal age, multiparity, obesity, a family history of deep vein thrombosis or pulmonary embolism (PE), varicose veins, smoking, known antiphospholipid syndrome or any other hypercoagulable state. Several obstetric complications have also been shown to be associated with increased risk of thromboembolic events, including prolonged bed rest, instrument-assisted delivery or surgical delivery, haemorrhage and sepsis.

Clinical suspicion is critical to the diagnosis of VTE in the pregnant woman. Many of the classic symptoms, such as tachycardia, tachypnoea, dyspnoea, and leg swelling, are similar to the symptoms experienced during late normal pregnancy. Therefore, the diagnosis can be confirmed only by objective testing.

The diagnosis of VTE disease during pregnancy is often impaired or delayed by a reluctance to expose a pregnant patient and the foetus to ionising radiation. However, epidemiological studies have demonstrated that for most diagnostic tests, foetal radiation exposure is minimal. Therefore, diagnosis should be made using the same tests as in the non-pregnant patient.

Treatment of acute VTE is similar to the non-pregnant patient and should be started whilst awaiting investigation [44]. Intravenous heparin is often initially used but many randomised trials and meta-analyses have shown that LMWH is as safe and effective as unfractionated heparin (UFH). Studies in non-pregnant patients have shown that long-term LMWH and UFH are as effective and safe as warfarin for the prevention of recurrent VTE. Consequently, warfarin tends to be avoided as it carries a significant teratogenic risk in pregnancy [45]. Higher doses of heparin are generally required in the pregnant population to achieve therapeutic anticoagulation. Heparin requirements increase during pregnancy due to increased circulating levels of heparin binding proteins, increased plasma volume, increased renal clearance, and increased heparin degradation by the placenta [46,47]. The dose requirements may be as high as two times the normal weight-based dose [47].

LMWH has several advantages over UFH: better bioavailabilty, a better safety profile with regard to osteoporosis and thrombocytopenia and the avoidance of frequent activated partial thromboplastin time monitoring. However, the main disadvantage of LMWHs is their longer half-life and so they are not as easily reversed with protamine. Therefore, regional analgesia/anaesthesia may be relatively contraindicated in their presence.

For pulmonary embolism, anticoagulation is the mainstay of therapy but in the event of massive PE, anticoagulation alone may be insufficient. In this situation, supportive care and intravenous anticoagulation should be undertaken without delay. Subsequent treatment options include thrombolytics or open embolectomy.

Inferior vena cava (IVC) filter placement has been described but is felt to be contraindicated in pregnancy by some authors as IVC filters are associated with a small but significant risk of complications. Risks include migration of the filter, perforation of the aorta, duodenum, or renal pelvis and penetration of nearby structures, including vertebrae and the retroperitoneum. For these reasons, retrievable filters may be a good option in the pregnant population who are young and have a higher risk of long-term complications from an indwelling filter. These retrievable filters must be removed within a short time period, although removal may cause a second embolic event.

24.5 Asthma

The incidence of asthma is increasing, and thus it is one of the most common medical conditions seen in pregnancy, occurring in approximately 1–7% of all pregnancies [48].

The effects of asthma on pregnancy are inconclusive. Some studies have found no difference in birth outcomes between asthmatic and non-asthmatic women [49] while other studies have demonstrated increased adverse outcomes, such as intrauterine growth restriction and preterm labour and delivery [50,51] with poorly controlled asthma. The effect of pregnancy on the course of asthma is also unpredictable [51]. Asthma has been reported to worsen, improve or remain unchanged during pregnancy.

Signs and symptoms and the treatment of an acute asthmatic attack in pregnancy are similar to that of a non-pregnant patient. Although an acute attack is unlikely during labour, regular inhaled drugs should be continued during this time. Furthermore, if the mother has been on long-term steroids, a parenteral dose of steroids should be given during labour. Certain drugs used to treat an acute attack, for example magnesium, may cause uterine relaxation and are relatively contraindicated. In contrast, high-dose β2 agonists and theophylline may delay delivery. Caution also should be exerted when administering drugs to contract the uterus as some drugs are associated with bronchospasm (for example prostaglandins). Intubation and mechanical ventilation may be needed in pregnant women with life-threatening asthma. The principles of mechanical ventilation in pregnant patients with severe acute asthma are similar to those for the non-pregnant patient.

24.6 Amniotic Fluid Embolism

The prevalence of amniotic fluid embolism has been quoted as 7.7 per 100,000 births with a fatality rate of 21% [52,53]. Risk factors for amniotic fluid embolism include induction of labour with oxytoxic drugs, for example syntocinon, multiparity, increased gestational age and male foetus.

Although the first case of amniotic fluid embolism (AFE) was described in 1926 [54], its pathophysiology still remains unclear. AFE usually occurs when there is a breach in the barrier between the maternal circulation and amniotic fluid. The route of entry is thought to be via the endocervical veins, either at the placental site or at a site where there has been uterine trauma [55]. The syndrome of AFE is now considered as an anaphylactoiod rather than an embolic process. Amniotic fluid has several components including desquamated skin cells, lanugo hair, prostaglandins and arachidonic acid metabolites [56]. It is the arachidonic acid metabolites which are thought to be involved in the inflammatory process of AFE, and are the same metabolites which have been associated in anaphylaxis [56]. Thus AFE is linked with a humoural mechanism.

AFE is a diagnosis of exclusion and presents with maternal collapse. Signs and symptoms include dyspnoea, cyanosis, hypotension, dysrhythmias or massive haemorrhage secondary to disseminated intravascular coagulopathy [56]. Signs of foetal distress may precede maternal collapse and may be a subtle indicator of AFE [56].

Management is supportive and requires maintenance of oxygenation, circulatory support and correction of the coagulopathy. In severe cases, the initial hypoxemia is often so profound that irreversible neurological injury may result despite appropriate resuscitative measures.

Treatment of hemodynamic instability includes optimisation of preload with fluids and restoring aortic perfusion pressure with vasopressors, such as norepinephrine, and inodilators, such as dobutamaine.

Disseminated intravascular coagulation (DIC) may cause massive haemorrhage and so replacement of blood loss with packed red blood cells is priority in order to maintain oxygenation of the tissues. Plasma and platelets are given as replacement therapy. Uterine atony is a common feature due to the associated DIC and should be managed with appropriate uterotonic drugs and surgery (see Section 24.3).

In 65% of cases of AFE, the baby has not been delivered [56]. Thus, delivery should be expedited to aid maternal resuscitation and to prevent further harm to the foetus.

Small case reports of newer techniques (e.g. intravenous high-dose steroids [57], inhaled nitric oxide [57], inhaled prostacyclin [57], cardiopulmonary bypass [58], extracorporeal membrane oxygenation [59] and plasma exchange transfusions [60]) have been described for the treatment of AFE.

The prognosis and mortality of AFE have improved significantly due to the earlier recognition of symptoms and prompt resuscitation. Although mortality rates have declined, there is still a significant morbidity (commonly hypoxic neurological impairment) associated with AFE, and the syndrome remains unpreventable.

References

[1] Hazelgrove, J.F., Price, C., Pappachan, J.V. *et al.* (2001). Multicenter study of obstetric admissions to 14 intensive care units in southern England, *Crit Care Med*, **29**, 770–775.

[2] Soubra, S.H. and Guntupalli, K.K. (2005). Critical illness in pregnancy: an overview, *Crit Care Med*, **33** (Suppl. 10), S248–S255.

[3] Pritchard, J.A. (1965). Changes in the blood volume during pregnancy and delivery, *Anesthesiology*, **26**, 393–399.

[4] Silver, H.M., Seebeck, M. and Carlson, R. (1998). Comparison of total blood in normal, preeclamptic, and nonproteinuric gestational hypertensive pregnancy by simultaneous measurement of red blood cell and plasma volumes, *Am J Obstet Gynecol*, **179**, 87–93.

[5] International Confederation of Midwives and International Federation of Gynecology and Obstetrics (2006). *Prevention and treatment of postpartum haemorrhage. New advances for low resource settings, joint statement*, ICM, The Hague/IFGO, London, [Online]. Available at: www.pphprevention.org/files/FIGO-ICM_Statement_November2006_Final.pdf [Accessed 31 January 2013].

[6] Confidential Enquiries into Maternal and Child Health (2007). *Saving Mothers' Lives: Reviewing Maternal Deaths to Make Motherhood Safer: 2003–2005*, Royal College of Obstetricians and Gynaecologists, London.

[7] Wise, A. and Clark, V. (2008). Strategies to manage major obstetric haemorrhage, *Curr Opin Anaesthesiol*, **21**, 281–287.

[8] European Project on obstetric Haemorrhage Reduction: Attitudes, Trial, and Early warning System (EUPHRATES) Group, European consensus on prevention and management of postpartum haemorrhage, [Online]. Available at: http://www.euphrates.inserm.fr/inserm/euphrates.nsf/AllDocumentsByUNID/95A14F46F31A5246C125707400485AED?OpenDocument&l=3.1. [Accessed 1 February 2013].

[9] Harber, C., Levy, D., Chidambaram, S. *et al.* (2007). Life threatening bronchospasm after intramuscular carboprost for postpartum haemorrhage, *BJOG*, **114**, 366–368.

[10] Sundaram, R., Brown, A.G., Koteeswaran, S.K. *et al.* (2006). Anaesthetic implications of uterine artery embolisation in management of massive obstetric haemorrhage, *Anaesthesia*, **61**, 248–252.

[11] Royal College of Obstetricians and Gynaecologists (2005). *Placenta praevia and placenta praevia accreta: diagnosis and management, The Royal College of Obstetricians and Gynaecologists Guideline, No. 27*, [Online]. Available at; http://www.aogm.org.mo/assets/Uploads/aogm/Guidelines/RCOG — UK/GT27-Placenta-Previa-Accreta-2005.pdf. [Accessed 1 February 2013].

[12] Royal College of Obstetricians and Gynaecologists, (2007). *The role of emergency and elective interventional radiology in postpartum haemorrhage Royal College of Obstetricians and Gynaecologists, Good Practice Guideline No. 6*, [Online]. Available at: http://www.rcog.org.uk/files/rcog-corp/uploaded-files/GoodPractice6RoleEmergency2007.pdf [Accessed 1 February 2013].

[13] Catling, S. and Joels, L. (2005). Cell salvage in obstetrics: the time has come, *BJOG*, **112**, 131–132.

[14] Franchini, M. (2007). The use of recombinant activated factor VII in obstetric and gynaecological haemorrhage, *BJOG*, **114**, 8–15.

[15] Haynes, J., Laffan, M. and Platt, F. (2007). Use of recombinant factor VIIa in massive postpartum haemorrhage, *Int J Obstet Anesth*, **16**, 40–49.

[16] Karalpillai, D. and Popham, P. (2007). Recombinant factor VIIa in massive postpartum haemorrhage, *Int J Obstet Anesth*, **16**, 29–34.

[17] Timmermans, S., Arjanneke, C. and Duvekot, J. (2007). Conservative management of abnormally invasive placentation, *Obstet Gynecol Surv*, **62**, 529–539.

[18] Malhotra, S. and Yentis, S.M. (2006). Reports on Confidential Enquiries into Maternal Deaths: management strategies based on trends in maternal cardiac deaths over 30 years, *Int J Obstet Anesth*, **15**, 223–226.

[19] Iserin, L. (2001). Management of pregnancy in women with congenital heart disease, *Heart*, **85**, 493–494.

[20] Ayoub, C., Jalbout, M. and Baraka, A. (2002). The pregnant cardiac woman, *Curr Opin Anaesthesiol*, **15**, 285–291.

[21] Lewis, G. (ed.). (2004). *Why Mothers Die 2000–2002. The Sixth Report on Confidential Enquiries into Maternal Deaths in the United Kingdom*, Royal College of Obstetricians and Gynaecologists, London.

[22] Royal College of Obstetricians and Gynaecologists (1998). *Why Mothers Die 1994–96. Report on Confidential Enquiries into Maternal Deaths in the United Kingdom*. Royal College of Obstetricians and Gynaecologists, London.

[23] Lewis, G. and Drife, J. (2001). *Why Mothers Die 1997–99. Report on Confidential Enquiries into Maternal Deaths in the United Kingdom*. Royal College of Obstetricians and Gynaecologists, London.

[24] James, A.H., Jamison, M.G., Biswas, M.S. *et al.* (2006). Acute myocardial infarction in pregnancy: a United States population-based study, *Circulation*, **113**, 1564–1571.

[25] Roos-Hesselink, J.W., Duvekot, J.J. and Thorne, S.A. (2009). Pregnancy in high risk cardiac conditions, *Heart*, **95**, 680–686.

[26] Niwa, K., Perloff, J.K., Bhuta, S.M. *et al.* (2001). Structural abnormalities of great arterial walls in congenital heart disease: light and electron microscopic analyses, *Circulation*, **103**, 393–400.

[27] Yentis, S.M., May, A. and Malhotra, S. (2007). *Analgesia Anaesthesia and Pregnancy*, second edition, Cambridge University Press, Cambridge.

[28] Steer, P.J., Gatzoulis, M.A. and Baker, P. (2006). *Heart Disease and Pregnancy*, Royal College of Obstetricians and Gynaecologists Press, London.

[29] Parry, A.J. and Westaby, S. (1996). Cardiopulmonary bypass during pregnancy, *Ann Thorac Surg*, **61**, 1865–1869.

[30] Chambers, C.E. and Clark, S.L. (1994). Cardiac surgery during pregnancy, *Clin Obstet Gynecol*, **37**, 316–323.

[31] Gouley, B.A., McMillan, T.M. and Bellet, S. (1937). Idiopathic myocardial degeneration associated with pregnancy and especially the peripartum, *Am J Med Sci*, **19**, 185–199.

[32] Pearson, G.D., Veille, J.C., Rahimtoola, S. *et al.* (2000). Peripartum cardiomyopathy: National Heart Lung and Blood Institute and Office of Rare Diseases (National Institutes of Health) workshop recommendations and review, *JAMA*, **283**, 1183–1188.

[33] Murali, S. and Baldisseri, M.R. (2005). Peripartum cardiomyopathy, *Crit Care Med*, **33**, S340–S346.

[34] Witlin, A.G., Mable, W.C. and Sibai, B.M. (1997). Peripartum cardiomyopathy: an ominous diagnosis, *Am J Obstet Gynecol*, **176**, 182–188.

[35] James, P.R. (2004). A review of peripartum cardiomyopathy, *Int J Clin Pract*, **58**, 363–365.
[36] Elkayam, U. Akhter, M.W., Singh, H. *et al.* (2005). Pregnancy-associated cardiomyopathy, Clinical characteristics and a comparison between early and late presentation, *Circulation*, **111**, 2050–2055.
[37] Demakis, J.G., Rahimtoola, S.H., Sutton, G.C. *et al.* (1971). Natural course of peripartum cardiomyopathy, *Circulation*, **44**,1053–1061.
[38] Weiss, B., Zemp, L., Seifert, B. *et al.* (1998). Outcome of pulmonary vascular disease in pregnancy: a systemic overview from 1978 through 1996, *J Am Coll Cardiol*, **31**, 1650–1657.
[39] Weiss, B. and Hess, O. (2000). Pulmonary vascular disease and pregnancy: current controversies, management strategies and perspectives, *Eur Heart J*, **21**, 104–115.
[40] La, Cassie, H., Germain, A., Valdes, G. *et al.* (2004). Management of Eisenmenger syndrome in pregnancy with sildenafil and l-arginine, *Obstet Gynecol*, **103**, 1118–20.
[41] Madden, B.P. (2009). Pulmonary hypertension and pregnancy, *Int J Obstet Anesth*, **18**, 156–164.
[42] Lam, G.K., Stafford, R.E., Thorp, J. *et al.* (2001). Inhaled nitric oxide for primary pulmonary hypertension in pregnancy, *Obstet Gynecol*, **98**, 895–898.
[43] Decoene, C., Bourzoufi, K., Moreau, D. *et al.* (2001). Use of inhaled nitric oxide for emergency, Cesarean section in a woman with unexpected primary pulmonary hypertension, *Can J Anaesth*, **48**, 584–587.
[44] Royal College of Obstetricians and Gynaecologists (2004). Thromboprophylaxis during pregnancy, labour and after vaginal delivery, Guideline no. 37, [Online]. Available at: http://www.neonatalformulary.com/pdfs/uk_guidelines/ENOXAPARIN-thromboprophylaxis_in_pregnancy_guideline.pdf. [Accessed 1 February 2013].
[45] Duhl, A.J., Paidas, M.J., Ural, S.H. *et al.* (2007). Antithrombotic therapy and pregnancy: consensus report and recommendations for prevention and treatment of venous thromboembolism and adverse pregnancy outcomes, *Am J Obstet Gynecol*, **197**, 457e1–457e21.
[46] Hirsh, J., Warkentin, T.E, Shaughnessy, S.G. *et al.* (2001). Heparin and low-molecular-weight heparin: mechanisms of action, pharmacokinetics, dosing, monitoring, efficacy, and safety, *Chest*, **119**, 64S–94S.
[47] Barbour, L.A., Smith, J.M. and Marlar, R.A. (1995). Heparin levels to guide thromboembolism prophylaxis during pregnancy, *Am J Obstet Gynecol*, **173**, 1869–1873.

[48] Kwon, H.L., Belanger, K. and Bracken, M.B. (2003). Asthma prevalence among pregnant and childbearing-aged women in the United States: Estimates from national health surveys, *Ann Epidemiol*, **13**, 317–324.
[49] Jana, N., Vasishta, K., Saha, S.C. *et al.* (1995). Effect of bronchial asthma on the course of pregnancy, labor and perinatal outcome, *J Obstet Gynaecol (Tokyo)*, **21**, 227–232.
[50] Lao, T.T. and Huengsburg, M. (1990). Labor and delivery in mothers with asthma, *Eur J Obstet Gynecol Reprod Biol*, **35**, 183–190.
[51] Liu, S., Wen, S.W., Demissie, K. *et al.* (2001). Maternal asthma and pregnancy outcomes: a retrospective cohort study, *Am J Obstet Gynecol*, **184**, 90–96.
[52] Burrows, A. and Khoo, S.K. (1995). The amniotic fluid embolism syndrome: 10 years' experience at a major teaching hospital, *Aust N Z J Obstet Gynaecol*, **35**, 245–250.
[53] Gilbert, W.M. and Danielsen, B. (1999). Amniotic fluid embolism: decreased mortality in a population-based study, *Obstet Gynecol*, **93**, 973–977.
[54] Meyer, J.R. (1926). Embolia pulmonar amnio caseosa, *Bras Med*, **2**, 301–303.
[55] Courtney, L.D. Amniotic fluid embolism, *Obstet Gynecol Surv*, (1974). **29**, 169–177.
[56] Moore, J. and Baldisseri, M.R. (2005). Amniotic fluid embolism, *Crit Care Med*, **33**, S279–S285.
[57] Davies, S. (2001). Amniotic fluid embolism: A review of the literature, *Can J Anaesth*, **48**, 88–98.
[58] Stanten, R.D., Iverson, L.I., Daugharty, T.M. *et al.* (2003). Amniotic fluid embolism causing catastrophic pulmonary vasoconstriction: Diagnosis by transesophageal echocardiogram and treatment by cardiopulmonary bypass, *Obstet Gynecol*, **102**, 496–498.
[59] Hsieh, Y.Y., Chang, C.C., Li, P.C. *et al.* (2000). Successful application of extracorporeal membrane oxygenation and intraaortic balloon counterpulsation as lifesaving therapy for a patient with amniotic fluid embolism, *Am J Obstet Gynecol*, **183**, 496–497.
[60] Awad, I.T. and Shorten, G.D. (2001). Amniotic fluid embolism and isolated coagulopathy: Atypical presentation of amniotic fluid embolism, *Eur J Anaesthesiol*, **18**, 410–413.

25
Paediatric Intensive Care

Simon Nadel

25.1 Principles of Paediatric Intensive Care

There is strong evidence that critically ill children should be cared for in regional, specialised paediatric intensive care units (PICUs) rather than in small local units or with adults in general units [1].

Patients admitted to PICUs represent a broad range of age groups and disease states. Optimal care for the unique needs of the critically ill infant, child or adolescent occurs best in an intensive care environment specifically designed for children, and separate from neonatal and adult facilities. It also requires coordinated multidisciplinary care by physicians, nurses, allied medical professions and others, including pharmacists, social workers, chaplains, nutritionists and therapists.

The speciality is young, and the first dedicated PICUs were founded in the 1970s and 1980s when this need for specialised care for critically ill children was recognised. The development of the speciality of paediatric critical care medicine paralleled the development and specialisation of the PICUs.

Although changes in paediatric care have paralleled many of the developments in medical care for adults, there have been some important differences:

- In most units in the developed world, the paediatric intensivist, rather than organ-specific specialists, takes primary responsibility for the care of the critically ill child in the PICU, with consultation from the organ

specialist. This has led the shift from an anaesthetic emphasis to a paediatric emphasis in the consultant-led delivery of the paediatric critical care service, particularly in the UK and USA.
- Because of the smaller number of critically ill children (approximately one PICU bed is required per 40,000 of the population, assuming an 80% occupancy rate), significant case-mix fluctuations occur throughout the year [2].
- Trauma is more common during school holidays and particularly the summer months. Medical admissions and respiratory complications are more common in the winter months, leading to a seasonal increase in the average length of stay. For this reason, organisation of paediatric critical care units is provided in a more centralised and coordinated fashion than with adult units, with a higher throughput and greater critical mass to ensure higher quality care and education and training opportunities for staff.
- The relatively smaller numbers of seriously ill children has resulted in more regionalised care, and possibly more collaborative interaction between medical and surgical paediatric specialists.

Paediatric intensivists are typically involved in the care, both medical and surgical, of all critically ill children in their institution and coordinate all aspects of their care. As a consequence, the PICU and its multidisciplinary team are major components of regional and hospital planning and operations. In this function, the PICU provides a resource for an entire health system, with inreach and outreach education, clinical training opportunities, coordination of care for all expected and unexpected paediatric critical illness within the whole health sector, from tertiary, secondary and primary care providers and other specialists [3].

25.2 Neonatal Sepsis

Generally, neonatal intensive care units (ICUs) admit newborns who have conditions related to prematurity or delivery, or who have congenital anatomical abnormalities.

The neonatal population (infants aged 0–28 days) is a very distinct group of patients, even when compared with other paediatric age groups.

They have unique physiology and pathology, hence the need for specialist neonatal ICUs.

Neonates are especially prone to infection, and sepsis is one of the leading causes of neonatal mortality. They have immature host-defence mechanisms, leading to infection with a unique range of pathogens. Infection in the neonate may present as systemic sepsis, or a localised infection such as pneumonia, meningitis or, more rarely, septic arthritis, osteomyelitis or cellulitis.

25.2.1 *Host defence*

Both the innate and specific components of the immune system start developing in foetal life. However, these are not yet fully mature by the time of birth.

Specific immunity is mediated via T and B lymphoid cells. At birth, the neonate has adequate numbers of T-cells, but a majority of these are 'naïve' having not had antigenic exposure [4,5]. These cells are also relatively poorly responsive in terms of cytotoxicity and cytokine production [6]. Neonates also have low levels of the major classes of immunoglobulins (Igs), and indeed the presence of IgM at, or soon after birth is suggestive of infection. IgG is transferred across the placenta, so the newborn infant will have high levels of maternal IgG conferring passive immunity, but these levels fall after birth. IgM is the first immunoglobulin to be produced, and there is comparatively slow class switching to IgG production. Adult levels of IgM, IgG and IgA are found by one year, five years and adolescence respectively [7].

Innate immunity is also immature at birth. The number of circulating neutrophils at birth is similar to adult levels, but there is low bone marrow reserve [8], explaining the neutropenia often observed in neonatal sepsis. Neonatal neutrophils are also relatively ineffective in phagocytosis and bacteriolysis. Complement levels are comparatively low at birth and activity is about 25–50% of maternal level, reducing effectiveness of opsonisation and bacteriolysis.

Therefore, the neonate is particularly prone to sepsis, and when infection occurs it can progress quickly [9].

25.2.2 *Presentation of neonatal sepsis*

Signs of early sepsis in the neonate are wide ranging and non-specific, and there needs to be a low threshold in these infants for further observation, investigation and treatment. Neonates are poor at localising their signs and symptoms, and in most cases systemic and localised infections cannot be distinguished on history and examination alone.

Symptoms include poor feeding, excessive sleepiness, vomiting, temperature instability, respiratory distress or a baby who is 'not quite their normal self'. The history should include specific questions about perinatal risk factors for sepsis. On examination the baby may be irritable, tachypnoeic with signs of respiratory distress and tachycardic with poor perfusion. Hypotension in any child is a late sign of shock, and care should be taken not to be overly reassured by a normal blood pressure.

25.2.3 *Early- and late-onset neonatal sepsis*

Neonatal sepsis can be divided into early-onset neonatal sepsis (EONS) and late-onset neonatal sepsis (LONS). There is little consensus whether EONS is defined as that occurring within the first 72 hours of life or within the first 7 days but whichever definition is used, a majority of cases present within the first 24 hours of life [10] whereas LONS is that occurring up to 28 days of age. EONS is usually caused by organisms that have been acquired from the mother's genital tract during birth (Table 25.1). It most often takes the form of septicaemia or pneumonia. In contrast, LONS presents more frequently as meningitis. However, the mortality rate in LONS is lower when compared with EONS.

25.2.4 *Investigations*

Blood work up should include a full blood count and C-reactive protein (CRP) measurement. In infants with sepsis, the neutrophil count may be elevated or reduced. There is often thrombocytopenia, and the CRP may be raised. Blood cultures should be taken. Active efforts should be made to look for focal infection, and chest X-ray, sterile urine collection and lumbar puncture should be done in all cases where there is suspected sepsis.

Table 25.1. Most common bacterial causes of neonatal sepsis.

Organism	Type of infection
Group B β-haemolytic streptococcus (Causes early- and late-onset sepsis)	Sepsis Meningitis Pneumonia Osteomyelitis Septic arthritis Cellulitis
Escherichia coli (Causes early- and late-onset sepsis)	Sepsis Meningitis Pneumonia Osteomyelitis Septic arthritis
Listeria monocytogenes (Causes early- and late-onset sepsis)	Sepsis Meningitis
Streptococcus pneumoniae	Sepsis Meningitis Pneumonia
Staphylococcus aureus	Sepsis Osteomyelitis Septic arthritis Cellulitis
Other Gram-negative organisms (including *Pseudomomas*, *Serratia*, *Klebsiella*, *Salmonella*, *Meningococcus*, *Haemophilus*) (Causes early- and late-onset sepsis)	Sepsis Meningitis Pneumonia Osteomyelitis Septic arthritis
Coagulase-negative *Staphylococcus*	Nosocomial infections due to indwelling catheters

These samples should preferably be taken prior to starting antibiotics unless their collection is going to delay the initiation of treatment.

25.2.5 *Treatment*

Antibiotics should be started as soon as suspicion of sepsis is raised, pending the results of investigations. Consideration should be made of the likely organism, but a common empiric regimen would be benzylpenicillin (a third-generation cephalosporin is a suitable alternative, especially if meningitis is suspected) together with an aminoglycoside such as Gentamicin.

25.2.6 *Group B β-haemolytic streptococcus (GBS)*

This is the commonest cause of neonatal sepsis, and has an incidence of nearly 1 in 1,000 live births in the UK [11]. The mortality rate is approximately 10%. Treatment is with intravenous benzylpenicillin, with gentamicin, or a third-generation cephalosporin; the length of treatment depending on the site of infection, with a longer treatment course being recommended for meningitis.

GBS is a commensal organism in the genital tract and perineal area of adults. Around 10–20% of pregnant women in Western Europe are colonised, although rates vary widely in other parts of the world [12]. Not all babies of colonised mothers become colonised, and only a proportion of these babies become infected. Table 25.2 shows some risk factors for babies becoming infected with GBS.

Intrapartum antibiotics are used to reduce the risk of neonatal sepsis in the presence of any of the above risk factors [13].

25.2.7 *Listeria monocyogenes*

Neonatal listeria is acquired tranplacentally, and has become rare in the UK since the introduction of advice to pregnant women to avoid eating unpasteurised foods. There are approximately 20 to 30 pregnancy-related cases in the UK annually [14].

Table 25.2. Risk factors for neonatal GBS sepsis.

Preterm delivery (< 37 weeks gestation)
Prolonged rupture of membranes (> 18 hours)
Maternal fever during labour (> 38°C)
Known vaginal carriage of GBS, or GBS bacteriuria during pregnancy
Birth of a previous infant infected with GBS

Listeriosis may be asymptomatic in the mother, or she may have a flu-like illness. Maternal listeria infection can result in preterm labour (often with meconium-stained liquor, an otherwise rare phenomenon in preterm labour) and severe EONS or meningitis, which is potentially fatal. The treatment is with amoxicillin (or ampicillin) together with an aminoglycoside.

25.2.8 *Herpes simplex virus (HSV) infection*

HSV can be acquired perinatally and is potentially fatal. It is sometimes transmitted transplacentally, but is more usually transmitted at the time of delivery from a mother with primary genital HSV infection. It can also be transmitted from a mother with recurrent genital HSV at the time of birth, or following delivery, although in this scenario neonatal HSV infection is less common due to passive immunity acquired by the infant transplacentally.

Neonatal HSV infection may present in three possible ways:

(i) Skin, eye or mouth disease.
(ii) Central nervous system involvement (Meningoencephalitis).
(iii) Disseminated HSV, with or without central nervous system involvement.

Skin eye or mouth disease, once treated, has a good outcome. The mortality of HSV encephalitis is around 15%, and among the survivors there is a high risk of neurological sequelae.

Disseminated HSV presents as systemic sepsis, usually in the second week of life with non-specific features of sepsis such as vomiting, poor feeding and lethargy. The typical skin lesions may be present, but by no means in every case. Shock may be present, and there is often lung (pneumonitis) and liver involvement (causing enzyme derangement and coagulopathy). There is not always a history of maternal HSV infection, so a high index of suspicion is needed in any neonate presenting with shock/sepsis. Treatment is with high-dose intravenous acyclovir. Even with aggressive treatment, disseminated HSV is often fatal.

25.2.9 *Necrotising enterocolitis (NEC)*

This is not strictly speaking an infection, but is considered here as it often presents with features similar to those of neonatal sepsis.

NEC is an inflammatory process in the bowel, with mucosal ulceration and, in some cases, bowel perforation. It is a disease unique to neonates, most commonly those born prematurely.

The cause of NEC is unknown, although there is an association with the type of feed, as it is very rare in the infant exclusively being fed breast milk. It presents with signs of neonatal sepsis, along with abdominal signs, such as abdominal distension and tenderness, bilious vomiting and rectal bleeding. Septicaemia from bowel flora occurs in 33% of cases. Abdominal radiography may reveal dilated bowel loops in early disease. As it progresses, pneumatosis coli (gas in the bowel wall), portal vein gas or signs of bowel perforation may be seen. Treatment is initially supportive with antibiotics and the withholding of enteral feeds. Intensive care with respiratory and cardiovascular support is often necessary. Surgical treatment is necessary if there are signs of bowel perforation.

25.2.10 *The preterm baby*

A majority of the workload in neonatal units in the developed world is due to preterm delivery. These babies are more prone to sepsis for a number of reasons. They have low levels of maternally acquired IgG [15], lower complement levels [9] and lower total neutrophil cell mass [8] when compared with term infants. They also have prolonged hospital admissions and often have indwelling central venous catheters to facilitate intravenous feeding, thus increasing the risk of nosocomial infection.

25.3 Advanced Ventilatory Techniques in Infants and Children

In this section we will discuss some less widely used methods of ventilatory support and adjuncts frequently used in critically ill infants and children.

25.3.1 *High frequency oscillatory ventilation (HFOV)*

HFOV is a useful alternative to conventional ventilation. There is most experience with its use in neonates, especially those with surfactant deficiency, and in these cases it is sometimes used as the first-line ventilatory strategy. In older children it is more usually used where excessively high ventilation pressures are needed to maintain adequate oxygenation or gas exchange on a conventional ventilator. It is also considered as a 'lung protective' ventilation mode as there is less pressure change throughout the respiratory cycle and less barotrauma and volutrauma when compared with conventional ventilation [16].

HFOV is based on a high airway pressure with small tidal volumes and a very high respiratory rate. The oscillation is created by rapidly alternating gas flow, which is forced in and withdrawn actively by a piston or diaphragm travelling backwards and forwards. It is unique in the fact that expiration as well as inspiration is active. The amplitude of the oscillation (known as delta Pressure) creates the tidal volume. This is small as compared with conventional ventilation, and approximates the dead space at 1–3 ml/kg. The frequency is high, at rates of between 3 and 20 Hz (180–1200 breaths/min). The inspiratory time is set at 33%, giving an inspiration:expiration ratio of 1:2. Using higher inspiratory times has been shown to cause distal alveolar pressure in excess of proximal pressure.

Alveolar ventilation (or minute volume) can be expressed as (rate) × (tidal volume) [17].

Thus, at such frequencies, the tidal volume influences carbon dioxide removal more than the rate. Therefore, in order to reduce arterial carbon dioxide levels, the amplitude should be increased. The equation would also suggest that increasing the rate would improve alveolar ventilation. However, at increasing rates, the inspiratory time decreases and oscillations become less efficient, thereby reducing tidal volume and reducing carbon dioxide clearance.

Oxygenation is determined primarily by the mean airway pressure, which leads to alveolar recruitment. Optimal mean airway pressure and lung volume is that at which there is the best oxygenation. This is achieved by gradually increasing the mean airway pressure. However, there is a possibility of overdistension, which causes worsening oxygenation.

25.3.2 *Negative-pressure ventilation*

This is a form of non-invasive ventilation. Negative pressure was initially used with the 'iron lung' in the 1950s for the treatment of muscle weakness associated with the polio epidemic.

Nowadays, negative-pressure respiratory support is most often delivered via a cuirass, a plastic jacket, which is worn over the torso. It can either be used as an aid to weaning from the ventilator or as a strategy to prevent the need for invasive ventilation. It can also be used as long-term home ventilation, most commonly in children with neuromuscular disorders.

Negative-pressure respiratory support can either be used as continuous negative pressure (CNEP) or in a biphasic mode. In the biphasic mode, inspiration is controlled by negative pressure and expiration is active, controlled by positive pressure.

Negative-pressure ventilation has been shown to improve pulmonary blood flow in patients following Fontan procedure [17]. In infants with respiratory distress syndrome, negative pressure has been shown to reduce respiratory rate and to increase lung compliance in the face of a low baseline compliance [18]. In this group of patients, negative pressure can reduce the rate of invasive ventilation and the total duration of oxygen therapy [19]. Currently, however, there is not enough evidence to support the use of CNEP in preference to non-invasive positive pressure ventilation in children with respiratory failure [20].

25.3.3 *Inhaled nitric oxide therapy*

Inhaled nitric oxide (iNO) is a potent, selective, pulmonary vasodilator that can be used in pulmonary hypertension to reduce pulmonary vascular resistance. Nitric oxide is synthesised by most cells in the human body and leads to decreased intracellular calcium, causing smooth muscle cell relaxation and pulmonary arteriolar vasodialtion.

iNO is generally used in conjunction with mechanical ventilation. It is used in doses of 5–20 parts per million (p.p.m.), and if effective should lead to an improvement in oxygenation. Doses of over 40 p.p.m. do not produce increased benefit, and increase the likelihood of toxicity. Toxicity can occur due to the production of nitrogen dioxide and methameoglobinaemia, and levels of both should be regularly monitored during iNO therapy.

iNO has been used in the acute respiratory distress syndrome (ARDS), where there is associated pulmonary hypertension, in order to produce initial improvement. However, there is no evidence of improvement in outcome associated with iNO use, but there are clearly individual cases which may benefit.

25.3.4 *Heliox therapy*

Heliox is a mixture of helium and oxygen and was first described by Barach in the 1930s for the treatment of respiratory failure [21].

Helium is biologically inert and insoluble in human tissues. It is also colourless and tasteless. It is seven times lighter than air. Heliox lowers airway resistance when it is inhaled, as airway resistance is a function of airway diameter and density of inspired gas. Lowering airway resistance causes the inspired gas to have a more laminar flow, which is more effective at delivering oxygen to the bronchial tree. Therefore, decreasing the airway resistance can decrease the work of breathing and improve oxygenation.

It is a reasonable hypothesis, therefore, that heliox is beneficial in conditions where the airway resistance is increased due to decrease in airway diameter, such as upper airway obstruction, asthma or bronchiolitis and croup. It should be noted that heliox has no bronchodilator or anti-inflammatory properties of its own and so can only be used as a holding measure while definitive treatments are having their effect [22].

There is some evidence that heliox is effective in improving work of breathing and gas exchange in children with severe asthma when used alongside bronchodilator treatment [23] A Cochrane review in 2006 stated that heliox may have a role to play in patients with more severe airway obstruction, but that the published studies involve small numbers of patients and should be interpreted with caution [24].

In bronchiolitis there is some evidence that the administration of heliox can improve severity of illness and carbon dioxide clearance, especially if used in combination with continuous positive airway pressure [25].

Other uses for heliox include croup, where there have been mixed reports of its benefit [26,27]. However, a recent systematic review concluded that there was not enough evidence to support its widespread use [28].

Upper airway obstruction, including post-extubation stridor is the most common indication for using heliox [22,29]. There are many published case series describing a rapid improvement in symptoms following heliox inhalation [22].

In summary, heliox has potential benefits in the treatment of upper and lower airways obstruction, but there is lack of good quality evidence to advocate its routine use.

25.4 Diagnosis and Management of Meningococcal Disease in Children

Meningococcal infection remains a significant health problem in children and young adults, with a significant mortality and morbidity.

Since the widespread introduction of the conjugated meningococcal serogroup C vaccine throughout the developed world, there has been an substantial and sustained reduction in the incidence of serogroup C meningococcal disease. However, in the absence of an effective serogroup B vaccine and without widespread use of vaccines against group A, W135 and Y meningococci, these remain an important cause of morbidity and mortality worldwide.

Prompt recognition and aggressive early treatment are the only effective measures against this invasive disease. This requires the immediate administration of antibiotic therapy and recognition and treatment of patients who may have complications of meningococcal infection such as shock, raised intracranial pressure (ICP) or both.

Encouragingly, mortality due to meningococcal infection has fallen in recent years. This is the result of several factors such as centralisation of the care of seriously ill children in PICUs, the establishment of specialised mobile intensive care teams, the development of protocols for the treatment of meningococcal infection and the dissemination by national bodies and charities of guidance about early recognition and management of meningococcal infection.

25.4.1 *Susceptibility to infection and severity of disease*

Approximately 10% of the population carry meningococci in their upper respiratory tract at any time, with higher rates of carriage amongst teenagers and young adults. Not all carriage is of highly virulent clones, and many commensal *Neisseria* are non-pathogenic and may confer an element of protection against highly virulent strains. By contrast, carriage in children under four years of age is rare.

Invasive disease usually occurs less than ten days after colonisation with a pathogenic strain in a susceptible individual. Risk factors for invasive disease include young age, winter or dry season, close contact with a carrier or case, overcrowding, moving into new communities, active or passive smoking and exposure to respiratory infection.

The most common age of infection is in young childhood (less than five years of age) with a secondary peak of disease in adolescents. The incidence of disease in the UK is about 4 per 100,000 of the population.

Whilst most individuals are colonised by pathogenic meningococci at some time in their lives, very few suffer invasive disease.

Even in those who do develop invasive infection, its severity varies considerably. These observations indicate that various host factors influence both susceptibility to infection and severity of disease. This is confirmed by the findings that complement deficiency, hypogammaglobulinaemia and hyposplenism all predispose to invasive meningococcal infection, while variations in cytokine responses and coagulation pathway control may lead to variations in severity [30].

In addition, real-time polymerase chain reaction (PCR) techniques have shown that the number of meningococci in plasma and cerebrospinal fluid (CSF) appears to be the main determinant of lipopolysaccharide levels, which have been shown to be associated with clinical presentation and outcome [31].

25.4.2 *Presentation and clinical features*

The classical presenting features of meningococcal disease include fever and a characteristic haemorrhagic rash, with features of meningitis and/or septicaemia.

A recent study on the clinical recognition of meningococcal disease in children and adolescents noted that the classical features developed later on in disease progression (median time of onset 13 to 22 hours after symptoms began), whereas early, less-specific features of sepsis, such as leg pain, cold hands and feet and abnormal skin colour, first develop after a median period of eight hours in the majority of children [32].

This suggests that recognition of these early symptoms of sepsis could increase the proportion of children identified by primary-care clinicians as likely to have sepsis, shorten the time to hospital admission and, potentially, save lives.

It seems that patients with meningitis are likely to present following a longer period of lower-grade bacteraemia than patients with fulminant meningococcal septicaemia, who will have higher levels of bacteraemia and thus higher levels of cytokinaemia than patients with a compartmentalised infection such as meningitis [33].

Of children with invasive meningococcal disease, 30–50% have meningitis alone (mortality 5%), 7–10% have features of septicaemia alone (mortality 5–40%) and 40% present a mixed picture of meningitis with septicaemia.

In the UK, mortality from meningococcal disease has fallen over the past 10 years. Even in the most severe cases, mortality rates are now reported to be around 5% for those treated in specialist PICUs [34,35].

Patients with the highest risk of death include those with a rapidly progressive purpuric rash, absence of meningism, coma, hypotension (mean arterial blood pressure two standard deviations below mean for age), low peripheral blood white cell count ($<10 \times 10^9$/l), low platelet count ($<100 \times 10^9$/l) and young age [36].

25.4.3 *Symptoms and signs of meningitis*

In patients with meningococcal meningitis the following symptoms and signs predominate: headache, fever, vomiting, photophobia, neck stiffness, positive Kernig's and Brudzinski's signs and lethargy. In infants and younger children, poor feeding, irritability, a high pitched cry and a bulging fontanelle are typical findings. Seizures may occur in up to 20% of cases and meningitis is a cause of the first episode of convulsive status epilepticus in 12% of cases [37].

25.4.4 *Symptoms and signs of septicaemia*

Patients with meningococcal septicaemia may present with fever, rash, headache, flu-like symptoms (especially myalgia), vomiting or abdominal pain. Clinical signs of shock including tachycardia, poor peripheral perfusion, tachypnoea, oliguria, confusion and hypotension may be present.

Rarely, invasive disease may take the form of focal infection, such as arthritis, pneumonia, conjunctivitis, pericarditis or endophthalmitis.

25.4.5 *Rash*

The presence of a characteristic haemorrhagic rash is highly variable, although 80% of bacteriologically proven cases of meningococcal disease develop a rash at some stage in their illness. Typically this is haemorrhagic (petechial or purpuric) in character, but around 15% of patients will present with an atypical, blanching, maculopapular rash, which may evolve into the more typical non-blanching form over anything from minutes to hours.

A small percentage of patients (around 7%) never develop a rash and their presentation is indistinguishable from other causes of sepsis. The extent and description of the rash does not always correlate with the severity of disease.

Whilst the presentation of a fulminant case of meningococcal disease should be unmistakable, many patients present with fever and a petechial rash but with no other features of severe infection. While a significant minority (between 2% and 11%) will turn out to have meningococcal infection, most such children have trivial viral illnesses. In addition, a haemorrhagic rash indistinguishable from that seen in meningococcal disease may also occur in other bacterial infections such as pneumococcal, staphylococcal or other Gram-negative septicaemia. However, in most series of petechial rashes in children, enterovirus infection predominates as the cause, while other viral infections (influenza and other respiratory viruses, parvovirus, Epstein–Barr virus, cytomegalovirus, measles, etc.), and rarer diagnoses such as Henoch–Schönlein purpura, connective tissue disorders, haematological disorders (notably protein C or S deficiency, platelet disorders (e.g., idiopathic thrombocytopaenic purpura), drug effects, bone marrow infiltration, etc.) and trauma (including non-accidental injury), need to be considered.

However, the presence of fever and a non-blanching haemorrhagic rash should always prompt a serious consideration of the diagnosis of meningococcal disease and lead to empiric antimicrobial therapy unless another diagnosis is apparent.

25.4.6 *Laboratory features*

Meningococcal disease should be suspected in the face of suggestive clinical features, and initial treatment with antimicrobials and the recognition and management of shock or raised ICP should not be delayed whilst waiting for the results of laboratory investigations. In any case, they may be misleading. Elevated white cell count and CRP are common features of invasive bacterial diseases. However, these acute phase responses may take 12 to 24 hours to develop following the onset of invasive meningococcal infection and are therefore not commonly raised early in the course of the disease, especially in severe or rapidly progressive cases [38].

In severe cases, biochemical and haematological derangements are common.

Microbiological confirmation is important for guiding public health management and in excluding other possible causes. Cultures of blood, secretions from the throat and CSF (in the absence of contraindications) may confirm a diagnosis and allow for antimicrobial sensitivity testing.

In many countries, PCR from samples of blood or CSF is now used to detect meningococcal DNA. This is particularly useful in patients who have received antimicrobial therapy prior to cultures being taken. It is likely that PCR-based techniques will replace serological methods for serotyping meningococcal outbreaks for epidemiological analysis and routine surveillance in the near future.

25.4.7 *Progression of disease*

Meningococcal disease may progress rapidly, even after appropriate treatment has commenced.

All patients admitted to hospital with suspected meningococcal disease should be closely monitored for signs of deterioration. Their outcome may critically depend on the prompt recognition of two important complications: shock or raised ICP. While patients with comparatively mild disease may have no complications, these two clinical problems may coexist in some cases, and present a formidable challenge in clinical management.

25.4.8 *The presence of shock*

Shock in meningococcal disease is multifactorial and results from a combination of hypovolaemia caused by capillary leak syndrome, myocardial dysfunction, altered vasomotor tone and impaired cellular metabolism.

The increased vascular permeability results from endothelial cell dysfunction, causing leakage of water and plasma proteins out of the intravascular compartment.

The vasoconstriction that occurs in shock reduces blood flow to the skin, to the peripheries and to some organs, especially the kidneys and gut. As a result, patients with meningococcal septicaemia may present with cold peripheries and prolonged capillary refill time, with sluggish or even absent blood flow to the skin, as well as oliguria. In the most severe cases, ischaemia of the skin or even a whole limb may occur, particularly if there is thrombosis in areas of vascular stasis. In addition, many patients with septic shock will develop renal dysfunction, often leading to acute renal failure.

Despite severe shock, preservation of brain perfusion and function is often present until decompensation occurs, so that the patient's relatively alert state may make observers underestimate the degree of cardiovascular collapse. Eventually a decreased level of consciousness indicates a loss of cerebral vascular homeostasis and reduced brain perfusion.

The onset of hypotension signifies a failure of the compensatory mechanisms. It should be remembered that the diagnosis of shock in children is not dependent on the presence of arterial hypotension. Children are able to compensate for the loss of up to 40% of their circulating volume without developing hypotension, and may therefore have a normal blood pressure until shock is advanced.

The presence of a haemorrhagic rash is pathognomonic of meningococcal disease and reflects coagulopathy. Coagulopathy is universal in severe sepsis, regardless of the cause. Both pro-coagulant and anticoagulant pathways of haemostasis are dysregulated as a consequence of activation of the inflammatory and coagulation cascades, in addition to endothelial dysfunction [39]. This results in intravascular clot formation, with a suppression of the normal mechanisms which degrade intravascular thrombi, and the clinical syndromes of disseminated intravascular coagulopathy (DIC) and purpura fulminans.

Myocardial dysfunction arises as a result of a number of the different pathological processes that are activated in septic shock. Hypovolaemia causes decreased ventricular filling, and metabolic derangements also affect myocardial contractility. Bacterial products and inflammatory cytokines, such as interleukin 6, also directly suppress myocardial contractility.

Myocardial contractility improves with volume resuscitation and correction of metabolic derangements, but patients with signs of ongoing shock despite adequate volume resuscitation require inotropic support to improve myocardial function.

25.4.9 *Initial assessment and management*

The use of pre-hospital parenteral antibiotic therapy is recommended in many countries following a provisional diagnosis of meningococcal disease. Observational studies that have attempted to assess the effects of such use in clinical practice, however, have reported conflicting results. However, it is likely that pre-hospital antibiotics are given to more severely ill children, and theoretically should be beneficial. Brandtzaeg *et al.* have shown that antibiotic therapy reduces endotoxin level on admission [40].

The initial assessment of any individual with potentially life-threatening illness follows the standard airway, breathing, circulation (ABC) algorithms that are widely taught in acute life support training.

Unless consciousness is impaired, the airway is usually patent in meningococcal disease, but breathing may be compromised by pulmonary oedema due to capillary leakage in the lungs and hypoxia may be present. Circulation is affected as described above.

Many prognostic scoring systems have been evaluated for use in patients with acute meningococcal disease. They all lack precision in their prediction of outcome, but the clinically based Glasgow Meningococcal Septicaemia Prognostic Score (GMSPS) has proven beneficial in determining whether patients are at high risk of poor outcome and should therefore be managed in an area which can offer a high level of support and monitoring (i.e., a high-dependency or intensive-care area).

25.4.10 *Management of shock*

The goal of circulatory support in shock is the maintenance of oxygenation and adequate tissue perfusion. The priority in achieving this goal is fluid resuscitation to restore intravascular volume. Early and aggressive fluid resuscitation is associated with an improved survival in paediatric septic shock [41]. In addition, inotropic support is frequently necessary in order to maintain cardiac output and organ perfusion.

The establishment of central venous access is a priority in the critically ill patient. This will aid and guide fluid resuscitation, and the measurement of central venous oxygen saturation ($ScvO_2$) has been a useful guide to the adequacy of oxygen delivery in shock, with the goal of achieving a central venous pressure (CVP) of 8–12 mmHg, and $ScvO_2 > 70\%$ [42].

An initial fluid bolus of 20 ml/kg should be given over 5 to 10 minutes to children with signs of shock. The expected response to volume replacement is a reduction in heart rate, a warming of the peripheries and a decrease in capillary refill time. In mild cases shock is rapidly reversed by this initial fluid bolus, but repeated review is mandatory as the disease may progress due to ongoing capillary leakage. Another marker of improvement in perfusion is increased urine output, and bladder catheterisation should be performed early to allow this to be accurately assessed.

When signs of shock persist after the initial fluid bolus, further 20 ml/kg fluid boluses should be given until signs of circulatory compromise improve. If signs of shock persist after 40 ml/kg of fluid resuscitation, there is a significant risk of pulmonary oedema developing. Elective tracheal intubation and mechanical ventilation is recommended at this stage, even in the absence of overt signs of respiratory failure. If performed early enough, before signs of pulmonary oedema are manifest, this procedure is associated with an improvement in outcome [38]. Early tracheal intubation and ventilation is thought to be beneficial by its reduction of myocardial and respiratory muscle oxygen consumption and by allowing the delivery of positive end-expiratory pressure (PEEP) to aid oxygenation. The sedation and muscle relaxation used in these circumstances additionally facilitates the placement of arterial and central venous catheters.

Fluid resuscitation therapy should be monitored continuously using heart rate, blood pressure, CVP, urine output, metabolic status and peripheral perfusion as indicators. There is evidence to suggest that the monitoring of mixed venous or central venous oxygen saturation may provide a surrogate indicator of cardiac output and help to guide fluid and inotrope requirements [42].

Some children with severe capillary leak syndrome are only stabilised after resuscitation with twice or more times their circulating volume of fluid, together with concurrent inotropic support.

Although there is controversy about the use of human albumin solution (HAS) for volume replacement, 4.5% HAS has been our preferred resuscitation fluid in children with sepsis, and its use has been associated with a reduction in morbidity and mortality [34,35].

A large randomised controlled study comparing 4% HAS with normal saline in critically ill adult patients in Australia and New Zealand has suggested that HAS may be beneficial in a subgroup analysis of patients with septic shock [43]. No such studies have been performed in children, however.

As myocardial depression is invariably a contributory feature of persistent shock, inotropic support should be initiated early, via a central vein. It is usually impractical to gain central venous access in children before intubation. Dilute solutions of vasoactive agents, such as dopamine or dobutamine, can be given as an infusion through a peripheral vein until central venous access is obtained.

In patients who are unresponsive to high doses of catecholamines, there are some anecdotal data that vasopressin or its analogues may be valuable in raising blood pressure. However, the use of vasoconstrictors, while increasing blood pressure, might not always be associated with improvement in cardiac output, and there is no evidence of any additional benefit over conventional vasopressors.

25.4.11 *Respiratory support*

High-flow facial oxygen should be delivered routinely from the outset during initial assessment. If no major problem in airway or breathing is present, priority is given to the assessment and treatment of circulatory failure.

Indications for immediate endotracheal intubation are hypoxia, with severe respiratory distress indicating a progression of pulmonary oedema, severe persistent shock, fluctuating or decreasing conscious level (Glasgow Coma Scale ≤ 8, or a decrease of 3 points within one hour) or other signs of raised ICP.

25.4.12 *Biochemical and haematological derangements*

Children with meningococcal sepsis may have profound derangements in blood chemistry including acidosis, hypoglycaemia, hypocalcaemia, hypokalaemia, hypomagnesaemia or hypophosphataemia. These can be detected by repeated blood testing and treated if present.

Hyperglycaemia may occur following resuscitation and stabilisation. Data from critically ill adults indicate that the control of blood glucose using insulin to maintain blood glucose within strictly defined limits may be associated with a reduction in mortality [44] and there appears to be a correlation between peak blood glucose level and outcome in meningococcal disease [45]. However, there are no data yet available for tightly controlling blood glucose in children with meningococcal disease.

DIC is common. There may be bleeding from mucosal surfaces and venepuncture sites. In addition, spontaneous pulmonary, gastric or cerebral haemorrhage may occur, particularly if there is associated thrombocytopenia. Correction of coagulopathy with fresh frozen plasma, platelets and, in severe cases, cryoprecipitate, may prevent life-threatening haemorrhage.

A recently completed study on the use of APC in children with severe sepsis, including some with purpura fulminans and meningococcal disease, has not shown survival benefit [47]. There is some suggestion that the use of APC may be more beneficial in the subgroup of children with DIC, but this remains to be confirmed.

The skin may be severely compromised in meningococcal disease through inadequate perfusion as a result of vasoconstriction and DIC. Decreased skin perfusion may predispose pressure areas to ischaemic damage, and tissue oedema from capillary leak may cause a compartment syndrome. The role of fasciotomy in treating ischaemic limbs is not clearly established, but it has been used in circumstances where there is evidence of an increase in compartment pressure. Multidisciplinary input from orthopaedic, vascular and plastic surgeons may be needed for limb salvage. Amputation should not be considered until it is felt to be absolutely necessary and only performed following extensive discussion.

25.4.13 *Raised intracranial pressure*

Raised ICP occurs due to inflammation of the meninges and capillary leak leading to cerebral oedema. Most patients with meningococcal meningitis have a mildly raised ICP, but clinically significantly raised ICP is uncommon. Although most critically ill children with meningococcal infection have shock as their primary clinical problem, a small proportion present primarily with signs of raised ICP as their predominant clinical manifestation.

Signs of raised ICP include a declining level of consciousness, focal neurological signs including unequal, dilated or poorly responsive pupils, relative hypertension and bradycardia. Papilloedema is a late finding in acutely raised ICP.

Patients without significant meningeal inflammation who have profound shock may also present with impaired consciousness as a result of cerebral hypoperfusion. Conversely, patients without shock who have raised ICP may have peripheral vasoconstriction and these signs may be confused with compensated shock. In this case, poor peripheral perfusion is associated with the absence of a metabolic acidosis in blood gases, together with relative bradycardia, normal or high blood pressure and a decrease in level of consciousness or other neurological signs. In these circumstances, it should be assumed that the abnormal neurology is due to raised ICP, and aggressive fluid resuscitation should be avoided, as excess fluid will exacerbate any cerebral oedema.

If raised ICP is suspected, an intravenous infusion of mannitol (0.25–0.5 g/kg over 5 minutes, or 3% saline 3 ml/kg over 5 minutes) may prevent brain-stem herniation and may be life-saving. Urgent tracheal intubation to protect the airway and control blood gases is indicated.

In the child with raised ICP from meningococcal infection, the initial assessment may reveal coexistent shock. In this case the priority is to correct the shock before addressing specific measures to control the ICP. An adequate or high blood pressure is necessary in order to maintain cerebral perfusion. In this situation fluid resuscitation may result in an improved level of consciousness.

In the absence of shock, cautious fluid restriction may be useful, but the fluid balance requires careful monitoring.

Seizures should be aggressively managed to avoid any further increases in ICP.

Neuro-intensive care should be instituted using a 30° head-up position, head midline, minimal suction, deep sedation, normothermia or moderate hypothermia and strict avoidance of hypercapnia.

25.4.14 *Lumbar puncture*

Lumbar puncture (LP) can yield rapid microbiological confirmation of meningococcal meningitis and exclude other diagnoses. However, the procedure may cause deterioration in patients who have raised ICP or who are shocked, as it may cause cerebral herniation or further compromise cardiovascular function.

The following are contraindications to LP:

- Cardiorespiratory insufficiency.
- Raised ICP (evidence for which includes fluctuating or deteriorating levels of consciousness).
- Normal or high blood pressure in the presence of a slow or normal heart rate.

- Unequal, dilated or poorly reacting pupils.
- Focal neurological signs or abnormal posturing.
- Seizures.
- Papilloedema.
- Coagulopathy.

In view of the rapid and unpredictable progression of the disease in some children, we have previously argued that LP should be avoided or deferred in the initial assessment of patients with clinically obvious meningococcal disease. This is because the additional information provided by the LP adds little to the diagnosis.

Clearly, microbiological confirmation is important, but with use of molecular diagnostics with a high sensitivity that can be deployed even after treatment has begun, it is unlikely that an LP at the outset will add vital information that will otherwise be lost. In a child with a haemorrhagic rash, with the most likely diagnosis of meningococcal infection, the routine use of broad-spectrum antibiotics such as the third-generation cephalosporins (which have excellent CSF penetration and little reported meningococcal resistance) further reduces the absolute dependence on early microbiological diagnosis. However, where the diagnosis is unclear, or in areas where resistant meningococci are emerging, important information may be obtained by carrying out a LP, but this should only be done in the absence of any of the contraindications described above.

Computed tomography (CT) brain imaging is frequently used in patients with depressed consciousness, and is particularly recommended in adult practice where there is a broader differential diagnosis in patients with presumed meningitis. However, urgent cranial imaging is rarely justified in children with meningitis and a haemorrhagic rash, unless there is abnormal focal neurology or a suspicion of neurosurgical emergency.

It is hazardous to take a critically ill patient to a radiology department before they have been adequately stabilised and monitored, and unjustifiable if it is unlikely that the scan will significantly alter clinical management. In any case, cranial CT scanning is not a sensitive way of ruling out raised ICP, and cannot therefore help in making the decision to perform a lumbar puncture, which must be made on a basis of clinical assessment.

25.4.15 *Antibiotic therapy*

Cefotaxime (80 mg/kg thrice daily) or ceftriaxone (50–80 mg/kg once daily) is preferred as the initial therapy in patients with a clinical diagnosis of meningococcal disease.

Penicillin resistance is rare amongst clinical isolates of *Neisseria meningitides* in the UK and therefore benzylpenicillin is the logical choice when the microbiological diagnosis has been made. However, until a positive identification is available, there remains the possibility of both penicillin resistance or alternative bacterial diagnoses that might not be adequately treated by penicillin therapy. Other rare bacterial causes of purpura fulminans include *Streptococcus pneumoniae*, *Staphylococcus aureus* and other Gram-negative bacteria.

The duration of antibiotic therapy for meningococcal disease does not need to be prolonged and most centres use a five to seven day course for both meningococcal meningitis and septicaemia.

25.4.16 *Adjunctive therapies*

Steroids given with the first dose of antibiotics appear to reduce the incidence of neurological sequelae in both *Haemophilus influenzae* type b and pneumococcal meningitis and there is a trend to improved outcome in meningococcal meningitis. In our opinion, based on data from other causes of bacterial meningitis and an extrapolation of those results, systemic high-dose dexamethasone should be given in cases of suspected bacterial meningitis with, or shortly before, the first dose of antibiotics [48]. A dose of 0.15 mg/kg four times daily for four days is recommended.

High-dose steroid use is contraindicated in meningococcal shock in the absence of meningitis, as it has been shown to worsen the outcome of adults with septic shock.

There is some evidence that refractory septic shock may be more common in children with impaired adrenal gland responsiveness in the acute phase of meningococcal disease [49]. In adults with septic shock and documented adrenal hyporesponsiveness, low-dose, replacement steroid supplementation may improve their chances of survival [50], but a more recent study has cast doubt on the utility of steroid replacement therapy [51].

There have only been two properly conducted randomised controlled studies of other adjunctive therapies in meningococcal disease: the anti-endotoxin antibody, HA-1A, was investigated in a randomised controlled trial as a treatment for children with meningococcal septicaemia.

This study showed that there was no significant reduction in mortality in the children treated with HA-1A when compared with placebo [52]. Subsequent studies in adults with Gram-negative septicaemia also showed no benefit of adjunctive therapy with HA-1A [53].

Recombinant bactericidal permeability-increasing protein (rBPI21), which binds to and neutralises endotoxin and blocks the inflammatory cascade, has been evaluated for use in meningococcal disease. In a large placebo-controlled randomised multicentre trial, there was evidence of improvement in outcome for a variety of parameters. Unfortunately, the study was not sufficiently powered to detect a reduction in mortality [54]. However, the patients treated with rBPI21 suffered fewer amputations, fewer blood-product transfusions and had improved functional outcome compared with those treated with placebo. In addition, fewer children died who had received a full 24-hour infusion of rBPI21 (2% rBPI21 versus 6% placebo, $p = 0.07$), compared with those who had not received the full infusion. This suggests that rBPI21 used earlier may be beneficial in children with meningococcal disease. However, the only published data at present would not support its routine use.

A randomised controlled trial of APC has been carried out in children with septic shock, with its primary endpoint being the reduction in time to resolve respiratory, cardiovascular and renal organ failure, as a surrogate indicator of mortality [47]. The study was terminated early as it was felt that it would be unlikely to reach its primary endpoint, with suggestions of an unfavourable risk/benefit profile.

25.4.17 *Transfer to intensive care or treatment on the general ward?*

Most patients with meningococcal disease will not require intensive care. However, those with persistent shock or signs of raised ICP should be managed in a specialist high-dependency unit or ICU.

For those who do not immediately require transfer to an ICU, management on the general ward should be undertaken, with careful and frequent monitoring of vital signs (pulse, blood pressure, transcutaneous oxygen saturation, respiratory rate, urine output, capillary refill time and consciousness level) for the first 24 to 48 hours. This is likely to be better facilitated by initial management in a high-dependency unit.

Failure to recognise deterioration following hospital admission is associated with increased mortality. A large case-control study of health-care delivery in children with meningococcal disease in the UK has demonstrated that suboptimal emergency care significantly increased the likelihood of death in children with meningococcal disease [55]. In 143 children with meningococcal disease who died, there were significantly more departures from optimal (per protocol) management compared with controls (children with meningococcal disease who survived). In this study, a multivariate analysis identified three factors independently associated with an increased risk of death: the failure of patients under the age of 16 years to be looked after by a paediatrician; inadequate supervision of junior medical staff; and failure to administer adequate inotrope doses. In addition, failure to recognise complications of the disease was a significant risk factor for death, although not independent of the absence of paediatric care. The authors concluded that suboptimal healthcare delivery significantly reduced the likelihood of survival in children with meningococcal disease and that improved training of medical and nursing staff, adherence to published protocols and increased supervision of junior staff by consultants may improve the outcome for these children as well as those with other life threatening illnesses.

The decision to transfer critically ill or unstable patients to a more specialised unit can be difficult. A prolonged period of resuscitation may be necessary in the emergency department before a child with severe shock is stable enough to move. Transporting patients before they are adequately resuscitated is hazardous and the patient should be fully stabilised, with monitoring equipment securely in place, before transfer to the ICU is undertaken.

Stabilisation includes provision of a secure airway, controlled mechanical ventilation, central venous, arterial and urinary catheterisation and cardiorespiratory monitoring. Transport-related morbidity and mortality can be reduced by the use of a specialist intensive care transfer team [56].

The benefits of transferring patients to specialised units for ongoing intensive care management have been borne out by a significant reduction in mortality of children with severe meningococcal infection [34,35]. It is likely that centralisation in the care of critically ill children with meningococcal sepsis into units with a large experience of dealing with such patients, has had a significant effect in reducing their mortality. The organisation of paediatric intensive care in the UK has necessitated the development of paediatric critical care transport teams, with a network of outreach education to district general hospitals. This should improve the initial resuscitation and stabilisation of all critically ill children.

The model of specialised tertiary centres giving telephone advice to district hospitals where the child presents has also been shown to improve outcome in meningococcal disease.

Whether health services can be organised in this way for adults as well as children with meningococcal infection presenting to their local hospital is a challenge for health service planners, but efforts to promote this should be made to improve the outcome of all patients with life-threatening infection.

25.5 Congenital Heart Disease

Congenital heart disease affects 8 of every 1,000 live born infants in the UK. About 30% of these are diagnosed on routine antenatal scanning [57,58]. Congenital heart disease is most commonly classified into cyanotic and acyanotic heart lesions (Table 25.3).

Most children with congenital heart disease will need antibiotic prophylaxis to prevent bacterial endocarditis when undergoing certain dental and surgical procedures.

25.5.1 *Aetiology of congenital heart disease*

In most cases congenital heart disease is sporadic and the cause is unknown. The incidence is increased by the presence of congenital heart disease in a first degree relative. There is also a strong association with certain chromosomal abnormalities, congenital infections and teratogens. These are shown in Table 25.4.

Table 25.3. Common congenital heart lesions and the frequency of occurrence (%).

Acyanotic lesions	Cyanotic lesions
Left-to-right shunts	• Tetralogy of Fallot — 5%
• Ventricular septal defects (VSD) —30%	• Transposition of the great arteries — 5%
• Patent ductus arteriosus (PDA) — 12%	
• Atrial septal defects (ASD) — 7%	
• Atrioventricular septal defects (AVSD) — 2%	
Outflow tract obstruction	
• Pulmonary stenosis — 7%	
• Aortic stenosis — 5%	
• Coarctation of the aorta — 5%	

Table 25.4. Associations of congenital heart disease.

Underlying condition	Cardiac abnormality
Maternal disorder	
• Diabetes	Hypertrophic cardiomyopathy, VSD, increase in all types of congenital heart disease
• Rubella infection	Peripheral pulmonary stenosis, PDA
• Systemic lupus erythematosus	Complete heart block
Maternal drug ingestion	
• Warfarin	Pulmonary stenosis, PDA
• Foetal alcohol syndrome	ASD, VSD, Tetralogy of Fallot
• Lithium	Ebstein's anomaly
Chromosomal abnormality	
• Down's Syndrome (Trisomy 21)	AVSD, VSD
• Turner's Syndrome (45 X,O)	Aortic valve stenosis, coarctation of the aorta
• William's Syndrome (chromosome 7 microdeletion)	Supravalvular aortic stenosis, peripheral pulmonary artery stenosis
• DiGeorge Syndrome (22q11 deletion)	Aortic arch abnormalities, tetralogy of Fallot
• Edward's Syndrome (Trisomy 18)	VSD, ASD, PDA, coarctation of the aorta
• Patau's Syndrome (Trisomy 13)	VSD, ASD, PDA, coarctation of the aorta

25.5.2 *Foetal circulation and circulatory changes at birth*

In the foetus blood is diverted away from the lungs as oxygenation occurs via the placenta. This is achieved by high pulmonary vascular resistance, and low left atrial pressure. Blood therefore travels in a right-to-left direction through a connection between the atria called the foramen ovale. The ductus arteriosus connects the aorta to the pulmonary artery. As the pulmonary pressure is high, and the aortic pressure relatively lower in foetal life blood flows through this duct from the pulmonary artery to the aorta. This has the effect of diverting blood away from the lungs.

At birth, the pulmonary vascular resistance falls, allowing blood to flow to the pulmonary vessels. This causes the pressure in the left atrium to increase above that of the right atrium, and the foramen ovale closes. The direction of flow through the ductus arteriosus reverses, and the duct usually closes within hours to days of birth.

Diagnosis of congenital heart disease may be by the following methods:

- Antenatal detection.
- Post-natal screening in children with known risk factors (e.g. chromosomal abnormality).
- Detection of murmur or abnormality on routine examination.
- Child with cardiac failure.
- Child with cardiogenic shock.
- Child with cyanosis.

While one can make deductions about the nature of the cardiac lesion based on the clinical examination of the child, the gold standard for definitive diagnosis remains echocardiography, and children with suspected congenital heart disease should be referred to a paediatric cardiologist for further evaluation.

25.5.3 *Cardiac failure*

Intracardiac shunts with high pulmonary blood flow, such as VSD and AVSD, tend to present as heart failure within the first few weeks of life. As pulmonary vascular resistance falls after birth, pulmonary blood flow increases and symptoms become progressively worse over time. Symptoms of cardiac failure in babies include tachypnoea, respiratory distress, tachycardia, poor feeding, sweating while feeding and failure to gain weight.

There may be hepatomegaly, and there is likely to be a murmur on auscultation, and possibly a gallop rhythm. Chest X-ray may reveal cardiomegaly and plethoric lung fields. PDA may present with bounding peripheral pulses — this is caused by a wide pulse pressure that is due to high left ventricular stroke volume causing systolic hypertension and a low diastolic blood pressure caused by arterial 'run off' of blood into the pulmonary artery.

Cardiac failure that presents in the first few days of life is more likely to be caused by outflow tract obstruction or cardiomyopathy, as opposed to high pulmonary blood flow.

The treatment of cardiac failure in infants in the first instance is to administer oxygen as appropriate and loop diuretics. In severe situations positive pressure ventilation may be required including the careful use of PEEP. If a duct-dependent lesion is thought possible, treatment with prostaglandin E1 should be initiated as soon as possible (see below).

Effects of positive-pressure ventilation in children with heart failure:

- Decreases work of breathing.
- Decreases systemic vascular resistance, leading to reduced right ventricular preload and improved cardiac function.
- Decreases left ventricular afterload, leading to improvement in stroke volume and ejection fraction.
- Reduces myocardial oxygen consumption.

If the child has reached the point of decompensation then inotropic support and correction of pH with bicarbonate may be needed.

25.5.4 *Cardiogenic shock*

Cardiogenic shock presents with signs of pulmonary oedema, cyanosis, hypotension and weak (or impalpable) peripheral pulses. This occurs in duct-dependent left ventricular outflow tract obstructive lesions such as critical aortic stenosis, critical coarctation or hypoplastic left heart syndrome. In these situations systemic blood flow is via the ductus arteriosus with shunting from pulmonary artery to the aorta. When this duct closes in the first few days of life the infant presents with sudden collapse. The emergency treatment is prostaglandin infusion at 2–20 ng/kg/min in order to maintain duct patency. A side effect of prostaglandin is apnoea, so intubation and positive-pressure ventilation may be required. Inotropic support and bicarbonate may also be needed. Transfer to a cardiac centre should be urgently arranged for definitive diagnosis and intervention. High inhaled oxygen concentration is a strong stimulus for duct closure. Therefore if mechanical ventilation is instituted, attempts to limit inhaled oxygen concentration should be made.

This clinical presentation is often confused with septic shock. In a young baby presenting with shock, a cardiac cause should always be considered. Starting a prostaglandin infusion until a cardiac diagnosis can be confidently excluded is unlikely to be harmful to the baby, and may indeed be life-saving.

25.5.5 *The infant with cyanosis*

Cyanosis is caused by reduced pulmonary blood flow (in which pulmonary circulation may be dependent on a PDA) or abnormal mixing between the pulmonary and systemic circulations. It is most commonly seen in the duct-dependent lesions that present as an emergency in the newborn, the most common of these being transposition of the great arteries (TGA). In a neonate with central cyanosis, especially in the absence of respiratory distress, cyanotic heart disease must be suspected. The immediate treatment is to start prostaglandin, as the ductus arteriosus may be the only route of blood flow to the lungs. Invasive ventilation may also be necessary. In cyanotic heart disease, oxygenation will not be normalised, even in spite of maximal fraction of inspired oxygen (FiO_2), and a normal arterial partial pressure of oxygen should not be aimed for. Indeed, oxygen administration may contribute to ductal closure.

If the baby is ventilated, in the absence of pulmonary oedema, the lungs are often very compliant and gentle ventilation must be used in order not to further reduce pulmonary blood flow.

Children with suspected congenital heart disease need urgent discussion and possible transfer to a cardiac centre for definitive diagnosis and intervention. In TGA, the first procedure will often be a balloon atrial septostomy, prior to an arterial switch procedure.

Some cyanotic lesions cause increased pulmonary blood flow, and therefore an element of cardiac failure may be seen. An example of this is truncus arteriosus, in which a single arterial trunk arises from both ventricles and provides both pulmonary and systemic circulations.

25.5.6 *Post-operative management of paediatric cardiac surgery*

Cardiac surgery that has involved bypass will lead to a systemic inflammatory response. Common problems that occur include:

- Temperature instability — this may include hypothermia due to bypass, or fever as part of the inflammatory response.
- Haemodynamic instability — hypovolaemia is common post-operatively, and there may be capillary leak. This needs to be countered by volume replacement and inotropic support.
- Myocardial dysfunction — this can be caused by the inflammatory response post bypass. The adequacy of cardiac output is assessed by markers of tissue perfusion such as blood pH, lactate and mixed venous saturations. Tamponade may be a post-operative complication.
- Dysrhythmias — these may be due to myocardial dysfunction. Metabolic disturbances may also contribute.
- Metabolic disturbances — potassium, calcium and glucose levels should be regularly monitored, and for any abnormalities the cause should be considered and the derangement corrected.

25.6 Paediatric Trauma

Care of the injured child requires a coordinated and organised approach by a team experienced in the management of this age group.

Clinicians dealing with the paediatric trauma patient are required to appreciate the anatomical and physiological differences between children and adults and different mechanisms of injury that may be experienced.

Trauma is the leading cause of death in children, accounting for 50% of deaths between the ages of 1 and 15 years in the USA [59].

Because of differences in patterns of behaviour in different age groups, younger children tend to suffer falls, non-accidental injuries, foreign body aspirations into the respiratory tract and drownings, whereas older children are more likely to be injured in pedestrian, motor vehicle and bicycle accidents.

The relatively large size of a child's head compared with their body makes head and neck injuries more common in children, with head injury accounting for 30% of the fatalities.

Penetrating injuries account for less than 10% of paediatric traumatic injury.

There is good evidence that accident prevention programmes lead to significant reduction in childhood injury mortality prevention. These include: education and public safety campaigns, such as helmet use for cyclists; legislation, such as child seats in cars, boundaries and fences for swimming pools; and initiatives, such as installation of safer playground surfaces and controlled school crossings [60]. In addition, education programmes directed at caregivers and the public, such as basic life support courses, advanced paediatric and trauma life support courses and the development of centres to deal with major trauma have all produced improvements in both morbidity and mortality.

25.6.1 *Initial approach to the child with trauma*

As seen in adults, there is a trimodal distribution of mortality in children with trauma.

(i) Immediate death at the scene of the accident due to airway obstruction, haemorrhage and head or spinal injury.
(ii) During the first hour (often called the platinum half hour, golden hour or golden hours. As in (i), appropriate immediate care to protect the airway, stop haemorrhage and deliver oxygen may have a significant effect on outcome.
(iii) Mortality in the following days and weeks results from intensive-care-related complications such as ARDS, sepsis and multiple

organ failure. Effective resuscitation and stabilisation in the minutes and hours following injury may significantly influence these complications.

25.6.2 *Principles of management*

The emphasis in paediatric pre-hospital trauma care is on aggressive support of vital functions during what has been called the 'platinum half hour'.

Because the most common paediatric traumatic injuries are blunt injuries involving the head, it is primarily a disease of airway and breathing rather than circulation (bleeding).

The primary survey (ABC and D (disability)) is addressed concurrently with the primary survey in a continuous cycle of assessment, intervention and then re-assessment. The primary survey is generally achieved by undressing the child to more fully assess injury, in an environment at room temperature, thus avoiding hypothermia.

The primary consideration is airway control and cervical spine immobilisation. The principles of management of airway and cervical spine control are the same as those which pertain to adults. There are, however, certain paediatric considerations:

- Nasal intubation is contraindicated in patients with severe facial and head injury, including particularly those with cerebrospinal fluid leak, and blind intubation is discouraged.
- Children should be assumed to have a full stomach, irrespective of the timing of their last meal.
- Children are more likely to develop respiratory failure than adults with equivalent injuries.
- The child's haemodynamic status will determine the most appropriate therapeutic approach (children with shock unresponsive to 40 ml/kg of fluid should be intubated and ventilated regardless of their respiratory status).
- A cuffed endotracheal tube is the airway of choice for intubation, particularly in severe thoracic injury with reduced lung compliance.

- The routine use of non-invasive ventilation, particularly in children with head, neck or facial injury, is contraindicated.
- As soon as a patent airway is established an FiO_2 of 1 should be delivered. Close assessment of the effectiveness of ventilation should be continued to prevent hypercarbia and reduce the risk of increased intracranial pressure.
- Decisions regarding drainage of pneumothoraces or adequacy of respiration should be on clinical grounds rather than waiting for chest radiography or blood gas evaluation.
- The basic steps in the management of haemorrhagic shock are control of active haemorrhage, placement of adequate venous access by the venous or intra-ossesous route, and adequate volume replacement.
- Most children who suffer haemorrhagic shock following traumatic injury have unrecognised haemorrhage, which is reversed only by prompt recognition and adequate treatment with blood transfusion and surgical intervention.
- Coagulopathy in injured children is typically related to dilution of platelets and clotting factors during extensive resuscitation and transfusion, although hypothermia may contribute.
- Consideration of empiric platelet and fresh frozen plasma transfusion is reasonable when more than two blood volumes have been replaced during resuscitation. Laboratory tests of coagulation should be used to guide specific replacement.
- Shock is less obvious in children and hypotension is not required to diagnose shock. The presence of tachycardia, cool peripheries, prolonged capillary refill time and altered mental status suggest hypovolaemia. Hypotension is a late sign and may not develop until 40% of blood volume is lost.
- Any injured child who is not stabilised by 20–40 ml of warmed isotonic saline/kg (or in a child with hypotension (systolic blood pressure = $70 + (2 \times \text{age in years})$ mmHg) the addition of 10–20 ml fresh warmed packed cells/kg), should be considered to have concealed haemorrhage and may need assessment for intrathoracic, intra-abdominal or intra-pelvic bleeding.

- If a child with shock has no signs of internal bleeding and fails to improve despite adequate fluid resuscitation, other forms of shock such as obstructive, cardiogenic or neurogenic should be considered [61].
- Once the primary survey is completed, resuscitation is ongoing, and shock, if present, is being effectively treated, a secondary survey is undertaken for definitive evaluation of the injured child. The primary survey and appropriate resuscitative efforts should be well advanced within 15 minutes. The secondary survey consists of a symptoms, allergies, medications, past illnesses, last meal, events and environment (SAMPLE) history from caregivers (if present).

A complete head-to-toe examination is then performed, along with a complete history of the injury. Continued reassessment and resuscitation continues during the secondary survey. The priority is to discover potential life-threatening injuries which may have been missed during the primary survey (i.e. tension pneumothorax). The neck is examined for tenderness, swelling, torticollis or spasm suggesting cervical spine injury (which may not be evident on lateral radiograph of the cervical spine, i.e. spinal cord injury without radiologic abnormality (SCIWORA)). SCIWORA is usually the result of high-energy injuries, usually associated with rapid acceleration/deceleration. Overall, traumatic spinal injuries are much less common in children compared with adults, with an incidence of < 2%. Most spinal injuries are the result of high-energy acceleration/deceleration injuries as with motor vehicle accidents, although falls and sports injuries are also common in younger children and adolescents respectively. Mortality in children with cervical spine (c-spine) injury is up to 20% because 50% of such injuries are associated with traumatic brain injury (TBI). In the presence of TBI, a c-spine injury should be assumed to be present until proven otherwise.

The age of the child influences the level of spinal injury; patients < 11 years more likely have high (cervical vertebrae C1–C4) c-spine injury, whereas patients > 11 years are more likely to have C5–C7 injuries.

There is no clear explanation for the different patterns of injury seen in children of differing ages, but anatomical and social differences appear the most likely. In younger children the head represents a greater proportion of body weight, resulting in the greater force of movement around C2–C3, rather than C5–C6 as in older children and adults. In addition, the c-spine is less able to support the greater weight due to increased muscle and ligamentous laxity in younger children. Clearance of the c-spine in children presents particular difficulties, since many children cannot reliably communicate if they have pain, let alone localise where it is present.

The most common method of c-spine clearance in children consists of absence of radiological evidence of injury and absence of neurological deficit. If doubt persists or the patient is unconscious, a magnetic resonance imaging scan to look for evidence of SCIWORA is the definitive investigation. In about 25% of c-spine injuries SCIWORA presents significantly later than the original injury [62].

Generally, patients with severe multiple trauma benefit from CT of the head, neck, thorax, abdomen and pelvis.

Focussed assessment by sonography in trauma (FAST) may be useful in detecting intra-abdominal bleeding but is not sufficiently reliable to exclude blunt abdominal trauma in haemodynamically stable children and adds little to management, as haemodynamically unstable children with suspected intra-abdominal bleeding are candidates for immediate operation, while stable children will be managed conservatively. However, a detailed ultrasound is useful where CT is not available [63].

Analgesia is essential and requires frequent titration. Most children with multiple injuries benefit from parenteral opiate therapy.

25.6.3 *Traumatic brain injury*

TBI is the most common injury in children following blunt trauma. It is rare for a child with significant injuries elsewhere not to also have TBI. The increased risk of TBI in children is largely due to the relatively larger size of the head in relation to the body in children compared with adults, less central nervous system myelination with younger age and more compliant bones.

Blunt trauma can result in significant acceleration/deceleration injury with cerebral contusion, intracranial haemorrhage and diffuse axonal injury (DAI). DAI is a common cause of long-term disability in TBI.

TBI should be assumed to be present even in the absence of obvious neurological deficits. Use of the modified Glasgow Coma Scale (GCS) for Children is helpful, either as a trend of progression, or as an absolute score. The modified GCS takes into account the child's age, and thus developmental level within the verbal and motor components. In general TBI is graded according to GCS: mild (GCS 13–15), moderate (GCS 9–12) and severe (GCS $\leq$ 8). The initial CT may show obvious injury (intracranial blood or contusions) but initially may be normal with DAI, until overt cerebral oedema develops.

Management of TBI is multifactorial, and current recommendations are extrapolated from adult studies.

Widely accepted guidelines recommend avoidance of hypoxia, hypo- and hypercarbia, maintenance of systolic blood pressure higher than fifth percentile for age and of cerebral perfusion pressure greater than 40 mmHg [62].

25.6.4 *Non-accidental injury (NAI)*

In the UK, about 2–3% of children suffer abuse each year, with serious injuries occurring in about 1 in 1,000 cases [62]. It is crucial that the possibility of NAI is considered in any child with unexplained or suspicious injury.

The presence of the following is suggestive of possible child abuse:

- Delay or failure to seek medical attention.
- Vague, inconsistent or changeable history.
- History incompatible with the child's injuries.
- Abnormal parental affect, including apparent lack of concern and hostility.
- Abnormal appearance of the child or unusual interaction with parents.
- Direct history from the child suggesting deliberate harm.
- Injuries of differing ages.

Some forms of injury are highly suggestive of NAI. These include finger-tip bruising, adult human bite marks, cigarette burns, lash marks and a torn frenulum. Unexplained subdural haematoma and retinal haemorrhages are pathognomonic, but there may be other explanations. Subdural haemorrhages occur when the infant has been shaken. They occur when the bridging subdural veins tear during acceleration/deceleration associated with violent shaking. This also causes diffuse axonal injury, which is the more likely cause of the severe mortality and morbidity associated with shaken baby syndrome — a term used to describe subdural and subarachnoid haemorrhage, retinal haemorrhages and associated changes in long bones (often metaphyseal-epiphyseal fractures are found).

Clinical presentation of shaken babies is non-specific and includes irritability, lethargy, seizures and apnoea. Parents may admit to shaking the baby because he or she has 'stopped breathing'. Retinal haemorrhages occur in about 70% of such children. Retinal haemorrhage may also be seen after accidental injury, after cardiopulmonary resuscitation, seizures, raised intracranial pressure and in other neurological or haematological conditions. Detailed fundoscopy should be performed by an experienced ophthalmologist where NAI is suspected.

Other injuries associated with shaken babies are rib fractures, which occur in up to 25% of such infants. If these are seen in children less than two years of age this should arouse a high index of suspicion for NAI.

A skeletal survey should be performed in all children less than two years of age with any features which make NAI a possibility. Expert radiological opinion is mandatory.

Clear and careful documentation is vital when assessing children with suspected NAI. A senior paediatrician should coordinate the care. Early involvement of social services, child protection teams and pastoral support is mandatory.

Any clinician dealing with the acute care of injured children must have adequate training in the detection and management of child abuse and NAI.

25.7 The Terminally Ill Child on the PICU

An inevitable part of paediatric intensive care is caring for the terminally ill and dying child. This is a sad and emotional time for all involved, and requires good communication between staff and parents, as well as adequate support for all involved. Around 5% of children admitted to

PICUs in the UK die [64], and approximately up to 75% of all childhood deaths occur on the PICU.

The paediatrician's role is to act in the best interests of the child. There are situations in which prolonging the child's life is no longer in their best interests. In order to assist clinicians with this difficult decision, the Royal College of Paediatrics and Child Health have published guidelines on the withholding and withdrawing of life-sustaining treatment in children [65].

According to these guidelines there are five situations in which it may be ethical and legal to consider withholding or withdrawing life-sustaining treatment.

These are:

(i) The 'brain dead' child — children who have fulfilled the criteria for brainstem death on testing by two qualified practitioners are legally dead, and therefore continuing cardiorespiratory support is futile.
(ii) The 'permanent vegetative' state — this is defined as complete unawareness of self and environment accompanied by sleep–wake cycles with either complete or part preservation of hypothalamic and brain stem functions [66]. The vegetative state is defined as permanent 12 months after traumatic brain injury and 6 months after other causes [67].
(iii) The 'no chance' situation — the child has such severe disease that life-sustaining treatment simply delays death without significant alleviation of suffering.
(iv) The 'no purpose' situation — the child may be able to survive with treatment, but the degree of physical or mental impairment will be so great that it is unreasonable to expect the child and family to bear it.
(v) The 'unbearable' situation — the child and/or family feel that in the face of progressive and irreversible illness further treatment is more than can be borne.

25.7.1 *Decision making in end of life issues*

The question often arises as to whose decision it is to make the decision to withdraw or withhold life-sustaining treatment — is it that of the child, the parents or medical staff? It has to be remembered that this is a decision led and advised by the medical team. However, it is a discussion that in some cases is initiated by the family. It is imperative that the religious and moral beliefs of the family are taken into consideration. There may be marked differences between families' views, especially when it comes to quality of life of disabled children. The 'unbearable situation' will be different for each individual, and it has to be remembered that there may be differences in what is an 'unbearable situation' between the child who has been born with a disability, and the child who has a disability acquired later in life. The child's best interest needs to be considered in the context of their family, including parents and siblings.

It is also important to give parents enough time to take on board the decisions that are being made, and for them to discuss and take counsel from family, friends and religious leaders. In most situations, given open and honest communication, and time, a decision can be agreed on by medical staff and the parents, and where appropriate the child themselves. This will usually take at least one meeting between the family and medical staff. In the rare cases where agreement cannot be reached it may be necessary to seek legal advice.

Once the decision has been taken to withdraw or withhold life-sustaining treatment it must be remembered that this is not stopping care. Indeed, good palliative care is often already in place, and if not it needs to be instituted. This should include consideration of the child's dignity, relief of pain and other symptoms, including seizure control.

25.7.2 *Withholding life-sustaining treatment and limitation to treatment plans*

In the UK, approximately 12 per 10,000 children are living with a life-threatening condition [68]. In some of these cases, the decision to withhold life-sustaining treatment may well have been discussed between the family, child and healthcare professionals prior to an acute deterioration in their condition. This may involve decisions such as not to initiate advanced respiratory support in the case of respiratory insufficiency, or to withhold antibiotics in the face of a life-threatening pneumonia. Children with a plan similar to this already in place are unlikely to come into contact with a PICU. However, they may present in the resuscitation room. In these situations it is important to fully communicate with parents about treatments being instigated or omitted. If there is any doubt about the appropriateness of a particular treatment then life-sustaining treatment should be instigated until the most senior clinician is available.

A limitation to a treatment plan may also be put in place, in full discussion with parents, while a child is on PICU. Decisions that may be made include: not to initiate cardiopulmonary resuscitation in the event of cardiac arrest or not to reintubate should a planned extubation be unsuccessful. In the PICU setting it is important that the limitations to treatment are frequently rediscussed, including when the child's clinical condition changes.

25.7.3 *Withdrawal of life-sustaining treatment*

In the PICU setting the most common mode of withdrawal of life-sustaining treatment is the removal of the child from the ventilator. Prior to this the family may wish a religious blessing. Ideally, the child and family should be cared for in an individual room to offer the maximum possible privacy. All unnecessary infusions, such as inotropes, should be stopped. It is imperative, however, to continue infusions of analgesics and sedatives in order to alleviate any potential suffering. The parents should be allowed to decide who else is in the room with them at the point of withdrawal of intensive care. Some parents wish to hold their child in their arms at the point of removing the endotracheal tube, and the parents' wishes should be accommodated as far as is possible. It should be explained to the parents what will happen, including the possibility of terminal gasping. They should be given as much time as they need with their child, and appropriate but not intrusive nursing care should be given. Parents should be given the opportunity to choose clothes for their child to be dressed in. They may also be offered mementoes, such as a lock of their child's hair, hand or footprints or a photo.

While death following withdrawal of life-sustaining treatment usually occurs within minutes to hours, in some situations the period prior to death may be prolonged. In these cases it may be appropriate to transfer the child to a lower-dependency ward or to a hospice.

The family or medical team may desire an autopsy if the cause of death is unclear or if it may have been due to an inherited condition, as there may be implications for future pregnancies.

25.7.4 *Support for the family following the death of a child on the PICU*

It goes without saying that the parents and family will need emotional support at the time of their child's death. The parents should be offered a follow-up appointment with a senior clinician within six to eight weeks following the child's death in order to discuss any outstanding questions they may have.

It is, however, important to remember that other people may need support following the death of a child on PICU. These include staff who have been involved in the child's care. Parents of other children on the unit at the time may also need support, as it may well raise concerns and anxieties about the future of their child.

When a child dies on PICU it is inevitably a sad time for all involved. But good quality care and communication can go a long way to making this time as easy as possible for the bereaved family.

25.8 Ethical Considerations

Improvements in medical expertise and technology have led to a significant reduction in infant and childhood mortality over the past few decades. Death among children aged 0 to 15 years has reduced over the last 30 years and is currently 1 per 1000 of the population [69]. With the exception of unexpected mortality resulting from injury or acute illness, a significant proportion of children die as a result of chronic complex conditions (CCCs) requiring prolonged medical care and repeated hospital admissions, such as acquired immunodeficiency syndrome, metabolic disorders, cancer, cystic fibrosis, extreme prematurity and severe congenital anomalies. In these children, early death is an inevitable outcome of their disease process, and the trajectory of their illness leading up to the terminal phase often follows a predictable pattern.

Over the past few decades the model of care during terminal illness has moved away from the traditional medical approach of aggressive treatment with curative intent to symptom care with palliative intent.

It is clear that many terminally ill adults prefer to die at home rather than in hospital, and that hospitalised adult patients often agree to waive invasive and painful life-sustaining treatments (LSTs) through 'advance directives' and do-not-attempt-resuscitation orders. Do-not-attempt-resuscitation orders remain uncommon in paediatric practice, and there is little information about what parental and, more importantly, children's choices are regarding the optimal nature and location of end-of-life care.

Only 17% of children with CCCs died at home in the state of Washington between 1980 and 1998; 75% of deaths occurred in hospital [70]. This study did suggest a trend towards more deaths at home in the above-one-year age group in recent years, indicating that parents of older children with terminal illnesses might prefer this option.

A number of recent studies have indicated that most children dying in hospital die in an intensive care environment [71]. Uncertainty among medical staff about when to withhold LST, and among parents regarding the nature of optimal end-of-life care, may lead to the initiation of intensive care in the face of deteriorating illness.

In most PICUs, withdrawal or limitation of life support has replaced failed resuscitation as the main pathway of death.

Currently, only 1 of 10 hospital deaths occur outside the ICU. The proportion of referrals from within the hospital contributing to ICU deaths has risen gradually. Infants represent a large proportion of children dying in an ICU; older children (1–14 years) constitute the majority in non-ICU settings. Most children with congenital malformations, perinatal conditions and injury seem to die in the ICU, whereas a significant number of children with malignancy experience their end-of-life in a non-ICU setting.

Irrespective of the reasons for changes in the nature of end-of-life care among hospitalised children their effects constitute important considerations.

For the individual child and parents, the experience of death is more unpleasant when it occurs within the circumstances of intensive care admission, multiple painful procedures, sedation, paralysis and other complications of ICU stay, despite significant improvements in end-of-life care in ICUs. This is especially true if the benefit of such LST was unclear at admission. By contrast, the management of grief is easier when parents are able to retain control over their child's end-of-life care, which is easier to achieve at home, in a hospice or even in-hospital outside the intensive care setting. There is also evidence that adverse psychological consequences among parents and siblings following the death of a child are diminished when it occurs as part of a home-care programme [72].

As the reasons leading to the frequent use of ICUs to manage end-of-life care may be multifactorial, one solution may be the creation of a multidisciplinary combined paediatric intensive care and palliative care team, consisting of hospital specialists, palliative care staff and intensive care clinicians. This team could be used to advise and assist a child's primary healthcare team during early discussions with parents regarding the optimal management of their child's predicted end-of-life care.

25.8.1 *Brain stem death in children*

A report of a working party of the British Paediatric Association of 1991 supported by the Council of the Royal College of Physicians suggested that, in children over the age of two months, the criteria used to establish death should be the same as those in adults [73].

Between 37 weeks of gestation and two months of age, it is rarely possible to diagnose death confidently as a result of cessation of brain-stem reflexes, and below 37 weeks of gestation the criteria to establish this cannot be applied.

25.8.1.1 *Infants 37 weeks gestation to two months of age*

In this age group coma may occur for a wide variety of reasons, the most common being hypoxic–ischaemic encephalopathy, especially when the cerebral insult occurred *in utero* or at the time of birth. Such infants are very difficult to assess. It may not be possible satisfactorily to demonstrate structural brain damage and the infant may have multi-system failure. On these grounds alone is could be argued that brain-stem death should not be diagnosed.

In the USA, the task force considers that in certain infants, after a period of observation, it may be possible to satisfy all the pre-conditions for the diagnosis of brain-stem death. They recommend two formal clinical examinations of brain-stem function at least 48 hours apart together with an isoelectric electroencephalogram (EEG) [74]. Whilst there is no evidence that the standard criteria of brain-stem death will falsely identify infants in this age group as brain-stem dead, there is no published evidence that if ventilation is continued asystole will follow in a few days. Such evidence was considered important in the development of the concept of brain-stem death in adults Therefore, given the current state of knowledge it is rarely possible confidently to diagnose brain-stem death at this age.

25.8.1.2 *Infants below 37 weeks gestation*

Apnoea and coma are common in this age group. It is extremely difficult to demonstrate irreversible brain damage in this age group, whilst hypoxia often is a complicating factor.

The development of brain-stem reflexes in the preterm infant has not been systematically studied. There are no data on the development of the caloric reflex, whilst the preterm infant may not respond to tracheal stimulation by suction. Thus, normal preterm infants may fail to respond to some of the diagnostic tests for brain-stem death. Because the pathways in the brain-stem are incompletely myelinated in very preterm infants, it is likely that major damage in this region will have different effects to those seen in older children or adults. Therefore the concept of brain-stem death is inappropriate for infants in this age group. Decisions on whether to continue intensive care should be based on an assessment of the likely outcome of the condition, after close discussion with the family.

25.8.2 *Electrophysiological measurements in infants and children*

Although the American guidelines accept an isoelectric EEG as supportive evidence of brain death, it is not certain that this investigation is of value in the diagnosis of brain death.

Radio-isotope or Doppler techniques for measuring cerebral blood flow are still being evaluated in children and neonates. They are only available in specialised centres and reports suggest that cerebral blood flow may be normal even when the child is brain-stem dead. Therefore it is unclear whether these investigations are a helpful addition to the diagnosis of brain-stem death in infants and children.

25.8.3 *Organ transplantation*

It is generally accepted that the concept of brain-stem death as a criterion of death is for the practical purpose of declaring that a heart-beating, haemodynamically-stable patient will die of multiple organ failure within a period of time that could vary from hours to days, or even longer. This creates a major ethical issue, particularly in religions or cultures which do not accept the concept of brain-stem death.

In addition, the concept of brain-stem death has been accepted as a means to procure healthy organs for transplantation from a heart-beating donor.

The more recent concept of non-heart-beating organ donation has been extended into paediatric practice. This allows for procurement of whole organs from dying patients whose parents consent to have life-support withdrawn. Following cessation of heart beat, and declaration of death, a few minutes are allowed to elapse before rapid organ procurement is performed.

The patient must be declared dead prior to removal of organs, and it is never permissible to allow someone to die in order that someone else may benefit from their organs. Ethically, in terms of scarce resources, it is also wrong to maintain a brain dead patient on a ventilator with no chance of benefit for that patient.

There is an argument that death of a child is somewhat ‘unnatural’ in the order of life, so that there is more acceptance that a ‘dead’ child should remain on mechanical ventilation for the sake of the family, to allow the time to come to terms with the tragic events, especially where there has been a rapid or unexpected critical event.

This must be balanced with the possibility that the family will have unrealistic or unreasonable expectations of continuation of intensive care support.

Skilled and compassionate ICU staff can make an extremely positive impact on what is a desperately tragic and difficult circumstance for the dying child's family.

References

[1] Ruttimann, U.E., Patel K.M. and Pollack, M.M. (2000). Relevance of diagnostic diversity and patient volumes for quality and length of stay in pediatric intensive care units, *Pediatr Crit Care Med*, **1**, 133–139.

[2] Paediatric Intensive Care Society (2001). *Paediatric Intensive Care Society Standards Document*, [Online]. Available at: www.ukpics.org/documents/PICS%20Standards%202001.pdf [Accessed 1 February 2013].

[3] Department of Health, Health Service Directorate (1997). *Paediatric Intensive Care, "Framework for the Future"* [Online]. Available at: http://www.longtermventilation.nhs.uk/_Rainbow/Documents/PICU%20Framework%20for%20the%20Future.pdf [Accessed 1 February 2013].

[4] Tsegaye, A., Wolday, D., Otto, S. *et al.* (2003). Immunophenotyping of blood lymphocytes at birth, during childhood, and during adulthood in HIV-1-uninfected Ethiopians, *Clin Immunol*, **109**, 338–346.

[5] D'Arena, G., Musto, P., Cascavilla, N. *et al.* (1998).Flow cytometric characterization of human umbilical cord blood lymphocytes: immunophenotypic features, *Haematologica*, **83**, 197–203.

[6] Wilson, C.B. and Lewis, D.B. (1990). Basis and implications of selectively diminished cytokine production in neonatal susceptibility to infection, *Rev Infect Dis*, **12** (Suppl. 4), S410–S420.

[7] Stoop, J.W., Zegers, B.J.M., Sander, P.C. *et al.* (1969). Serum immunoglobulin levels in healthy children and adults, *Clin Exp Immunol*, **4**, 101–112.

[8] Carr, R. (2000). Neutrophil production and function in newborn infants, *Brit J Haem*, **110**, 18–28.

[9] Davies, E.G. (2008). 'The immunology of infants and children and its relationship to susceptibility to infection', in Nadel, S. (ed.), *Infectious Diseases in the Pediatric Intensive Care Unit*, Springer-Verlag, London, pp. 1–58.

[10] Bromberger, P., Lawrence, J.M., Braun, D. *et al.* (2000). The influence of intrapartum antibiotics on the clinical spectrum of early-onset Group B streptococcal infection in term infants, *Pediatrics*, **106**, 244–250.

[11] Moses, L.M., Heath, P.T., Wilkinson, A.R. *et al.* (1998). Early onset group B streptococcal neonatal infection in Oxford 1985–96, *Arch Dis Child*, **79**, F148–F149.

[12] Barcaite, E., Bartusevicius, A., Tameliene, R. *et al.* (2008). Prevalence of maternal group B streptococcal colonisation in European countries, *Acta Obstet Gynecol Scand*, **87**, 260–271.

[13] Smaill, F. (2002). Intrapartum antibiotics for group B streptococcal colonization, *Cochrane Database Syst Rev*, CD000115.

[14] Cases in England and Wales (2013). *Listeria monocytogenes: Human cases in England and Wales reported to the Health Protection Agency Centre for Infections, 1983–2007*, Public Health Agency, London.

[15] Ahmad, P., Hameed, F. and Ahmad, K.N. (1986). Serum IgG levels in full term preterm and SFD neonates, *Ind J Ped*, **53**, 405–407.

[16] Arnold, J.H., Hanson, J.H., Toro-Fiquero, L.O. *et al.* (1994). Prospective randomized comparison of high-frequency oscillatory ventilation and conventional mechanical ventilation in pediatric respiratory failure, *Crit Care Med*, **22**, 1530–1539.

[17] Penny, D.J., Hayek, Z., Reddington, A.N. (1991). The effects of positive and negative extrathoracic pressure ventilation on pulmonary blood flow after the total cavopulmonary shunt procedure, *Int J Cardiol*, **30**, 128–130.

[18] Gappa, M., Costeloe, K., Southall, D.P. *et al.* (1994). Effect of continuous negative extrathoracic pressure on respiratory mechanics and timing in infants recovering from neonatal respiratory distress syndrome, *Pediatr Res*, **36**, 364–372.

[19] Samuels, M.P., Raine, J., Wright, T. *et al.* (1996). Continuous negative extrathoracic pressure in neonatal respiratory failure, *Pediatrics*, **98**, 1154–1160.

[20] Shah, P.S., Ohlsson, A. and Shah, J.P. (2008). Continuous negative extrathoracic pressure or continuous positive airway pressure for acute hypoxemic respiratory failure in children, *Cochrane Database Syst Rev*, CD0036999.

[21] Barach AL, Eckman M (January 1936). The effects of inhalation of helium mixed with oxygen on the mechanics of respiration, *J Clin Invest*, **15(1)**, 47–61.

[22] Reuben, A.D. and Harris, A.R. (2004). Heliox for asthma in the emergency department: a review of the literature, *Emerg Med J*, **21**, 131–135.

[23] Kim, I.K., Phrampus, E., Venkataraman, S. *et al.* (2005). Helium/oxygen-driven albuterol nebulization in the treatment of children with moderate to severe asthma: a randomized controlled trial, *Pediatrics*, **116**, 1127–1133.

[24] Rodrigo, G.J.J., Pollack, C.V., Rodrigo, C. *et al.* (2006). Heliox for nonintubated acute asthma patients, *Cochrane Database Syst Rev*, CD002884.

[25] Martinon-Torres, F., Rodriguez-Nunez, A. and Martinon-Sanchez, J.M. (2008). Nasal continuous positive airway pressure with heliox versus air oxygen in infants with acute bronchiolitis:a crossover study, *Pediatrics*, **121**, e1190–e1195.

[26] Duncan, P.G. (1979). Efficacy of helium-oxygen mixtures in the management of severe viral and post extubation croup, *Can J Anaeasth*, **26**, 206–212.

[27] Weber, J.E., Chudnofsky, C.G., Younger, J.G. *et al.* (2001). A randomized comparison of helium-oxygen mixture (Heliox) and racemic epinephrine for the treatment of moderate to severe croup, *Pediatrics*, **107**, E96.

[28] Vorwerk, C. and Coats, T.J. (2008). Use of helium-oxygen mixtures in the treatment of croup: a systematic review, *Emerg Med J*, **25**, 547–550.

[29] Myers, T.R. (2006). Use of heliox in children, *Respir Care*, **6**, 619–631.

[30] Nadel, S. and Kroll, J.S. (2007). Diagnosis and management of meningococcal disease: the need for centralized care, *FEMS Microbiol Rev*, **31**, 71–83.

[31] Ovstebo, R., Brandtzaeg, P., Brusletto, B. *et al.* (2004). Use of robotized DNA isolation and real-time PCR to quantify and identify close correlation between levels of *Neisseria meningitidis* DNA and lipopolysaccharides in plasma and cerebrospinal fluid from patients with systemic meningococcal disease, *J Clin Microbiol*, **42**, 2980–2987.

[32] Thompson, M.J., Ninis, N., Perera, R. *et al.* (2006). Clinical recognition of meningococcal disease in children and adolescents, *Lancet*, **367**, 397–403.

[33] van Deuren, M., Brandtzaeg, P. and van der Meer, J.W. (2000). Update on meningococcal disease with emphasis on pathogenesis and clinical management, *Clin Microbiol Rev*, **13**, 144–166.

[34] Booy, R., Habibi, P., Nadel, S. *et al.* (2001). Reduction in case fatality rate from meningococcal disease associated with improved healthcare delivery, *Arch Dis Child*, **85**, 386–390.

[35] Thorburn, K., Baines, P., Thomson, A. *et al.* (2001). Mortality in severe meningococcal disease, *Arch Dis Child*, **85**, 382–385.

[36] Lodder, M.C., Schildkamp, R.L., Bijlmer, H.A. *et al.* (1996). Prognostic indicators of the outcome of meningococcal disease: a study of 562 patients, *J Med Microbiol*, **45**, 16–20.

[37] Chin, R.F., Neville, B.G., Peckham, C. *et al.* (2006). Incidence, cause, and short-term outcome of convulsive status epilepticus in childhood: prospective population-based study, *Lancet*, **368**, 222–229.

[38] Pollard, A.J., Nadel, S., Ninis, N. *et al.* (2007). Emergency management of meningococcal disease: eight years on, *Arch Dis Child*, **92**, 283–286.

[39] Pathan, N., Faust, S.N. and Levin, M. (2003). Pathophysiology of meningococcal meningitis and septicaemia. *Arch Dis Child*, **88**, 601–607.

[40] Brandtzaeg, P., Kierulf, P., Gaustad, P. *et al.* (1989). Plasma endotoxin as a predictor of multiple organ failure and death in systemic meningococcal disease, *J Infect Dis*, **159**, 195–204.

[41] Carcillo, J.A., Davis, A.L. and Zaritsky, A. (1991). Role of early fluid resuscitation in pediatric septic shock, *JAMA*, **266**, 1242–1245.

[42] Rivers, E., Nguyen, B., Havstad, S. *et al.* (2001). Early goal-directed therapy in the treatment of severe sepsis and septic shock, *N Engl J Med*, **345**, 1368–1377.

[43] Finfer, S., Bellomo, R., Boyce, N. *et al.* (2004). A comparison of albumin and saline for fluid resuscitation in the intensive care unit, *N Engl J Med*, **350**, 2247–2256.

[44] van den Berghe, G., Wouters, P., Weekers, F. *et al.* (2001). Intensive insulin therapy in the critically ill patients, *N Engl J Med*, **345**, 1359–1367.

[45] Day, K.M., Haub, N., Betts, H. *et al.* (2008). Hyperglycemia is associated with morbidity in critically ill children with meningococcal sepsis, *Pediatr Crit Care Med*, **9**, 636–640.

[46] Bernard, G.R., Vincent, J.L., Laterre P.F. *et al.* (2001). Efficacy and safety of recombinant human activated protein C for severe sepsis, *N Engl J Med*, **344**, 699–709.

[47] Nadel, S., Goldstein, B., Williams, M.D. *et al.* (2007). Drotrecogin alfa (activated) in children with severe sepsis: a multicentre phase III randomised controlled trial, *Lancet*, **369**, 836–843.

[48] McIntyre, P.B., Berkey, C.S., King, S.M. *et al.* (1997). Dexamethasone as adjunctive therapy in bacterial meningitis. A meta-analysis of randomized clinical trials since 1988, *JAMA*, **278**, 925–931.

[49] Hatherill, M., Tibby S.M., Hilliard, T. *et al.* (1999). Adrenal insufficiency in septic shock, *Arch Dis Child*, **80**, 51–55.

[50] Annane, D., Sebille, V., Charpentier, C. *et al.* (2002). Effect of treatment with low doses of hydrocortisone and fludrocortisone on mortality in patients with septic shock, *JAMA*, **288**, 862–871.

[51] Sprung, C.L., Annane, D., Keh, D. *et al.* (2008). Hydrocortisone therapy for patients with septic shock, *N Engl J Med*, **358**, 111–124.

[52] Derkx, B., Wittes, J. and McCloskey, R. (1999). Randomized, placebo-controlled trial of HA-1A, a human monoclonal antibody to endotoxin, in children with meningococcal septic shock, *Clin Infect Dis*, **28**, 770–777.

[53] McCloskey, R.V., Straube, R.C., Sanders, C. *et al.* (1994). Treatment of septic shock with human monoclonal antibody HA-1A. A randomized, double-blind, placebo-controlled trial, *Ann Intern Med*, **121**, 1–5.

[54] Levin, M., Quint, P.A., Goldstein, B. *et al.* (2000). Recombinant bactericidal/permeability-increasing protein (rBPI21) as adjunctive treatment for children with severe meningococcal sepsis: a randomised trial, *Lancet*, **356**, 961–967.

[55] Ninis, N., Phillips, C., Bailey, L. *et al.* (2005). The role of healthcare delivery in the outcome of meningococcal disease in children: case-control study of fatal and non-fatal cases, *BMJ*, **330**, 1475–1480.

[56] Britto, J., Nadel, S., Maconochie, I. *et al.* (1995). Morbidity and severity of illness during interhospital transfer: impact of a specialised paediatric retrieval team, *BMJ*, **311**, 836–839.

[57] Chew, C., Halliday, J.L., Riley, M.M. *et al.* (2007). Population-based study of antenatal detection of congenital heart disease by ultrasound examination, *Ultrasound Obstet Gynecol*, **29**, 619–624.

[58] McBrien, A., Sands, A., Craig, B. *et al.* (2009). Major congenital heart disease: antenatal detection, patient characteristics and outcomes, *J Mat-Fet & Neo Medicine*, **22**, 101–105.

[59] Lau, S.T. and Brisseau, G.F. (2006). 'Evaluation, stabilization and initial management after multiple trauma', in Fuhrman, B.P. and Zimmerman, J. (eds), *Pediatric Critical Care*, third edition, Mosby Elsevier, Philadelphia, pp. 1579–1585.

[60] Bergman, A.B. and Rivara, F.P. (1991). Sweden's experience in reducing childhood injuries, *Pediatrics*, **88**, 69–74.

[61] Committee on Trauma, American College of Surgeons (2004). *Advanced trauma life support for doctors, student course manual*, seventh edition, American College of Surgeons, Chicago.

[62] Tasker, R.C. (2008). 'Head and spinal cord trauma', in Nichols, D.G. (ed.), *Rogers' Textbook of Pediatric Intensive Care*, fourth edition, Lippincot Williams and Wilkins, Philadelphia, pp. 887–911.

[63] Baird, J.S. and Cooper, A. (2008). 'Multiple trauma', in Nichols, D.G. (ed.), *Rogers' Textbook of Pediatric Intensive Care*, fourth edition, Lippincot Williams and Wilkins, Philadelphia, pp. 385–407.

[64] Parslow, R.C., Tasker, R.C., Draper, E.S. *et al.* (2009). Epidemiology of critically ill children in England and Wales: incidence, mortality, deprivation and ethnicity, *Arch Dis Child*, **94**, 210–215.

[65] Royal College of Paediatrics and Child Health (2004). *Witholding or Withdrawing Life Sustaining Treatment in Children: A Framework for Practice*, second Edition, [Online]. Available at: www.gmc-uk.org/Witholding.pdf_40818793.pdf [Accessed 1February 2013].

[66] The Multisociety Task Force on PVS (1994). Medical aspects of the persistent vegetative state, *N Engl J Med*, **330**, 1499–1508.

[67] Royal College of Physicians (2003).*The Vegetative State — Guidance on Diagnosis and Management, Report of a Working Party of the Royal College of Physicians*, [Online]. Available at: http://bookshop.rcplondon.ac.uk/contents/pub165–9e4092a9–85fb-4b27–8121–261045b1aac2.pdf.

[68] Goldman, A. (2001). Recent advances in palliative care. Importance of palliative care for children is being increasingly recognised, *BMJ*, **322**, 234.

[69] Office for National Statistics (2013). *Childhood, infant and perinatal mortality in England and Wales, 2011* [Online]. Available at: http://www.ons.gov.uk/ons/dcp171778_300596.pdf [Accessed 17 October 2013].

[70] Feudtner, C., Silveira, M.J. and Christakis, D.A. (2002). Where do children with complex chronic conditions die? Patterns in Washington State, 1980–1998, *Pediatrics*, **109**, 656–660.

[71] Ramnarayan, P., Craig, F., Petros, A. *et al.* (2007). Characteristics of deaths occurring in hospitalised children: changing trends, *J Med Ethics*, **33**, 255–260.

[72] Burns, J.P. and Rushton, C.H. (2004). End-of-life care in the pediatric intensive care unit: research review and recommendations, *Crit Care Clin*, **20**, 467–485.

[73] British Paediatric Association (1991). *Working Party Report, Diagnosis of brain stem death in infants and children,* British Paediatric Association, London 1991.

[74] Taskforce for the Determination of Brain Death in Children (1987). Guidelines for the determination of brain death in children, *Pediatr Neurol*, **3**, 242–243.

26
Trauma Intensive Care

Peter J. Shirley

26.1 Introduction

Despite significant advances in management over the last 20 years, trauma remains the chief cause of death and disability in individuals under 40 years of age. Trauma is a worldwide phenomenon with profound public health implications and numerous challenges, including the need for an increased emphasis on accident prevention and rehabilitation, particularly in the developing world. The Essential Trauma Care Project has defined and promoted core essential trauma care services that every injured person in the world should be able to receive. This project is a collaborative effort of the World Health Organization and the International Society of Surgery [1].

Patients requiring intensive care for severe trauma often pose particular challenges. The treatment of these patients can be protracted (commonly referred to as the prolonged-care phase) and the initial injury may become of secondary importance to the effects of systemic inflammatory response syndrome, acute lung injury (ALI), nosocomial infection and inter-current multiple organ dysfunction syndrome (MODS). Multiply injured patients often require lengthy periods of mechanical ventilation and a variety of therapeutic interventions may have to be considered during the management of the disease process.

The issues raised by those involved in the intensive care management of trauma patients include:

(i) Consideration of the injury mechanisms and potential structures at risk in blunt and penetrating trauma.
(ii) Pre-operative management of the trauma patient, including indications for intubation and approaches to fluid management.
(iii) Clearance of the cervical spine in a sedated and ventilated trauma patient.
(iv) Timing of fracture fixation and damage control surgery.
(v) Ventilation strategies and analgesia in patients with multiple injuries.
(vi) Use of inotropic support for maintenance of blood pressure.
(vii) Rehabilitation from injury.

26.2 Initial Management

As always in trauma, management begins with airway, breathing and circulation. Ideally, the intensive care unit (ICU) should be represented within the trauma team. This role is often filled by an anaesthetist, whose role goes beyond assessment of the airway. Provision of advanced airway interventions and ventilatory support is often necessary. If the patient is awake, the ICU doctor needs to take a full history, including when they last ate or drank, allergies, medications and any other co-morbidities.

In all trauma patients at risk of cervical spine injury who require urgent intubation and ventilation, cervical spine immobilisation must be maintained during intubation. The cervical hard collar may need removal to allow adequate mouth opening but a suitable assistant must apply manual in-line immobilisation. A second assistant will be required to maintain cricoid pressure if this is required. Additionally they need to ensure that spinal immobilisation is maintained and, in conjunction with the trauma team leader, assess circulation and co-ordinate fluid, blood and blood-product replacement as necessary They need to assist with large-bore peripheral or central venous access as required and establish intra-arterial blood pressure and central venous pressure monitoring as soon as practicable. The ICU doctor needs to co-ordinate patient transfer in conjunction with the team leader, whether to the computed tomography (CT) scanner, operating theatre or ICU.

A nominated scribe must be advised of all therapeutic interventions undertaken and encouraged to document vital signs, blood results and other relevant information.

Discussion of the need for intensive/high-dependency care after resuscitation must be done earlier rather than later and the necessary communication made with both the trauma team leader and ICU staff.

26.3 Acute Fluid Resuscitation

Volume replacement is the accepted method for treating hypovolaemia but it can also significantly compromise other organ systems. Continuous infusions of even blood or normotonic fluids can cause significant peripheral tissue oedema, frank acute respiratory distress syndrome (ARDS) or an increase in lung water with impairment of both gas exchange and cardiac function. Traditionally multi-trauma patients have been given aggressive fluid resuscitation and blood pressure support to maintain vital organ perfusion. There is now a view that fluid resuscitation should be limited until haemostasis is achieved, and that delays in the emergency department when surgical intervention to stop bleeding is required are a cause of increased mortality [2]. Most experimental studies have looked at models of pure vascular bleeding and there are few reliable clinical studies; the only prospective randomised ones have been done in penetrating trauma. In the case of head injuries, however, a low systemic arterial blood pressure (SABP) relates to a poor outcome; the patient with an altered mental status with multiple injuries (that are bleeding) presents a dilemma. Aggressive fluid administration could exacerbate bleeding from an occult injury or inadequately splinted femur but blood pressure support in terms of maintaining cerebral perfusion would be considered to be a key therapeutic intervention [3]. The current consensus view in pre-hospital care is that fluid should not be administered to the trauma victims prior to haemorrhage control if a radial pulse can be felt. Judicious aliquots of 250 ml should be titrated for other patients. If the radial pulse returns, fluid resuscitation can be suspended for the present and the situation monitored. In penetrating injury, the presence of a central pulse should be considered adequate [4]. It is recognised that patients with head injuries are a special group and may require higher blood pressure to maintain cerebral perfusion (systolic blood pressure >100 mmHg). The continued application of this protocol in the hospital setting is still not established [5]. Rather controversially, some have pointed out that the amount of fluid to be used in resuscitation has been overshadowed by questions about the choice of fluid and have suggested that this is driven by commercial interests of pharmaceutical companies looking for a market share [6]. The use of artificial colloids is not without risk, due to the pathophysiological processes (capillary leak and inflammation) involved in the response to tissue trauma [7]. The use of lower volumes of resuscitation fluid would seem sensible in the case of chest trauma in particular and the use of hypertonic saline may have some place, although it has certainly not gained universal acceptance [8]. It should be remembered that the presence of non-response shock in blunt trauma may be due to direct myocardial injury. Transoesophageal echocardiography (TOE) is an effective tool in the assessment of cardiac trauma in conjunction with electrocardiogram and cardiac enzyme measurements. It can also be used in the early assessment of aortic injuries. A high index of suspicion must be retained, even in the face of normal TOE findings [9]. With a negative TOE but with a high index of suspicion (mediastinal widening on plain X-ray remains the most reliable sign), then the patient should have a contrast-enhanced spiral CT of the thorax as part of the initial management [10]. Regardless of the treatment or monitoring methods used, the goal of resuscitation is to fully restore homeostasis and prevent end organ damage. Current resuscitation approaches (of which there are many) support the notion that hypoperfusion results in metabolic acidosis, from the production of lactate. The initial resuscitation and management priorities in the emergency department are somewhat different from those in the operating theatre (or ICU) but the ultimate endpoints of resuscitation are the same. Fluid requirements (or their absence) serve as an imprecise endpoint of resuscitation. Invasive haemodynamic monitoring provides the clinician with systemic or global values but might not currently have the ability to detail regional or microcirculatory flow. While bolus infusions of crystalloid or colloid solutions are still recommended for patients in extremis and for patients with isolated extremity injuries, patients who have a strong potential for ongoing internal haemorrhage should now be managed with a deliberate hypotensive approach until definitive haemostasis has been achieved [11]. While this approach remains controversial in the setting of severe head injury, recent experimental evidence has still favoured a slow infusion technique. The most appropriate fluid for resuscitation remains the subject of debate, but trials of hypertonic saline, colloid and blood-substitute solutions have all been recently conducted or are under way. Topical and systemic haemostatic agents and new types of tourniquets all have the potential to improve outcomes and simultaneous 1:1 ratios of red blood cell and plasma infusions may also enhance survival rates [12].

26.4 Clearance of the Cervical Spine

Cervical spine injury occurs in 5–10% of blunt polytrauma patients. Despite several published clinical guidelines this is a controversial topic. The application of these guidelines to the obtunded trauma patient is limited. The presence of a severe head injury increases the relative risk of a cervical spine injury by as much as 8.5 times and a focal neurological deficit by 58 times. When the patient is unlikely to be evaluated fully within 24 hours, prolonged immobilisation shifts the risk–benefit analysis from waiting for an opportunity to do a full clinical evaluation, to a non-clinical clearance, given that the vast majority (95%) will not have a cervical injury. Some units combine cervical plain films (lateral, antero-posterior and odontoid views) with saggital reconstructions of the entire cervical spine CT [13].

A protocol using CT scanning alone for blunt trauma patients who were obtunded has shown that the risk of missing a cervical spine injury is 0.04% [14].

Current practice at the Royal London Hospital is whole-cervical-spine helical CT scanning for assessment of cervical spine injury in the unconscious trauma patient. CT scanning had a sensitivity of 98.1%, a specificity of 98.8%, and a negative predictive value of 99.7%. There were no missed unstable injuries. In contrast, an adequate lateral cervical spine film had a sensitivity of 53.3%, and unstable injuries will be missed. It must be remembered though that no imaging modality will have 100% sensitivity, and there will always be injuries missed by any given protocol [15].

26.5 Timing of Fracture Fixation and Surgery (Damage Control)

The two main surgical goals for the critically injured trauma patient undergoing a damage control operation are haemorrhage and source (contamination) control. It is increasingly clear that the coagulopathy stems from both low temperature and acidosis working together (coagulopathy, acidosis, hypothermia — the 'triad of death'). The concept of damage-control surgery is now well established and has become the accepted method of management of unstable trauma patients over the last decade [16]. This refers to a three-phase surgical approach taken on the basis of patient physiology, the response to fluid loading and level of blood loss. Its application has been shown to be of benefit both in penetrating abdominal injury and severe chest trauma [17]. The optimal timing of fracture fixation in the multiply injured is still widely debated. There is no doubt that early fixation of fractures reduces inflammation at the site of injury and thus decreases pain and opiate requirements. There is also evidence that this approach reduces overall pulmonary complications and promotes early mobilisation [18].

Larger studies are tending to indicate that the early stabilisation of femoral fractures with definitive intramedullary mailing appears to be the treatment of choice even for patients with combined head and chest injuries [19]. However, it must be remembered that the initial fixation can only take place if the multi-trauma patient is adequately resuscitated. Also, the effect of fatigue on outcome, if surgery is performed in the middle of the night, must not be dismissed [20]. For all the reasons outlined above, it must not be assumed that definitive fracture fixation will necessarily be carried out prior to ICU admission. Indeed it is recognised now that damage control is not just a surgical concept but really applies to the whole of the patient management and particularly whenever the patient is admitted (or readmitted after surgery) to the ICU [21].

26.6 Admission to the ICU

A secondary survey should have been completed in the emergency department but, if the patient has been expedited to the operating theatre, then this may not have been completed prior to ICU admission.

For all patients, even if a secondary survey has been completed, a tertiary survey must be performed. When the patient first arrives in the ICU, continued resuscitation and further evaluation of possible injuries must proceed simultaneously. As in the emergency department, ongoing resuscitation takes precedence over fine detail. Nonetheless, the patient needs to be fully evaluated as quickly as possible so that all injuries and concurrent medical conditions are recognised. This complete re-evaluation of the trauma patient that typically occurs in the ICU has been called the tertiary survey [22]. This should be performed in all trauma patients, regardless of whether or not they require critical care management. The goal is to identify all injuries. Missed injuries can have a significant effect on morbidity, as well as on mortality, from trauma. The more severely injured patients, particularly those with traumatic brain injury (TBI), are at the greatest risk of having occult lesions.

A common pitfall is to focus only on the immediately life-threatening wounds, while inadvertently ignoring less obvious but potentially debilitating injuries. The specific components of the tertiary survey include a thorough review of all previously learned information and completion of all abbreviated or deferred elements of the primary and secondary surveys.

Items to be specifically included are an acquisition of a complete and accurate history, performing a thorough physical examination, review of all imaging studies and laboratory data, and ordering of additional tests as indicated.

Repeated limb compartment checks and continued presence of distal pulses must be recorded in all those with limb injuries. Clinical vigilance (and rising serum creatinine kinase levels) at this stage can prevent limb loss later.

A thorough examination of the eyes and ears is also indicated; this is an often overlooked aspect of the trauma examination.

26.7 Respiratory Support and Ventilation Strategies

Mechanical ventilation is often necessary in severe trauma and particularly blunt chest trauma. Chest CT is known to be superior to chest radiography in assessing the extent of lung contusions. In patients sustaining multiple traumatic injuries the development of ALI and ARDS is not uncommon. The use of mechanical ventilation is often inevitable in these circumstances and in fact their development is more likely in patients with prolonged ventilation. Current clinical care has moved towards low-tidal-volume ventilation and higher positive end-expiratory pressures, following the publication of the ARDS-net study [23]. Characteristically, established ARDS has refractory hypoxaemia, intrapulmonary shunting and a respiratory and metabolic acidosis. Marked inflammatory infiltrates and capillary leakage, along with fibrosis and atelectasis (resulting from loss of surfactant), leads to a loss of compliance. The use of the ARDS criteria in trauma patients has been questioned on the basis that some patients seem to behave very differently to others. Some patients have rapid resolution of their symptoms and early weaning from mechanical ventilation, whereas others go on to have ARDS-related pulmonary fibrosis and prolonged weaning. High minute ventilation is characteristic of the long-term ARDS patients, indicating increased dead-space, along with higher peak inspiratory pressures and poorer lung compliance, when initially ventilated. It is accepted, however, that the lower-tidal-volume ventilation strategies described earlier should still be applied to both subsets of patients [24]. At alveolar level, alterations in the mechanics may account for some of these differences in ventilated patients. Repetitive alveolar collapse and expansion with ventilation occurs throughout the lung but differences between alveoli do occur, some totally collapsing and re-expanding with each breath and others remaining patent at the end of expiration [25]. The mechanisms behind longer-term lung injury may be explained by alveoli behaving differently in different patients, with some patients' lungs being potentially more affected by direct trauma and the stretch effect of mechanical ventilation.

Novalung (Hechingen, Germany) has developed a new system (lung assist device (LAD)) using an arteriovenous shunt and a low-resistance membrane such that the patient's arteriovenous pressure gradient can be used as the driving force. The membrane is based on heparin-coated hollow fibre technology with optimised blood flow by reduction of resistance. The LAD is connected to the patient via arterial and venous cannulae inserted by Seldinger technique. The system runs with a low-dose heparin infusion. Recent studies have suggested a survival benefit as this device allows less aggressive lung ventilation to achieve CO_2 clearance and maintain blood pH [26]. It has been used successfully to facilitate transfer of trauma patients with early acute lung injury over long distances for specialised care [27].

Prone ventilation, high-frequency oscillatory ventilation and extra-corporeal membrane oxygenation have been tried with varying success in trauma and are discussed comprehensively in Chapters 7, 19 and 20.

Early tracheostomy (before day eight) has also been shown to be beneficial in multiple trauma patients and may reduce the incidence of pneumonia and decrease the time to weaning from mechanical ventilation [28].

Recently, a multicentre randomised study in the UK comparing early and late tracheostomy (Trachman) has reported results which do not suggest a trend towards better outcome in early tracheostomies [29].

The Advanced Trauma Life Support algorithm of intubating hypoxic patients with isolated chest contusions has been challenged. It has been shown that patients with significant pulmonary contusion (arterial partial pressure of oxygen:inspired oxygen fraction (PaO_2:FiO_2) ratio < 300) can be treated safely with non-invasive ventilation alone and instances with patients requiring intubation were not for reasons of respiratory failure [30].

In patients with unilateral chest trauma, ventilator-associated lung injury is a distinct possibility in the healthy lung, as this more compliant lung may be preferentially ventilated, leading to excessive stretching and shearing. A double-lumen endotracheal tube and independent lung ventilation using two ventilators is sometimes employed to protect the healthy lung. Most reports of this technique are in the form of case reports but these do suggest merit in patients with significant unilateral chest trauma [31].

26.8 Cardiovascular Support

The optimal management of fluid balance in severe trauma involving mechanically ventilated patients is widely debated. Questions revolve around whether patients should be kept 'dry' to help prevent pulmonary oedema, or whether the development of oedema is inevitable due to the underlying condition and therefore fluids should be used to optimise the circulation with the aim of improving cardiac output, oxygen delivery and vital organ perfusion. In all cases the objective is to restore oxygen delivery to the tissues while correcting the underlying cause (for example, surgical intervention to arrest haemorrhage or eradicate infection). Speed is essential. Delays in making the diagnosis and initiating treatment, as well as sub-optimal resuscitation, contribute to the development of peripheral vascular failure and irreversible defects in oxygen use which can culminate in vital organ dysfunction [32].

The first priority is to secure the airway and, if necessary, to provide mechanical ventilation. Because mechanical ventilation abolishes or minimises the work of breathing, reduces oxygen consumption and improves oxygenation, early respiratory support benefits patients with severe shock. Tissue blood flow must be restored by achieving and maintaining an adequate cardiac output and by ensuring that systemic blood pressure is sufficient to maintain perfusion of vital organs. Traditionally, a mean arterial pressure of 60 mmHg (or systolic blood pressure of 80 mmHg) has been considered sufficient, but some evidence suggests that a mean pressure of 80 mmHg may be more appropriate. It may be contended that the patient's normal blood pressure should be targeted. Circulatory support, therefore, involves manipulation of the three determinants of stroke volume — namely preload, myocardial contractility and afterload — as well as heart rate. Blood transfusions are not without risk and this must be borne in mind when considering the relative benefits of transfusion in terms of oxygen carriage [33]. The use of goal-orientated resuscitation in trauma (as has been advocated in severe septic shock) is gaining support, using the oxygen delivery index (DO_2I) but the results from studies are by no means conclusive. Measurement of central venous oxygen saturation ($ScvO_2$) as an indicator of cardiac output ($ScvO_2 > 70\%$ being optimal) and directing the use of fluid resuscitation and ionotropic support has a place in the trauma population. Measurements of base deficit and lactate are also of use [34]. The circulating volume must be replaced within minutes, since rapid restoration of cardiac output and tissue perfusion pressure reduces the chances of serious organ damage, particularly acute renal failure. There is no longer any place for the use of dopamine or diuretic infusions to maintain urine output in renal impairment; these manoeuvres have been shown to do nothing to prevent subsequent renal failure. Efforts should be concentrated on maintaining perfusion via adequate fluid input and use of vasopressors as necessary to prevent sustained hypotension [35]. It has been recognised for some time, however, that early depression of cardiac function is associated with poor outcome in patients with trauma [36]. With the decline in the use of the pulmonary artery catheter (PAC), less invasive forms of cardiac monitoring are now being used (such as oesophageal Doppler), with the potential to get haemodynamic variables measured much earlier. In intensive care circles there has been an ongoing debate about crystalloid versus colloid and the outcome on patients. It has been reported in a large prospective multicentre trial that the use of albumin or normal saline in the ICU shows similar outcomes at 28 days [37]. Although resuscitation has conventionally aimed at achieving normal haemodynamic values, survival of many critically ill patients is associated with raised values for cardiac output, oxygen delivery and oxygen consumption. In reality a balanced approach is the norm; fluids are managed with close monitoring of numerous parameters, including peripheral perfusion, pulse rate, central venous pressure response to fluid challenges and stroke volume response to fluids, oesophageal Doppler probe or lithium-dilution continuous cardiac output monitoring. Adequate volume resuscitation and ionotropic support improves survival in systemic inflammatory response syndrome whilst achieving the same level of cardiac support with ionotropes alone does not [38].

26.9 Traumatic Brain Injury

Primary brain injury is caused directly by the initial impact and this damage is generally referred to the pathology existing immediately following the trauma; secondary injury refers to the destructive changes that evolve over time (hours to days) following the primary event. Direct injury can occur to the brain parenchyma, as well as to the skull, meninges, dura or blood vessels, which result in space-occupying lesions or haematomas. Intensive care treatment is aimed at lessening the impact of secondary injury by controlling intracranial pressure (ICP) and modification of cerebral perfusion pressure (CPP). Maintenance of a CPP greater than 70 mmHg is now widely recognised as a vital component of management of traumatic brain injury.

A systolic blood pressure of less than 90 mmHg occurring between the time of TBI and completion of resuscitation is associated with a 33% increase in mortality. The highest blood sugar occurring in the first

24 hours of ICU care is linearly correlated with mortality. Fever should be prevented in TBI patients as it will merely increase the cerebral metabolic requirement for oxygen.

For the patient with TBI, a CPP of 60–70 mmHg is generally sufficient to maintain cerebral oxygenation. Excessive hyperventilation of patients with TBI will cause ischemia if CO_2 reactivity is preserved. The interpretation of a given ICP measurement must be made in the light of the underlying pathology and the speed of its evolution. Current evidence suggests that 20–25 mmHg is the upper threshold above which treatment to lower ICP should be started. The management of hypotension must include not only fluid replacement but also identification of the cause. There is minimal evidence for the routine use of anticonvulsants to prevent seizures.

A standardised protocol for the management of ICP appears to provide more consistent control. Protocols need to be agreed jointly between the neurosurgical and intensive care medical team. There are a number of protocols for the prevention of secondary brain injury following major trauma. They are generally directed at the maintenance of CPP to ensure adequate cerebral blood flow. The Brain Trauma Foundation found that mortality increased as the average CPP fell below 70 mmHg, and that aggressive therapy was required to control ICP and systemic arterial pressure. A number of historical trials have suggested that the ICU and ward mortality for patients with head injuries on a neurosurgical ICU is reduced by the implementation of a target CPP-guided protocol but there are no prospective randomised trials comparing goal-directed therapy with previous conventional head injury management. The evidence suggests that patients with head injuries in the following groups should undergo ICP monitoring [39]:

(i) Those with a Glasgow Coma Scale score less than 11.
(ii) Those requiring prolonged non-neurosurgical surgery.
(iii) Those with head injury and abnormal CT brain scan.

26.10 Chest Trauma

By far the most important cause of significant blunt chest trauma is road traffic accidents (RTAs). RTAs account for 70–80% of such injuries. Falls and acts of violence are other causative mechanisms. Blast injuries can also result in significant blunt thoracic trauma [38]. Blunt trauma commonly results in chest wall injuries. The pain associated with these injuries may compromise ventilation. Pulmonary contusions are frequently associated with major chest trauma and may impair ventilation by a similar mechanism. Shunting and dead space ventilation produced by these injuries can also impair oxygenation. Blunt trauma that causes significant cardiac injuries (e.g., rupture of a chamber) or severe great vessel injuries (e.g., thoracic aortic disruption) frequently results in death before adequate treatment can be instituted. The clinical presentation of patients with blunt chest trauma is dependent on the mechanism of injury and other organ systems involved [41].

The management of the pain associated with chest injuries has also come under scrutiny and is worth considering; especially if the patient is managed with non-invasive ventilation (compared with those who are mechanically ventilated and more likely to have intravenous sedation and analgesia). The pain from rib fractures is known to decrease pulmonary function. Comparisons of intravenous patient-controlled analgesia with morphine and epidural infusions of bupivacaine plus fentanyl have shown superior analgesia via the epidural route [42]. Moreover epidural analgesia has demonstrated improvements in pulmonary function and modifications of the immune response (as measured by lower levels of interleukin IL-8), as compared with patient-controlled analgesia [43]. The use of epidurals can be difficult, however, especially in patients with coagulopathy, non-radiologically cleared thoracic spines and those that are already mechanically ventilated. As such there is limited use of epidural analgesia in the emergency trauma patient. It has been shown to reduce nosocomial infection rates and shorten mechanical ventilation in patients with more than three rib fractures [44]. Elderly patients with rib fractures have twice the morbidity and mortality of younger patients. For each additional rib fracture in the elderly, mortality increases by 19% and the risk of pneumonia by 27%. Improvements in terms of hospital stay or mortality have not been shown in patients treated using epidural analgesia, especially in the elderly population [45]. Penetrating chest trauma comprises a broad spectrum of injuries and severity. The clinical consequences depend on the mechanism of the injury, the location of the injury, associated injuries and underlying illnesses. Organs at risk, in addition to the intrathoracic contents, include the intraperitoneal viscera, the retroperitoneal space and the neck. A patient with combined intrathoracic and intra-abdominal wounds has a markedly greater chance of dying. These patients present a particular challenge for the surgical team [46].

26.11 Extremity Trauma

Extremity injuries pose a complex problem to the multiply injured trauma patient. Additionally, special consideration should be given to patients with injuries isolated to the extremity but who require extensive resuscitation and/or operative intervention. Consultation with orthopaedic, vascular, plastic surgery and anaesthetic teams is essential to the expeditious care of patients and improving outcomes. In this setting of polytrauma with severe mangled extremities intubation, fluid resuscitation and proximal vascular control are required during initial resuscitation. Once stabilised, treatment of the injuries to the extremities is staged. In muscle compartments, the muscle damage may result in myoglobinuria and acute renal failure in the acute phase; the long-term effects are of muscle damage and contractures (Volkmann's contracture). The prevention of the syndrome depends on recognising conditions that may lead to compartment syndrome and measuring intra-compartmental pressure. A similar syndrome can occur in muscle compartments through any form of injury or trauma that causes muscle swelling. The rise in compartment pressure initially causes extrinsic compression of the venous circulation, and reduces transcapillary flow. The renewed use of tourniquets in the initial treatment of severe peripheral injuries has lead to fears that limbs may be lost due to muscle compartment ischaemia as a result of this treatment [47].

26.12 Abdominal Compartment Syndrome

Theoretically, compartment syndrome can develop in any compartment where swelling within the compartment results in a rise in intra-compartmental pressure. This may be within the abdomen, where trauma, ileus, retroperitoneal bleeding, mesenteric oedema and intra-abdominal fluid can all contribute to a rise in abdominal pressure. Once the pressure rises above arterial pressure, ischaemia occurs in the compartment. In the abdomen, this may manifest as acute renal failure or bowel ischaemia, giving rise to a progressive metabolic acidosis. Abdominal compartment syndrome often occurs in severely injured patients, especially those who undergo laparotomy with abdominal packing. Early recognition with decompressive laparotomy, leaving an open abdomen with a temporary covering (such as the Bogotá bag) provides immediate improvement in organ function and physiologic status.

Abdominal compartment syndrome may be recognised by the presence of a tensely distended abdomen, elevated peak airway pressures, inadequate ventilation and decreased urine output. However, these findings are relatively non-specific. Intra-abdominal pressure can be monitored by instilling 100 ml of saline into the catheterised bladder, which at that volume remains a passive reservoir. The intra-abdominal portion of the bladder can then serve as a transducer to record abdominal pressure, without any contribution from its own musculature. The tubing is held parallel to the patient at the level of the pubis until urine forms a meniscus distal to the sampling port. A clamp is placed distal to the port and a needle is inserted through the port and connected to a water manometer or electronic pressure transducer. A pressure greater than 30 mmHg is associated with oliguria due to a decreased renal blood flow associated with increased renal venous pressure and a calculated increase in renal vascular resistance. Abdominal compartment syndrome is also associated with an intra-abdominal pressure of 25 mmHg and can also cause elevation in ICP, presumably by increasing central venous pressure, therefore resulting in significant decreases in cerebral perfusion [48].

26.13 Pelvic Trauma

The management of unstable pelvic fractures has evolved over the last two decades. Radiographic signs of pelvic instability include more than 5 mm of displacement of the posterior sacroiliac complex, the presence of a posterior fracture gap (as opposed to impaction) and avulsion fractures of the posterior iliac spine, sacrum, ischial tuberosity or transverse process of the fifth lumbar vertebra. The first major goal of the trauma practitioner in controlling pelvic bleeding is stabilisation of the unstable pelvic injury.

This can be achieved immediately through the use of a pelvic binder applied around the pelvis, often (but not always) followed by application of an external fixation device, and subsequent delayed surgical repair once haemorrhage control is satisfactory. Pelvic trauma patients should have intravenous access placed via tributaries that drain into the superior vena cava. Evolving protocols for the haemodynamically unstable patient suggests that initial management should be aimed at the detection of intra-abdominal bleeding using focussed assessment by sonography in trauma (FAST) or diagnostic peritoneal lavage within 30 minutes of arrival. Patients with intra-abdominal bleeding should undergo laparotomy immediately, with concomitant pelvic stabilisation, to control pelvic venous bleeding. In patients with no intra-abdominal bleeding, or those in whom pelvic arterial bleeding persists after laparotomy, the patient should receive pelvic angiography no more than 45 minutes after arrival. Optimum bleeding control can usually be achieved with coil embolisation [49]. The risk of deep vein thrombosis is as high as 60% in trauma patients with pelvic fractures and there may be a subsequent need for insertion of an inferior vena cava filter for the prevention of pulmonary embolus.

26.14 Other Considerations

As with all ICU patients, general supportive measures are essential and trauma patients are no exception. Sepsis is the main cause of death in this group and efforts should be made to prevent and treat nosocomial infections. Infection control and hand washing in particular have a major role to play in this respect. Early enteral feeding and thrombo-embolic prophylaxis are also important. Range of motion checks of all joints should be performed at least daily on patients who are unconscious or unable to conduct their own exercises in conjunction with the normal daily respiratory physiotherapy.

Trauma patients tend to be young. Successful outcome is often measured in terms of mortality but from the patients perspective a return to a functionally useful life is usually what they want. Intensive care only forms one link in the chain of survival and as such the goal should be viewed as enabling the patient to benefit from the rehabilitation phase, which follows discharge from the ICU [50].

Previously it had been considered that trauma patients without intracranial haemorrhage or focal neurologic deficits were typically low-risk for lasting neuropsychological and emotional deficits. However it has been demonstrated that the majority of trauma survivors without intracranial haemorrhage display persistent cognitive impairment, which is nearly twice as likely in those with skull fractures or concussions. This cognitive impairment was associated with functional defects, poor quality of life, and an inability to return to work [51]. The increased use of follow-up clinics for survivors of intensive care will hopefully help with the identification of patients requiring ongoing help and support more than has been the case in the past [52].

26.15 Summary

Improved trauma care systems have resulted in an increasing number of multiply injured patients surviving their initial trauma. Patients requiring intensive care for trauma are at risk from sepsis and multiple organ failure. Attention to detail is important, as is preservation of organ function, infection control and nutrition in order to maintain muscle strength and allow normal metabolic function to return.

Trauma management involves good pre-hospital, emergency, surgical, anaesthetic and intensive care decision-making. Optimal outcome depends on keeping abreast of the latest thinking in an ever-changing and increasingly technology-rich environment. Of concern for UK intensive care are suggestions that the relative lack of intensive care bed provision compared with other countries may have an influence on survival of multi-trauma patients. Mortality in this country has been shown to be up to 9% higher in a case-matched group of severely injured patients with chest injury (Injury Severity Score > 16) in comparison with Germany. The reasons for this may be varied and in some respects related to differing treatment strategies but non-intubated patients in Germany are more likely to be admitted to intensive care rather than a high-dependency unit or regular ward in the UK [53]. Only with continued audit of the service delivery to trauma patients in intensive care in the UK can standards be maintained and morbidity and mortality improve in the future.

26.16 Clinical Case

An otherwise fit and healthy 35-year-old male car driver was involved in a road traffic accident. He lost control at speed, colliding with a lamp post at approximately 50 mph. He was attended by a paramedical ambulance crew and found to be hypoxic and combative at the scene with a Glasgow Coma Scale score of 13 and oxygen saturation of 90% on pulse oximetry. He had obvious blunt chest injuries bilaterally and there was clinical evidence of a closed femoral fracture on the right

He was given nalbuphine intravenously at the scene and a femoral traction splint was applied prior to transport to hospital. On admission to A&E he was noted to have equal pupillary reactions with no obvious head injury. He had severe bruising over his chest wall anteriorly on both sides and a centrally mobile flail segment. He had mild inspiratory noise on auscultation on the right and an intercostal drain was sited through the thoracostomy incision. An intercostal drain was also sited on the left. His abdomen was soft and he had a normal FAST scan in the emergency department. There was no evidence of pelvic injury or other long-bone fractures. He had received 700 ml of crystalloid pre-hospital in line with a policy of low-volume resuscitation. His mean arterial pressure on admission was 80 mmHg. He had impaired gas exchange, the FiO_2 was 0.5 with a pH 7.29 PaO_2 9.6 kPa arterial partial pressure of carbon dioxide ($PaCO_2$) 5.6 kPa base excess (BE) –5.1 oxygen saturation (SaO_2) 94%.

Initial cervical spine and pelvic radiographs were unremarkable. His chest X-ray revealed fractured ribs 3–7 anteriorly on the left and 5/6 on the right and an area of contusion in the right mid-zone. He was taken for a CT scan of the head and neck (including saggital reconstruction views of the cervical spine), which were reported as normal. In view of the impairment of gas exchange and evidence of contusion on chest X-ray, helical CT scanning of the chest and abdomen was performed at this time. He was noted to have a contained rupture of the spleen. After discussion with the orthopaedic team he was transferred to the operating theatre and had internal fixation of his femoral fracture by a consultant orthopaedic surgeon. He was subsequently transferred to the ICU (FiO_2 0.6, pH 7.30 PaO_2 9.4 $PaCO_2$ 6.8 BE–6.0 temperature 34.5°C). He was actively warmed and his acidosis corrected. His sedation was reduced and he responded appropriately to command. However, his condition subsequently deteriorated and his oxygen requirements increased. He required ionotropic support for maintenance of blood pressure and vital organ perfusion. Both transthoracic and transoesohageal echocardiography were normal. On day three of intensive care he required an emergency laparotomy due to obvious bleeding and a splenectomy was performed. Subsequent recovery was hampered by the development of ventilator-associated pneumonia. Protective ventilation strategies were employed over the next few days but ARDS developed. He responded to intermittent prone-ventilation. He had a percutaneous tracheostomy performed at day ten and was eventually weaned from ventilation at day 18. He was transferred to the high-dependency unit 22 days after admission.

References

[1] Mock, C., Kobusingye, O., Joshipura, M. *et al.* (2005). Strengthening trauma and critical care globally, *Curr Opin Crit Care*, **11**, 568–575.

[2] Clarke, J.R., Trooskin, S.Z., Doshi, P.J. *et al.* (2002). Time to laparotomy for intra-abdominal bleeding from trauma does affect survival for delays up to 90 minutes, *J Trauma*, **52**, 420–425.

[3] Fowler, R. and Pepe, P.E. (2002). Fluid resuscitation of the patient with major trauma, *Curr Opin Anaesthesiol*, **15**, 173–178.

[4] Revell, M.P., Porter, K.M. and Greaves, I. (2002). Fluid resuscitation in prehospital trauma care: a consensus view, *Trauma*, **4**, 21–28.

[5] Dutton, R.P., Mackenzie, C.F. and Scalea, T.M. (2002). Hypotensive resuscitation during active hemorrhage: impact on in-hospital mortality, *J Trauma*, **52**, 1141–1146.

[6] Roberts, I., Evans, P., Bunn, F. *et al.* (2001). Is the normalisation of blood pressure in bleeding trauma patients harmful? *Lancet*, **357**, 385–387.

[7] Parkhouse, D. (2005). Sugar solutions used in resuscitation, *J R Army Med Corps*, **151**, 5–10.

[8] Myers, C. (1997). Fluid resuscitation, *Eur J Emerg Med*, **4**, 224–232.

[9] Porembka, D.T. (1997). Transesophageal echocardiography in the trauma patient, *Curr Opin Anaesthesiol*, **10**, 130–141.

[10] O'Conor, C.E. (2004). Diagnosing traumatic rupture of the thoracic aorta in the emergency department, *Emerg Med J*, **21**, 414–419.

[11] Pepe, P.E., Dutton, R.P. and Fowler, R.L. (2008). Preoperative resuscitation of the trauma patient, *Curr Opin Anaesthesiol*, **21**, 216–221.

[12] Moore, E.E., Johnson, J.L., Cheng, A.M. *et al.* (2005). Insights from studies of blood substitutes in trauma, *Shock*, **24**, 197–205.

[13] Morris, C.G.T. and McCoy, E. (2004). Clearing the cervical spine in unconscious polytrauma victims, *Anaesthesia*, **59**, 464–482.

[14] Sanchez, B., Waxman, K., Jones, T. *et al.* (2005). Cervical spine clearance in blunt trauma: evaluation of a computed tomography-based protocol, *J Trauma*, **59**, 179–183.

[15] Brohi, K., Healy, M., Fotheringham, T. *et al.* (2005). Helical computed tomographic scanning for the evaluation of the cervical spine in the unconscious, intubated trauma patient, *J Trauma*, **58**, 897–901.

[16] Loveland, J.A. and Boffard, K.D. (2004). Damage control surgery in the abdomen and beyond, *Br J Surg*, **91**, 1095–1101.

[17] Gillham, M.J. and Parr, M.J.A. (2002). Resuscitation for major trauma, *Curr Opin Anaesthesiol*, **15**, 167–172.

[18] Roberts, C.S., Pape, H.-C., Jones, A.L. *et al.* (2005). Damage control orthopaedics: evolving concepts in the treatment of patients who have sustained orthopaedic trauma, *J Bone Joint Surg Am.* **87**, 434–449.

[19] Nau, T., Aldrian, S., Koenig, F. *et al.* (2003). Fixation of femoral fractures in multiple-injury patients with combined chest and head injuries, *ANZ J Surg*, **73**, 1018–1021.

[20] Revell, M.P. and Porter, K.M.(2002). When is the best time to fix fractures? *Trauma*, **4**, 159–167.

[21] Sagraves, S.G., Toschlog, E.A. and Rotondo, M.F. (2006). Damage control surgery — the intensivist's role, *J Intensive Care Med*, **21**, 5–16.

[22] Enderson, B.L., Reath, D.B., Meadors, J. *et al.* (1990). The tertiary trauma survey: a prospective study of missed injury, *J Trauma*, **30**, 666–669.

[23] The Acute Respiratory Distress Syndrome Network (2000). Ventilation with lower tidal volumes as compared with traditional tidal volumes for acute lung injury and the acute respiratory distress syndrome, *N Engl J Med*, 342, 1301–1308.

[24] Dicker, R.A., Morabito, D.J., Pittet, J.-F. *et al.* (2004). Acute respiratory distress syndrome criteria in trauma patients: why the definitions do not work, *J Trauma*, **57**, 522–528.

[25] Schiller, H.J., McCann, U.G., Carney, D.E. *et al.* (2001). Altered alveolar mechanics in the acutely injured lung, *Crit Care Med*, **29**, 1049–1055.

[26] Bein, T., Weber, F., Philipp, A. *et al.* (2006). A new pumpless extracorporeal interventional lung assist in critical hypoxemia/hypercapnia, *Crit Care Med*, **34**, 1372–1377.

[27] Zimmermann, M., Philipp, A., Schmid, F.-X. *et al.* (2007). From Baghdad to Germany: Use of a new pumpless extracorporeal lung assist system in two severely injured US soldiers, *ASAIO Journal.* **53**, e4–e6.

[28] Dimopoulou, I., Anthi, A., Lignos, M. *et al.* (2003). Prediction of prolonged ventilatory support in blunt thoracic trauma patients, *Intens Care Med* **29**, 1101–1105.

[29] Young, D., Harrison, D.A., Cuthbertson, B.H. *et al.* (2013). Effect of early vs. late tracheostomy placement on survival in patients receiving mechanical ventilation: the TracMan randomized trial, *JAMA*, **309**, 2121–2129.

[30] Vidhani, K., Kause, J., and Parr, M. (2002). Should we follow ATLS guidelines for the management of traumatic pulmonary contusion: the role of non-invasive ventilatory support, *Resuscitation*, **52**, 265–268.

[31] Katsaragakis, S., Stamou, K.M., Androulakis, G. (2005). Independent lung ventilation for asymmetrical chest trauma: effect on ventilatory and haemodynamic parameters, *Injury*, **36**, 501–504.

[32] Tisherman, S.A, Barie, P., Bokhari, F. *et al.* (2003). *Clinical practice guidelines: endpoints of resuscitation*, [Online]. Available at: http://www.east.org/Content/documents/practicemanagementguidelines/resuscitation-endpoints.pdf [Accessed 11 January 2012].

[33] McIntyre, L. and Hebert, P.C. (2002). To transfuse or not in trauma patients: a presentation of the evidence and rationale, *Curr Opin Anaesthesiol*, **15**, 179–185.

[34] McKinley, B.A., Valdiva, A. and Moore, F.A. (2003). Goal-orientated shock resuscitation for major torso trauma: what are we learning? *Curr Opin Crit Care*, **9**, 292–299.

[35] Durham, R.M., Moran, J.J., Mazuski, J.E. *et al.* (2003). Multiple organ failure in trauma patients, *J Trauma*, **55**, 608–616.

[36] Rady, M.Y., Edwards, J.D. and Nightingale, P. (1992). Early cardiorespiratory findings after severe blunt thoracic trauma and their relation to outcome, *Br J Surg*, **79**, 65–68.

[37] SAFE Study Investigators. (2004). A comparison of albumin and saline for fluid resuscitation in the intensive care unit, *N Engl J Med*, **350**, 2247–2256.

[38] Tomlinson, L. and Bellingan, G.J. (2002). Trauma and acute lung injury, *Trauma*, **4**, 147–157.

[39] Fakhry, S.M., Trask, A.L., Waller, M.A. *et al.* (2004). Management of brain-injured patients by an evidence-based medicine protocol improves outcomes and decreases hospital charges, *J Trauma*, **56**, 492–499.

[40] Lavery, G.G. and, Lowry, K.G. (2004). Management of blast injuries and shock lung, *Curr Opin Anaesthesiol*, **17**, 151–157.

[41] Sayman, A.G. and Findlay, G.P. (2003). The management of blunt thoracic trauma, *BJA — CEPD Review*, **6**, 171–174.

[42] Wu, C.L., Perkins, F.M. and Barquist, E. (1999). Thoracic epidural analgesia versus intravenous patient-controlled analgesia for the treatment of rib fracture pain after motor vehicle crash, *J Trauma*, **47**, 564–567.

[43] Moon, M.R. Luchette, F.A., Gibson, S.W. *et al.* (1999). Prospective randomized comparison of epidural versus parentaral opioid analgesia in thoracic trauma, *Ann Surg*, **229**, 684–691. Discussion 691–692.

[44] Bulger, E.M., Edwards, T., Klotz, P. *et al.* (2004). Epidural analgesia improves outcome after multiple rib fractures, *Surgery*, **136**, 426–430.

[45] Bulger, E.M., Arnneson, M.A., Mock, C.N. *et al.* (2000). Rib fractures in the elderly, *J Trauma*, **48**, 1040–1046.

[46] Asensio, J.A., Arroyo, H., Veloz, W. *et al.* (2002). Penetrating thoracoabdominal injuries: ongoing dilemma — which cavity and when? *World J Surg*, **26**, 539–543.

[47] Parker, P.J. and Clasper, J. (2007). The military tourniquet, *JR Army Med Corps*, **153**,10–15.

[48] Gentilello, L.M. and Pierson, D.J. (2001). Trauma critical care, *Am J Respir Crit Care Med*, **163**, 604–607.

[49] Fangio, P., Asehnoune, K., Edouard, A. *et al.* (2005). Early embolization and vasopressor administration for management of life-threatening hemorrhage from pelvic fracture, *J Trauma*, **58**, 978–984.

[50] Moecke, H. and von Knobelsdorff, G. (2008). The anesthesiologist in prehospital and hospital emergency medicine, *Curr Opin Anaesthesiol*, **21**, 228–232.

[51] Jackson, J.C., Obremskey, W.B., Bauer, R. *et al.* (2007). Long-term cognitive, emotional, and functional outcomes in trauma intensive care unit survivors without intracranial hemorrhage, *J Trauma*, **62**, 80–88.

[52] Griffiths, J.A., Barber, V.S., Cuthbertson, B.H. *et al.* (2006). A national survey of intensive care follow-up clinics, *Anaesthesia*, **61**, 950–955.

[53] Hildebrand, F., Giannoudis, P.V., van Griensven, M. *et al.* (2005). Management of polytraumatised patients with associated blunt chest trauma: a comparison of two European countries, *Injury*, **36**, 293–302.

27

Intensive Care of Burns Patients

Lena C. Andersson, Hans C. Nettelblad and Folke Sjoeberg

27.1 Introduction

The treatment of burns has improved dramatically over the last 25 years. During this period the incidence of burns has decreased in industrialised countries, as has the hospital mortality, but the number of patients dying before reaching hospital has remained static. There is an over-representation of the elderly, patients with psychological or physiological handicaps and patients suffering from drug abuse amongst those who die prior to reaching hospital. The hospitalisation times have more than halved during this period and there has been a rapid increase in ambulatory management of even the larger burns [1]. The improved results are due to a better understanding of the pathology and physiology of burns, occurring simultaneously with and contributing to a generalised improvement of intensive care [2]. Important factors that have contributed to better results include:

- Improved early fluid resuscitation, which has reduced the incidence of burn shock, secondary renal insufficiency and fluid overload.
- Early surgical intervention with improved wound care using more efficient topical antibiotic treatments has reduced the number of infections which might have otherwise led to sepsis.
- New systemic antibiotics.

- Improved nutrition, which strengthens the immune system and promotes better healing.

Despite these improvements in burn care there are still many areas in the world where the survival of patients with burns of more than 40% of the total body surface is rare [3]. In contrast, in many developed countries even patients with severe burns can survive to have a relatively good quality of life. It is wrong to assume that acute burn care involves a high number of large burns. Extensive burns are in fact quite rare, as reported in 2005 by the American Burn Association, where 62% of burns with recorded extent involved less than 10% of the total body surface [4]. Modern burns units today function as multidisciplinary teams encompassing specialists from intensive care to psychosocial rehabilitation. In order to maintain high standards of care with decreasing numbers of burns presenting, it has become vital for the supervising medical teams to undergo continuous professional development.

27.2 Clinical Presentation of Burn Injuries and Management Strategies

A burn is defined as a tissue injury caused by open fire, hot fluids, contact with a hot item, electrical current, or exposure to chemicals or radiation. Burn injuries are characterised by an initial cardiovascular and pulmonary instability due to increase in total body capillary permeability [5]. Unless adequately treated, this progresses into burn shock. For those with severe injuries the burn shock may be so powerful during the first 48 hours after the initial injury that the patient dies [6]. This initial primary treatment (resuscitation phase) is followed by a second phase, the post-resuscitation period, when infections, septicaemia and multiple organ failure remain the major problems. During this period, which focuses on the healing of the patient's open wounds, the majority of inpatient deaths occur [7]. The next phase is the rehabilitation period when medical care is focussed on minimising the scar contractures that can lead to severe handicaps and many surgical reconstructive procedures will be performed. Physical rehabilitation and psychosocial re-integration also occur during this phase. With respect to intensive care, it is the primary phase and the post-resuscitation period, which are the most important. Further discussion in this chapter is therefore focussed around these two phases.

Every burns patient needs an individualised treatment protocol after initial assessment. After stabilising the respiratory and circulatory functions the aim should be the treatment of the burned skin in order to close open portals of entry before microorganisms invade. Burns patients are usually treated within specific burns units, which allow both intensive care and surgical treatments to be performed in a temperature-controlled secluded individual patient room. It is of vital importance to adhere to infection-control policies and to prevent unnecessary patient movement within the hospital, where microorganisms could be contracted or spread [8].

27.3 Initial Assessment of Injuries and Treatment Principles — The Resuscitation (Initial 48-Hour) Phase

The initial treatment of a burn injury follows the same protocols as with normal trauma patients described in Advanced Trauma Life Support [9] or, alternatively, the more specific Advanced Burn Life Support [10]. It is important to establish the extent of the burnt area as a percentage of total body surface area (% TBSA) affected (Fig. 27.1) and to assess the burn's depth [11] in order to formulate a treatment plan and to start the individually estimated fluid resuscitation. To understand the actual management of a burn one has to be familiar with the anatomy and function of the skin (Fig. 27.2). The burn's estimation (extent and depth) is a major prognostic indicator of survival, which, together with the age and further complicating conditions, determines the patient's survival chances.

27.3.1 *Primary assessment*

(i) Airway

- Assess the risk of airway obstruction, due to decreased level of consciousness (intoxication, head trauma) or a thermally induced mucosal oedema.
- Assess the adequacy of breathing (restrictive chest defect due to circumferential thoracic burn and the possible need for escharotomies).

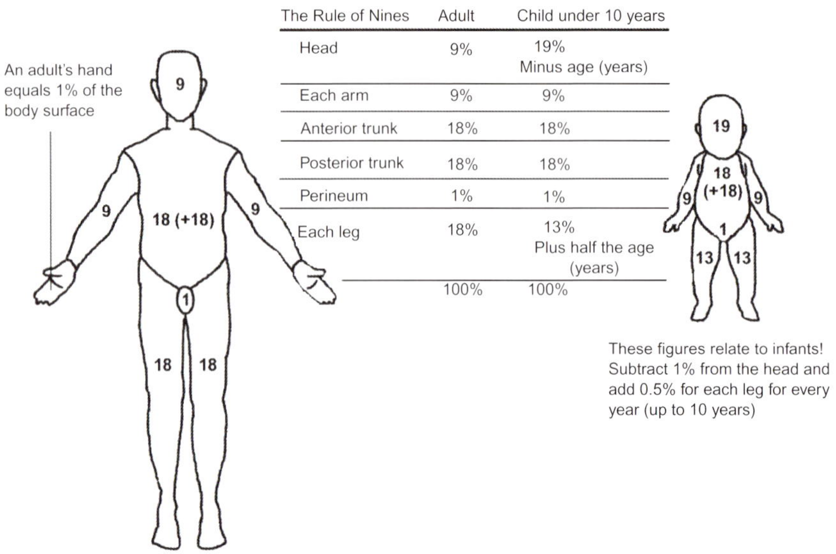

The Rule of Nines	Adult	Child under 10 years
Head	9%	19% Minus age (years)
Each arm	9%	9%
Anterior trunk	18%	18%
Posterior trunk	18%	18%
Perineum	1%	1%
Each leg	18%	13% Plus half the age (years)
	100%	100%

Figure 27.1. The Rule of Nines, which aids a quick, approximate calculation of the burn size (expressed as % TBSA).

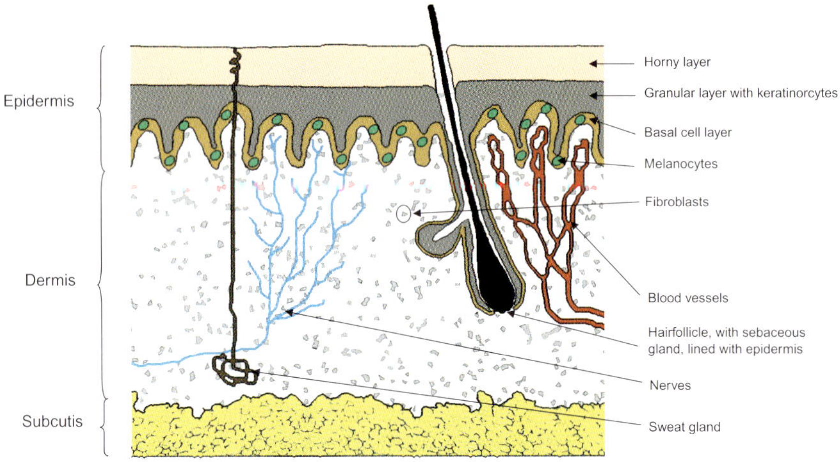

Figure 27.2. Anatomy of the skin.

- Administer 100% oxygen, via continuous positive airway pressure (CPAP) if necessary.
- Assess need for intubation.

(ii) Neck/cervical spine

- Stabilisation of the cervical spine may be necessary if a cervical spine injury cannot be excluded.

(iii) Circulation

- Continuous assessment of heart rate, perfusion and blood pressure.
- Examine for peripheral ischaemia due to circumferential extremity burns and consider the need for escharotomies and fasciotomies.

(iv) Level of consciousness/awareness

- Assessment of Glasgow Coma Scale (GCS) score.
- Look for carbon monoxide or cyanide poisoning.
- Is there associated head trauma, drug abuse or intoxication?

(v) Total body examination

- Expose and examine the whole patient quickly in order to prevent hypothermia and document the burn's extent. In children under ten, it is necessary to correct for the larger head and the smaller extremities (Fig. 27.1).
- Clothing stuck onto burns wounds, may be left *in situ* and removed at the first wound debridement.
- Rings and jewellery must be removed, as when tissue oedema develops they will restrict blood flow causing ischaemia.

(vi) Fluid resuscitation

- Start fluid resuscitation with a crystalloid solution such as Ringers' lactate (Fig. 27.3). Peripheral lines can be inserted through healthy or burnt skin.

(vii) Nutrition

- In patients with large burns, after intubation, a nasogastric tube should be passed and enteral nutrition started as soon as possible.

(viii) Tetanus prophylaxis — Further Immunisation

(ix) Pain relief

The referral criteria to a specific burns unit may have to be considered after the primary assessment [10].

Fluid resuscitation–the first 24 hours:

50 % of the fluid should be given during the first 8 hours and 50% during the next 16 hours

ADULTS
Ringer lactate, 2–4 ml/kg × %TBSA

CHILDREN
Ringer lactate, 3–4 ml/kg × %TBSA
Maintenance fluids need to be added due to evaporation

Up to 10 kg:	add 100 ml/kg/24 hours
11–20 kg:	add 50 ml/kg/24 hours
Over 20 kg:	add 20 ml/kg/24 hours

For example: Maintenance fluids for a child of 22 kg:
1,000 ml + 500 ml, + 40 = a total of 1,540 ml.

Figure 27.3. Fluid resuscitation.

27.3.2 *Referral criteria*

If the patient is initially treated in a hospital which lacks a burns unit and has little experience in the treatment of burns, the patient should be referred to a burns centre. These criteria, according to the American Burn Association, are as follows [11]:

- Second-degree burns over 10% TBSA.
- Second- and third-degree burns involving the face, hands, genitalia, perineum or overlying the large joints.
- Third-degree burns over 5% of TBSA in all age groups.
- Electrical burns and lightning strikes.
- Chemical burns.
- Inhalation burns.
- Burns patients with additional complex medical conditions which would increase treatment time and management.
- Patients with a burn and an additional trauma where the burn itself carries the largest risk for morbidity and mortality.
- Children with burns where there are no paediatric facilities.
- Burns patients with a further need for psychosocial or emotional support with prolonged rehabilitation (suspected child abuse, drug abuse or severe psychiatric diseases).

27.3.3 *Clinical monitoring*

Monitoring should normally be the same as for other intensive care patients, but there are specific demands of good venous access due to the need for the infusion of large volumes of fluids. Also it can be difficult to maintain non-invasive monitoring because the facial tissues are damaged and oedematous. It is therefore important to initiate invasive monitoring early with arterial lines and urinary catheters in order to secure continuous monitoring of the circulation. A further, full-body examination of the patient should be repeated in order to identify injuries, which could have been missed at the initial assessment [9,13].

27.3.4 *Transport of a burns patient*

It is important to assess a burns patient before transportation, specifically with regards to a secured airway, intravenous access, urinary catheter and possibly a nasogastric tube if the patient has been intubated. Check that the temperature within the transporting vehicle is adequate in order to prevent hypothermia. Fluid resuscitation should be started prior to transport. Treatment documentation, sent with the patient, must include how the injuries have happened, drugs administered and time and quantity of fluids given [14].

27.4 Further Clinical Assessment of Injuries and Treatment Principles

27.4.1 *Airway and lung problems*

The treating team must obtain and maintain a secure airway and respiratory function. There are usually four well-defined processes, which threaten the airway/lungs/respiration [8,15]:

- Carbon monoxide and cyanide poisoning.
- Upper airway obstruction due to oedema of the airway.
- Inhalation injury (chemical/inflammatory lung damage).
- Restricted ventilation due to circumferential burns of the thorax.

27.4.1.1 *Inhalation poisoning*

Respiratory insufficiency resulting from carbon monoxide [16–18] is common at the time of the injury at indoor fires, but symptoms due to carbon monoxide poisoning are rarely present when the carboxy-haemoglobin (COHb) is below 15%. The symptoms during medium intoxication (10–30% COHb) have been described as neurological hypoxic symptoms of nausea, headache and difficulties in concentration. Findings show tachycardia, hypotension and tachypnoea without cyanosis due to a pink colouration by CO involving all tissues. At COHb levels of 30% to 50%, patients are affected by changes of eyesight, arrhythmias, syncope, agitation, convulsions and coma. Blood gases can usually confirm the diagnosis. The symptoms of cyanide poisoning are similar, but the diagnosis is more difficult to confirm due to cyanide being more difficult to analyse. The typical clinical picture presents with a metabolic acidosis of the patient with normal oxygenation and absence of COHb. Cyanokit or hydroxicobolamin (Vitamin B12) should be given intravenously with wide indications if cyanide poisoning is suspected (adults: 5 g over 15–30 minutes, children: 70 mg per kg weight). The dose can be repeated if symptoms persist [19]. It is very important to treat carbon monoxide and cyanide intoxication with 100% oxygen, administered by high oxygen flow, CPAP or endotracheal intubation. It is recommended that oxygen treatment should be continued even after the carbon monoxide has been eliminated from the blood in order to minimise any late neurological residual symptoms. This is particularly important for pregnant women, children and those with neurological symptoms and when the COHb has been higher than 25%. Hyperbaric oxygen treatment does increase the elimination of CO and is therefore recommended [20]. From a practical point of view though, it is usually difficult to move a severely burnt patient.

27.4.1.2 *Thermal injuries and upper airway obstruction*

Burns which involve the head and neck, can lead to airway compromise [21]. The same applies if the patient has inhaled hot gases or steam, which can lead to direct injuries on the mucosa. Maximum swelling can occur up to

48 hours from the initial injury and this is exacerbated by the fluid resuscitation. If there is any risk that airway obstruction could occur the airway should be secured by intubation and ventilation. It is particularly important to protect the airway during transport. Oedema usually decreases after three to seven days when most of the excess fluid has been eliminated from the body. If chemical damage could have occurred lower down the airway it may be necessary to clean/clear this by endotracheal suction or via fibre-bronchoscopy, and intubation is then indicated.

27.4.1.3 *Inhalation injury*

This is a large problem which arises mostly after major burns [22–25]. After body surface area, inhalation injury and advanced age are the most important prognostic factors [26]. Lung inhalation injury develops after exchange between toxic components in the actual smoke and the inflammation in the lung. This respiratory insufficiency develops slowly; it manifests during the first three to five days and the patient can be symptom-free on admission to hospital. Inhalation difficulties are rarely encountered after smoke exposure without skin burns. The skin burn does therefore play an important roll in the development of inhalation injury. It is also possible that the patient may have suffered soot deposition and an irritated airway, but without later developing respiratory insufficiency. The pathology and physiology of respiratory insufficiency is caused by the ventilation–perfusion mismatch rather than oedema of the pulmonary tissue. Some investigations show that smoke has an effect on the production of surfactant. Also, recent work shows that patients who have most criteria for inhalation injury and who have received large volumes of fluid during fluid resuscitation do not get an increased amount of pulmonary oedema [27].

Treatment strategies for inhalation injury [28,29]:

(i) Keep the airway clear and clean by regular suctioning. If necessary, perform bronchial cleaning via fibre-bronchoscope. In order to make the secretions less viscid and easier to suction, saline can be inserted via the endotrachael tube. Mucolytic substances can be added e.g. Acetylcystein.

(ii) Add beta-2-agonists if bronchospasm occurs.
(iii) Stabilise the circulation and keep the patient well hydrated rather than too dry.
(iv) The ventilation treatment should follow the same guidelines as in acute lung insufficiency with low tidal volumes (6–8 ml/kg) and adequate positive end-expiratory pressure.

27.4.1.4 *Reduced ventilation due to circumferential skin burns of thorax*

This type of restriction develops slowly with increasing oedema and a hard skin eschar, especially in third-degree burns. The actual extent may be so severe that it can be impossible to mechanically establish an acceptable tidal volume. The treatment consists of early escharotomies in the anterior axillary lines and possibly horizontally to connect the two together [30]. The escharotomies can be performed with or without light sedation, or under extra morphine, since deeply burnt skin lacks sensation. It is important that the excisions are extended into the subcutaneous fat in order to fully remove the restrictiveness around the chest. Both blood pressure and airway pressure are usually normalised after the escharotomies.

27.4.2 *Circulatory problems — monitoring and treatment*

27.4.2.1 *Burns pathophysiology*

Burns lead to large physiological and pathological changes [31–33]. If untreated in the early stages, the feared burn shock will develop. Physiologically significant intravascular fluid is lost by burnt and non-burnt tissue even in burns of only 6–8% of the total body surface. In order to avoid hypovolaemia it is necessary to initiate fluid resuscitation. Those patients that can re-hydrate themselves orally usually do not have more than 15% of the total body surface burnt. If a patient has more than 15% TBSA affected then intravenous fluid resuscitation will be needed. This fluid loss develops due to the severe negative pressure in the burnt tissue and the permeability also increases in the post-capillary venulae. The increase of permeability causes fluid and protein to leak out of the vessels.

This general tissue oedema also involves the healthy tissue. The permeability changes occur during the first 24 hours and are at maximum during the first 12 hours. Colloids should not be administered [34] before the permeability in the vessels is considered to be normal. This avoids further proteins leaking out into the tissue where they will continue to exert yet more osmotic pressure, leading to further oedema.

27.4.2.2 *Intravenous access*

The fluid resuscitation should preferably be given via peripheral venous access through non-burnt skin, but can be inserted through burnt tissue as necessary in some severely burnt patients [35,36]. This is also true of arterial and central venous access. Due to the risk of infection, one should minimise the use of central cannulation, but monitoring of the circulation should not be compromised.

In order to minimise the risk of central catheter infections, it is recommend that the central line is renewed every three to four days. The risk of systemic spread of bacteria due to central line catheters in burns is substantial.

27.4.2.3 *Fluid resuscitation and haemodynamic stability*

Due to the enormous loss of intravascular fluids and due to vessel dilation, it is necessary to replace the fluid losses in acute burns patients in order to maintain satisfactory organ perfusion and to reduce the risk of organ failure [37,38]. The resuscitation fluid should contain the same amount of sodium as plasma. Numerous treatment protocols for fluid resuscitation have been described in the literature and they have all proven efficacy. Hypertonic solutions have been used in some burns centres with success, but should be used with caution [39,40]. Crystalloid solutions are the most commonly used. Charles Baxter described the first to gain international recognition: the Parkland formula of 2–4 ml/kg/% TBSA, 50% of which is given within the first eight hours with the remaining volume given over the following 16 hours (Fig. 27.3)[41]. Many other protocols have been described since and it is important to point out that the treatment suggestions in the formulae are only early guidelines for fluid resuscitation and may require adjustments. The fluid administration during the second 24 hours is usually half of the initial amount. The urine production during the initial phase needs to be kept between 0.5 and 1 ml/kg/hour [42]. In order to maintain a mean arterial pressure of above 70 mmHg it is sometimes necessary to consider additional treatment with colloids, blood or vasopressors. It is often wise to administer plasma prior to early debridement/surgery in order to reduce potential blood loss [43,44].

27.4.3 *Analgesia*

Burns are associated with considerable pain and good analgesia [45] is a cornerstone in the management of burns. Pain can be divided into resting and activity pain. Resting pain is treated with a combination of opiate and non-opiate analgesics. An opiate such as morphine can be given intermittently, via continuous infusion or patient-controlled analgesia. The advantage of the latter is that the patient can vary the dose depending on their activity/pain level. Slow-release oral preparations of morphine can be used after the acute phase. Oramorph can be used to treat breakthrough pain or to cover moderately painful procedures such as dressing changes. Patients with burns often require very large doses of opiates for a prolonged period of time and usually develop opiate tolerance.

27.5 Specific Assessment and Management of Burnt Areas

27.5.1 *Assessment of burn depth*

The depth of the burn will depend on the amount of heat which has been transferred to the tissues [46–50]. The actual amount of energy will depend on temperature and duration of exposure. The skin varies in thickness all over the body and this will also influence the burn depth. Burn injuries are classified by size and how deeply the epidermis and dermis are damaged (Fig. 27.4). Clinically this is assessed by examining the skin's appearance, sensation and blood perfusion. A first-degree burn only involves the epidermis and no blistering is seen e.g. light sunburn. The damaged skin is reddish, swollen and sensitive and this type of damage heals fast within a couple of days. Second-degree burns involve the

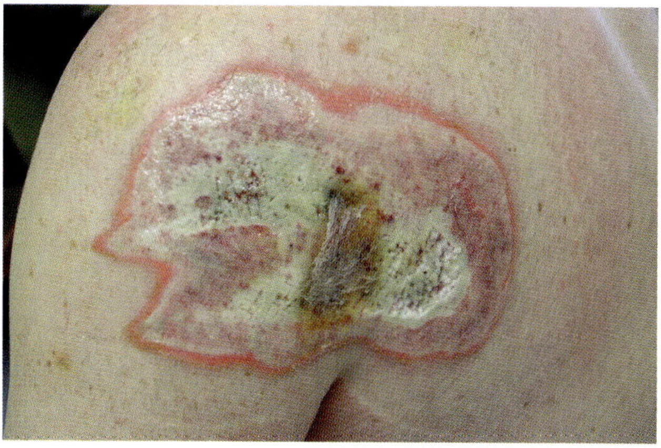

Figure 27.4. Friction burn to shoulder with all burn depths. The outer edge of the wound is a first-degree burn, the centre is a third-degree burn and the remainder is a second-degree burn.

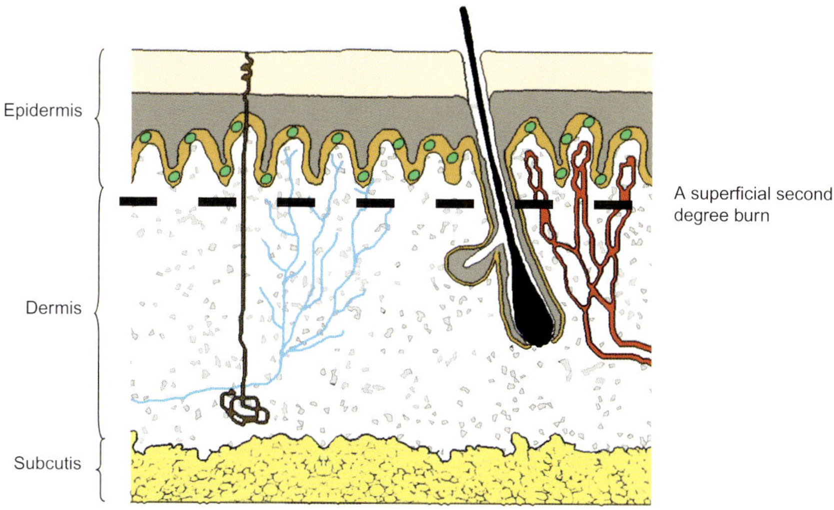

Figure 27.5. A superficial second-degree burn.

epidermis as well as parts of the dermis. Superficial second-degree burns involve the epidermis as well as the upper third of the dermis (Fig. 27.5). Damage to capillaries with vessel leakage and the formation of clinical blistering is seen. Even if large areas of epidermis have been damaged, most of these injuries heal within 7 to 14 days. The deeper second-degree burns extend deeper into the dermis, leaving very few epidermal cells to re-epithelialise (Fig. 27.6). The burnt area appears red-whitish with no capillary refill on pressure. The re-epithelialisation process takes longer and can extend to several weeks/months if skin grafting is not performed. The microcirculation may also be reduced in these injuries and the depth of the burn may deepen with time. A third-degree burn involves the whole of the epidermis and dermis; there is no potential for spontaneous re-epithelialisation (Fig. 27.7). Injured areas of third-degree burns have to be covered with skin grafts in order to heal without severe infections and scar contractions. The depth of the burn is certainly not static; it can change with time and treatment. Increasing tissue oedema and/or an infection may deepen the amount of tissue injury and stop potential healing.

27.5.2 *Assessment of the burns extent*

The initial estimate of a burn's extent [9] does not include first-degree burns, but only second- and third-degree burns with at least a sign of epidermal blistering. There are several methods to estimate the burn extent, the most common and most simple is the '9% rule'. The adult body is divided into regions of approximately 9% (arms, 9%: legs 18%, upper torso front and back, 18%) (Fig. 27.1). If the patient has scattered burns, the patient's palm including the fingers can be used in order to estimate a burnt area and this area corresponds to approximately 1% TBSA.

27.5.3 *Initial debridement, wound care and infection control*

The initial wound care should be started at the place of injury. The aims of treatment are a reduction in exposure time to heat through, for example, flushing the wounds with cold water. It is however important to avoid hypothermia. In large injuries it may be necessary to keep the patient warm and the wounds dry to reduce fluid loss. In order to assess and debride larger wounds the patient may require sedation or anaesthesia to facilitate removal of burnt clothes and escharotomies. The aim is to remove dead tissue, either by excision or by secondary intent. Non-excised burn areas should be treated with appropriate dressings using local antimicrobial

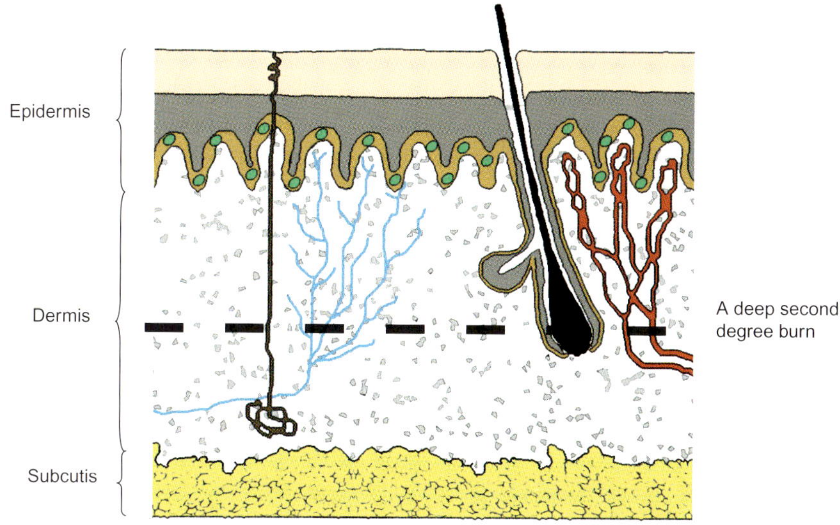

Figure 27.6. A deep second-degree burn.

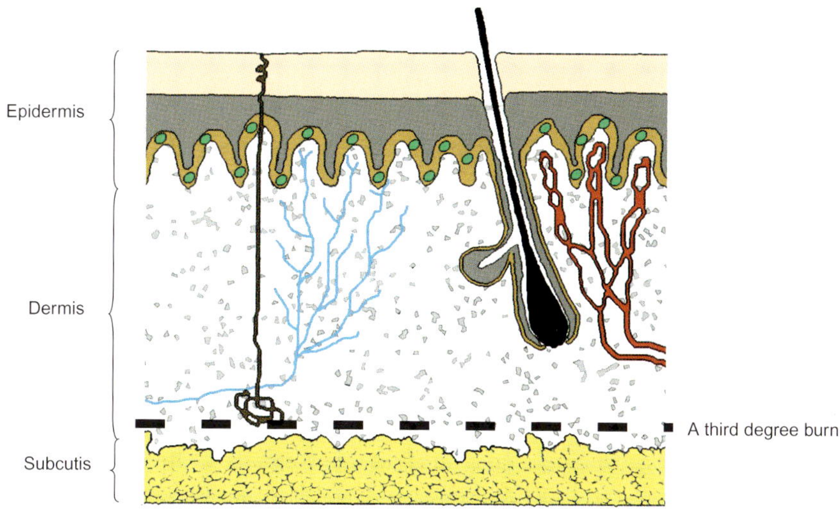

Figure 27.7. A third-degree burn.

agents. The most efficacious creams contain silver ions that are released into the wounds and have a direct toxic effect on any bacteria. The silver ions are not damaging to the patient, but they may delay wound healing [51,52]. Prophylactic systemic antibiotic treatment is not indicated and it increases the risk of the development of resistant bacterial infections.

27.5.4 *Early surgical treatment of deep second- and third-degree burns*

Evidence has proven that early surgical intervention for full–thickness burns reduces the risk of infection and septicaemia that can lead to further complications, including multiple organ failure and death [53–55]. It has been shown that if the wounds are not closed within two to three weeks the ongoing healing process will be complicated by infections and development of severe scarring [56]. Early surgical excision enables removal of burn eschar and replacement with split skin grafts from non-burnt skin areas [57]. Allografts/xenografts or other tissue-engineered skin substitutes can be used, particularly in burns greater than 50% TBSA. The use of cultivated keratinocytes as well as other types of tissue engineered products, e.g. dermal matrixes (Intregra/Alloderm) is well described [58–63]

The problems which can be anticipated peri-operatively can be summarised as follows:

(i) Risk of hypovolaemia [64].

Surgical debridements/excisions in burns patients can lead to profound hypovolaemia due to substantial blood loss. At this early stage the burns patient is additionally at risk of hypovolaemia from burn shock. One can estimate the surgical blood loss at one-third of a blood unit per %TBSA which is to be excised. Multiple techniques can be employed in order to reduce the blood loss, these include: hot gauzes with adrenalin, the use of tourniquets on extremities, subcutaneous injections of adrenalin, application of tissue glues into the wound. Adequate large-bore intravenous access is essential. The use of cardiovascular monitoring in the peri-operative period such as oesophageal Doppler or non-invasive cardiac output measurement may be helpful.

(ii) Risk of hypothermia.

The risk of hypothermia is high in these patients due to large areas of skin/wounds exposed during surgery which leads to massive heat loss from evaporation [65]. Surgery must be performed in a heated environment or under adequate roof heaters or hot air blankets. Infusion warmers for infusions or transfusions are mandatory.

27.6 The Post-Resuscitation Period

27.6.1 *Post-resuscitation fluid balance*

After the initial phase of resuscitation there is usually an excess of extravascular fluid [66]. Some have suggested the use of albumin or artificial colloids and diuretics. In patients with a large burn it may be necessary to give additional blood, because of bone marrow depression and haemolysis, and bleeding from the wounds after surgery may also need substitution. Repeated surgical treatments with debridements and skin grafting will be needed to close all open areas. During this part of the treatment monitoring is as in any other intensive care patient. The amount of fluid needed for each individual patient in the post-resuscitation period is variable, depending on specific patient factors such as: the extent of the burn, age, sex and severity of septicaemia. It can be difficult to manage fluid balance in burns due to unmeasurable large fluid losses into dressings and via evaporation. The best way to determine the fluid balance is to weigh the patient. Patients who loose a lot of fluids due to wound secretions in the bandages also loose a substantial amount of protein. This can clearly be seen in reduced serum protein levels. Experts continue to debate as to whether to replace this protein loss or not.

27.6.2 *Complications with infections and sepsis*

Burns patients are particularly susceptible to infections due to the loss of a normal skin barrier which protects the internal body from the outer world, and burns patients have a suppressed immune system [67,68]. Infection parameters need to be monitored in order to detect septicaemia early and allow treatment to be initiated if complications with infection or

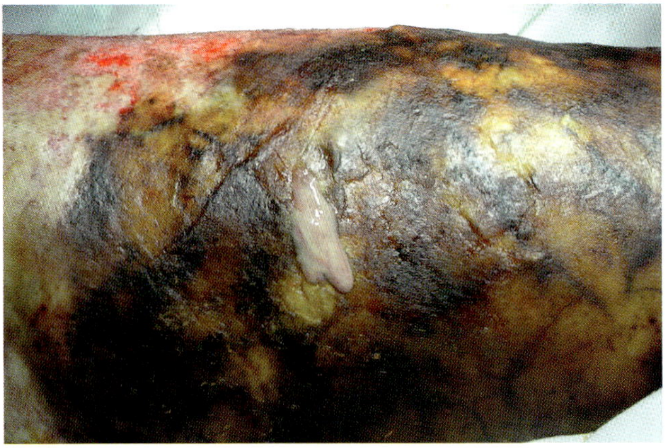

Figure 27.8. Burn eschar with discharging pus.

septicaemia arise. Infection parameters that should be monitored routinely are: C-reactive protein, white blood cells and platelets; microbiology swabs and cultures should be taken from blood, airways, urine and wounds (Fig. 27.8). Selected systemic antibiotics may be administered if sepsis arises.

27.6.3 *Continued ventilation*

It can be necessary for the patient to remain intubated and ventilated due to severe pain and the need for a large amount of opiates. It is important to point out that intubation and ventilation increase the risk of infection for these immune-suppressed patients and they should be weaned off ventilation as soon as possible.

27.6.4 *Metabolic effects and nutrition*

There is a characteristic hypermetabolism seen after a burn injury, which reaches its full effect after approximately five days. The reason for the increase in metabolism is not entirely clear but it is believed that it is caused by a combination of factors relating to the open wounds. Nutrition is important to optimise the wound healing, avoid infections and prevent severe cachexia [69]. Nutritional assessment of the patient should include indirect calorimetry in order to establish the necessary nutritional need. As a guide, patients will require 35 kcal/kg/day for medium to large injuries (below 40% TBSA), and 40–45 kcal/kg/day for injuries below 40% TBSA. Protein, fat and trace elements as well as vitamins have to be given in large quantities. The nutritional composition should be: fat, 50%; carbohydrates, 50%; protein: 1.5–2.0 g/kg, vitamins and minerals, ten times the normal need. Many burns centres in the USA use oxydronolone (anabolic steroid) [70] and non-selective β-blockers today in larger burns in order to stop the protein catabolism.

27.6.5 *Associated complications*

It is very important to prevent stress-related ulcers, cholecystitis, thromboembolic complications and multiple organ failures during this phase.

27.7 Burns Treatment in Children

Most of the burns in children are scalds, and children affected are usually below the age of three. Flame burns are more common in older children. The management of burns in children follows the principles used in adults but there are a few points which are important to bear in mind in the management of children's burns [71].

27.7.1 *The child's relatively larger body surface area and thinner skin*

Children have a relatively larger body surface in comparison to their body weight and a child's skin is also thinner than an adult's (especially below the age of two), which means that children get deeper burns for the same degree of heat and the extent of the burn is larger in comparison to the body's volume (Fig. 27.1). Children therefore need increased fluid resuscitation compared with adults (Fig. 27.3).

27.7.2 *Temperature regulation and temperature sensitivity*

A child's capability to maintain body temperature is influenced by the larger body surface, which increases the risk of hypothermia.

27.7.3 *Child abuse*

Many burns in the paediatric population can be attributed to poor parenting skills, neglect or child abuse.

27.7.4 *Airway*

For the child, as for the adult, one must have a very low threshold for endotracheal intubation, if there is any suspicion that an upper airway problem may develop and this also applies to scalds that involve the head and neck.

27.7.5 *Specific monitoring*

Hypoglycaemia may be seen in children due to their reduced glucose deposits. Blood sugar should therefore be monitored and if hypoglycaemia presents, a drip with 5% glucose should be started. Urine production has to be kept above 1 ml/kg/hour.

27.8 Electrical Burns and Lightning Strikes

Electrical injuries are normally divided into different groups depending on the voltage to which the patient has been exposed; low-voltage injuries are described as up to 1,000 volts; high-voltage injuries are of 10,000–20,000 volts and even up to a million volts. Approximately 10% of patients treated in hospital for specialist care have been exposed to electrical burns and an increase of 50% have been seen in statistics for these injuries over the last ten years. Low-voltage injuries may be similar to minor burns in which the skin has been damaged with only minor injuries to the deeper tissues. There is a big contrast to high-voltage injuries where the electricity has passed in and out of the tissue leaving skin burns at the entrance and exit points, but in between these points there are wide complex injuries in the deeper tissues. The apparent extent of these injuries is extremely difficult to determine on external inspection. The extent of the injury usually increases as time passes, which furthermore makes fluid resuscitation very difficult. It may be necessary for cardiopulmonary resuscitation to be performed due to arrhythmias and cardiorespiratory arrest. Full cardiac monitoring must be maintained for at least 24 hours after the accident due to the risk of late-developing arrhythmias. Specifically in the management of high-voltage injuries there is a risk of renal failure due to the release of myoglobin and haemoglobin from injured tissues. In order to reduce the risk of renal failure a diuresis to above 200–300 ml/hour should be maintained. It may also be necessary to increase the alkalinity of the urine via administration of sodium bicarbonate if the urine pH is below seven. Skin grafting is more often necessary in deep high-voltage injuries than in conventional burns and there is a greater need for fasciotomies due to the extent of the injuries within the deeper tissues. The short passage of electricity after a lightning strike (direct current) rarely leads to deep-tissue injury and if the patient did not suffer skin burns, there is usually no need for fluid resuscitation [72].

References

[1] Pruitt Jr, B.A., Wolf, S.E. and Mason Jr, A.D. (2007). 'Epidemiological, demographic and outcome characteristics of burn injury', in Herndon, D.N. (ed.), *Total Burn Care*, third edition, Saunders Elsevier, Philadelphia, pp. 14–32.

[2] Kramer, G.C., Lund, T. and Beckum, O.K. (2007). 'Pathophysiology of burn shock and burn edema', in Herndon, D.N. (ed.), *Total Burn Care*, third edition, Saunders Elsevier, Philadelphia, pp. 93–106.

[3] Pruitt Jr, B.A., Wolf, S.E. and Mason Jr, A.D. (2007). 'Epidermiological, demographic, and outcome characteristics of burn injury', in Herndon, D.N. (ed.), *Total Burn Care*, third edition, Saunders Elsevier, Philadelphia, p. 29.

[4] American Burn Association (2006). *National Burn Repository. 2005 report. Data set version 2.0.* American Burn Association, Chicago, [Online]. Available at: http://www.ameriburn.org/NBR2005.pdf [Accessed 2 February 2013].

[5] Cope, O. and Moore, F.D. (1947). The redistribution of body water and fluid therapy of the burned patient, *Ann Surg*, **126**, 1010–1045.

[6] Muller, M.J. and Herndon, D.M. (1994). The challenge of burns, *Lancet*, **343**, 216.

[7] Warden, G.D. (2007). 'Fluid resuscitation and management', in Herndon, D.N. (ed.), *Total Burn Care*, third edition, Saunders Elsevier, Philadelphia, pp. 107–118.

[8] Sjoberg, F. (2005). 'Intensivvård av brännskadade (Intensive Care of Burns)', in Larsson, A. and Runertsson, S. (eds), *Intensivvård* (*Intensive Care*), Liber, Stockholm, pp. 501–519.

[9] Committee on Trauma, American College of Surgeons (1984). 'Burns', in *Advanced Trauma Life Support Course Book*. American College of Surgeons, Chicago, pp. 155–163.

[10] American Burn Association (2007). *Advanced Burn Life Support Providers Manual*. American Burn Association, Chicago, [Online]. Available at: http://www.scribd.com/doc/83859073/ABLS-Advanced-Burn-Life-Support-Provider-Manual [Accessed 15 March 2013].

[11] American Burn Association (2006). *Burn Center Referral Guide*. American Burn Association, Chicago, [Online]. Available at: http://www.ameriburn.org/BurnCenterReferralCriteria.pdf?PHPSESSID=305bb37ee94d4710494e0722abb790cd [Accessed 15 March 2013].

[12] Initial Assessment and Management, Chapter 1 In: Advanced Burn Life Support course book. American Burn Association, Chicago, 2004:22.

[13] Boswick, J.A. (ed.) (1987). *The Art and Science of Burn Care*, Aspen Publishers, Rockville, MD.

[14] Mlcak, R.P. and Buffalo, M.C. (2007). 'Pre-hospital management, transportation and emergency care', in Herndon, D.N. (ed.), *Total Burn Care*, third edition, Saunders Elsevier, Philadelphia, p. 91.

[15] Wachtel, T.L. (1989). Initial care of major burns, *Postgrad Med*, **85**, 178–196.

[16] Schulte J.H. (1963). Effects of mild carbon monoxide intoxication, *Arch Environ Health*, **7**, 524–530.

[17] Clark, C.J., Campbell, D. and Reid, W.H. (1981). Blood carboxyhaemoglobin and cyanide levels in fire survivors, *Lancet*, **1**, 332–1335.

[18] Crapo R.O. (1981). Smoke-inhalation injuries, *JAMA*, **246**, 1694–1696.

[19] European Medicines Agency. Annex I: Summary of Product Characteristics. Usage of Cyanokit [Online]. Available at: http://www.ema.europa.eu/docs/en_GB/document_library/EPAR_-_Product_Information/human/000806/WC500036429.pdf [Accessed 15 October 2013].

[20] Myers, R.A., Snyder, S.K., Linberg, A. *et al.* (1981). Value of hyperbaric oxygen in suspected carbon monoxide poisoning, *JAMA*, **246**, 2478–2480.

[21] Haponic, E.F., Myers, D.A. Munster, A.M. *et al.* (1987). Acute upper airway injury in burn patients: serial changes of flow-volume curves and nasopharyngoscopy, *Am Rev Respir Dis*, **135**, 360–366.

[22] Thompson, P.B., Herndon, D.N., Broemeling L. *et al.* (1986). Effect on mortality of inhalation injury, *J Trauma*, **26**, 163–165.

[23] Navar, P.D., Saffle, J.R. and Warden, G.D. (1985). Effect of inhalation injury on fluid resuscitation requirements after thermal injury, *Am J Surg*, **150**, 716–720.

[24] Fitzpatrick J. and Cioffi Jr, W.G. (1997). Ventilatory support following burns and smoke-inhalation injury, *Respir Care Clin N Am*, **3**, 21–49.

[25] Reper, P., Dankaert, R., van Hille, F. *et al.* (1998). The usefulness of combined high-frequency percussive ventilation during acute respiratory failure after smoke inhalation, *Burns*, **24**, 34–38.

[26] Shirani, K.Z., Pruitt Jr, B.A. and Mason Jr, A.D. (1987). The influence of inhalation injury and pneumonia on burn mortality, *Am Surg*, **205**, 82–87.

[27] Herndon, D.N., Barrow, R.E., Traber, D.L. *et al.* (1987). Extravascular lung water changes following smoke inhalation and massive burn injury, *Surgery*, **102**, 341–349.

[28] Cioffi Jr, W.G., Rue III, L.W., Graves, T.A. *et al.* (1991). Prophylactic use of high-frequency percussive ventilation in patients with inhalation injury, *Am Surg*, **213**, 575–582.

[29] Muller, M. J. and Herndon, D. M. (1994). The challenge of burns, *Lancet*, **343**, 217.

[30] Herndon, D.M., Desai M.A., Abston S. *et al.* (1992). *Residents Manual*, Shriners Burns Hospital, and the University of Texas Medical Branch, Galveston, 1–17.

[31] Deitch, E.A. (1990). The management of burns, *N Engl J Med*, **323**, 1249–1253.

[32] Horton, J.W., Baxter, C.R. and White, D.J. (1989). Differences in cardiac responses to resuscitation from burn shock, *Surg Gynecol Obstet*, **168**, 201–213.

[33] Zetterstrom, H. and Arturson, G. (1980). Plasma oncotic pressure and plasma protein concentration in patients following thermal injury, *Acta Anaesthesiiol Scand*, **24**, 288–294.

[34] Duncan, R. and Dunn, K. (2008). 'Physiological responses to burn injury and resuscitation protocols for adult major burns', in, Stone, C. (ed.), *The Evidence for Plastic Surgery*, TFM Publishing Ltd, Harley, p. 75.

[35] Purdue, G.F. and Hunt, J.L. (1986). Vascular access through the femoral vessels: indications and complications, *J Burn Care Rehabil*, **7**, 448–450.

[36] Norwood S.H., Cormier B., McMahon N.G. *et al.* (1988). Prospective study of catheter-related infection during prolonged arterial catheterisation, *Crit Care Med*, **16**, 127–131.

[37] Moyer, C.A., Margraf H.W. and Monafo, W.W. (1965). Burn shock and extravascular sodium deficiency: treatment with Ringer's solution with lactate, *Arch Surg*, **90**, 799–811.

[38] Baxter, C.R. and Shires, G.T. (1968). Physiological responses to crystalloid resuscitation of severe burns, *Ann NY Acad Sci*, **150**, 874–894.

[39] Duncan, R. and Dunn, K. (2008). 'Physiological responses to burn injury and resuscitation protocols for adult major burns', Stone, C. (ed.), *The Evidence for Plastic Surgery*, TFM Publishing Ltd, Harley, p. 80.

[40] Duncan, R. and Dunn, K. (2008). 'Physiological responses to burn injury and resuscitation protocols for adult major burns', in, Stone, C. (ed.), *The Evidence for Plastic Surgery*, TFM Publishing Ltd, Harley, p. 87.

[41] Warden, G.D. (1992). Burn shock resuscitation, *World J Surg*, **16**, 21–23.

[42] Artz, C.P. (1976). Burns updated, *J Trauma*, **16**, 2–15.

[43] American Society of Anesthesiologists (1996). Practice guidelines for blood component therapy: a report by the American Society of Anaesthesiologists Task Force on Blood Component Therapy, *Anesthesiology*, **84**, 732–747.

[44] O'Mara, M.S., Hayetian, F., Slater, H. *et al.* (2005). Results of a protocol of transfusion threshold and surgical techniques on transfusion requirements in burn patients, *Burns*, **31**, 558–561.

[45] Choinière, M., Melzack, R., Rondeau, J. *et al.* (1989). The pain of burns: characteristics and correlates, *J Trauma*, **29**, 1531–1539.

[46] Southwood, W.F. (1955). The thickness of the skin, *Plast Reconstr Surg*, **15**, 423–429.

[47] Randolph, R. and Ballantyne Jr, D.L. (1990). 'Skin grafts', in McCarthy, J. (ed.), *Plastic Surgery*, WB Saunders, Philadelphia, pp. 221–274.

[48] Hlava, P., Moserova, J. and Konigova, R. (1983). Validity of clinical assessment of the depth of a thermal injury, *Acta Chir Plast*, **25**, 202–208.

[49] Boykin, J.V., Eriksson, E. and Pittman, R.N. (1980). In vivo microcirculation of a scald burn and the progression of postburn dermal ischemia, *Plast Reconstr Surg*, **66**, 191–198.

[50] Jackson, D.M. (1953). The diagnosis of the depth of burning, *Br J Surg*, **40**, 588–596.

[51] Moyer, C.A., Brentano, L., Gravens, D.L. *et al.* (1965). Treatment of large human burns with 0.5 per cent silver nitrate solution, *Arch Surg*, **90**, 812–867.

[52] Klasen, H.J. (2000). A historical review of the use of silver in the treatment of burns. II. Renewed interest for silver, *Burns*, **26**, 131–138.

[53] Burke, J.K., Bondoc, C.C. and Quinby, W.C. (1974). Primary burn excision and immediate grafting: a method shortening illness, *J Trauma*, **14**, 389–395.

[54] Engrav, L.H., Heimback, D.M., Reus, J.L. *et al.* (1983). Early excision and grafting vs. nonoperative treatment of burns of indeterminate depth: a randomized prospective study, *J Trauma*, **23**, 1001–1004.

[55] Thompson, P., Herndon, D.N., Abston, S. *et al.* (1987). Effect of early excision on patients with major thermal injury, *J Trauma*, **27**, 205–207.
[56] Deitch, E.A., Wheelahan, T.M., Rose, M.P. *et al.* (1983). Hypertrophic burn scars: analysis of variables, *J Trauma*, **23**, 895–898.
[57] Janzekovic Z. (1970). A new concept in the early excision and immediate grafting of burns, *J Trauma*, **10**, 1103–1108.
[58] Wainwright, D.J. (1995). Use of an acellular allograft dermal matrix (Alloderm) in the management of full-thickness burns, *Burns*, **21**, 243–248.
[59] Munster, A.M., Smith-Meek, M. and Shalom, A. (2001). Acellular allograft dermal matrix: immediate or delayed epidermal coverage? *Burns*, **27**, 150–153.
[60] Sheridan, R., Choucair, R., Donelan, M. *et al.* (1998). Acellularallodermis in burns surgery: 1-year results of a pilot trial, *J Burn Care Rehabil*, **19**, 528–530.
[61] Grzesiak, J.J., Pierschbacher, M.D., Amodeo, M.F. *et al.* (1997). Enhancement of cell interactions with collagen/gylcosaminoglycan matrices by RGD derivatization, *Biomaterials*, **18**, 1625–1632.
[62] Stern, R., McPherson, M. and Longaker, M.T (1990). Histologic study of artificial skin used in the treatment of full-thickness thermal injury, *J Burn Care Rehabil*, **11**, 7–13.
[63] Chiu, T. and Burd, A. (2005). "Xenograft" dressing in the treatment of burns, *Clin Dermatol*, **23**, 419–423.
[64] Woodson, L.C., Sherwood, E.R., Aarsland, A. *et al.* (2007). 'Anesthesia for burns patients', in Herndon, D.N. (ed.), *Total Burn Care*, third edition, Saunders Elsevier, Philadelphia, pp. 201–203.
[65] Woodson, L.C., Sherwood, E.R., Aarsland A. *et al.* (2007). 'Anesthesia for burns patients', in Herndon, D.N. (ed.), *Total Burn Care*, third edition, Saunders Elsevier, Philadelphia, p. 221.
[66] Pruitt Jr, B.A. (1981). Fluid resuscitation of extensively burned patients, *J Trauma*, **21**, 690–692.
[67] Linares, H.A. (1981). A report of 115 consecutive autopsies in burned children 1966–80, *Burns*, **8**, 263–270.
[68] Gallagher, J.J., Williams-Bouyer, N., Villarreal C. *et al.* (2007). 'Treatment of infection in burns' in Herndon, D.N. (ed.), *Total Burn Care*, third edition, Saunders Elsevier, Philadelphia, Chapter 12, pp. 136–174.
[69] Saffle, J.R. and Graves, C. 'Nutritional support of the burned patient', in Herndon, D.N. (ed.), *Total Burn Care*, third edition, Saunders Elsevier, Philadelphia, pp. 398–416.
[70] Demling, R.H. and DeSanti, L. (1997). Oxandrolone, an anabolic steroid, significantly increases the rate of weight gain in the recovering phase after major burns, *J Trauma*, **43**, 47–50.

[71] Lee. J.O. and Herndon, D.M. (2007). 'The pediatric burned patient', in Herndon, D.N. (ed.), *Total Burn Care*, third edition, Saunders Elsevier, Philadelphia, pp. 485–494.
[72] Purdue, G.F., Arnoldo, B.D. and Hunt, J.L. (2007). 'Electrical injuries', in Herndon, D.N. (ed.), *Total Burn Care*, third edition, Saunders Elsevier, Philadelphia, pp. 513–519.

28
Poisoning

David J. Watson

28.1 Introduction

In the UK, patients admitted to hospital suffering from the effects of acute poisoning account for up to 15 to 20% of all medical admissions. Although only a proportion of poisoning victims require intensive observation and supportive care (with or without active treatment), management of such patients may account for up to one-third of admissions to a multidisciplinary intensive care unit. The total number of deaths from poisoning in the United Kingdom remains unchanged at approximately 4,000 per year. The commonest cause of death by poisoning in the United Kingdom is currently carbon monoxide [1].

28.2 Types of Poisoning

28.2.1 *Self-poisoning*

The vast majority of adult cases of acute poisoning are self-administered. Most of these are manipulative or represent 'a cry for help' rather than a genuine attempt at suicide and there is often a history of previous similar episodes. The mean age of patients admitted to hospital with an overdose is approximately 25 years, with a female: male ratio of 1.3:1, whereas the mean age of successful suicide is about 50 years. In females the peak incidence is in those less than 25 years of age, whereas in males self-poisoning is commonest between the ages of 20 and 35 years.

28.2.2 *Accidental poisoning*

Accidental poisoning is most common in children between one and five years of age who ingest medicinal, domestic or cosmetic agents. In only a minority of such cases presenting to a hospital does the child develop symptoms, and fatalities are unusual. Accidental poisoning may also be the result of industrial or agricultural mishaps.

28.2.3 *Non-accidental poisoning*

Non-accidental poisoning may be related to experimentation with drugs or solvents (usually in young adults) or may represent part of the syndrome of child abuse, in which case poisoning is more often fatal than in accidental cases. Homicidal poisoning is rarely encountered in clinical practice.

Because the hospital mortality of acute poisoning is generally low, active measures to hasten the elimination of the poison (which can be associated with a significant morbidity and, in some cases, mortality) is recommended only in a few exceptional instances; indeed, the 'Scandinavian method' of elective supportive care was originally introduced because of the dangers associated with the use of analeptics in patients in barbiturate coma.

Above all else, therefore, the management of acute poisoning involves the application of the principles of supportive care, including:

- Maintenance and protection of the airway.
- Respiratory support.
- Expansion of the circulating volume.
- Maintenance of fluid and electrolyte balance.
- Correction of acid-base disturbances.
- Occasionally the use of inotropes and/or vasopressors.
- Provision of nutritional support.
- Thrombo-embolic and stress ulcer.
- Control of body temperature
- Skilled nursing care.

28.3 Diagnosis and Assessment

28.3.1 *History*

The diagnosis can often be established from the history, which may need to be supported by circumstantial evidence. The quantity and nature of the substances taken must be determined. In most cases, a history can be obtained from the patient, although this is frequently misleading and about half will exaggerate or, less often, minimise the severity of poisoning. Currently self-poisoning episodes in the UK most commonly involve the ingestion of benzodiazepines, paracetamol, aspirin or tricyclic antidepressants or the inhalation of motor exhaust fumes. In many cases a mixture of drugs will have been ingested, often including alcohol and a benzodiazepine. Sometimes patients refuse to divulge any information, while others are incoherent or unconscious. In all cases, therefore, the history should be corroborated by interviewing witnesses such as patients, carers or relatives, friends and paramedics, as well as by contacting the general practitioner when appropriate. Bottles, pills or other substances found on or about the patient may provide important clues as to the nature of the poisoning, although they can also be misleading (e.g. drugs may have been stored in incorrectly labelled bottles). Tablets can often be identified using the Chemist and Druggist Directory, or a computer-aided tablet and capsule identification system such as 'TicTac'. In the UK this is available to authorised users, such as poisons information centres. In some cases it may be appropriate to send a sample of the substance ingested to the laboratory for analysis. Clear documentation of all relevant information is essential.

TOXBASE is the primary clinical toxicology database of the National Poisons Information Service in the United Kingdom. It is also available on the Internet to registered users (http://www.toxbase.org/) and provides information about routine diagnosis, treatment and management of patients exposed to drugs, household products and agricultural chemicals.

Other important aspects of the initial enquiry include a history of previous psychiatric disorders and self-poisoning episodes, as well as evidence of complicating illnesses such as liver or renal disease, which might impair the patient's ability to handle poisons.

Table 28.1. Clinical grading of consciousness level in acute poisoning.

Grade 0	Fully conscious
Grade I	Drowsy, but responsive to verbal commands
Grade II	Unconscious, but responding to painful stimuli
Grade III	Unconscious, but responding only to maximal painful stimulus
Grade IV	Unconscious, not responding to pain

28.3.2 *Examination*

A detailed physical examination should be performed and should include a search for associated injuries (e.g. pressure necrosis, compartment syndrome) as well as medical conditions that might have precipitated the overdose (e.g. depression or psychosis) or could be responsible for coma. When indicated, body temperature should be recorded with a low-reading rectal thermometer. An assessment of the patient's consciousness level is particularly important; this should be repeated at regular intervals to follow progress and, in some cases, indicate the need for active intervention. A simple clinical grading of consciousness level suitable for use in cases of acute poisoning is shown in Table 28.1.

Organic brain damage should be suspected when there is no improvement in the depth of the coma within 24 hours, especially when the history of poisoning is dubious. Although the signs and symptoms may suggest intoxication with a specific poison there is, in practice, often little relationship between the drugs suspected on admission and those detected in the blood.

28.3.3 *Investigations*

When possible, samples of gastric contents (50 ml of vomit, aspirate or first portion of gastric lavage), blood (10 ml lithium-heparinised blood, 10 ml clotted sample, 2 ml of fluoride blood for ethanol assay) and urine (50 ml of the first sample voided after admission) should be obtained for laboratory identification of the poisons involved. Preferably these samples should be collected before the administration of medications, which might complicate toxicological analysis.

Table 28.2. Recommended investigations in acute poisoning.

Toxicological analysis
Gastric contents
Blood
Urine
Haemoglobin, white cell count
Blood sugar
Urea, creatinine and electrolytes
Liver function tests
Blood gas analysis
Chest radiograph

Since about 50% of those presenting to the emergency department with coma of unknown cause are suffering from self-poisoning it is often advisable to perform a toxicological screen in all such cases. Automated devices for measuring blood levels of some of the common poisons are now available and can be positioned within, or close to, the intensive care unit. Meticulous maintenance and quality control is, however, essential, and purchase of such a device can only be recommended when the unit admits large numbers of poisoned patients. Assistance is always available from the poisons information centre or TOXBASE (see above).

Baseline determinations of haemoglobin concentration, blood sugar, urea and electrolyte levels and liver function tests should be performed in all cases. Blood gas analysis is also routine and may reveal hypercarbia due to respiratory depression or hypoxaemia related to pulmonary pathology such as infection, atelectasis, aspiration or oedema. A chest radiograph should also be obtained (Table 28.2).

28.4 Principles of Management

The principles of management are listed in Table 28.3.

Table 28.3. Principles of management of acute poisoning.

Immediate management
Secure and protect airway
Respiratory support
Expand circulating volume
Occasionally inotropes and/or vasopressors
Treat arrhythmias
Pass nasogastric tube
Control seizures
Supportive care
Cardiovascular support
Respiratory support
Renal support
Prevent and treat neurological complications
Skilled nursing care
Physiotherapy
Stress ulcer prophylaxis
Enteral nutrition (rarely parenteral)
Antithrombotic/antiembolic prophylaxis
Control body temperature
Prevent further absorption of poison
Activated charcoal
Gastric aspiration and lavage
Whole gut irrigation
Accelerated elimination of poison
Repeated dose activated charcoal
Enhanced urinary excretion
Haemodialysis and/or haemoperfusion
Treat liver failure
Specific antidotes

28.4.1 *Immediate management*

It is worth reiterating that the majority of patients require only supportive treatment. This should include immediate life-saving measures and prevention of complications such as hypotension, pulmonary aspiration, acid-base disturbances, fluid and electrolyte imbalance and hypothermia.

28.4.1.1 *Airway*

Patients with impaired cough and gag reflexes, as well as those with borderline airway protection needing gastric lavage, require immediate tracheal intubation to secure their airway and prevent aspiration. All patients should be given supplemental oxygen.

28.4.1.2 *Breathing*

Mechanical ventilation should be instituted without delay in those with respiratory depression. Because hypoxia and hypercarbia can exacerbate intracranial hypertension and may cause or potentiate cardiac arrhythmias, prompt treatment is essential. Some patients may have developed aspiration or hypostatic pneumonia before admission.

28.4.1.3 *Circulation*

Acutely poisoned patients are frequently hypotensive, usually as a result of peripheral vasodilatation. Fluid depletion is also common with prolonged stupor or coma and is often exacerbated by vomiting, sweating and hyperventilation. In most cases blood pressure can be restored by intravascular volume expansion, although occasionally vasopressors will be indicated, and in a few cases inotropic support may be required to counteract myocardial depression. Hypertension occurs less frequently than hypotension but may be associated with poisoning by sympathomimentic drugs such as amphetamines, phencyclidine and cocaine.

Cardiac arrhythmias are common and may be due to hypoxia, hypercarbia, acid–base disturbances or electrolyte imbalance, as well as the direct effects of the toxin or drug (e.g. tricyclic antidepressants, some antipsychotics, some antihistamines and co-proxamol). A 12-lead electrocardiogram (ECG) should be obtained and the ECG should then be continuously monitored. Ventricular arrhythmias associated with significant hypotension may require treatment. If the QT interval is prolonged, specialist advice should be sought because the use of some anti-arrhythmic drugs may be contraindicated. Should cardiac arrest occur it is often resistant to attempts to restore sinus rhythm. It is therefore important to persist with cardiopulmonary resuscitation, (if necessary using a mechanical support device), especially since fixed dilated pupils may be attributable to the direct effects of the toxin. When toxicity is likely to be prolonged (e.g. with tricyclic antidepressants or calcium antagonists), cardiovascular support, in the form of intra-aortic balloon counterpulsation or cardiopulmonary bypass, may be life-saving [2].

28.4.1.4 *Gastrointestinal*

Gastric stasis is common in comatose patients and may be exacerbated by the effects of opiates or drugs with anticholinergic properties. A nasogastric tube should therefore be passed to decompress the stomach and reduce the risk of regurgitation.

28.4.1.5 *Neurological*

Prolonged or recurrent convulsions should be treated with lorazepam (up to 4 mg) or diazepam (preferably as emulsion, up to 10 mg) by slow intravenous injection in the first instance.

28.4.2 *Supportive care*

As well as continued cardiovascular and respiratory support, subsequent management involves the institution of measures to prevent and treat complications. Intensive nursing care and physiotherapy are essential in prolonged coma. It is important to document the presence or absence of neuropraxias, corneal abrasions and injury to pressure areas on admission to the intensive care unit.

28.4.2.1 *Gastrointestinal*

Stress ulcer prophylaxis should be instituted in the most seriously ill patients. Enteral nutrition should be established early; if this is not possible parenteral nutrition should be considered.

28.4.2.2 *Thrombo-embolic prophylaxis*

28.4.2.2.1 Neurological

Neurological complications may include:

- Coma.
- Seizures (related to cerebral hypoxia, metabolic disturbances or the direct effects of the poison).
- Cerebral oedema (due to severe hypoxia, cardiac arrest, profound hypotension, severe carbon monoxide (CO) poisoning).
- Peripheral nerve injuries (due to prolonged pressure).

The possibility that neurological abnormalities are unrelated to poisoning should be considered when:

- The reduction in consciousness level is out of proportion to the severity of poisoning.
- The consciousness level fails to improve.
- There are lateralising signs.

In such cases further investigations, including a cerebral computed tomography (CT) scan are warranted to exclude, for example, an intracranial haemorrhage.

28.4.2.2.2 Renal

Renal failure may be related to the direct effects of the toxin (e.g. in those poisoned with non-steroidal antiinflammatory drugs (NSAIDs) or heavy metals), to prolonged hypotension or to sepsis/septic shock (e.g. in patients with pneumonia). Rhabdomyolysis is a common cause of renal failure in patients with poisoning and should be suspected in those who have been immobile for a prolonged period before admission, especially when pressure areas are seen to be discoloured with poor capillary refill. Rhabdomyolysis may also be precipitated by the combination of prolonged seizures, hyperthermia, hypokalaemia and extreme tissue hypoxia.

A urinary catheter should be inserted in at-risk patients and measures instituted to reverse oliguria and prevent renal failure. Those who progress to established renal failure will require renal support.

28.4.2.3 *Temperature regulation*

Hypothermia is a common complication of prolonged coma outside hospital in patients of any age and is particularly likely in those poisoned with drugs that prevent vasoconstriction and shivering (e.g. barbiturates and phenothiazines). Usually passive rewarming is sufficient, but occasionally active measures are warranted.

Hyperthermia may complicate intoxication with tricyclic antidepressants, monoamine oxidase inhibitors, cocaine, amphetamines or ecstasy, and is an important feature of the neuroleptic malignant syndrome. Children and the elderly are also at risk of raised body temperature when taking drugs with anticholinergic properties in therapeutic doses.

Initial management involves removing all unnecessary clothing and using a fan. Sponging with tepid water will also promote evaporation; iced water should not be used. In the severest cases active cooling measures with sedation, muscle relaxation and mechanical ventilation with unheated gases may be required. Advice should be sought from a poisons information centre on the management of severe hyperthermia.

28.4.3 *Prevention of absorption of poison*

28.4.3.1 *Activated charcoal*

Activated charcoal is a powerful non-specific adsorbent that can bind many drugs and poisons within the gastrointestinal tract, thereby reducing absorption. It seems to provide a relatively safe and effective means of limiting drug absorption when given soon after ingestion of the poison.

Drugs that are well adsorbed to activated charcoal include:

- Benzodiazepines.
- Barbiturates.
- Anticonvulsants, e.g. carbamazepine, phenytoin.
- Theophylline.
- Antidepressants.
- Quinine.
- Dapsone.

Salicylates and paracetamol are only moderately well adsorbed. Substances not well adsorbed to activated charcoal are listed in Table 28.4. Current recommendations are that 50 g of activated charcoal should be given to adults who have taken a substantial overdose of a toxic substance no more than one hour previously — longer in the case of modified-release preparations or drugs with anticholinergic properties [3]. Charcoal should not be given if the airway cannot be protected. Repeated doses can be used for sustained-release preparations such as propranolol or theophylline, as well as for salicylates, phenobarbitone and carbamazepine (see below).

Table 28.4. Substances not effectively adsorbed by activated charcoal.

Ferrous salts
Lithium preparations
Potassium salts
Ethanol
Methanol
Ethylene glycol
Acids
Alkalis
Fluorides
Organic solvents
Mercury and its salts
Lead and its salts

28.4.3.2 *Gastric aspiration and lavage*

When performed in seriously poisoned patients, gastric aspiration and lavage is associated with a considerable risk of complications, including:

- Pulmonary aspiration.
- Seizures.
- Arrhythmias.
- Perforation of the stomach.

The procedure should therefore only be undertaken by experienced personnel with the facilities available to treat any complications, and then only if potentially life-threatening amounts of a toxic substance have been ingested within the preceding hour [4]. This time limit can be extended in cases of poisoning with agents that delay gastric emptying, such as salicylates and tricyclic antidepressants. It may also occasionally be considered in patients who have ingested drugs that are not adsorbed by charcoal, such as iron or lithium. On the other hand, in those who have ingested agents that do not delay gastric emptying and are rapidly absorbed from the gastrointestinal tract (e.g. paracetamol), gastric aspiration and lavage may prove ineffective, even when performed early.

Gastric aspiration and lavage is contraindicated when corrosive substances or a petroleum distillate have been taken. Aspiration of kerosene or its derivatives can produce a particularly destructive form of lipoid pneumonia.

28.4.3.2.1 Procedure

Gastric aspiration and lavage should only be performed if the patient has adequate laryngeal and pharyngeal reflexes or has an endotracheal tube in place with the cuff inflated. The use of an intravenous anaesthetic agent and muscle relaxation to allow tracheal intubation of a semi-comatose patient is only justified when gastric lavage is clearly indicated; in the majority of cases it is not. The semi-conscious patient should be positioned head down, lying on the left side. Facilities for pharyngeal suction must be immediately available. Foreign matter should be removed from the mouth, and pharynx before introducing a wide-bore tube into the mouth, which the patient is then persuaded to swallow (a large tube is less likely to enter the trachea and allows aspiration of particulate matter). The stomach contents are then aspirated and retained for analysis, following which lavage is performed with 250 ml warmed tap water. This procedure is repeated until the aspirate is clear of debris. Subsequently, the wide-bore tube is replaced by a Ryle's tube, which is aspirated hourly.

28.4.3.3 *Whole-gut irrigation*

Whole-bowel irrigation has been used in poisoning with certain sustained-release medications, in severe poisoning with heavy metals, iron and lithium salts, button batteries and illicit drug packets. The procedure involves isotonic polyethylene glycol administration (e.g. KleenPrep) (2 litres per hour) orally or via a nasogastric tube for three to five hours in adults to flush out gastrointestinal contents but it is not yet clear whether outcome is improved. Advice should be sought from a poisons information centre. This technique is contraindicated in patients with bowel obstruction, perforation, ileus, haemodynamic instability or where the airway cannot be protected [5]. Polyethylene glycol or laxatives are sometimes used in 'body packers' to remove packets that are beyond the pylorus, although one report described the death of a body packer when ingested condoms dissolved after paraffin was given [6]. Packets in the stomach are best removed endoscopically [7] and packets in the small or large intestine that contain potentially lethal amounts of drugs may be removed surgically [8].

28.4.3.4 *Induction of vomiting*

Induction of emesis (e.g. with ipecacuanha) is not now recommended because there is no evidence that it affects absorption or systemic toxicity [9] and it may increase the risk of aspiration. It is also difficult to give activated charcoal after an emetic [10].

28.4.4 *Accelerated elimination of poison*

Active measures to increase the elimination of a poison are indicated if the patient is seriously ill and deteriorating, if significant amounts of the poison can be removed and if this is likely to produce worthwhile improvement. In fact only a small proportion of acutely poisoned patients merit such treatment and it is sensible to first obtain the advice of a poisons information centre.

28.4.4.1 *Activated charcoal*

Repeated administration of activated charcoal is a cheap, safe and effective means of reducing drug levels by creating a negative diffusion gradient between the gut lumen and blood — so called 'gastrointestinal dialysis' [11]. Nevertheless, pulmonary aspiration of activated charcoal can have serious consequences [12]. There is also a risk of gastrointestinal obstruction and hypernatraemia from the sodium load.

Severely poisoned adults should be given 50 g orally or via a nasogastric tube then every 4 hours as repeated doses (Table 28.5).

In cases of intolerance the dose may be reduced and the frequency increased e.g. 25 g every two hours or 12.5 g every hour. Vomiting and dose reductions may, however, compromise the efficacy of charcoal treatment. Other techniques intended to enhance the elimination of poisons after their absorption are only indicated for a small number of severely poisoned patients.

28.4.4.2 *Renal elimination*

Urinary excretion can be enhanced by altering the pH of the urine to increase the degree of ionisation of the substance and reduce its lipid

Table 28.5. Indications for multiple-dose activated charcoal.

Modified release preparations such as theophylline (but not lithium)
Carbamazepine
Dapsone
Digoxin
Paraquat
Phenobarbitone
Quinine
The fungus *Amanita phalloides*

solubility. In aspirin overdose, alkalinisation of the urine increases salicylate elimination, but forced alkaline diuresis is no longer recommended. In severe chlorpromazine poisoning maintaining acidic urine may be appropriate.

28.4.4.3 *Haemodialysis and haemoperfusion*

Haemodialysis and haemoperfusion [13] are of dubious value, but are likely to be most effective when:

- The poison diffuses readily across the dialysis membrane or is avidly taken up by the adsorbent.
- The pharmacological effect of the toxin is closely related to blood levels.
- Dialysis or haemoperfusion adds significantly to other routes of drug elimination.

On the other hand, drugs that are highly lipid-soluble and have a large volume of distribution are difficult to eliminate.

Haemodialysis may be of value in the management of severe salicylate overdose and poisoning with death cap mushrooms (*Amanita phalloides*). Clearance of barbiturates, anticonvulsants, benzodiazepines, lithium, cardiac glycosides and many other less-commonly encountered poisons can certainly be enhanced with these techniques, but it is uncertain whether morbidity or mortality are reduced. In severe methyl alcohol (methanol) and ethylene glycol ingestion, it is logical to attempt removal of these water-soluble poisons before they are metabolised to potentially lethal formaldehyde and formic acid or glycollic and oxalic acids respectively. Large molecules and poisons that are highly protein-bound cannot be cleared efficiently by haemodialysis and in such cases haemoperfusion is preferred e.g. chloral hydrate, theophylline. Such extracorporeal techniques are relatively complex and can be associated with a significant risk of complications. Clearance of paracetamol, paraquat and tricyclic antidepressants is not significantly enhanced.

Haemodialysis or haemofiltration may also be considered for renal failure or refractory acid–base disturbances. It is occasionally indicated when a patient is deteriorating, despite adequate supportive care, as a result of poisoning with a dialysable substance. Peritoneal dialysis has no established role in the management of poisoning.

28.4.5 *Specific antidotes*

An antidote can be defined as any substance that can favourably influence the onset, severity or duration of the toxic effects of a poison [14]. Only a few specific antidotes are available and some may themselves have toxic effects. They may act by:

- Competing for drug receptor sites (e.g. flumazenil, naloxone).
- Binding with the toxin to form less toxic chelates that are more easily excreted (e.g. digoxin-specific antibody fragments, snake anti-venoms).
- Influencing metabolism of a poison to prevent or reduce the formation of harmful metabolites (e.g. *N*-acetylcysteine in paracetamol overdose; ethanol or fomepizole in methanol or ethylene glycol poisoning).

The use of specific antagonists such as naloxone and flumazenil to reverse central nervous system (CNS) depression is controversial and is discussed later in this chapter. Analeptics should never be used.

28.5 Management of Specific Poisonings

28.5.1 *Alcohols*

28.5.1.1 *Ethanol*

Acute intoxication with alcohol (ethanol) is seen most commonly in adults but also is occasionally encountered in children. Aspiration of vomitus, hypothermia and non-traumatic rhabdomyolysis are special risks accompanying alcohol-induced coma, and hypoglycaemia may occur in children and some adults. Management is supportive. Glucose can be given if indicated.

28.5.1.2 *Methanol*

Acute methanol (methyl alcohol) poisoning occurs most frequently in vagrants, although cases of accidental ingestion are occasionally encountered.

Methanol is a constituent of antifreeze (alone or with ethylene glycol), paint removers and varnish and is produced in some home-made beverages. Methylated spirit, however, is composed largely of ethanol with only 5% methanol. Methanol is metabolised to formic acid and formaldehyde, both of which are extremely toxic.

28.5.1.2.1 Clinical features

The central effects of acute methanol intoxication may be delayed for 12 to 36 hours after ingestion, at which time nausea, vomiting, abdominal pain, headache and ataxia can occur and may progress to coma. There is often, a profound metabolic acidosis with Kussmaul respiration. If poisoning is severe (blood methanol >500 mg/l, marked acidosis), the patient may develop an acute optic nerve papillitis with blurring of vision that can progress to blindness, dilatation of the pupils and papilloedema.

28.5.1.2.2 Treatment

Advice on the treatment of methanol or ethylene glycol poisoning should be obtained from a poisons information centre.

Gastric aspiration and lavage should be performed if the patient is seen within one hour of ingestion and any metabolic acidosis should be corrected. Because ethanol competes with methanol for the enzyme alcohol dehydrogenase, administration of the former (by mouth or intravenous infusion) can limit the production of formic acid. Haemodialysis has also been recommended if the patient fails to respond to these measures and has visual impairment, a severe metabolic acidosis or a blood methanol level greater than 1 g/l. There is no evidence, however, that dialysis is more effective than standard measures. Fomepizole (Antizol), available from poisons information centres, has also been used for the treatment of methanol or ethylene glycol poisoning [15]. Like ethanol, fomepizole (4-methylpyrazole) is a competitive inhibitor of alcohol dehydrogenase. Compared with treatment with ethanol (by mouth or intravenous infusion) 4-methylpyrazole has the advantage of reduced CNS depression, although haemodialysis may still be required for the management of renal failure.

28.5.2 *Analgesics*

28.5.2.1 *Salicylates*

The increased use of paracetamol as a mild analgesic has resulted in a reduction in the incidence of salicylate poisoning. Nevertheless, it remains a relatively common cause of poisoning in children and adults. Many readily available salicylate preparations do not mention that they contain aspirin. Oil of wintergreen, for example, contains methyl salicylate and is potentially highly toxic.

28.5.2.1.1 Mechanisms of toxicity

Aspirin is normally deacetylated by plasma esterases and is eliminated by conjugation. Following overdose, however, the conjugation pathway is saturated, free salicylate has to be eliminated via the kidneys and excretion is prolonged.

Aspirin uncouples oxidative phosphorylation, leading to increased metabolism of glucose and fats with a rise in oxygen consumption (VO_2) and carbon dioxide production. The respiratory centre is stimulated both directly and by the increased carbon dioxide production, thereby producing respiratory alkalosis. If salicylate levels are very high, however, respiratory depression may supervene. Blood levels of pyruvate, lactate and ketone bodies are increased and, combined with the fact that aspirin is itself an organic acid, this produces a metabolic acidosis.

28.5.2.1.2 Clinical features

The majority of patients present within six hours of ingestion and are conscious, alert and orientated, although some are restless, irritable and confused. Hallucinations may occur. Coma is rare and in adults, drowsiness indicates severe poisoning. Confusion and drowsiness are more frequently seen in children.

Other clinical features include:

- Sweating.
- Tinnitus and deafness.
- Blurred vision.

- Tachycardia.
- Hyperventilation.

Initially there is a respiratory alkalosis, although in severe cases respiratory acidosis may occur as a terminal event, whilst in children a metabolic acidosis can develop rapidly and usually becomes the dominant abnormality.

Less commonly, patients poisoned with aspirin have epigastric pain and vomiting with severe dehydration and oliguria. Rarely, they may develop acute renal failure. Gastrointestinal bleeding is uncommon, but may be related to gastric erosions and a coagulopathy. The latter is usually due to hypoprothrombinaemia, which can be corrected with fresh frozen plasma and vitamin K, but may also be due to thrombocytopenia, decreased production of factor VII or impaired platelet function.

In some cases, pulmonary oedema develops in association with an increase in capillary permeability, proteinuria and hypoproteinaemia. These patients may also be hypotensive and hypovolaemic. Administration of colloidal solutions is appropriate but care is required to avoid precipitating or worsening pulmonary oedema.

Salicylate poisoning may also be associated with hypokalaemia, hyperglycaemia or hypoglycaemia; the latter may be particularly severe in children. Some patients develop an encephalopathy and hyperthermia.

28.5.2.1.3 Investigations

Investigations should include:

- Blood gas and acid–base analysis.
- Urea and electrolytes.
- Coagulation studies.
- Blood glucose.

In severe poisoning, protein and calcium levels should be determined and liver function tests should be performed.

The diagnosis should be confirmed, and the severity of poisoning assessed, by measuring plasma salicylate levels. This should be related to the time of ingestion, bearing in mind that after an overdose absorption of aspirin continues for some time and peak levels may not be attained for eight hours or more. Therefore, a level of 350 mg/l (2.5 mmol/l) may be significant 12 hours after ingestion but is almost within the therapeutic range at four to six hours. Active treatment, including sodium bicarbonate (1.26%) given to enhance urinary salicylate excretion, should be considered if the level is more than 500 mg/l (3.6 mmol/l) within 12 hours of ingestion and if it is over 350 mg/l (2.5 mmol/l) beyond this time. In children, measures to hasten elimination are indicated when the level is more than 350 mg/l (2.5 mmol/l) at 12 hours. Respiratory depression is a common mode of death when the plasma salicylate level exceeds 1000 mg/l (7.2 mmol/l).

28.5.2.1.4 Treatment

Gastric aspiration and lavage should be performed if the patient presents within one hour of ingestion. Activated charcoal should be administered in repeated doses via the nasogastric tube (although see comments earlier in this chapter).

When active treatment is indicated, it should be instituted immediately, since death can occur suddenly and unexpectedly. Intravascular volume must be replenished and any significant metabolic acidosis should be corrected. In selected cases, invasive monitoring may be indicated to guide volume replacement and avoid fluid overload. The clearance of salicylates is pH-dependent, increasing ten-fold when blood pH rises from 6.0 to 7.5. Salicylate levels and acid–base status should be measured repeatedly. If a moderate salicylate level has increased to greater than 700 mg/l (5.1 mmol/l), if a severe metabolic acidosis persists or the salicylate level has failed to decrease, haemodialysis is appropriate. If the salicylate level has fallen, however, activated charcoal with or without sodium bicarbonate (1.26%) treatment should be continued.

28.5.2.2 *Paracetamol*

The incidence of poisoning with paracetamol has gradually increased over the last 20 to 30 years and is now one of the commonest causes of fulminant hepatic failure (FHF) [16]; see also Chapter 22.

28.5.2.2.1 Clinical features

Patients who have taken a paracetamol overdose normally remain fully conscious. Clinical features may include pallor, perspiration, epigastric pain, nausea and vomiting. Occasionally, a massive paracetamol overdose may directly damage the myocardium and cause peripheral vasodilatation with shock. In such cases metabolic acidosis may be severe.

The early symptoms are not a reliable indication of the severity of poisoning and there is a wide individual variability in tolerance to paracetamol, as well as in susceptibility to hepatotoxicity. When liver damage does occur, the signs of hepatic failure are not usually apparent until 48 hours after the overdose. At this time, the patient may become jaundiced with an enlarged and tender liver. Liver function tests are most abnormal three to five days after ingestion. In severe, but non-fatal, hepatotoxicity a cholestatic picture is usually seen, and in the most serious cases FHF develops about three to seven days after ingestion.

28.5.2.2.2 Mechanisms of hepatotoxicity

Paracetamol hepatotoxicity is due to a toxic metabolite, which is formed via an oxidative pathway dependent on cytochrome P2E1 and is normally scavenged by intracellular glutathione. Following an overdose, this mechanism may be overwhelmed and the highly reactive metabolite combines with sulphydryl groups of liver cell proteins, producing a centrilobular necrosis. Increased intracellular concentrations of calcium appear to play an important role in causing cellular injury. Paracetamol-induced liver damage is likely to be more severe in patients exposed to hepatic-enzyme-inducing agents such as barbiturates, carbamazepine, isoniazid, phenytoin, rifampicin, ethanol and St. John's wort. In patients who are malnourished (e.g. in anorexia, chronic alcoholism or those who are human-immunodeficiency-virus(HIV)-positive), however, increased susceptibility to paracetamol poisoning is probably related to decreased plasma and liver concentrations of glutathione.

28.5.2.2.3 Investigations

Plasma levels of paracetamol must be determined in any patient suspected of being poisoned with this agent. When related to the time since ingestion, they correlate closely with the subsequent risk of liver damage, provided this time interval is not less than 4 hours. Therefore, in the absence of treatment, a level of more than 200 mg/l (1.32 mmol/l) at four hours or more than 50 mg/l (0.33 mmol/l) at 12 hours is usually hepatotoxic (Fig. 28.1), while a level less than 100 mg/l (0.66 mmol/l) at four hours should be regarded as carrying a low risk of liver damage. It is worth noting that large overdoses of paracetamol can triple its plasma half-life from

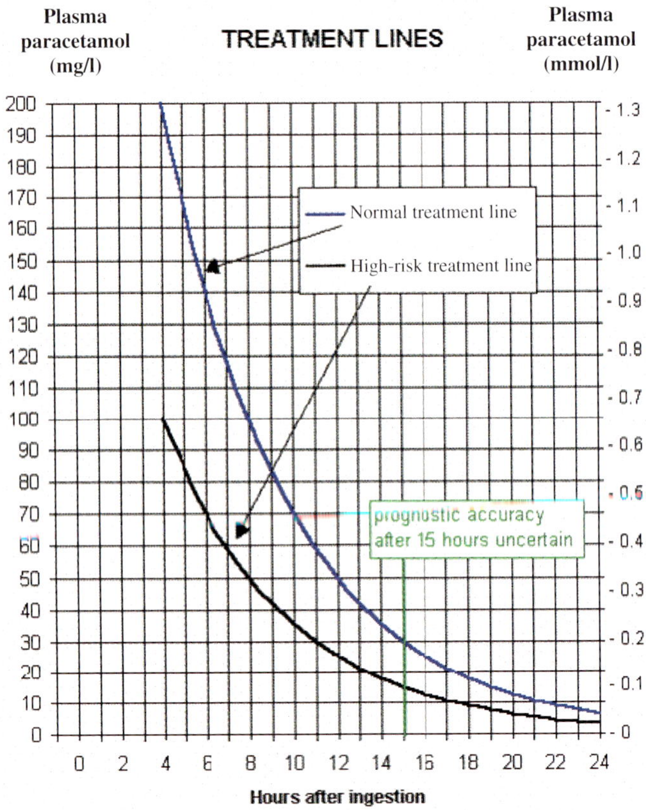

Figure 28.1. Plasma paracetamol concentrations related to time since ingestion. Liver damage is likely to be severe above the upper line, severe to mild between the lines and clinically insignificant below the lower line (which joins points that are 50% of the plasma paracetamol concentrations of the normal treatment line).

2.4 to 7.3 hours. Plasma paracetamol concentrations measured earlier than four hours from ingestion may be misleading. Furthermore, the prognostic accuracy of plasma paracetamol concentrations 15 hours or more after ingestion is uncertain, although values above the relevant treatment lines should be regarded as carrying a serious risk of significant liver damage. Plasma paracetamol concentrations may also be difficult to interpret when the history is unreliable or when paracetamol has been ingested over several hours. If there is any doubt the patient should be treated with an antidote (see below).

Laboratory investigations should include:

- Urea and electrolytes.
- Coagulation studies.
- Blood sugar level.
- Liver function tests.

Blood glucose levels should be determined hourly.

28.5.2.2.4 Treatment

Gastric lavage is recommended if the patient is seen within one hour of ingestion. Intravenous glucose should be administered if required. Administration of activated charcoal should also be considered if paracetamol in excess of 150 mg/kg or 12 g (whichever is the smaller) is thought to have been ingested within the previous hour. Intravenous glucose should be administered if required. Early renal replacement therapy may also be necessary.

Preventive treatment is based on the principle that by providing an alternative supply of sulphydryl groups, unstable precursors can be displaced from either glutathione or liver cell protein. Antidotes such as acetylcysteine and methionine protect the liver if given within 10 to 12 hours of ingestion; acetylcysteine is thought to be effective up to, and possibly beyond, 48 hours.

Oral methionine (2.5 g immediately followed by three further doses at four-hourly intervals) may be used if acetylcysteine is not available in those who present within 10 to 12 hours of ingestion and are not vomiting.

Acetylcysteine, which repletes gluthathione stores, has fewer side effects and is now the treatment of choice [17]. This agent should be given in a dose of 150 mg/kg intravenously over 15 minutes, followed by 50 mg/kg in 500 ml 5% dextrose over four hours and then 100 mg/kg in 1 l of 5% dextrose over 16 hours.

Currently it is recommended that acetylcysteine is administered by intravenous infusion to all high-risk patients whose plasma paracetamol concentrations are above the lower line of treatment threshold (Fig. 28.1). Treatment is still indicated at least as late as 24 hours after ingestion [18] and there is evidence to suggest that acetylcysteine can improve outcome even when administered after the onset of paracetamol-induced FHF, possibly by improving oxygen delivery (DO_2) and VO_2 and limiting the extent of vital organ dysfunction [17]. Acetylcysteine is also a potent antioxidant, an action that partly underlies its protective effect in paracetamol overdose. Very occasionally acetylcysteine may precipitate a histamine-mediated reaction.

Referral to a centre specialising in the management of paracetamol intoxication should be considered when:

- pH is less than 7.3 more than 24 hours after ingestion.
- Prothrombin time is longer than 45 seconds at 48 hours, or longer than 50 seconds at 72 hours.
- Creatinine concentration is increasing.
- There is rapid development of grade II encephalopathy.

Liver transplantation may be considered when:

- pH is less than 7.3 (irrespective of grade of encephalopathy).
- Prothrombin time is longer than 100 seconds.
- Serum creatinine is higher than 300 µmol/l.
- There is grade III or IV encephalopathy (see Chapter 22).

28.5.2.3 *Opiates*

Opiate poisoning is usually encountered in drug abusers who have taken an overdose, either intentionally or accidentally. Overdose may also occur with inexperienced users, when there has been a change in the purity of the supplied drug or when loss of tolerance has occurred during a period of abstinence. Drug 'couriers' who swallow opiates in containers (e.g. a condom or plastic bag) may develop severe toxicity if the package leaks ('body packers' — see earlier in this chapter). An abdominal radiograph often reveals the package, which may require surgical removal.

28.5.2.3.1 Clinical features

The triad of coma, respiratory depression (infrequent deep respirations) and pinpoint pupils (which are equal and reactive) is virtually diagnostic of opiate poisoning. Cardiovascular depression also occurs.

Physical examination may reveal evidence of addiction, such as venepuncture scars, or the complications of intravenous drug abuse, such as hepatitis and sepsis. Acute heroin intoxication can be complicated by non-cardiogenic pulmonary oedema, which may be related to hypoxia, hypersensitivity to the heroin or a contaminant, or to a direct toxic effect. Profound sedation may be associated with muscular compression which, especially when aggravated by hypoxia, acidosis and hypovolaemia, can precipitate rhabdomyolysis.

Death is usually due to respiratory depression, often combined with pulmonary aspiration.

28.5.2.3.2 Treatment

Coma and respiratory depression can be reversed by naloxone (0.4–1.2 mg intravenously or intra-muscularly (in children 5–10 μg/kg)). Because the half-life of naloxone is short (opiate reversal persists for only 15 to 30 minutes), repeated doses or an infusion may be required. Naloxone can precipitate an acute withdrawal syndrome in addicts and may cause laryngeal spasm. In addition, a number of adverse reactions to naloxone have been described, including ventricular fibrillation, hypertension and pulmonary oedema. These are presumably related to sympathetic nervous system responses to opiate withdrawal. Caution is therefore required in those with known cardiovascular disease and in some cases it may be safer to intubate the trachea and institute mechanical ventilation until the opiate effects have resolved spontaneously. Non-cardiogenic pulmonary oedema usually responds rapidly to mechanical ventilation with a positive end-expiratory pressure.

It is important to recognise that some opioids, such as methadone, have a very long duration of action. Methadone also has cardiotoxic effects, which may require treatment with sodium bicarbonate or magnesium sulphate or both: arrhythmias may occur for up to 12 hours.

28.5.3 *Antidepressants*

28.5.3.1 *Tricyclic and related antidepressants*

Tricyclic and related antidepressants are extensively prescribed for an 'at-risk' population of depressed patients. Furthermore, improvement in mood is often delayed for up to two weeks after the start of treatment. Consequently, acute poisoning with tricyclic antidepressants is common.

28.5.3.1.1 Clinical features

The features of tricyclic antidepressant overdose are due to a mixture of central excitation and depression combined with anticholinergic effects. Although the conscious level may be decreased, coma is not common unless the overdose is large. Both pyramidal and extrapyramidal disturbances may occur and convulsions are common. Some patients hallucinate, and rapid distorted speech is characteristic. Respiration is frequently depressed. Anticholinergic effects are manifested as:

- Dilated pupils.
- Dry mouth.
- Tachycardia.
- Absent sweating.
- Urine retention.
- Paralytic ileus.

The combination of central depression and an inability to sweat impairs temperature regulation and may lead to hyperthermia. Examination may reveal hyperreflexia and extensor plantar responses. The diagnosis can be confirmed by detecting the drug in the urine.

The cardiovascular effects of tricyclic antidepressants are complex. Sinus tachycardia is common, and both hypertension and hypotension may occur. Terminally, hypotension may become refractory, culminating in pulseless electrical activity (PEA). The ECG changes include a dose-related prolongation of the QT interval, widening of the QRS complex, atrioventricular block, and intraventricular conduction disturbances; right bundle branch block is characteristic. When the QRS complex is longer than 0.1 seconds, convulsions are likely; when prolonged to more than 0.16 s there is a considerable risk of ventricular arrhythmias [19]. Although in one case death occurred five days after the overdose [20], a review of 72 consecutive cases of tricyclic antidepressant overdose suggested that late unexpected complications are very rare and in practice a two-day period of intensive observation is probably sufficient [21].

28.5.3.1.2 Treatment

Because stomach emptying may be delayed following an overdose of tricyclic antidepressants, gastric aspiration/lavage and administration of activated charcoal may be worthwhile in an attempt to prevent absorption even many hours after ingestion. Measures to hasten elimination of tricyclic antidepressants are however ineffective because these drugs are highly lipid-soluble, they are also strongly protein-bound and only small amounts are excreted in the urine. Management is therefore supportive.

The ECG should be monitored continuously following a serious overdose. It has been recommended that all patients with respiratory depression, twitching or cardiac arrhythmias should be intubated and mechanically ventilated [14]. In this way hypercarbia and hypoxia, which may precipitate cardiac arrhythmias, and acidosis (respiratory or metabolic), which enhances cardiotoxicity, can be avoided. Also tracheal intubation secures the airway, thereby allowing the safe use of anticonvulsants. Provided the patient is well oxygenated and the pH is maintained above 7.4 cardiac arrhythmias usually resolve. If hyperventilation alone fails to raise the pH above this level it has been suggested that small (50 mmol) doses of bicarbonate should be given.

If ventricular arrhythmias do occur, they may be resistant to conventional treatment, although some claim that they have experienced no difficulty in defibrillating such patients and that the subsequent infusion of amiodarone or lidocaine successfully prevents recurrence. Prophylactic antiarrhythmics have also been recommended for those with ventricular ectopics. Phenytoin may be useful since it can control both the ventricular arrhythmias and any accompanying convulsions, although it is a negative inotrope and as such could precipitate PEA.

Although it might seem logical to administer an anticholinesterase, such as physostigmine, this is unwise in the acute phase since such treatment may precipitate seizures, bradycardia and cardiac failure. Similarly, administration of a β-blocker may cause extreme bradycardia and even asystole. Although a DC shock should be used when clearly indicated, there is a risk of precipitating asystole or PEA.

A few patients may be hypotensive in the absence of arrhythmias, but expansion of the circulating volume will usually restore the blood pressure. Inotropes should, in general, be avoided because of the danger of precipitating arrhythmias. If inotropic support is required, dobutamine is a suitable agent. Pulmonary artery catheterisation should be avoided because of the risk of precipitating arrhythmias.

Cardiac toxicity generally resolves quite rapidly, within about six hours, and mechanical ventilation for convulsions is rarely required for more than 24 hours.

Extrapyramidal symptoms can be controlled with benztropine (1–2 mg intramuscularly or intravenously), while the agitation and convulsions that may occur during the recovery phase are best treated with diazepam or lorazepam, either orally or by intravenous administration.

28.5.3.2 *Selective serotonin reuptake inhibitors (SSRIs)*

These antidepressants act by inhibiting serotonin reuptake but lack the antimuscarinic actions of tricyclics.

28.5.3.2.1 Clinical features

Even large overdoses of SSRIs appear to be relatively safe, unless combined with alcohol. In most patients there are no signs of toxicity. Drowsiness, nausea, diarrhoea, sinus tachycardia and influenza-like symptoms have been reported. Seizures, hypertension and functional bradycardia are rare. A 'serotonin syndrome' (confusion, sweating, diarrhoea and cardiovascular instability — see Chapter 18) usually only occurs as a result of an interaction with another drug, rather than from an overdose of the SSRI alone.

28.5.3.2.2 Treatment

Management is supportive.

28.5.3.3 *Monoamine oxidase inhibitors*

An isolated overdose of these agents may produce a severe serotonin syndrome, and severe toxicity may occur when they are taken in combination with foods containing precursors of biogenic amines or with drugs such as amphetamines and sympathomimetic amines.

28.5.3.3.1 Clinical features

Signs and symptoms of toxicity include:

- Tachycardia.
- Fluctuating blood pressure.
- Warm peripheries.
- Sweating.
- Pyrexia.
- Dilated pupils.

Muscle twitching may progress to diffuse muscle spasm, trismus and opisthotonos. As with amphetamine analogues, severe cases may be complicated by rhabdomyolysis, disseminated intravascular coagulopathy and renal failure.

The interaction between a monoamine oxidase inhibitor and another drug or food (the 'cheese' reaction) consists of a hypertensive crisis with headache, vomiting, abdominal pain and possibly heart failure.

28.5.3.3.2 Treatment

Management is supportive combined with cooling, sedation and administration of muscle relaxants when core temperature is 39 °C or more. A hypertensive crisis can be managed with phentolamine.

28.5.3.4 *Lithium intoxication*

Toxicity may be precipitated by an overdose, dehydration, concomitant administration of NSAIDs or diuretics and, because lithium is cleared via the kidney, renal failure.

28.5.3.4.1 Clinical features

Features of intoxication include:

- Confusion.
- Agitation.
- Hypertonia.
- Hyperreflexia.
- Ataxia and tremor.
- Convulsions.
- Vomiting.

Patients may also develop hyponatraemia, diabetes insipidus and renal failure.

28.5.3.4.2 Investigations

In acute lithium poisoning the plasma level is usually higher than 2 mmol/l (therapeutic range 0.4–1.0 mmol/l).

28.5.3.4.3 Treatment

Management should include gastric lavage up to one hour after ingestion and measures to increase urine output. Haemodialysis is indicated in those with neurological symptoms, renal failure or both. Whole-bowel irrigation should be considered for significant ingestion of a delayed-release formulation but advice should be sought from a poisons centre.

28.5.4 *Cardiovascular drugs*

28.5.4.1 β-*blocking drugs*

β-blockers are extensively prescribed and readily available; poisoning with β-blockers is therefore relatively common.

28.5.4.1.1 Clinical features

Manifestations of profound β-blockade include lassitude, drowsiness, bradycardia and hypotension. Peripheral vasospasm and Raynaud's phenomenon may occur. Bronchospasm may be precipitated, particularly in those with asthma or chronic obstructive pulmonary disease.

28.5.4.1.2 Treatment

Gastric aspiration and lavage should be performed if the patient is seen within one hour of ingestion. Intravenous atropine (1–3 mg) and an isoprenaline infusion can be given in an attempt to counteract the hypotension and bradycardia. Cardiogenic shock unresponsive to atropine is probably best treated with an intravenous injection of glucagon (2–10 mg) (unlicensed indication and dose) followed by an intravenous infusion of 50 mg/kg/h in 5% glucose (with precautions to protect the airway in case of vomiting). The mechanism of action of glucagon is thought not to involve the β-adrenoreceptor. Some recommend dopamine or dobutamine as alternatives to isoprenaline. Ideally, cardiac pacing should be instituted in those with extreme bradycardia. Severe bronchospasm should be treated with salbutamol.

28.5.4.2 *Calcium channel blockers*

28.5.4.2.1 Clinical features

Calcium channel blocking drugs (CCBs) can cause fatal cardiovascular toxicity in overdose. They slow sinoatrial and atrioventricular nodal conduction, decrease myocardial contractility and cause vasodilatation. CCBs also decrease insulin secretion and cause peripheral insulin resistance, leading to lactic acidosis and hyperglycaemia and depriving the myocardium of carbohydrate substrate.

28.5.4.2.2 Treatment

Treatment of CCB poisoning is challenging as patients can deteriorate suddenly, with prolonged hypotension and bradyarrhythmias resistant to conventional treatments; inotropic and antiarrhythmic agents are largely ineffective. These drugs are well absorbed enterally, are highly protein-bound and have large volumes of distribution, so that extracorporeal removal is not effective. Aggressive supportive care has been the mainstay of treatment. The most effective specific treatment to date appears to be the use of high doses of insulin. Hyperinsulinaemic euglycaemia therapy involves the infusion of high doses of insulin (range 0.1–2.0 IU/kg/h) together with appropriate amounts of dextrose to maintain normal blood glucose levels. Because insulin drives potassium into cells, potassium supplements may also be necessary [22].

28.5.4.3 *Digoxin*

Digoxin has a narrow therapeutic index and is therefore particularly liable to produce life-threatening complications after accidental or deliberate overdose. Serious overdoses are frequently fatal, mortality being around 18% following ingestion of 15 mg digoxin and approximately 95% when more than 35 mg are taken. In general plasma levels do not correlate closely with the severity of poisoning but the likelihood of toxicity increases progressively through the range 1.5 to 3 μg/l.

28.5.4.3.1 Clinical features

Nausea and vomiting are constant features, while diarrhoea is less common. There may be anorexia and abdominal pain.

Digoxin overdose is associated with hyperkalaemia due to inhibition of Na^+/K^+ ATPase, the extent of the rise in plasma potassium being correlated with the clinical course. Any patient with a plasma potassium of over 5.3 mmol/l should be considered at high risk.

Cardiac toxicity may be associated with:

- Bradycardia.
- Varying degrees of atrioventricular block.
- Supraventricular arrhythmias (with or without heart block).
- Less commonly, ventricular arrhythmias including ventricular tachycardia/ventricular fibrillation.

Other features of toxicity may include extreme fatigue, weakness and visual disturbances, often with abnormal red–green colour perception. Some patients complain of headaches, dizziness and abnormal dreams.

28.5.4.3.2 Management

Gastric lavage, when indicated, should only be performed with extreme care because of the risk that increased vagal tone will precipitate cardiac arrest. Tissue stores of cardiac glycosides are large; measures to enhance their elimination, such as enhanced diuresis, haemodialysis or haemoperfusion are therefore generally ineffective and the risks outweigh the benefits.

Bradycardia should be treated with atropine or transvenous pacing. Infusion of catecholamines should be avoided.

Hypokalaemia, which is most likely in those receiving chronic diuretic therapy, should be corrected.

Hyperkalaemia may be treated with intravenous dextrose and insulin (see Chapter 12), but inhibition of Na^+/K^+ ATPase may limit its efficacy.

Lidocaine can be administered for the treatment of ventricular arrhythmias. In cases of paroxysmal supraventricular tachycardia with block intravenous administration of a β-blocker may be useful following specialist advice.

Severe digitalis intoxication should be treated with digoxin-specific antibody fragments [23]. These have a greater affinity for digoxin than digoxin does for its receptors, they do not fix complement and they are not susceptible to immune degradation. The antibody fragments easily pass into the interstitial spaces where they bind to molecules of digitalis glycoside, leading to an improvement in signs and symptoms within about 30 minutes. At this time plasma digoxin levels rise, although, because the drug is now bound, it is pharmacologically inactive. Plasma potassium levels fall. The digoxin–antibody complex is then eliminated via the kidneys. The plasma half-life after intravenous administration of digoxin-specific antibody fragments is 16 to 34 hours in those with normal renal function. There is little experience of using digoxin-specific antibody fragments in renal failure and there is at least a theoretical danger that retained complex might be metabolised to release free digoxin, with recurrence of toxicity.

Suggested indications for digoxin-specific antibody treatment are:

- Life-threatening cardiac arrhythmias.
- Plasma digoxin concentration higher than 20 μg/l.
- Rising or uncontrollable potassium levels.

28.5.5 *Hypnotics and sedatives*

28.5.5.1 *Benzodiazepines*

28.5.5.1.1 Mechanisms

Many of the effects of benzodiazepines are mediated by occupation of specific receptor sites, thereby enhancing the effects of gamma-aminobutyric acid (GABA), an inhibitory neurotransmitter.

28.5.5.1.2 Clinical features

When taken alone, benzodiazepines can produce drowsiness, dizziness, ataxia and slurred speech. More serious manifestations of overdose, such as coma or hypotension, are infrequently seen, and death due to isolated benzodiazepine poisoning, which is usually related to respiratory depression and pulmonary aspiration, is unusual. Many cases of self-poisoning, however, involve ingestion of a number of drugs, and benzodiazepines are often one of these. Under these circumstances the clinical picture is often confusing and additive effects may aggravate or precipitate respiratory failure and hypotension.

Benzodiazepines are absorbed relatively slowly from the gastrointestinal tract and elimination of their active metabolites, as well as the parent compound, may take several days. In general, less than 5% of the ingested dose is recovered unchanged in the urine. However, acute tolerance occurs after an overdose and clinical recovery within hours is the rule. Nevertheless the performance of skilled tasks (e.g. driving a car or operating machinery) can be impaired for weeks after apparent recovery from benzodiazepine poisoning.

28.5.5.1.3 Treatment

In general, management of benzodiazepine poisoning involves supportive care only. Although the benzodiazepine antagonist flumazenil can reverse coma in such cases [24], its value in clinical practice is uncertain. It has been suggested that following isolated benzodiazepine overdose, flumazenil might speed recovery, reduce after-effects and shorten hospital stay, while in multiple self-poisoning it could reverse respiratory depression and facilitate diagnosis. Flumazenil can be given in aliquots of 100 μg to a dose of 1.0 mg and has a rapid onset of action in less than a minute, with a maximal effect at five minutes. Because it has a relatively short half-life (54 minutes), repeated administration or a continuous infusion at 100–400 μg/h may be required. Moreover, there is a danger of precipitating acute withdrawal symptoms. Convulsions may be produced, especially in epileptics and in the presence of proconvulsant agents such as tricyclic antidepressants, and rapid reversal may also precipitate ventricular fibrillation. Many therefore now believe that flumazenil has little or no place in the management of benzodiazepine overdose. Others, however, have suggested that flumazenil is a safe aid to diagnosis in cases of multiple drug overdose and that this agent reduces the requirement for interventions such as gastric lavage, tracheal intubation, mechanical ventilation and CT scan of the brain [25]. Flumazenil should, therefore, be used on expert advice only.

28.5.5.2 *Phenothiazines and related drugs*

Although these major tranquillisers are often prescribed for the 'at-risk' population of patients with psychotic illnesses, they are a relatively uncommon cause of self-poisoning.

28.5.5.2.1 Clinical features

Following an overdose, the patient may becomes drowsy or comatose with respiratory depression and hypotensive with a tachycardia. Arrhythmias may occur (particularly with thioridazine) and the ECG may show prolongation of the QT interval and flattening of the T waves. Sudden death is a possibility, probably as a result of *torsades de pointes.* Impaired hypothalamic function combined with cardiovascular depression makes the patient susceptible to hypothermia. Extrapyramidal disturbances such as oculogyric crises, dystonia (particularly with prochlorperazine and trifluoperazine) and convulsions may also occur. Some may develop neuroleptic malignant syndrome.

28.5.5.2.2 Treatment

Methods to speed elimination are ineffective, and treatment is therefore supportive. Plasma potassium should be maintained within the normal range and the pH should be kept above 7.4. Extrapyramidal disturbances can be treated with repeated intravenous administration of benzatropine mesilate (1–2 mg) or diazepam (emulsion preferred). Acute dystonia is generally relieved by procyclidine (5–10 mg intravenously). Arrhythmias may respond to correction of hypoxia, acidosis and other biochemical abnormalities, otherwise specialist advice should be sought. If hypotension requires specific treatment an α-adrenoreceptor stimulant should be used.

28.5.5.3 *Barbiturates*

These drugs are now rarely prescribed as anticonvulsants. Consequently, barbiturate overdose is uncommon.

28.5.5.3.1 Clinical features

Barbiturate overdose produces generalised depression of the CNS. The consciousness level is reduced and this may progress to deep coma with flaccidity and hyporeflexia. The corneal reflex is often absent. The pupillary response to light is sluggish or absent and conjugate eye movement is lost. Unequal pupils suggest hypoxic cerebral damage, a diagnosis that is supported by the presence of other focal neurological signs, sometimes accompanied by seizures.

Profound cardiovascular depression may occur and is caused by a reduction in central vasomotor activity, a decrease in arteriolar tone and myocardial depression. Cardiac output and blood pressure are low, while central venous pressure (CVP) may be high (in those with myocardial failure) or low (in the presence of relative hypovolaemia). There may be a metabolic acidosis.

Respiratory depression causes hypoventilation with hypercarbia and hypoxaemia. The latter may be exacerbated by increased capillary permeability leading to the development of acute respiratory distress syndrome (see Chapters 7 and 20) and/or ventilation–perfusion mismatch [26].

The reduction in muscle tone combined with cardiovascular depression causes vascular stasis and tissue hypoxia. Ischaemic muscle damage may lead to rhabdomyolysis, which may in the long term be followed by muscle calcification. Local hypoxia may also be responsible for the development of skin blisters, which are seen in approximately 5% of patients with barbiturate poisoning. Although these blisters often develop over pressure areas, they are not necessarily related to trauma and may occasionally complicate even a relatively trivial overdose.

Gastrointestinal motility is often depressed. It is thought that the fluctuations in consciousness level that sometimes occur in barbiturate poisoning are due to the intermittent recovery of intestinal function leading to further absorption of the drug.

Hypothermia is a common complication of barbiturate overdose and is a result of impaired hypothalamic function, a reduction in muscle tone and vasodilatation.

28.5.5.3.2 Treatment

The vast majority of those who reach hospital alive will survive with aggressive supportive care, provided they have not suffered irreversible cerebral damage. CVP, and in some cases cardiac output monitoring, is required in seriously poisoned patients to guide intravenous volume replacement. Hypothermia must be prevented or treated.

Repeated doses of activated charcoal may be used for barbiturate poisoning, combined, in severe cases, with haemodialysis. Charcoal haemoperfusion has been recommended for those who are deeply unconscious and failing to improve following a massive overdose of a long-acting barbiturate.

28.5.6 *Iron salts*

Iron tablets are most frequently prescribed to young women and they, or their children, therefore account for the majority of cases of poisoning.

28.5.6.1 *Clinical features*

Within the first six hours, symptoms are mainly due to gastrointestinal irritation with abdominal pain, nausea, vomiting, haematemesis, melaena and even gastric perforation. Some complain of a metallic taste. Those who are seriously poisoned become hypovolaemic and shocked. There is usually an asymptomatic interval from 8 to 24 hours after ingestion. Convulsions, coma, hepatic necrosis, hypoglycaemia and metabolic acidosis may supervene later due to the toxic effects of iron on the liver and other organs.

28.5.6.2 *Treatment*

Iron is slowly absorbed. Gastric aspiration and lavage should be performed within 1 hour of ingesting a significant quantity of iron or if radiography reveals tablets in the stomach. Whole-bowel irrigation may be considered in severe poisoning.

The severity of poisoning can be assessed by measuring the serum iron level, and if this is more than twice the upper limit of normal, 1–2 g of desferrioxamine, which chelates iron, should be administered intramuscularly and repeated 3 to 12 hours later. In severe toxicity or if the patient is shocked, this agent should be given intravenously (15 mg/kg/h up to a total dose of 80 mg/kg in 24 hours — in severe cases higher doses may be used on advice from a poisons centre).

28.5.7 *Stimulants and drugs of misuse*

28.5.7.1 *Amphetamines*

Amphetamines are now rarely prescribed, and episodes of poisoning are therefore usually related to illicit use. Amphetamines can be injected, inhaled or taken orally.

28.5.7.1.1 Clinical features

In overdose, amphetamines produce:

- Confusion and hallucinations.
- Anxiety.
- Restlessness and wakefulness.
- Tremor.
- Irritability.

The patient may be hyperreflexic with dilated pupils. An initial pallor is followed by flushing, tachycardia and arrhythmias. Hypertension may be associated with convulsions, hyperthermia and coma.

28.5.7.1.2 Treatment

Treatment is supportive and includes sedation with a benzodiazepine or, if this fails, a phenothiazine. Advice should be sought from a poisons information centre on the management of hypertension, convulsions and hyperpyrexia. Elimination of amphetamines can be enhanced by inducing an acid diuresis, although this is rarely necessary.

28.5.7.2 *MDA and MDMA (ecstasy)*

Methylenedioxyamphetamine (MDA) and methylenedioxymethamphetamine (MDMA) — known as ecstasy — are synthetic amphetamine derivatives with a mild amphetamine-like stimulant effect. They also induce a feeling of euphoria and increased sociability, as well as enhanced perception. Their hallucinogenic potential is low [27] although many substances are added to ecstasy including caffeine and ketamine [28]. Side effects include:

- Loss of appetite, nausea.
- Trismus and teeth grinding.
- Muscle aches and stiffness.
- Ataxia.
- Sweating, dehydration.
- Tachycardia, hypertension.
- Hyponatraemia and catatonic stupor [29].

The pharmacological effects of the drug can be compounded by relentless drug-stimulated physical exertion in a hot environment such as a nightclub. Afterwards there may be fatigue and insomnia. Under these circumstances acute severe complications may occur unpredictably and can include:

- Hyperpyrexia.
- Delirium, collapse, hyperreflexia, convulsions.
- Rhabdomyolysis.
- Disseminated intravascular coagulation (DIC).
- Acute renal failure.
- Acute hepatitis.
- Ventricular arrhythmias, hypotension.
- Acute respiratory distress syndrome.
- Cerebral haemorrhage or infarction due to uncontrolled hypertension or vasculitis.
- Self-induced water intoxication.

The hyperthermic syndrome resembles malignant hyperpyrexia and heat stroke. Serotonin syndrome may occur.

28.5.7.2.1 Management

Management is urgent and should include:

- Control of agitation and convulsions with diazepam (emulsion preferred).
- Rapid rehydration.
- Measurement of core temperature and active cooling measures if rectal temperature exceeds 40°C.
- Paralysis and ventilation if muscle spasm is continuing to generate heat.
- Cardiovascular and respiratory support.
- Management of rhabdomyolysis, DIC and renal failure as described elsewhere.

The extent to which dantrolene is of value [30] is in doubt [31] and dose-dependent adverse effects such as hepatitis are a cause for concern. Hepatotoxicity has also occurred with ecstasy poisoning and has been successfully treated with liver transplantation [32]. Advice should be sought from a poisons centre.

28.5.7.3 *Cocaine*

The recreational use of cocaine has increased dramatically. It can be taken intravenously, by intranasal insufflation or smoked. 'Crack' (so-called because it crackles when burnt) is a more potent alkaloid of cocaine that is suitable for smoking and is very rapidly absorbed. Abuse of 'crack' has now reached epidemic proportions.

28.5.7.3.1 Mechanisms

Unlike other local anaesthetics, cocaine also impairs the presynaptic uptake of catecholamines and upregulates postsynaptic receptors. It also has other poorly understood actions within the central nervous system. When mixed with alcohol, cocaine may be metabolised in the liver to a longer lasting, more lethal metabolite, cocaethylene [33]. Street cocaine is frequently contaminated with adulterants such as amphetamines, LSD, quinine and heroin.

28.5.7.3.2 Clinical features

The clinical features of cocaine intoxication are related to peripheral and central nervous system stimulation and include:

- Euphoria (the effect desired by the user).
- Dysphoria.
- Chest pain.
- Agitation, hyperactivity, confusion, headaches, aggression.
- Delirium.
- Paranoia.
- Hallucinations.
- Hyper-reflexia, tremors, fasciculation, seizures.
- Hyperthermia.
- Dilated pupils.

Increased peripheral sympathetic activity may cause tachycardia, cardiac arrhythmias and hypertension associated with marked vasoconstriction [34]. Complications include myocardial infarction, dilated cardiomyopathy, cerebrovascular accidents and rhabdomyolysis with or without renal failure [35].

When taken intravenously, impurities are filtered by the lungs, but all forms of cocaine abuse can be associated with non-cardiogenic pulmonary oedema. Bronchiolitis obliterans has also been reported. 'Crack lung' is characterised by bronchospasm, fever and transient pulmonary infiltrates. Because it is associated with elevated serum immunoglobulin E levels and eosinophilia it has been attributed to a hypersensitivity reaction. Those who smoke cocaine may perform a deep, prolonged and forceful Valsalva manoeuvre, which can also be complicated by subcutaneous emphysema, pneumomediastinum and pneumothorax. Cocaine can also cause pulmonary haemorrhage.

Cocaine use in pregnancy has been associated with serious maternal and foetal complications, including abruptio placentae, spontaneous abortion and preterm labour. It may also cause placental ischaemia, as well as myocardial or cerebral infarction in the foetus.

28.5.7.3.3 Diagnosis and investigations

The clinical features of cocaine toxicity are similar to those of neuroleptic malignant syndrome, acute withdrawal from alcohol, sedatives or hypnotics, and an overdose of anticholinergics, hallucinogens or amphetamine.

Investigations should include:

- ECG.
- Blood glucose.
- Creatine phosphokinase and troponin levels, urinary myoglobin.
- Blood and urine cultures.
- In selected cases, cerebral CT scan and occasionally lumbar puncture.
- Core temperature (should be measured frequently).

The metabolites of cocaine can be detected in the urine.

28.5.7.3.4 Management

The circulating volume should be expanded and adequate oxygenation ensured. Tracheal intubation and mechanical ventilation may be indicated in those with:

- Extreme agitation.
- Deep coma.
- Seizures.
- Hyperthermia.

Agitation should be controlled with an intravenous benzodiazepine. This will limit the severity of the cardiovascular disturbance as well as helping to prevent hyperthermia and acidosis. A benzodiazepine, such as lorazepam, is also indicated in those with seizures. More resistant cases will require a benzodiazepine infusion, usually combined with tracheal intubation and mechanical ventilation. In general, phenytoin is not a particularly effective anticonvulsant in those with cocaine toxicity and barbiturates are preferred. Dantrolene may have a place in the management of severe hyperthermia (core temperature >40°C). Neuroleptic agents should be avoided.

Supraventricular tachyarrhythmias may not require specific treatment. Importantly, lidocaine can aggravate cocaine toxicity. Severe hypertension can be treated with an infusion of sodium nitroprusside or, possibly, labetalol. Pure β-blockers should be avoided because there is a danger that the unopposed α-activity will precipitate extreme vasoconstriction, hypertension and a fall in cardiac output.

Myocardial ischaemia should be treated with nitrates and morphine. Surprisingly, calcium channel blockers have not proved useful and thrombolytic therapy can be dangerous.

Non-cardiogenic pulmonary oedema should be managed as outlined elsewhere, while steroids may be indicated in patients with bronchiolitis obliterans and 'crack lung'.

28.5.7.4 *Gamma hydroxybutyric acid (GHB)*

Also known as liquid ecstasy or liquid X, this is a substance of misuse which is increasing in popularity, especially amongst participants in the dance rave scene and individuals using it for its 'date rape' potential. GHB is a four-carbon metabolite, similar in structure to GABA. It is found naturally in the human body, in areas like the basal ganglia, cortex, midbrain, substantia nigra and the hippocampus. GHB increases dopamine levels in the brain. It is sold by dealers 'on the street' and can be purchased readily via internet sites. GHB is available either as a powder form that is easily soluble, or a liquid that is clear, odourless and tasteless.

28.5.7.4.1 Mechanism of toxicity

GHB has a depressant effect on the brain, most probably mediated via its action at GABA receptors. Feelings of inhibitions are depressed, leading to a sensation of euphoria, 'warmth' and ease of conversation. The drug is most commonly ingested orally with a rapid onset time of 15 to 30 minutes and an elimination half-life of 20 to 30 minutes. When the desired effects have worn off, a further dose of the drug can be taken by the individual.

Consequently, several doses may be ingested by the individual during the course of an evening. GHB readily crosses the blood–brain barrier and placental membrane.

28.5.7.4.2 Clinical features

Mild to moderate effects include nausea, vomiting, diarrhoea, dizziness, euphoria, anterograde amnesia, confusion, agitation, urinary incontinence, tremor, myoclonus and hypotonia. In severe toxicity there may be coma, convulsions, bradycardia, hypotension (or rarely hypertension after intravenous use) and respiratory depression leading to respiratory arrest. These effects are potentiated by co-ingestion of other sedative agents like alcohol and benzodiazepines. For chronic abusers of GHB, withdrawal symptoms include insomnia, anxiety, tremors, nausea and vomiting. This presentation is similar to the alcohol withdrawal syndrome.

28.5.7.4.3 Investigations

As GHB is readily metabolised into CO_2 and H_2O and excreted as such, it is extremely difficult to trace its prior use. There is no laboratory test available to measure toxicity levels.

28.5.7.4.4 Treatment

The adequacy of the airway, breathing and circulation should be assessed and appropriate management instituted immediately. Activated charcoal should be considered in patients who present within one hour of ingestion. Observation of the patient for at least two hours post-overdose is indicated; patients asymptomatic after this period are unlikely to develop further symptoms. Recurrent or prolonged convulsions should be treated as described earlier in the chapter. Respiratory depression can be treated with either intravenous naloxone or managed by a period of mechanical ventilation. Patients who exhibit severe agitation as part of their symptomatology may also require mechanical ventilation to facilitate ongoing supportive care.

28.5.8 *Other poisons*

28.5.8.1 *Carbon monoxide (CO)*

The commonest sources of CO poisoning are motor vehicle exhaust fumes, incorrectly maintained and ventilated heating systems and smoke from fires. Approximately 300 people die from CO poisoning in England and Wales every year and CO is a common cause of death from poisoning in children. Carbon monoxide is a complex poison and the diagnosis is often difficult [36].

28.5.8.1.1 Mechanisms

The affinity of CO for haemoglobin is some 200 to 250 times greater than that of oxygen, which it therefore displaces. It also shifts the oxyhaemoglobin dissociation curve to the left and may inhibit cellular respiration as a result of binding to other haem-containing proteins. Although CO only combines with cytochromes under hypoxic conditions, once binding occurs it is difficult to reverse with conventional oxygen therapy. These tissue effects may be the major cause of clinical toxicity and this may explain the discrepancy between clinical consequences and carboxyhaemoglobin (COHb) levels. The net effect is cellular hypoxia, which may be fatal.

28.5.8.1.2 Clinical features

The clinical course of CO toxicity is directly related to the degree and duration of exposure [37].The diagnosis can be confirmed by estimating the percentage of COHb present in the blood, but this should be taken as only an approximate indication of severity, as clinical findings are a better guide. In general COHb levels less than 10% produce no symptoms, whereas levels above 50–60% are associated with coma and a risk of cardiovascular collapse and cardiac arrest. Arterial oxygen tension is usually normal.

Manifestations of acute poisoning include headaches, dizziness, hyperventilation, confusion, disorientation and, in severe cases, coma. Nausea, vomiting and faecal incontinence may also occur, as may hyperreflexia, convulsions and cardiac arrhythmias. Later, pulmonary oedema and respiratory depression may supervene, while extreme hypoxia may produce cerebral oedema and hyperpyrexia. Myocardial injury is common and is a predictor of long term mortality [38]. Some patients develop rhabdomyolysis and renal failure. The pink discoloration of the skin caused by the presence of large amounts of COHb is generally only seen in post-mortem cases. Cyanosis and skin pallor is more usual. Skin blisters may occur as a result of tissue hypoxia. Delayed sequelae may include neuropsychiatric disturbances such as memory loss, impaired intellect and cerebellar damage, which may appear several weeks after exposure. Repeated exposure may lead to headaches, poor concentration, dizziness, visual disturbances, paraesthesiae, chest pain, abdominal pain and diarrhoea. Repeated chronic exposure or a severe single exposure may be followed by fatigue, poor memory, impaired concentration and a change in personality.

28.5.8.1.3 Treatment

Administration of oxygen in high concentrations and mechanical ventilation, if indicated, should be instituted immediately. Cerebral oedema should be anticipated in severe poisoning and is treated with an intravenous infusion of mannitol.

28.5.8.1.4 Hyperbaric oxygen

The elimination half-life of CO is reduced from 250 minutes when breathing air to 59 minutes when 100% oxygen is administered and to 22 minutes when 100% oxygen is breathed at 2.2 atmospheric pressure. To date, however, the authors of several randomised trials have disagreed as to whether treatment with hyperbaric oxygen is effective in clinical practice [39–42]. Limitations of these trials have included too few patients, inclusion of patients exposed to other toxins in fires and differing protocols for delivering hyperbaric oxygen therapy.

Current recommendations for considering hyperbaric oxygen therapy include:

- Recovery of consciousness after an initial high COHb concentration.
- Neurological or psychiatric features other than headache.
- Evidence of myocardial ischaemia.
- Pregnancy (in view of the greater susceptibility of the foetus to carbon monoxide).

Contraindications to hyperbaric oxygen are in the main related to the practical difficulties of managing patients in single-person (monoplace) chambers and include:

- Mechanical ventilation.
- Inability to maintain an airway.
- Hypovolaemic or vasopressor-dependent patients.
- Cardiac arrhythmias potentially requiring urgent intervention.
- Asthma.

Larger (multiplace) chambers in which medical attendants can also be accommodated overcome most of these difficulties but are not widely available. The logistical difficulties of transporting patients to distant hyperbaric oxygen chambers should not be underestimated.

28.5.8.2 *Cyanide*

Cyanides are used industrially in electroplating and to clean or harden metals as well as in some chemical laboratories. Most cases of poisoning encountered in clinical practice are caused by ingestion or inhalation of sodium or potassium cyanide; free hydrocyanic acid (prussic acid) is almost instantaneously fatal if taken orally. The effects of inhaled prussic acid depend on the concentration of the vapour. The direct-acting vasodilator sodium nitroprusside is a complex cyanide that releases free hydrogen cyanide (HCN) *in vivo* and may produce related toxic effects when a large amount has been administered.

28.5.8.2.1 Mechanisms

Cyanide produces its toxic effects by reacting with cytochrome oxidase, thereby inhibiting the final steps in oxidative phosphorylation.

28.5.8.2.2 Clinical features

If large quantities (1–2 g) are ingested, there is a rapid loss of consciousness, followed by convulsions and death. Lesser amounts produce drowsiness, dizziness, breathlessness, confusion, nausea, vomiting and shock. Coma and death may follow. Severe lactic acidosis and a reduced arterial–venous O_2 content difference are characteristic. Some individuals are able to detect an odour of bitter almonds on the breath of the victim. For obvious reasons expired air resuscitation must not be given.

28.5.8.2.3 Treatment

When an unconscious patient is known to have ingested or inhaled cyanide, immediate treatment is imperative. A heparinised blood sample should be obtained for blood gas analysis and cyanide assay. General supportive measures, including the administration of oxygen in high concentrations, should be instituted and a specific antidote given. Immediately following massive exposure to cyanide (e.g. following an industrial accident) intravenous dicobalt edetate (300 mg over one minute), should be administered by intravenous injection followed immediately by an infusion of 50 ml of 50% glucose (dicobalt edetate can cause hypoglycaemia). If the response is inadequate a second dose of both may be given. If there is still no response after a further five minutes a third dose of both may be administered. Dicobalt edetate is an effective antidote because it has a rapid action and although it is itself toxic, in the presence of HCN a stable non-toxic complex is formed. If the patient is conscious or has minimal symptoms after assumed exposure to cyanide, dicobalt edetate should not be given since in the absence of HCN it is likely to produce an anaphylactoid reaction, sometimes with severe laryngeal oedema. Dicobalt edetate may also precipitate atrial fibrillation, hypocalcaemia and hypomagnesaemia. Therefore, when some time has elapsed between ingestion and arrival in hospital or when there is doubt as to the nature of the poisoning, sodium nitrite followed by sodium thiosulphate are the antidotes of choice.

Sodium nitrite acts by converting haemoglobin to methaemoglobin, the ferric iron of which then combines with HCN. Sodium nitrite (300 mg) should be given intravenously in order to convert approximately 25% of the haemoglobin to methaemoglobin. However, this clearly reduces the amount of haemoglobin available for oxygen transport and is potentially hazardous, especially in children. In addition, nitrites can precipitate or exacerbate hypotension.

Sodium thiosulphate enables natural detoxification mechanisms to convert cyanide to thiocyanate. A sodium thiosulphate injection (500 mg/ml) should be administered in a dose of 12.5 g every 10 minutes. Both sodium nitrite and sodium thiosulphate are special order (unlicensed) products used without restriction when administered to save life in an emergency. Advice should be sought from a poisons information centre, drug manufacturer or regional hospital manufacturing unit. Hydroxocobalamin is an alternative antidote for cyanide poisoning but its use should ideally be discussed with a poisons information centre. The usual dose is 70 mg/kg by intravenous infusion (repeated once or twice according to severity).

28.5.9 *Pesticides*

28.5.9.1 *Paraquat*

Paraquat [43] is a herbicide that is available commercially as a 10–20% concentrated liquid (e.g. Gramoxone) and to the general public in the form of solid granules containing 2.5% paraquat (e.g. Weedol).

28.5.9.1.1 Clinical features

Paraquat is a strong cytotoxin that will burn the skin, tongue, mouth and oesophagus. This may not be apparent until 24 to 48 hours after ingestion when large white necrotic areas develop; these are often painless. Inhalation of spray, mist or dust containing paraquat may cause nose bleeding and sore throat. Eye contamination will cause extreme irritation with ulceration of the conjunctivae and cornea. Sweating, nausea, repeated vomiting and diarrhoea are usual, and in some cases the vomitus will contain gastric and oesophageal epithelial cells. Tremor and convulsions may occur.

Ingestion of large amounts of paraquat may be associated with the development of multiple organ failure and death within 72 hours. When poisoning is less severe, evidence of myocardial, liver and renal dysfunction may be delayed for several days. Paraquat can, however, accumulate progressively in the lungs by an energy-dependent process [44] even when plasma concentrations are relatively low. Subsequently, the alveolar epithelial lining is destroyed and this is followed by progressive pulmonary fibrosis, culminating in hypoxaemic respiratory failure. Although this lung lesion may take two to three weeks to develop, it is irreversible and death is inevitable.

28.5.9.1.2 Investigations

The diagnosis of paraquat poisoning can be confirmed by a simple qualitative urine test. Moreover, there is a good correlation between early blood levels and the severity of poisoning.

28.5.9.1.3 Treatment

Treatment with activated charcoal should be started immediately, although severe vomiting may complicate its administration and an anti-emetic may be required. Intravenous fluids and analgesics are given as necessary. Unduly high inspired oxygen levels should be avoided in the early stages of management since this may accentuate the lung damage, although high concentrations may be required later to palliate symptoms. Further measures to enhance elimination of absorbed paraquat should be discussed with poisons centres and guidance obtained on predicting the likely outcome based on plasma concentrations.

28.5.9.1.4 Prognosis

An oral dose of approximately 2–3 g is likely to be fatal if untreated. Although the ingestion of granular preparations for garden use has caused few deaths, the mortality from poisoning with the concentrated solution is approximately 90%.

28.5.9.2 *Organophosphorus insecticides*

Organophosphorus insecticides are usually supplied as powders or dissolved in organic solvents.

28.5.9.2.1 Mechanisms

Most of the organophosphorus compounds are highly lipid-soluble and are therefore well absorbed via all routes, including the bronchi and intact skin. They form very stable links with acetylcholinesterase, thereby prolonging and intensifying the effects of acetylcholine. Recovery of anti-cholinergic activity is therefore delayed until sufficient quantities of enzyme have been manufactured. This may take days or even months.

28.5.9.2.2 Clinical features

Poisoning with cholinesterase inhibitors causes:

- An increase in postganglionic parasympathetic nervous activity.
- Muscle fasciculation followed by paralysis.
- Central nervous stimulation followed by depression.

There is anorexia, salivation, rhinorrhoea, vomiting, abdominal colic and diarrhoea. The patient is restless with constricted pupils; coma and convulsions may occur. Later, respiratory depression supervenes with paralysis of respiratory and ocular muscles, laryngobronchospasm and increased tracheobronchial secretions. Cardiovascular manifestations include bradycardia and hypotension. Hyperglycaemia and glycosuria without ketonuria may also be present.

28.5.9.2.3 Treatment

Immediate management must include measures to prevent further exposure to the poison, including the removal of contaminated clothing and thorough washing of contaminated skin with soap and water. Gastric lavage should be considered provided the airway is protected. Atropine should be administered in large doses (2 mg) repeated every 5 to 10 minutes until the skin becomes flushed and dry, the pupils dilate and tachycardia develops. Prolonged administration (two to three days) may be required. Pralidoxime mesilate, a cholinesterase reactivator, is used as an adjunct to atropine in moderate or severe poisoning. It improves muscle tone within 30 minutes following intravenous injection in an initial dose of 30 mg/kg (repeated every four to six hours or intravenous infusion at 8 mg/kg/h in severe case). Otherwise, treatment is supportive and may include mechanical ventilation.

28.5.10 *Nerve agents*

The course of nerve-agent poisoning is shorter than that of organophosphorus insecticide poisoning, and although treatment is similar, patients reaching hospital alive have generally already recovered. In emergencies involving the release of nerve agents, kits which contain pralidoxime may be obtained from designated centres (see TOXBASE http://www.toxbase.org/) or contact the UK National Poisons Information Service on 0870 600 6266). In very rare circumstances, when exposure to tabun is suspected, obidoxime will also be supplied. In all instances involving nerve agents the risk of cross contamination is significant and protective clothing and adequate decontamination are essential.

28.5.11 *Corrosives*

28.5.11.1 *Clinical features*

28.5.11.1.1 Acids and alkalis

Acids and alkalis are used for cleaning, both domestically and industrially, as well as being involved in chemical manufacturing processes. When swallowed, they can cause extensive burns of the mouth, tongue, pharynx, oesophagus and stomach. These are extremely painful and may lead to perforation of the oesophagus or stomach. Oedema of the epiglottis and larynx can produce severe upper airway obstruction, necessitating tracheal intubation. Systemic absorption produces profound acid–base disturbances and shock. Delayed deaths may be associated with necrosis and superimposed infection.

Long-term complications in survivors include gastrointestinal scarring and stenosis.

28.5.11.1.2 Phenolic compounds

Phenolic compounds are commonly found in antiseptics, disinfectants and preservatives. If swallowed, they cause blanching or erythema around the mouth and chin followed by intense thirst, nausea, vomiting, diarrhoea and sweating. Those who are severely poisoned may develop abdominal pain, convulsions and coma. Acute renal failure is common and hepatic damage may occur.

28.5.11.1.3 Treatment

Gastric lavage should probably be avoided because of the risk of aspiration, although some recommend this technique as a means of diluting the corrosive. Surgical intervention is required if there are signs of perforation. Otherwise, treatment is supportive and may include total parenteral nutrition. Prognosis is poor in severe cases.

28.5.12 *Mushroom poisoning*

Over 90% of those who die as a result of fungal poisoning have eaten *A. phalloides*. Earlier recognition of mushroom poisoning combined with aggressive treatment before liver failure has developed has been associated with mortality rates of 10–15% [45].

28.5.12.1 *Amanita phalloides (death cap)*

28.5.12.1.1 Mechanisms

This fungus contains two toxins. The phallotoxins (heptopeptides) produce violent nausea, vomiting and diarrhoea, while the amatoxins (octapeptides) cause a fatal hepatorenal syndrome. The latter produce severe cellular damage by binding to the nuclear RNA polymerase B of eukaryotic cells, inhibiting enzyme activity and precipitating cell necrosis. In humans, amatoxins are specifically toxic to hepatocytes, intestinal epithelium and possibly the kidney.

28.5.12.1.2 Clinical features

Nearly all patients poisoned by *A. phalloides* first develop gastrointestinal symptoms some 6 to 18 hours after ingestion. There is vomiting and abdominal pain. Diarrhoea can be severe ('cholera like') leading to hypovolaemia, dehydration and hypokalaemia.

The signs of hepatocellular necrosis become evident about 36 hours after ingestion with elevated transaminase levels and, a little later, prolongation of the prothrombin time.

28.5.12.1.3 Treatment

The patient should be rehydrated and the circulating volume should be expanded. Removal of circulating toxins by inducing a diuresis is the most effective, safest and cheapest immediate intervention.

Although other techniques such as haemodialysis, haemofiltration and haemoperfusion are effective, they should probably only be used when it proves impossible to produce an enhanced diuresis. Activated charcoal can be given to bind toxins within the gastrointestinal tract.

No specific antidotes are available, although high-dose penicillin has been recommended. The mechanism of action of penicillin in this situation is unclear, but it may reduce hepatic uptake of amatoxins.

FHF should be managed as outlined elsewhere. Liver transplantation has been performed in patients with FHF associated with mushroom poisoning.

28.5.12.2 *Other rare mushrooms*

Other rare mushrooms include:

- *Gyromitra*, the effects of which are similar to those produced by amatoxins, except that it also produces neurological symptoms such as restlessness, stupor, dizziness, tremor, seizures, diplopia and nystagmus.
- *Orellanus*, which rarely causes initial gastrointestinal symptoms; patients may develop renal failure 7 to 17 days after ingesting the mushrooms.

28.5.13 *Snake bites and animal stings*

Envenoming from snake bites is unusual in the UK but common worldwide. The only indigenous venomous snake in the British Isles is the adder (*Vipera berus*).

28.5.13.1 *Clinical features*

The bite may cause local and systemic effects, including early anaphylactoid symptoms and later persistent hypotension, ECG abnormalities, coagulopathy with spontaneous systemic bleeding, acute respiratory distress syndrome and acute renal failure.

28.5.13.2 *Treatment*

Early anaphylactoid symptoms should be treated with adrenaline. Indications for antivenom treatment include systemic envenoming and marked local envenoming with increasing swelling and erythema within four hours of the bite. For both adults and children the contents of one vial (10 ml) of European viper venom antiserum is given by intravenous injection over 10 to 15 minutes or by intravenous infusion over 30 minutes after diluting in sodium chloride 0.9% (5 ml diluent/kg body-weight). The dose can be repeated in one to two hours if symptoms of systemic envenoming persist. Adrenaline may be required for management of anaphylactic reactions to the antivenom.

Antivenom is available for certain foreign snakes, spiders and scorpions. Specialist information will be required on identification, management and antivenom supply and administration (e.g. Arizona Poison & Drug Information Center http://www.pharmacy.arizona.edu/centers/arizona-poison-drug-information center; Rocky Mountain Poisons Center http://www.rmpdc.org/).

References

[1] Jones, A.L. and Volans, G. (2005). Recent advances: management of self-poisoning, *BMJ*, **319**, 1414–1417.

[2] Purkayastha, S., Bhangoo, P., Athanasiou, T. *et al.* (2006). Treatment of poisoning induced cardiac impairment using cardiopulmonary bypass: a review, *Emergency Med J*, **23** (4), 246–50.

[3] American Academy of Clinical Toxicology and European Association of Poisons Centres (1997). Position statement: Single-dose activated charcoal, *J Toxicol Clin Toxicol*, **35**, 721–741.

[4] American Academy of Clinical Toxicology and European Association of Poisons Centres (1997). Gastric lavage, *J Toxicol Clin Toxicol*, **35**, 711–719.
[5] American Academy of Clinical Toxicology and European Association of Poisons Centres (1997). Whole bowel irrigation, *J Toxicol Clin Toxicol*, **35**, 699–709.
[6] Visser, L., Stricker, B., Hoogendoorn, M. *et al.* (1998). Do not give paraffin to packers, *Lancet*, **352**, 1352.
[7] Choudhary, A.M., Taubin, H., Gupta, T. *et al.* (1998). Endoscopic removal of a cocaine packet from the stomach, *J Clin Gastroenterol*, **27**, 155–156.
[8] Lancashire, M.J.R., Legg, P.K., Lowe, M. *et al.* (1988). Surgical aspects of international drug smuggling, *BMJ*, **296**, 1035–1037.
[9] Vale, J.A., Meredith, T.J. and Proudfoot, A.T (1986). Syrup of ipecacuanha: is it really useful? *BMJ*, **293**, 1321–1322.
[10] American Academy of Clinical Toxicology and European Association of Poisons Centres (1997). Position statement: ipecac syrup. *J Toxicol Clin Toxicol*, **35**, 699–709.
[11] Levy, G. (1982). Gastrointestinal clearance of drugs with activated charcoal, *N Engl J Med*, **307**, 676–678.
[12] Menzies, D.G., Busuttil, A. and Prescott, L.F. (1988). Fatal pulmonary aspiration of oral activated charcoal, *BMJ*, **297**, 459–460.
[13] Cutler, R.E., Forland, S.C., St John Hammond, P.G. *et al.* (1987). Extracorporeal removal of drugs and poisons by hemodialysis and hemoperfusion. *Annu Rev Pharmacol Toxicol*, **27**, 169–191.
[14] Collee, G.G. and Hanson, G.C. (1993). The management of acute poisoning, *Br J Anaesth*, **70**, 562–573.
[15] Brent, J., McMartin, K., Phillips, S. *et al.* (1999). Fomepizole for the treatment of ethylene glycol poisoning, *N Engl J Med*, **340**, 8832–8838.
[16] Routledge, P.A., Vale, J.A., Bateman, D.N. *et al.* (1998). Paracetamol (acetominophen) poisoning, *BMJ*, **317**, 1609–1610.
[17] Keays, R., Harrison, P.M., Wendon, J.A. *et al.* (1991). Intravenous acetylcysteine in paracetamol-induced fulminant hepatic failure: a prospective controlled trial, *BMJ*, **303**, 1026–1029.
[18] Smilkstein, M.J., Knapp, G.L., Kulig, K.W. *et al.* (1988). Efficacy of oral, N-acetylcysteine in the treatment of acetaminophen overdose. Analysis of the national multicentre study (1976 to 1985), *N Engl J Med*, **319**, 1557–1562.
[19] Boehnert, M.T. and Lovejoy Jr, F.H. (1985). Value of the QRS duration versus the serum drug level in predicting seizures and ventricular arrhythmias after an acute overdose of tricyclic antidepressants, *N Engl J Med*, **313**, 474–479.

[20] Masters, A.B. (1967). Delayed death in imipramine poisoning, *BMJ*, **3**, 866–867.

[21] Stern, T.A., O'Gara, P.T., Mulley, A.G. *et al.* (1985). Complications after overdose with tricyclic antidepressants, *Crit Care Med*, **13**, 672–674.

[22] Lheureux, P.E., Zahir, S., Gris, M. *et al.* (2006). Bench-to-bedside review: hyperinsulinaemia/euglycaemia therapy in the management of overdose of calcium-channel blockers, *Crit Care*, **10**, 212.

[23] Martiny, S.S., Phelps, S.J and Massey, K.L. (1988). Treatment of severe digitalis intoxication with digoxin-specific antibody fragments: a clinical review, *Crit Care Med*, **16**, 629–635.

[24] Ashton, C.H. (1985). Benzodiazepine overdose: are specific antagonists useful? *BMJ*, **290**, 805–806.

[25] Höjer J., Baehrendtz, S., Matell, G. *et al.* (1990). Diagnostic utility of flumazenil in coma with suspected poisoning: a double-blind, randomised controlled study, *BMJ*, **301**, 1308–1311.

[26] Sutherland, G.R., Park, J. and Proudfoot, A.T. (1977). Ventilation and acid–base changes in deep coma due to barbiturate or tricyclic antidepressant poisoning, *Clin Toxicol*, **11**, 403–412.

[27] Henry, J.A. (1992). Ecstasy and the dance of death, *BMJ*, **305**, 5–6.

[28] Winstock, A.R. and King, L.A. (1996). Ecstasy and neurodegeneration. Tablets often contain substances in addition to, or instead of, ecstasy, *BMJ*, **313**, 423–424.

[29] Maxwell, D.L., Polkey, M.I. and Henry, J.A. (1993). Hyponatraemia and catatonic stupor after taking 'ecstasy', *BMJ*, **307**, 1399.

[30] Denborough, M.A. and Hopkinson, K.C. (1997). Dantrolene and "ecstasy", *Med J Aust*, **166**, 165–166.

[31] Watson, J.D., Ferguson, C., Hinds, C.J. *et al.* (1993). Exertional heat stroke induced by amphetamine analogues. Does dantrolene have a place? *Anaesthesia* **48**, 1057–1060.

[32] Henry, J.A., Jeffreys, K.J. and Dawling, S. (1992). Toxicity and deaths from 3, 4 methylenedioxymetamphetamine ("Ecstasy"), *Lancet*, **340**, 384–387.

[33] Randall, T. (1992). Cocaine, alcohol mix in body to form even longer lasting, more lethal drug, *JAMA*, **267**, 1043–1044.

[34] Cregler, L.L, and, Mark, H. (1986). Medical complications of cocaine abuse, *N Engl J Med*, **317**, 1495–1500.

[35] Steingrub, J.S., Sweet, S. and Teres, D. (1989). Crack-induced rhabdomyolysis, *Crit Care Med*, **17**, 1073–1074.

[36] Wright, J. (2002). Chronic and occult carbon monoxide poisoning: we don't know what we're missing, *Emerg Med J*, **19**, 386–390.

[37] Meredith, T. and Vale, A. (1988). Carbon monoxide poisoning, *BMJ*, **296**, 77–79.

[38] Henry, C.R., Satran, D., Lindgren, B. *et al.* (2006). Myocardial injury and long-term mortality following moderate to severe carbon monoxide poisoning, *JAMA*, **295**, 398–402.

[39] Raphael, J.-C., Elkarrat, D., Jars-Guincestre, M.C. *et al.* (1989). Trial of normobaric and hyperbaric oxygen for acute carbon monoxide intoxication, *Lancet*, **2**, 414–419.

[40] Ducasse, J.L., Celsius, P. and Marc-Vergnes, J.P. (1995). Non-comatose patients with acute carbon monoxide poisoning: hyperbaric or normobaric oxygenation? *Undersea Hyperb Med*, **22**, 1–9.

[41] Thom, S.R., Taber, R.L., Mendiguren, H. *et al.* (1995). Delayed neuropsychologic sequelae after carbon monoxide poisoning: prevention by treatment with hyperbaric oxygen, *Ann Emerg Med*, **25**, 474–480.

[42] Scheinkestel, C.D., Bailey, M., Myles, P.S. *et al.* (1999). Hyperbaric or normobaric oxygen for acute carbon monoxide poisoning: a randomised controlled clinical trial, *Med J Aust*, **170**, 203–210.

[43] Editorial (1976). Paraquat poisoning, *Lancet*, **1**, 1057.

[44] Rose, M.S., Smith, L.L. and Wyatt, I. (1974). Evidence for energy-dependent accumulation of paraquat into rat lung, *Nature*, **252**, 314–315.

[45] Vesconi, S., Langer, M., Iapichino, G. *et al.* (1985). Therapy of cytotoxic mushroom intoxication, *Crit Care Med*, **13**, 402–406.

29

Transfer of the Critically Ill

Harriet Wordsworth

29.1 Introduction

Transferring the critically ill presents a number of problems. Patients are often unstable, space is restricted, monitoring is inaccurate, noise makes communication difficult, there are environmental hazards and the health care professional commonly feels isolated. High-profile cases in the 1990s involving long distance transfers resulted in poor outcomes [1]. This led to the release of formal guidance on patient transfer by the UK Department of Health [2] and the Intensive Care Society [3]. The Intensive Care National Audit and Research Centre estimated that 4,500 inter-hospital transfers occur annually between British intensive care units [3]. However, this is a huge underestimation as it does not include transfers from emergency departments. Accurate national data does not exist for these types of transfers, although regional networks collect local information. Critically ill patients are also transferred every day within hospitals for investigations and interventions, and the same principles apply whether the transfer is 100 metres or 1,000 km.

29.2 Physiological Factors Important in Patient Transfer

29.2.1 *Road transfer*

The main physiological disruptions encountered in road transfers are due to dynamic hazards. As acceleration or deceleration occurs, 'inertial' forces

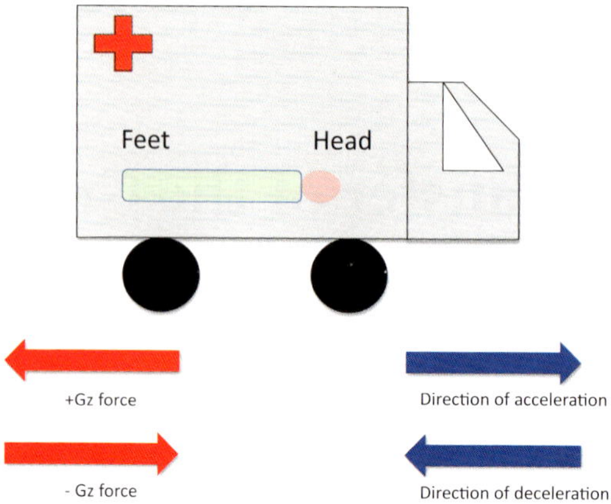

Figure 29.1. Effects of acceleration and deceleration on Gz forces experienced by a patient.

act on solid organs and blood in the opposite direction to the movement of the vehicle (Fig. 29.1). This can be explained by Newton's Third Law which states that 'for every action there is an equal and opposite reaction'. Such inertial forces can be termed Gz and can be negative or positive depending on the direction of acceleration [4].

Positive Gz forces of around 0.25 G are experienced when a road ambulance accelerates. Blood will pool in the feet, which decreases venous return, reducing preload and causing a drop in cardiac output. Healthy people can compensate quickly by an increase in contractility, heart rate and vasomotor tone but such responses are blunted in the critically ill. The best way to prevent such problems is to optimise preload [5]. Positive Gz forces also have neurological effects [6], blood pooling in the lower limbs causes a reduction in blood flow to the brain and, in extreme circumstances, can cause a loss of consciousness.

Negative Gz forces of between –0.25 G and –1 G occur during fast braking and deceleration. Such negative forces cause blood to move into the head and thorax, resulting in an increase in preload and right atrial distension. This would usually be compensated by an increase in cardiac contractility and heart rate but in the critically ill it can lead to arrhythmias and pulmonary oedema. Negative Gz forces can also lead to raised intracranial pressure, decreased cerebral flow and cerebral haemorrhage.

The gastrointestinal system is also affected; the risk of gastro-oesophageal reflux is reduced by inserting a nasogastric tube and intubating high-risk patients.

Negative Gz forces are usually more detrimental than positive forces. Therefore patients are usually positioned with the head tilted up, if there are no contraindications, to limit the cardiovascular and neurological sequelae. These dynamic forces can also be problematic if spinal injury is suspected, since axial forces, shearing and vibration can potentially disrupt spinal stabilisation. The main way to minimise all of these dynamic hazards is to limit hard braking and acceleration and provide a smooth journey.

29.2.2 *Air transfer*

Rotary-wing transfers (helicopters) usually fly at around 1,000 feet whilst fixed-wing aircraft fly considerably higher. Propellor-driven planes cruise at around 15,000 feet and jet-powered planes at 30,000 to 40,000 feet [7]. High altitude has three main effects when transferring the critically ill.

- Gas Expansion — Boyle's Law states that, at a constant temperature, the volume of a gas is inversely proportional to pressure. Therefore as a plane ascends, the barometric pressure decreases and the volume of any enclosed gas increases. Gas-filled cavities within the body of particular concern include ears, teeth, the bowel, pneumothoraces, post-laparotomy gas and air emboli in the blood. This means that a pneumothorax must be decompressed prior to transfer and that chest drains must not be clamped [8]. Close monitoring of any suspected gas-filled cavities is essential and pneumoperitoneum and intracranial air may be considered to be contraindications to air transport [3]. The cuff of the endotracheal tube is also subject to changes in pressure, and cuff pressure should be monitored during ascent and descent as the volume will change. Alternatively, the cuff can be filled with saline.
- Partial pressure of inspired oxygen and consequently alveolar partial pressure of oxygen are altered with altitude due to changes in barometric pressure. Since oxygen constitutes approximately 21% of inspired air:

$$PiO_2 = 0.21 \times (B.P.-SVP) \tag{29.1}$$

PiO_2 = partial pressure of inspired oxygen
B.P. = barometric pressure
SVP = saturated vapour pressure (47 mmHg at body temperature)

The drop in barometric pressure from 760 mmHg at sea level to 140 mmHg at 40,000 feet causes a reduction in PiO_2 which is incompatible with life. As a result, high-altitude flights use cabins pressurised to a pressure equivalent to flying at 7,000 feet [9] and an unsupported PiO_2 of 107 mmHg (14 kPa) is achieved. It has been shown that partial pressure of oxygen in arterial blood decreases from 98 mmHg (13 kPa) to 55 mmHg (7.3 kPa) in healthy subjects at 7,000 feet. One study showed a mean drop of oxygen saturations of 5.5% in cardiac patients transferred at a cabin pressurised to 6,900 feet [10]. Physiological compensation to hypoxia occurs by increasing minute ventilation and cardiac output. Since critically ill patients may not be able to manipulate their ventilation, a dramatic increase in cardiac output could lead to arrhythmias and a decrease in the ischaemic threshold.

Compensation for changes in barometric pressure is achieved by altering the inspired concentration of oxygen delivered. To calculate the new inspired oxygen concentration (fraction of inspired oxygen (FiO_2)) at altitude for an equivalent partial pressure of oxygen as at sea level, the following formula can be used: [11]:

$$FiO_2 \text{ at altitude} = (\text{B.P. at referring centre} \times FiO_2)/\text{B.P. at flight altitude} \tag{29.2}$$

- Temperature — An increase in altitude leads to a decrease in temperature. It is conservatively estimated that 20% of patients become hypothermic during helicopter transfer [12] and that those with a low Glasgow Coma Scale (GCS) score and/or requiring neuromuscular blockade are most at risk.

29.3 General Principles

29.3.1 *Indications for inter-hospital transfer*

Ideally, transfer should only be considered if it is likely to improve a patient's clinical outcome [3]. The most common reason for inter-hospital transfer is for specialist care; for example to neurosurgical, burns, cardiothoracic or vascular centres [13], or for specialist investigation such as angiography. However, pressure on limited intensive care beds inevitably means that patients are transferred for non-clinical reasons. In some regions, it is estimated that up to 50% of transfers are due to lack of staffing or beds [14]. Patients may also be transferred as a repatriation, so that family members can visit more easily or for financial reasons. The decision to transfer a patient, whatever the indication, should be made by the supervising consultant, in conjunction with speciality consultants from both referring and receiving hospitals [3].

The Intensive Care Society suggests dividing up preparation for transfer into patient, personnel, equipment, logistics and departure [3]. First however, the mode of transport must be decided upon as this will affect how the transfer is managed and who will accompany the patient, and may change clinical decisions.

29.3.2 *Modes of transport*

Geographical terrain and distance, traffic and weather conditions, cost and availability of air transfer, and patient condition and stability all need to be considered (Table 29.1).

In general, air transfer should be considered if the distance to be travelled is over 80 kilometres or if transfer time is expected to be longer than 90 minutes [15]. For transfers over 240 kilometres, a fixed wing aircraft, preferably pressurised, should be used rather than a helicopter.

The most important thing to consider is the size, capabilities and limitations of the vehicle performing the transfer.

In the UK, traffic more than geographical factors will limit the speed of transfer but this is very different in countries such as Australia, where air transfer is the norm. It is difficult to prove whether any particular mode is beneficial when compared with another with respect to reduced mortality or morbidity. A Norwegian expert panel assessed 370 inter-hospital transfers and showed that patients arrived, on average, 69 minutes earlier if transported by air ambulances but that only 11% of patients 'benefited' from earlier arrival [16] and that the benefit was greatest amongst paediatric patients.

Table 29.1. Advantages and disadvantages of various modes of transport.

Road	Rotary wing (helicopter)	Fixed wing
Readily available	Variable availability	Requires prior arrangement
Operates in most weather conditions	Can only operate in certain weather conditions	Can only operate in certain weather conditions
Operates at any time of dazy	Maybe limited to daylight missions	Usually can operate 24 hours a day
Slow and traffic-dependent	Usually faster	Faster for long distances
Does not require specialised medical crew	Usually requires medical crew with aeromedical training	Usually requires medical crew with aeromedical training
Some noise and vibration	A great deal of noise and vibration which can hamper communication	Level of noise and vibration dependent on aircraft
Acceleration/deceleration effects on patient physiology	Also need to consider altitude effects on physiology	Also need to consider altitude effects on physiology
Readily available transfer equipment	Civil Aviation Authority-approved equipment only	Civil Aviation Authority-approved equipment only
Usually enough space to operate	Cramped conditions for any practical procedures	Varying amounts of space to operate
No restriction on type of patient condition that can be transferred	Certain conditions may not be suitable for air transfer	Certain conditions may not be suitable for air transfer
Able to transfer patient door-to-door	Secondary transfer maybe required	Secondary transfer maybe required
Cheap	Expensive	Expensive

Potential contraindications to air transfer include clinical reasons, such as pneumoperitoneum or pneumocranium, or safety and ethical factors, such as an uncontrollable combative patient or patient refusal.

Cardiac patients were traditionally regarded as being high-risk for aeromedical transfer because of concerns over hypoxia-induced ischaemic events, arrhythmias, and anxiety-induced sympathetic stimulation [9]. However, a recent randomised trial has compared on-site thrombolysis with transfer by air or road, to a centre for primary angioplasty for the treatment of acute myocardial infarction. This showed a decreased length of stay and a 38% reduction of major cardiac events in the transferred group [17]. In this study and several other audits, no difference in mortality or cardiac events was observed between road and air transfers [8].

29.3.3 *Patient stabilisation*

The length of time spent preparing for transfer is a balance between resuscitation and stabilisation and a requirement for specialist intervention. It has been shown that patients who require resuscitation at the receiving hospital have worse outcomes [18]; however, on the other hand, in some conditions such as an intracerebral haemorrhage, delays in transfer can adversely affect outcome [19].

All staff involved in the transfer must familiarise themselves with the patient's history, and at the very least an 'AMPLE' history [20] (which includes knowledge of allergies, medications, past medical history, last oral intake and events leading up to the transfer). A full physical examination and review of investigations should be conducted in a systematic way. Many checklists exist to aid reviewing patients prior to transfer (Fig. 29.2).

29.3.3.1 *Airway*

If there is any doubt that the patient may need to be intubated during the transfer, this should be done before departure, as this may be technically difficult in cramped conditions with unfamiliar equipment. Generally, it is advised that patients with a GCS of 8 or less or a fluctuating level of consciousness should be intubated. Arterial partial pressures of oxygen of less than 8 kPa or respiratory acidosis may also be indications for invasive ventilation. Once intubated, the endotracheal tube should be secured and documentation made of the level of the tube at the teeth. Ideally chest X-ray confirmation of the tube position should be obtained.

Cervical spine protection must also be considered in trauma patients. Computed tomography (CT) scans of the spine should be reviewed by a consultant radiologist and a report taken to the receiving centre. It may not be possible to 'clear' the cervical spine clinically if the patient has a decreased level of consciousness, in which case protective measures should be continued, i.e. neutral position, a rigid collar, sandbags and tape.

Imperial College Healthcare **NHS**
NHS Trust

Major Trauma Patient Transfer Checklist

Patient name and ID number

Pre Transfer

Team Leader:
Transfer From:
Transfer Time:
Transfer To:

Action	**Confirmed**	**N/A or reason for variance**
Incubated	☐	
C-spine cleared/continued immobilisation	☐	
Plain film trauma series completed	☐	
Primary survey completed	☐	
Secondary survey completed	☐	
Transport bag and equipment checked	☐	
Oxygen cylinder checked	☐	
Airway secure and stable for transport	☐	
Central line	☐	
Arterial line	☐	
Chest drain	☐	
Catheter in situ	☐	
Blood products location		
Blood pressure pre transfer		
Heart rate pre transfer		
Respiratory rate pre transfer		
Receiving area informed of transfer	☐	
Notes completed and signed	☐	
Notes scanned	☐	
List additional equipment transferred with patient **(Equipment to be collected post transfer)**	☐ Donway ☐ Kendrick ☐ Pelvic splint ☐ Syringe driver ☐ Other – please state	

Post Transfer

Receiving team:
Receiving team senior signature:
COMPLETED & SIGNED FORM TO BE RETURNED TO RESUS ROOM MAJOR TRAUMA FOLDER

Created on 10/28/2010 6:06:00 PM \\dirone\root\Departments\Accident & Emergency - Clinical Documents\ED DOCUMENTS - MASTER COPIES\SHOPFLOOR PROFORMAS\TRANSFER CHECKLIST.doc

Figure 29.2. Pre-transfer patient checklist.

29.3.3.2 *Breathing*

If the patient is to be invasively ventilated, they should be established on the ventilator for at least 15 minutes before departure. Inspired oxygen and ventilator settings should be guided by arterial blood gas analysis and end-tidal carbon dioxide monitoring [3]. A pneumothorax must be ruled out or treated with a chest drain, left unclamped. A recent chest X-ray should be reviewed.

29.3.3.3 *Circulation*

Every effort should be made to establish haemodynamic stability. In actively bleeding patients, permissive hypotension in certain carefully considered situations could be acceptable [21] but other causes of hypovolaemia should be corrected. The mantra 'full patients travel better' must be remembered [22]. Inotrope infusions should be established in advance of departure with continuous central venous pressure and invasive blood pressure monitoring. At least two wide-bore intravenous cannulae should be inserted and flushed. Remember that line extensions and three-way taps cause dead space, which can be important when compensating for slow-running infusions. A baseline electrocardiogram (ECG) or a series of ECGs should be reviewed.

29.3.3.4 *Disability*

Make sure that the best GCS and neurological and motor status are recorded for the receiving unit; reassess pupil response and GCS prior to departure. Intubated patients should always be sedated for transfer and, unless there is a contraindication, muscle relaxants should be administered as close to time of departure as possible. If there is evidence of raised intracranial pressure, sedation level should be optimised, mean arterial pressure maintained above 90 mmHg and neurosurgical advice sought in case of worsening neurological symptoms which may require treatment *en route*.

29.3.3.5 *Exposure*

Patients usually become hypothermic to some extent during transfer. It is best to optimise core temperature prior to departure as it may be difficult to rectify once *en route*. Hypothermia can cause peripheral vasoconstriction and coagulopathy, therefore worsening cardiovascular stability. Patients requiring lots of infusions and equipment can get pressure injuries as pumps and monitoring equipment is piled on top of them due to lack of space. Pressure areas must be protected as vibration during transfer can worsen tissue damage. A secondary survey should be documented and fractures stabilised to minimise pain and blood loss.

29.3.3.6 *Fluids and electrolytes*

A record of resuscitation fluids or a 24-hourly fluid balance should be noted along with a general overview of recent urine output. Electrolyte disturbances should be corrected, ideally prior to departure, especially potassium and magnesium. Glucose levels should be within the normal range and, if appropriate, metabolic acidosis corrected with a bicarbonate infusion.

29.3.3.7 *Gastro-intestinal*

Nasogastric or orogastric tubes should be inserted and a repeat abdominal examination performed to appreciate a baseline and rule out pathologies that need to be treated prior to transfer. Any focussed assessment by sonography in trauma or CT scan results should be recorded and a copy taken to the receiving hospital.

29.3.3.8 *Haemotology*

A recent full blood count should be reviewed. A haemoglobin of 7 g/dl is acceptable in a stable patient but the target of 10 g/dl is more appropriate in actively bleeding patients or those with ischaemic heart disease [23]. A formal test of coagulation or at least a near-patient test (such as thromboelastography) should be performed to guide blood-product administration. Adequate blood products should be released from haematology, checked, signed for and stored appropriately. Time of removal from blood fridge should be noted and the time of expiry for safe administration calculated.

29.3.3.9 *Infection*

Microbiology results should be collated and a history of antibiotics used noted. Any multi-resistant or hospital-acquired infections should be discussed with the receiving unit.

29.3.4 *Personnel*

In the UK, 90% of adult inter-hospital transfers are conducted by the referring hospital [15]. However, in many countries, such as Australia, it is normal for critically ill patients to be transferred by a dedicated retrieval team [24]. Retrieval team transfer has been advocated by some studies [25] and guidelines, [2] highlighting the advantages of specialised equipment and transfer vehicles, higher training and skill of accompanying staff, and better pre-transfer stabilisation. In the UK, paediatric retrieval networks exist for critically ill children and have been shown to reduce morbidity [26], but such strong evidence does not exist for the transfer of adult patients.

A critically ill patient should be accompanied by a minimum of two attendants as well as the vehicle crew. For a Level 2 or 3 patient this should be a doctor, competent in airway care, resuscitation and intensive care medicine, and usually a nurse, from an intensive care or emergency department background [15]. The level of training and seniority of the accompanying physician has been a source of much debate. One survey showed that 26% of transfers from emergency departments were conducted by an anaesthetic senior house officer and 53% by an anaesthetic registrar [27]. In one region, only 33% of doctors performing transfers had attended a specific transfer course and 39% had been asked to transfer a patient when they felt that it was beyond their level of experience [28]. It is now advised that staff should have obtained their transfer competencies as set out by the Royal College curriculums [29,30] before transferring a patient unsupervised.

29.3.5 *Equipment*

As highlighted by the National Patient Safety Agency (NPSA), equipment failures contribute to many adverse events during transfers [31]. It is therefore essential that equipment is checked in a methodical manner, using a kit check list and that dedicated transfer equipment is available 24 hours a day. Transport trolleys for use in land ambulances must comply with European Committee for Standardisation (CEN) regulations and be able to withstand a 10 G deceleration [32]. Electrical equipment used in air transfers must have a certificate of safety from the Civil Aviation Authority. The weight of equipment will also need to be estimated for air transfer, to allow for fuel calculations by the air crew, and therefore monitoring and ventilator equipment should be as light as possible.

Equipment for securing and maintaining an airway should be stored in an easily accessible manner and checked for date of expiry and battery power. A portable suction unit is required for all intra- and inter-hospital transfers [33]. Transfer ventilator design is dependent on gas supplies, electrical sources and on the modes of ventilation required by the patient. Minimum requirements for a transfer ventilator include disconnection and high-pressure alarms, variable FiO_2 concentration and the ability to set inspiration:expiration ratio, tidal volume, respiratory rate and positive end-expiratory pressure [3]. Traditionally gas-powered ventilators, such as the ventiPAC, have been used. These time-cycled flow generators utilise the pneumatic power of pressurised oxygen cylinders but can deliver unreliable tidal volumes [34]. Microprocessor-controlled ventilators such as the Oxylog 3000, have enabled most modes of ventilation used on the intensive care unit to be replicated [35] and these ventilators are more suitable for air transfer as they contain transducers which can compensate for changes in barometric pressure (Fig. 29.3).

The Association of Anaesthetists of Great Britain and Ireland (AAGBI) has defined minimum standards for monitoring during all types of transfer [36]. This should include oxygen saturations, ECG, blood pressure, core temperature and, for ventilated patients, end tidal carbon dioxide, airway pressure, tidal volume and respiratory rate. It is important to secure monitoring equipment before departure and to set alarm volumes to higher than normal levels so that they can be heard above external noise levels.

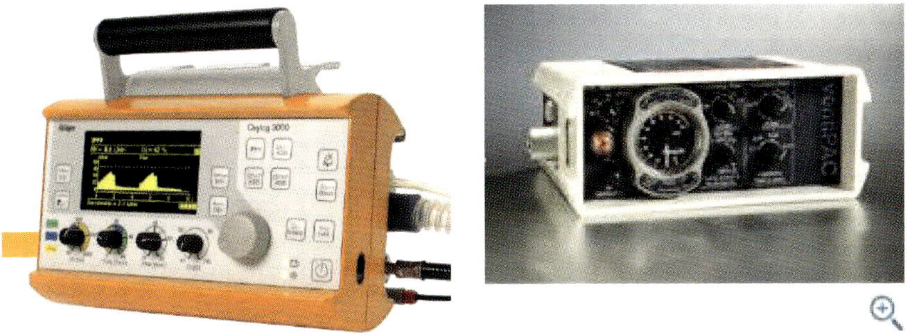

(A) (B)

Figure 29.3. VentiPAC and Oxylog 3000 transfer ventilators.

In general, transfer equipment must be battery-powered and a protocol should be established for charging batteries after transfer. Spare batteries should be taken in case of failure. Some, but not all, ambulances have inverters which can convert DC current produced from the vehicle battery to the 240V AC supply suitable for hospital equipment [35]. The type of electricity source available should be determined when booking a vehicle.

Infusions should be delivered by syringe drivers only. The Medical Devices Agency has produced performance parameters required for infusion devices based on the type of drug to be infused [37]. These dictate the degree of accuracy as well as the need for occlusion and air emboli alarms. Pressure changes occur with ascent to altitude, and therefore bags, not bottles, of fluids should be used to maximise control over speed of fluid administration. Pressure bags will also change in volume causing the pressure exerted on the fluid bag to increase or decrease depending on altitude.

Packaging of equipment is important to ensure safe travel. Ideally pumps and ventilators should be attached below the patient to ensure the lowest possible centre of gravity. Infusion pumps can become hazardous missiles *en route* and so should be secured to the trolley or vehicle. Care should be taken to pad any portion of the equipment which could possibly come into contact with the patient so as to reduce pressure damage.

Oxygen requirements must be calculated for transfer. A buffer should also be included in case of patient deterioration or delays in journey time.

$$\text{In general the volume of oxygen} = \text{Patient consumption} \times \text{Ventilator consumption} \times \text{Transport time} \times 2 \text{ (for safety)} \quad (29.3)$$

Patient consumption = Minute ventilation × FiO_2

Ventilator consumption for Oxylog 3000 = 1 l/min

For example a patient with a minute ventilation of 8 l/min on FiO_2 of 0.5 to be transferred for 60 minutes:

$$\text{Volume of } O_2 \text{ required} = (8 \times 0.5) \times 1 \times 60 \times 2 = 480 \text{ litres.} \quad (29.4)$$

However, it is normally assumed that a patient will need an FiO_2 of 1 'just in case'; therefore 960 litres should be available.

The amount of stored oxygen available from ambulance reservoirs should not be assumed and keys required to open new cylinders (Table 29.2) must be kept with the cylinders.

29.3.6 *Logistics*

Communication is essential to the smooth running of a transfer. Whilst organising the transfer, a lead clinician at both referring and receiving hospital must be identified. If the patient is a transfer from an intensive care unit, an intensivist as well as the lead specialty consultant must be nominated. Ideally, a nursing communication between units should be conducted prior to departure to allow for preparation of the bed. The receiving hospital should be notified of time of actual departure and kept updated of delays *en route*.

Table 29.2. Cylinder sizes and stored oxygen volume.

Cylinder size	Volume of oxygen stored in litres
C	170
D	340
E	460
F	680
G	1360

A calculation of distance between units should be estimated to aid decisions about mode of transport and equipment preparation.

The ambulance service should be notified as early as possible and the urgency of transfer specified. In many services, an emergency or 'time critical' ambulance will be available within 15 minutes. This means that the next double-manned ambulance will be dispatched and will take priority over community emergencies [38] — this should be reserved for true emergencies. It is common for the ambulance operators to ask if a paramedic crew is required but usually they will be unable to guarantee one, so it should not be relied upon.

All patient notes and investigations should be photocopied and a transfer letter from the referring hospital produced. Often a transfer checklist is completed pre-departure to ensure patient and equipment readiness. A transfer form must be completed and this process will start at the referring hospital, continue during the transfer and finish with handover in the receiving hospital. Timings of referrals, contact with ambulance service, arrival of vehicle, departure and arrival should be recorded. Transfer forms also usually include a pre-departure assessment of the patient which should be filled in by the accompanying clinician.

Personal mobile phones should be taken *en route* with pre-programmed phone numbers for referring and receiving units and direct numbers for on-call speciality doctors, such as neurosurgeons, in case advice is required. Warm and preferably high-visibility clothing should be worn in case of delays or vehicle mishap and to protect against cold temperatures in both air and road vehicles. Preparation for return to base hospital should be made well in advance as ambulance services cannot guarantee an ambulance transfer back to the base hospital.

Relatives should also be informed of the transfer and given details about time of departure and exact location of the receiving unit. Relatives should not be advised to 'follow the ambulance' as this could put them at risk of accident.

29.3.7 *During the transfer*

The aim of careful stabilisation and pre-departure planning is to limit the need for active intervention whilst *en route*. Monitoring and recording of observations should be performed as in theatre for Level 2 or 3 patients [36].

Conversion to ambulance supplies of electricity and oxygen should be done as soon as possible and all equipment secured before the vehicle moves. Noise and vibration can limit communication, particularly during air transfer. Poor communication has been highlighted by the NPSA for being responsible for adverse events such as drug errors during transfers [39]. Seat belts must be worn whenever the ambulance is in motion — the Department of Transport statistics show that 81 ambulance passengers were admitted to hospital for treatment following collisions between 1999 and 2008 [38].

Adverse events (Table 29.3) must be documented and resolved as quickly as possible and included in the handover at the receiving hospital. A prospective audit of nearly 300 inter-hospital transfers from the emergency department to intensive care showed 9% of transfers were associated with equipment failure, 7% of patients became hypothermic and 6% had a cardiac event. Delays were very common with 38% of patients waiting more than 20 minutes and 14% being delayed by more than an hour [40].

Neurosurgical patients are at particular risk from transfer as commonly occurring adverse events, such as hypoxia and hypotension, can lead to secondary brain injury [41]. Such adverse events during transfer have been correlated with poor outcomes — one study showed that even one episode of hypotension or hypoxaemia could double patient mortality [42] in traumatic brain injury. To minimise such complications the AAGBI produced guidelines for the care of patients with brain injury, highlighting the importance of stabilisation and monitoring [43].

Table 29.3. Adverse events reported during transfer.

Patient problems	Equipment problems	Logistical problems
Extubation	Battery exhaustion	Delays in vehicle arrival
Hypoxia	Oxygen exhaustion	Getting lost *en route* to hospital or receiving unit
Hypotension	Drug errors	Delayed return to base hospital
Hypothermia	Loss of intravenous access	Personal injury to clinicians
Arrhythmias	Lack of suction	
Pressure damage to skin		

29.3.8 *Handover*

A formal handover should take place on arrival at the receiving unit and once this has been done, receiving staff are assumed to have taken responsibility for the patient care. Normally this is done using an 'airway, breathing, circulation' approach and events that have occurred on transfer should be explained clearly. A contact number for the referring team should be left so that further questions can be answered. Usually transfer forms have three carbon copies; one should be left in patient notes at the receiving hospital, one should be returned to the referring hospital and one given to the transfer network for audit purposes.

29.3.9 *Ethical and medicolegal considerations*

The four pillars of medical ethics must be considered when transferring a patient: beneficence, non-maleficence, justice and autonomy [44]. It is usually easy to demonstrate beneficence in cases of transfer for specialty services or investigations but this is harder to show for non-clinical transfers. It has been argued that the transfer of a patient for the sole reason of making space for a more unstable patient is not in the patient's best interest and is therefore unethical. However, in such cases, the principle of justice, or fair treatment for all, may be debated.

Respect for the patient's wishes, or autonomy, is important even if the patient is unable to communicate their wishes. Consent and explanation with the patient should be documented. Assent from the next of kin is desirable but, in the UK, not an essential or legally binding requirement unless the patient is below the age of consent [45].

Insurance is advised for all medical staff conducting a transfer. For example, the AAGBI and Intensive Care Society offer worldwide personal injury insurance for their members during transfers. In the UK, employers must ensure that adequate medical indemnity insurance is in place for staff involved in transfers and it is also advised that the clinicians are members of a medical defence organisation. This is because it is assumed that the transfer team has full responsibility of the patient during transfer, from leaving the referral unit until verbal and written handover to the receiving unit [43].

References

[1] Easby, J., Clarke, F.C., Bonner, S. *et al.* (2002). Secondary inter-hospital transfers of critically ill patients: completing the audit cycle, *Br J Anaesth*, **89**, 354.

[2] Department of Health (2000). *Comprehensive Critical Care: A review of adult critical care services*, Online. Available at: http://www.dh.gov.uk/prod_consum_dh/groups/dh_digitalassets/@dh/@en/documents/digitalasset/dh_4082872.pdf [Accessed 4 February 2013].

[3] Whiteley, S., Mcartney, I, Mark, J. *et al.* (2011). *Guidelines for the Transfer of the Critically Ill Adult*, third edition, The Intensive Care Society, London.

[4] Handy, J. (2005). The physiological effects of transferring critically ill patients, *Clin Inten Care*, **16**, 65–69.

[5] Handy, J. and van Zwanenberg, G. (2007). Secondary transfer of the critically ill patient, *Curr Anaes Crit Care*, **18**, 303–307.

[6] Houghton, J., McBride, D.K. and Hannah, K. (1985). Performance and physiological effects of acceleration-induced (+Gz) loss of consciousness, *Aviat Space Environ Med*, **56**, 956–965.

[7] American Medical Association (1982). Medical aspects of transportation aboard commercial aircraft, *JAMA*, **247**, 1007–1100.

[8] Essebag, F., Halabi A.R., Churchill-Smith M., *et al.* (2003). Air medical transport of cardiac patients, *Chest*, **124**, 1937–1943.

[9] Gong Jr, H. (1992). Air travel and oxygen therapy in cardiopulmonary disorders, *Chest*, **101**, 1104–1113.

[10] Bendrik, G., Nicolas, D.K., Krause, B.A. *et al.* (1995). Inflight oxygen saturation decrements in aeromedical evacuation patients, *Aviat Space Environ Med*, **66**, 40–44.

[11] Nehrenz, G. (2000). Altitude and oxygenation, *Internet Journal of Aeromed Transp*, **1** (1), doi: 10.5580/215e.

[12] Fiege, A., Rutherford, W. F. and Nelson, D. R. *et al.* (1996). Factors influencing patient thermoregulation in flight, *Air Med J*, **15**, 18–23.

[13] Gray, A., Gill, S., Airey M. *et al.* (2003). Descriptive epidemiology of adult critical care transfers from the emergency department, *Emerg Med J*, **20**, 242–246.

[14] Jameson, P. and Lawler, P.G. *et al.* (2000). Transfer of critically ill patients in the Northern region, *Anaesthesia*, **55**, 489–518.

[15] Wallace, P. and Ridley S.A. (1999). ABC of intensive care. Transport of critically ill patients, *BMJ*, **319**, 368–371.

[16] Stevenson, A., Fiddler, C., Craig, M. *et al.* (2005). Emergency department organisation of critical care transfers in the UK, *Emerg Med J*, **22**, 795–798.

[17] Grines, C., Westerhausen Jr, D.R., Grines, L.L. *et al.* (2002). A randomized trial of transfer for primary angioplasty versus on-site thrombolysis in patients with high-risk myocardial infarction: the Air Primary Angioplasty in Myocardial Infarction study, *J Am Coll Cardiol*, **39**, 1713–1719.

[18] Gray, A., Bush, S. and Whiteley, S. (2004).Secondary transfer of the critically ill and injured adult, *Emer Med J*, **21**, 281–285.

[19] Gentleman, D. and Jennett, B. (1990). Audit of transfer of unconscious head-injured patients to a neurosurgical unit, *Lancet*, **335**, 330–334.

[20] American College of Surgeons (2008). *Advanced Trauma Life Support*, eighth edition, American College of Surgeons, Chicago.

[21] Dutton, R., Mackenzie, C.F. and Scalea, T.M. (2002). Hypotensive resuscitation during active haemorrhage: impact on in-hospital mortality, *J Trauma*, **52**, 1141–1146.

[22] Ashworth, S. (2007). *Inter-hospital Transfer of Level 3 Patients, St Mary's Hospital Anaesthetic Department Guidelines*, [Online]. Available at: http://www.st-marys-anaesthesia.co.uk/Guidelines/Transfer%20notes%20and%20FAQ%20for%20SMH%20trainees-2007.pdf [Accessed 4 February 2013].

[23] British Committee for Standards in Haematology, Stainsby, D., MacLennan, S. *et al.* (2006). Guidelines on the management of massive blood loss, *Br J Haem*, **135**, 634–641.

[24] Shirley, P. and Heams, S. (2006). Retrieval Medicine: a review and guide for UK practitioners, Part 1: clinical guidelines and evidence base, *Emerg Med J*, **23**, 937–942.

[25] Bellingham, G., Olivier, T., Batson, S. *et al.* (2000). Comparison of a specialist retrieval team with current United Kingdom practice for the transport of critically ill patients, *Intens Care Med*, **26**, 740–744.

[26] Edge, W., Kanter, R.K., Weigle, C.G. *et al.* (1994). Reduction of morbidity in interhospital transport by specialised paediatric staff, *Crit Care Med*, **22**, 1186–1191.

[27] Stevenson, A., Fiddler, C., Craig, M. *et al.* (2005). Emergency department organisation of critical care transfers in the UK, *Emerg Med J*, **22**, 795–798.

[28] Cook, C. and Allan, C. (2008). Are trainees equipped to transfer critically ill patients? *JICS*, **9**, 145–147.

[29] The Royal College of Anaesthetists (2010). *Curriculum for a CCT in Anaesthetics*, second edition, The Royal College of Anaesthetists, London.

[30] The Intercollegiate Board for Training in Intensive Care Medicine (2010). *Curriculum for a CCT in Intensive Care Medicine*, second edition, The Intercollegiate Board for Training in Intensive Care Medicine, London.

[31] Thomas, A. and Galvin, I. (2008). Patient safety incidents associated with equipment in critical care: a review of reports to the UK National Patient Safety Agency, *Anaesthesia*, **63**, 726–733.

[32] British Standards Institution (2007). *British and European Standards: Medical Vehicles and their Equipment- Road Ambulances*, BS EN 1789:2007.

[33] Shirley, P. (2004). Transportation of the critically ill and injured patient, Update, *Anaesthesia*, **18**, (Article 2), 1–2.

[34] McCluskey, A. and Gwinutt, C.L. (1995). Evaluation of the Pneupac Ventipac portable ventilator: comparison of performance in a mechanical lung and anesthetized patients, *Br J Anaesth*, **75**, 645–650.

[35] Fludger, S. and Klein, A. (2008). Portable ventilators, *BJA:CEACCAP*, **8**, 199–202.

[36] Association of Anaesthetists of Great Britain and Ireland (2007). *Recommendations for Standards of Monitoring during Anaesthesia and Recovery*, fourth edition, AAGBI, London.

[37] Keay, S. and Callender, C. (2004). The safety of infusion devices, *BJA: CEACCAP*, **4**, 81–85.

[38] Black, J., Thompson, F. and Stephens, L. (2010). *Hospital Guidance on South Central Ambulance Service Protocol for Emergency Inter-hospital Transfer Decision Flow Chart*, South Central Ambulance Service, Bicester.

[39] Thomas, A. and Panchagnula, U. (2008). Medication-related patient safety incidents in critical care: a review of reports to the UK National Patient Safety Agency, *Anaesthesia*, **63**, 726–733.

[40] Gillman, L., Leslie, G., Williams, T. *et al.* (2006). Adverse events experiences while transferring the critically ill patient from the emergency department to the intensive care unit, *Emerg Med J*, **23**, 858–861.

[41] Gentleman, D. and Jennett, B. (1981). Hazards of interhospital transfer of comatose head injured patients, *Lancet*, **2**, 853–854.

[42] Gentleman, D. and Jennett, B. (1990). Audit of transfer of unconscious patients to a neurosurgical unit, *Lancet*, **335**, 330–334.

[43] Association of Anaesthetists of Great Britain and Ireland (2006). *Recommendations for the Safe Transfer of Patients with Brain Injury*, AAGBI, London.

[44] Pekkegrino, E. (1993). The metamorphosis of medical ethics. A 30-year retrospective, *JAMA*, **269**, 1158–1162.

[45] Parekh, S. (2007). Child consent and the law: an insight and discussion into the law relating to consent and competence, *Child Care Health Dev*, **33**, 78–82.

30
Ethics in Critical Care

Simon Munk and Andrew Hartle

30.1 Introduction

Critical care medicine has changed enormously from its origins in treating single-organ failure to its current state of increasingly developed technology and pharmacology able to treat multiple organ failure. Patients survive now that would not have done so in the past. These changes have been paralleled by demographic and socio-cultural changes in the population. People are living longer, but also with more obesity, and other comorbidities associated with ageing. At the same time there has been a change from more paternalistic practice of medicine to a patient-focussed, inclusive and transparent system. Society's expectations have been mirrored by legislative changes such as the Human Rights [1] and the Mental Capacity [2] Acts.

Just because we can do something — treat someone, keep them alive — does not mean we should. How then do we make the 'right' decision? Medical ethics is a system of values which helps guide decision making. It may be codified, for example in the Hippocratic Oath or the Declaration of Geneva, or form the basis of professional regulation such as guidance issued by a regulatory body like the General Medical Council. Ultimately, medical practice is constrained by the law, however it is important not to confuse the two; what may be legal may not be ethical and *vice versa*.

It is self-evident that decisions in critical care medicine are emotive ones concerning matters of life and death; patients are not referred for critical care unless they are at risk of dying. Doctors, nurses, patients and their families will have strongly held personal moral and religious views about death and dying. These must be respected and may strongly influence decision making. There will often be several options available. Ethics will not reveal the 'right' answer, but will guide the process, help identify any 'wrong' answer and help chose the 'best' (or often, 'least worst') option.

30.2 Ethical Principles

Many philosophical theories contribute to medical ethics. Deontology focuses on the rightness or wrongness of an action, whilst consequentialism, as espoused by Bentham, focuses on the outcome of an action and the extent to which it maximises happiness. More familiar to most and of more practical use is Beauchamp and Childress' concept of principlism [3]. This proposes that decision making can be aided by reference to four basic ethical principles: respect for autonomy (the individual has a right to choose), beneficence (doing good), non-maleficence (avoiding harm) and justice (treating people fairly). Principlism is easy to understand and apply, but there is no 'weighting' to the principles, although as will be discussed later, autonomy has become almost pre-eminent, particularly in legal changes, and weighing up the relative merits of the different principles can be challenging.

30.2.1 *Autonomy*

Individuals, once adults, have the right to make decisions about what happens to them within the limits set by society. Nowhere is this principle more important than in medicine, where it is manifested by the requirement for patients to consent to treatment. Valid consent requires that the patient has capacity to make the decision, is free from duress, and has all the information necessary to make that decision themselves. Consent to critical care is possibly only obtained from those patients whose admission to an intensive care unit is planned after elective surgery, and even then it can be questioned whether it is truly voluntary; rather like anaesthesia it is only consented to in order to have another procedure that the patient wants or needs, rather than as the primary therapeutic manoeuvre. More frequently, one or more of the elements will be missing; the patient will have reduced or no capacity because of the underlying treatment or condition, treatment will be needed urgently to preserve life, and there will be no opportunity to exchange information.

30.2.1.1 *Capacity*

For an adult to have capacity (different rules apply to children, and vary between jurisdictions) they must be able to:

- Understand information relevant to the decision.
- Retain information related to the decision to be made.
- Use or weigh up that information as part of the process of making the decision.
- Communicate the decision, whether by talking, using sign language or any other means.

Capacity is decision-specific, and the person proposing a particular action or course of treatment is responsible for assessing capacity. It will be self evident that patients who are sedated and ventilated will lack capacity, failing all the above tests, but at lower levels of critical care, patients must be involved with treatment decisions if they meet these criteria.

30.2.1.2 *Patients without capacity*

Until recently adults who lacked capacity were left in a legal limbo, with no other adult being able to consent or refuse consent on their behalf. Doctors and others were forced to act in the patient's best interests, and only slowly did professional guidance develop to support that process. Recent legislative changes (Adult with Incapacity (Scotland) Act 2001 and Mental Capacity Act 2005) have codified previous common law and best practice into statute law.

30.2.1.3 *Lasting powers of attorney*

A person who loses capacity can continue to exercise it in two ways, by giving someone power of attorney, or by forming an advanced decision.

An attorney may consent on behalf of another if appointed, and the power is registered with the Court of Protection (rules vary in Scotland; more detailed advice may be obtained from the General Medical Council guidance [4]). The attorney is able to make decisions about life-sustaining treatment that needs specific authorisation; at all times the power of attorney must be exercised in the patient's best interests. Doctors are not obliged to comply with requests which are not in the patient's best interests. Although the Mental Capacity Act has been in force for several years, lasting powers of attorney are still rare.

30.2.1.4 *Advanced decisions*

Previously known as 'living wills' or 'advanced directives', advanced decisions are statements of the person's wishes and expectations, and should be complied with. If an advanced decision refuses life-sustaining treatment (the commonest example is probably a refusal of blood products in a patient who is a Jehovah's Witness) it must be written, signed and witnessed. Poorly written living wills may cause as many problems as poorly written wills. A lay person's terminology may not fit well with the nuances of critical care medicine (for example what is a 'life support machine'?). Doctors must also be certain that the advanced decision applies in the circumstances at hand, since there may have been significant changes since it was executed that may mean the patient had changed their views.

Where there is no lasting power of attorney or relevant advanced decision then the treating doctor must decide what course to take acting in the patient's best interests. In law the doctor is the decision maker, but they are legally and professionally bound to consult with others.

30.2.2 *Best interests*

It has been accepted for many years that best interests may not be the same as best medical interest; merely being alive, but suffering, may not be better than dying in comfort and dignity. The Mental Capacity Act now specifies how a best interest decision should be reached (although without specifying what best interests are!).

This is more than just a balancing act of the pros and cons of a course of treatment (although this was the common-law approach). Decisions must only be made that have to; if it is likely that the patient will recover capacity in a time frame that allows them to decide then this should be waited for. Any treatment must also leave as many options open for the patient should they recover capacity (for example medical rather than surgical treatment if this is possible). Doctors must consider what the patient's wishes, feelings, values or beliefs were when they had capacity, or would be now if they had capacity. If the patient still has limited capacity then their current wishes and feelings must be considered, and all reasonable steps must be taken to involve them in the decision.

When practicable and appropriate (bearing in mind at all times the ongoing duty of confidentiality) the doctor must consult anyone named by the patient (e.g. next of kin), anyone caring for the patient or concerned with their welfare, and anyone holding a lasting power of attorney or appointed by the court as a deputy.

Best interest decisions are some of the most difficult to make as there are so many variables and unknowns. Although scoring systems (such as the Acute Physiology and Chronic Health Evaluation) may give some indication of the likelihood of survival, extrapolation of population statistics to individuals is fraught with problems. As Sokol once commented, life would be much easier with a 'best interests meter' [5].

30.2.2.1 *Independent mental capacity advocates (IMCAs)*

Again when appropriate and practicable, for patients who are 'unbefriended' (have no family, friends or unpaid carers) then an IMCA should be instructed. IMCAs act as advocates, not attorneys, and so they have no decision-making authority, but they may see the patient and their notes and ask for a second opinion. Their role is to ensure that the best-interests process has been complied with. However, IMCAs provide a working-hours-only service, and life-saving and other time-sensitive decisions should not be deferred if this will be detrimental; the main aim of the act is that those without capacity should not be treated adversely.

30.2.3 *Futility*

Futility is a concept much used when considering critical care, but it is a term which should be used cautiously, particularly with friends and family as it may be misinterpreted, suggesting that something is not worth trying (or too expensive). Futility has most usefully been described as '...a treatment which cannot provide a minimum likelihood or quality of benefit should be regarded as futile and is not owed to the patient as a matter of moral duty' [6]. Treatments may be futile if they don't work at all, don't confer any benefit in terms of survival, or would not allow the patient's own wishes to be achieved in terms of outcome.

In general terms for critical care to be appropriate there must be the possibility of recovery (although the extent of that recovery will vary). There must be some reversible and/or treatable element to the patient's condition. Even if this condition is met, the patient must be able to survive long enough for the treatment to be effective; critical care may make them better eventually but they have to survive long enough to let this happen.

30.3 Practical Aspects

30.3.1 *Appropriate referral*

Responsibility for deciding the appropriateness of critical care rests not just with the critical care team, but with the referring team; they are more likely to know more about a patient's functional status, wishes and desires and prognosis from their underlying condition and comorbidities. Early, senior involvement is always preferable to the middle-of-the-night referral of a patient in a peri-arrest state, when the time for careful review is limited.

Where possible the patient must be involved in any decisions and their wishes, views and feelings taken into account, either directly or by consultation with those family members and carers who are able to assist.

It is rarely appropriate to make a 'not for critical care' decision, particularly now that many interventions previously the sole reserve of the (Level 3) intensive care unit, such as invasive monitoring, inotropes and non-invasive ventilation, may be administered in other (Level 2) critical care units. Rather, for each patient, appropriate ceilings of intervention should be set, which should also be reviewed regularly at senior level depending on changes in the patient's condition, responsiveness to treatment or the discovery of more diagnostic or prognostic information.

In particular, decisions to withdraw or withhold aspects of critical care should be made by senior doctors, ideally in discussion with others in a multidisciplinary setting, whether formal or otherwise, with consistent communication with the patient and/or relatives and carers. Unilateral, poorly communicated decisions can lead to terrible legal and professional consequences.

30.4 Conclusion

Critical care medicine saves lives, but it can also prolong death and cause suffering to patients, their friends, families and carers. Deciding when and when not to embark on critical care, and when to stop, is one of the most challenging skills to learn, and is made easier by a basic understanding of ethical principles and the ever-changing law.

References

[1] *Human Rights Act 1998* (c. 42), HMSO, London.
[2] *Mental Capacity Act 2005* (c. 9), HMSO, London.
[3] Beauchamp, T.L. and Childress, J.F. (2008). *Principles of Biomedical Ethics*, sixth edition, Oxford University Press, Oxford.
[4] General Medical Council (2008). *Consent: Patients and Doctors Making Decisions Together*, General Medical Council, London.
[5] Schneiderman, L.J. and Jecker, N.S. (1993). Futility in Practice, *Arch Intern Med*, **153**, 437–441.
[6] Mason, J.K. and Laurie, G.T. (2010). *Mason and McCall Smith's Law and Medical Ethics*, Oxford University Press, Oxford.

31
Leadership and Management in Critical Care

Andrew R. Webb

31.1 Introduction

The critical care unit is a complex environment, where public expectation, technological innovation, funding challenges, increasing age of patients and co-morbidity, health quality and patient safety, information technology and intra-professional rivalry all place demands on staff. In order to negotiate one's way through these issues the critical care clinician needs to develop appropriate leadership behaviours and understand the principles of management [1,2].

Critical care is a clinical service providing care to patients originating from other hospital-based specialties, such as medicine and surgery. As a clinical service, critical care is responsible for identifying and meeting the needs of specialties it supports. Critical care management has two distinct relationships in the hospital. The traditional managerial hierarchy includes vertical relationships describing the lines of accountability for delivering objectives and responsibilities. However, the service nature of the critical care unit requires the development of horizontal relationships between departments. A horizontal relationship requires that the manager is particularly adept at inter- and intra-professional collaboration.

Management and leadership skills need to be learnt. They are not the same thing. The manager is an individual who holds an office that includes several roles; leadership is one of those roles but is not exclusive to the manager.

31.2 Leading

Effective managers must be leaders and leaders must manage. At the heart of good leadership is the ability to influence followers through interpreting events, organising objectives, motivating and maintaining relationships [3]. In critical care, motivating the unit's multi-professional team, building enthusiasm and creating momentum towards the agreed vision is a key leadership skill. High-quality leaders are especially adept at managing change. The successful leader has been described as one who makes things happen, faces reality and mobilises resources [4]. Collins described exemplary leaders as ambitious for their organisation rather than themselves, and as modest, understated and attributing success to others whilst accepting responsibility when things go wrong [5]. High-performing leaders think of the whole system, have a vision and articulate that vision in a compelling way, create priorities and direction, facilitate continuous learning in preparation for dealing with future challenges and empower followers to be creative while being sensitive to their needs [6–8]. Successful leaders understand the importance of creating team-orientated approaches to providing patient care focussed on improving quality and patient safety. They keep the critical care team focussed on problem-solving. However, while the team may be empowered to create a decision, the leader remains accountable for outcomes of the group's decisions.

31.2.1 *Leadership styles*

There are many behavioural styles used by leaders, most of which will depend on the situation. The most effective leader can use several styles to the benefit of those he is leading (known as situational leadership) rather than using a one-size-fits-all approach. Amongst the classical leadership styles are those described as charismatic, transformational, transactional and participative [9].

A charismatic leader uses influence based not on formal authority but on his ability to inspire while remaining approachable. Charismatic leadership may create a radical vision for change and it is the vision that attracts followers because they believe in it.

A transformational leader appeals to the followers' values and emotions. The transformational leader convinces followers to go beyond individual self-interest for the sake of the team.

A transactional leader recognises what the follower wants and exchanges reward for followership. This style, while sometimes necessary has more to do with managing than leading.

A participative leader encourages the team to develop ideas and solutions to problems rather than simply directing the team. This approach creates a forum for colleagues to help both with problem-solving and implementation of solutions. Using the collective intellect of the team to solve problems creates a better solution, and one that is easier to implement as it has involved the people to be affected by change in the development of the solution.

31.2.2 *Leading change*

Many will question the need for the change, yet the complex environment of critical care must always adapt to changing demands, changing technologies or changing evidence. Without understanding the effect(s) of proposed change on the critical care staff it is difficult to achieve benefits of the proposed change. Muir-Gray stated the most important step in facilitating change is to ensure that clinicians want to change. The most effective way of encouraging this is to help them see evidence-based decision-making not as a management imperative, but as an intellectual challenge [10]. Changing clinician behaviours and practices requires a leader to be prepared to implement a combination of different strategies simultaneously [11].

The aim of the changes proposed must be communicated to all members of the critical care team who will be affected. Not everything will be clear at the outset, and all participants in the change process need to understand that ambiguity is a normal part of any change process. The leader must demonstrate his commitment to change and encourage commitment at all levels in order to make the proposed change. The leader must ensure resources are available to deliver the change.

Communicate, communicate, communicate! In any change process, it is essential to make sure that communication is open so that all members of the team feel comfortable in providing their views and opinions about the proposed change.

31.2.3 *Power*

While leadership is the ability to influence followers, power is the potential to exert influence, and thus, be it directly or indirectly, cause a change in the behaviour of another individual or group [12]. Arguably, influence is power that is translated into action. Leaders need to understand the different types of power and be especially aware of their sources of power.

Legitimate power exists when it is derived from a leader's position in the hospital's managerial hierarchy. Reward-based power exists when the leader is able to reward desirable behaviours whereas coercive power occurs when the leader has the ability to prevent a colleague from achieving rewards they want. Expert power occurs when the leader has knowledge that is considered important to the unit's objectives. Thus, power is the tool of transactional leadership.

Creating power happens through a leader's ability to create opportunities, control resources and/or assist in successfully dealing with challenges. Exerting influence should be reserved only for issues of high priority. In other situations, transformational or participative styles are usually more appropriate.

31.2.4 *Teamwork*

Creating teams and encouraging teamwork are essential ingredients of successful management and leadership. A team is a high-performing task group whose members are interdependent and share a common performance objective [13].

Teamwork occurs when staff work together in such a way that their collective skills are integrated to achieve a common goal. In creating a team, the workload is delegated and team members are encouraged, developed and empowered to participate. A clinician in a team leadership role is most effective when he defines the objectives of the task and allows team members to contribute to creating solutions (participative leadership). Team building is always more successful when the team leader provides role modelling of the types of behaviour expected from staff members.

A team is most effective when collaboration (rather than competition) is promoted and team members are encouraged to assume leadership roles themselves. The collective brainpower of a team exceeds the capability or capacity of one individual. The more inclusive the team, the greater will be the talents and viewpoints available to deal with problems.

In critical care, teamwork is especially important for delivering high-quality and safe patient care. The critical care clinical team has grown to include many professionals who collectively contribute to patient care. The impact of good teamwork on ICU clinical outcomes is now accepted. When the whole team concerned with a patient's care (doctors, residents, nurses, attending physicians, pharmacists and others) participated in rounds together both communication and professional job satisfaction were improved. There was also better resource use measured as a decrease in critical care stay [14].

31.3 Managing

The manager provides five key functions: planning, organising, staffing, directing and controlling [15]. Good planning begins with analysis, e.g. trends in service delivery and includes objectives, policies and procedures to guide daily activities. Organising might involve determining how clinical authority and responsibility are divided between different professionals (e.g. physicians, nurses, physiotherapists) and ensuring everyone understands their roles. The critical care unit's most important resource is its staff. The manager is responsible for ensuring appropriate staff are recruited and opportunities for professional development are provided. Directing is influencing behaviour through motivation, communication leadership and discipline.

Performance must be measured and reported in terms of clinical, academic, budgeting and resource utilisation. These are important parts of the controlling function. If performance is inadequate (e.g. against national benchmarks) the manager must implement the necessary changes.

The critical care manager typically adopts three roles. An interpersonal role sees the manager acting as a figurehead for the critical care team, liaising with internal and external stakeholders and influencing decision-making. In an informing role the manager monitors and disseminates knowledge to the team. In a decision-making role, the manager manages conflict, allocates resources to support the department's objectives and negotiates with other decision-makers both inside and outside the hospital.

Critical care managers are responsible for decisions that affect the quality and costs of patient care. Within a climate of scarce healthcare resources, difficult decisions are made about complex issues such as allocation of resources (e.g. creating and managing admission/discharge policies) and organisation of care processes (e.g. protocols, nurse:patient ratios).

31.3.1 *Planning*

Planning for the critical care department involves creating objectives and designing and implementing strategies to achieve them [16]. Developing a plan is an iterative process that provides direction, prepares for change and helps the department deal with uncertainty. It must focus on outputs such that effort is directed to achieving the predefined objectives. In order to achieve the objectives, the plan requires a clear statement of priorities to allow better decisions on allocating and using available resources. It must be measurable so that progress can be plotted. Planning is never complete. Ongoing monitoring is necessary to identify factors that might require a change in the plan.

31.3.1.1 *Strategic planning*

A strategic plan defines the longer-term direction of travel. Shorter-term goals and objectives are often set annually as part of the department's progression towards its strategic objectives. Strategic planning is focussed on both the external and internal environment and will include the development of a vision, objectives and policies and procedures. It involves choices based on a strategic assessment and objectives.

Table 31.1. SWOT matrix.

	Helpful to achieving goals	**Unhelpful to achieving goals**
Internal factors controlled by critical care	**Strengths** Things that are good now	**Weaknesses** Things that are bad now
External factors not controlled by critical care	**Opportunities** Things that may become good	**Threats** Things that might become bad

A strategic assessment compiles information from several sources for evaluation. Assumptions are made about the future based on interpretation of, for example, current position, trends, emerging technologies and political factors. These assumptions, depicted in Table 31.1, are collectively known as an environmental analysis, and categorised into strengths, weaknesses, opportunities and threats (SWOT analysis).

When undertaking the environmental analysis, an (honest) examination of the department's strengths (e.g. its reputation for high-quality care, staff qualifications, its capacity to do research, the range of life-support technologies available) and opportunities (e.g. development of new research funding, development of new technologies) must be made. It is easy to put greater focus on the strengths and opportunities than the weaknesses and threats, but failure to understand issues with negative impact fully is a key reason for the failure of a strategic plan. Weakness might include outdated equipment, poor reputation or excessive staff turnover. Threats might include changes in funding streams (with potential negative impact) or the introduction of new technologies that divert patients away from critical care. This latter example is both a threat to the critical care department and an opportunity for patients or other departments to whom they may go.

After completing an environmental analysis, the planning process should include the creation of a vision and objectives. The vision describes the purposes for which the department exists and what it aspires to achieve. A compelling vision is essential to motivate the critical care team, focussing energies towards the goal.

Objectives are statements of the results that a department seeks to achieve. They describe how the vision will be accomplished and give direction to the department's activities. Objectives must be specific, measurable, achievable, realistic and have a clear timescale for delivery (SMART). They enable work towards specific endpoints, provide criteria for prioritising decision-making, provide a sense of direction and provide criteria for use in control processes.

Once the vision and objectives are defined, the planning process identifies strategies to achieve the objectives. These are broad work programmes involving choices dependent on, and in response to, the expected impact of the environmental analysis.

31.3.2 *The budget*

The budget is a short-term plan describing the financial roadmap to achieving the objectives required for the current year. Thus, the budget is a numerical expression of the plan. It is a statement of expected revenues and expenses over a defined time period. Most hospital budgets are based on the previous year's budget with additional costs identified to deliver the key objectives, cost pressures identified (e.g. staff pay awards, increases in consumable and drug prices, adoption of new technologies) and cost reductions identified as part of an annual cost-improvement plan.

In a cost-improvement plan unit costs may be reduced by providing more activity for the same budget or providing the same amount of activity for less cost. A cost-improvement programme encourages the development of new ways of providing care and should, therefore, be seen as synonymous with quality improvement. It is important to remember cost improvement might require investment prior to delivery.

Whereas the hospital budget will be developed within the total income derived from its services, departments within the hospital often do not receive all the income related to their services. This is because the cost of overheads and corporate functions are usually not devolved to service units. This is a fixed budget model where resources are committed to the critical care department for the budget period and are based on planned workload. In this model, expenditure control is the only way of managing the budget.

A variable budget means that resources change with activity. In this model the revenue budget flexes with activity, allowing the budget to keep pace. There is also the possibility of volume efficiency as more activity may be delivered at a lower unit cost. With the development of service line reporting, each service unit, such as the critical care department, is considered as a subsidiary profit centre. In this model, income is fully attributed to the service line earning it. A revenue budget describes the income apportioned to the critical care department, generated by patient care, education and research. This income may be derived by recharging users of the critical care service based on a price tariff that aims to recover full costs. Alternatively, critical care may be reimbursed directly by the agency funding the hospital. The full cost of the service, including the reasonable share of overheads attributable to the service, is within an operating expense budget. An operating expense budget includes costs of day-to-day critical care operations, e.g. pay, consumables and drugs. Expenses in critical care operating budgets can be direct (critical care staffing costs) or indirect (costs that must be shared between different cost centres). Indirect costs may be attributable to activity, for example the cost of physiotherapy, or may be considered as an overhead, for example the cost of utilities.

Service line reporting provides for reinvestment for growth and quality initiatives in a profitable service. It enables resources to be allocated efficiently to ensure the highest-quality outcome for patients and helps identify the highest-priority areas for improvement.

31.3.3 *Staffing*

Critical care medical staff, assisted by senior nursing and pharmacy colleagues, take primary responsibility for the structural and financial management of the unit. It is through their actions that treatment of the critically ill is initiated and perpetuated; they are ultimately responsible for the activity of the unit and patient outcome. Senior medical staff must have a number of skills (see Table 31.2).

Critically ill patients require close nursing supervision. Many will require high-intensity nursing throughout a 24-hour period while others are of a lower dependency and can share nurses. In addition to the bedside nurses, the department needs additional staff to manage the day-to-day running of the unit, to assist in lifting and handling of patients, to relieve bedside nurses for rest periods, and to collect drugs and equipment. Maintaining the nurse to patient ratio is associated with

Table 31.2. Required skills of senior medical staff.

Decision-making

Most decisions are made by team consensus. Clinical decisions fall into three categories: (i) decisions relating to common or routine problems for which a unit policy exists; (ii) decisions relating to uncommon problems requiring discussion with all staff currently involved and (iii) decisions of an urgent nature taken by critical care staff without delay.

Practical skills

Expertise in the management of complex equipment, monitoring procedures and performance of invasive procedures are required.

Clinical experience

Medical staff require experience in the recognition, prevention and management of critical illness, infection control, anaesthesia, analgesia and organ support.

Technical knowledge

The critical care specialist has an important role in the choice of equipment used in the unit. Advice should be sought from non-medical colleagues.

Pharmacological knowledge

Drug therapy regimens are clearly open to the problems of drug interactions, while pharmacokinetics are often severely altered by the effects of major organ system dysfunction, particularly involving the liver and kidneys. Adverse reactions are common.

Teaching and training

The modern critical care specialist has acquired skills that cannot be gained outside the critical care unit. It is therefore necessary to impart this knowledge to doctors training in the speciality.

better outcomes [17–19]. Critical care staffing needs are determined by employee turnover and growth (increased demand for services, higher occupancy, expansion and the addition or enhancement of services).

Each member of the workforce must have a job description of specific duties and responsibilities, working conditions and qualifications. Job descriptions should also describe requirements for staff involvement in quality improvement and continuing education. On starting a new job it is essential employees are provided with an orientation programme that includes:

- Information about the department and its organisational structure.
- Information on the hospital's fire procedures.
- Information on the occupational health service.

- Explanation of key policies and benefits.
- Information about the philosophy, vision and values of the hospital and the department.

Staff should receive a performance appraisal at least annually. They provide feedback about progress within the team and identify areas where coaching for improvement may be required. During performance appraisals development plans for individual staff can be constructed and training proposed.

Staff can be provided with career counselling and health education and promotion. Educating staff can enable them to better manage their own health. Health education might include stress management, nutrition counselling and weight reduction and smoking cessation advice. Health education improves productivity and contributes to staff retention.

31.3.4 *Managing conflict*

Conflict is inevitable in critical care. Although conflict research in critical care is scant, a recent study gave an evaluation of 248 conflicts involving 209 patients. The different types of conflict described included: team–family disputes, intra-team disputes, and intra-family conflict. The leading sources of conflict were disagreements or uncertainty over life-sustaining treatments, poor communication, the (lack of) availability of family decision-makers and the surrogates' (perceived) inability to make decisions [20]. Examples of 'uncertainty' in critical care include the suddenness of patient admissions and patient-related complications.

As the coping strategy of critical care staff members differs substantially, conflict management is an important skill for the critical care leader [21–23].

Conflict resolution requires the maintenance of objectivity in reviewing the circumstances of the conflict issue. It is important to remove emotion from the problem's analysis. Aschenbrener and Siders listed the following strategies in conflict resolution [24]:

- Minimise defensiveness because it only serves as a barrier to communication.
- Separate fact from emotion because individuals in conflict need to state their version of the events.

- Gather facts from both sides of a conflict situation and remember conflict often arises from a simple misunderstanding.
- Deal with conflict in a timely manner. If left alone a small misunderstanding might build into a substantial problem that will distract the entire critical care team.

31.3.5 *Controlling*

Monitoring performance against the budget is one of the most common control methods a manger uses. Both control and auditing are related to planning. Controlling refers to the processes set up to ensure that what is planned actually occurs. It requires monitoring of performance, comparing actual and expected results and intervening to take corrective action when results are not as predicted or planned [25]. In controlling the budget the manager is required to review the budget statement, identify reasons for variance and identify the actions that will be instituted to bring the budget back in line with what was predicted. In order to ensure that objectives are delivered, managers similarly monitor performance and intervene with change strategies when needed [15].

There are three types of control: output control, process control and input control [26]. Output control is also called feedback control, a retrospective process that involves measuring issues such as quantity and quality of care in the critical care unit. Process control monitors processes that generate outputs. With regard to quality improvement, monitoring the use of clinical practice guidelines by clinicians would be an example of process monitoring. Input control is also called feed-forward control. With input control, the manager measures inputs as a means of controlling objectives. Pronovost *et al.* demonstrated that clinicians with critical care training provided better critical care outcomes [27]. The closed unit, managed by the critical care team with consultation from other parties, has been shown to be more efficient [28–30] and have better outcomes [31–33]. A closed unit uses input control for care provision.

31.3.6 *Clinical governance*

Clinical governance is a framework through which organisations are accountable for continuously improving the quality of their services and safeguarding high standards of care by creating an environment in which excellence in clinical care will flourish [34]. As such, it is a system of controlling clinical quality. Quality in critical care is the degree to which patient care processes increase the probability of the desired patient outcome and reduce the probability of undesired outcomes [35]. Continuous quality improvement aims to meet and exceed patient and family satisfaction by continuously examining and improving systems and work processes [36]. Quality may be evaluated in terms of structure, process and outcome [37], or what you have, how you use it and what you achieve with it [38]. Aspects of the structure of critical care that may be relevant include having enough trained staff, cleanliness or having enough appropriate equipment. Process measures might include admission, discharge and transfer protocols, communication systems or evidence-based clinical protocols. The impact of evidence-based protocols was evaluated in 13 adult critical care units [14] with reduced length of stay as a positive benefit.

While risk-adjusted mortality is an important outcome measure, it is only one of many. For many patients, morbidity may be equally important. Quality-of-life-adjusted mortality in the months following discharge is more relevant to patients than the crude or risk-adjusted mortality [39]. Given the time and resources invested in the delivery of critical care, post-discharge mortality is probably an inappropriate outcome measure.

Clinical governance requires commitment to the assurance of health-care quality using the components listed in Table 31.3. There must be systems in place to recognise and act upon poor performance within each of these components.

The critical care unit interfaces with most of the rest of the hospital and its clinical governance arrangements must contribute to patient care throughout the hospital. Some aspects of critical illness are managed outside the critical care unit yet the critical care team retain a responsibility for ensuring quality and safety of this care.

Based on data collected on almost 18,000 patients in 42 critical care units, Shortell and colleagues [40] found that good management practice was associated with:

- A patient-centred culture.
- Strong medical and nursing leadership.
- Effective communication and co-ordination.

Table 31.3. Essential components of clinical governance.

Clear management arrangements	
Everyone must know who they are accountable to, the limits of their decision-making and who must be informed in the decision-making process.	
Quality improvement	
Through the process of clinical audit the standard of practice is monitored and changes are effected to improve quality.	
Clinical effectiveness	
Evidence-based practice is essential where sound evidence exists to support clinical decisions. Protocols and guidelines standardise practice.	
Risk assessment and management	
A register of clinical risks should be kept, to which new risks are appended as they are assessed. An action plan should be developed for managing each risk and the implementation of the plan monitored.	
Staff and organisational development	
Including continued professional education, clinical supervision and professional regulation.	
Patient input	
Complaint monitoring should be used to learn lessons and improve practice within critical care. Patient and relative suggestions and surveys can be used to adapt quality initiatives to the needs of patients.	

- Open, collaborative approaches to problem-solving and conflict management.
- Lower risk-adjusted length of stay.
- Lower nurse turnover.
- Greater ability to meet needs of family members.

These represent high performance within a clinical governance framework.

31.3.7 *Clinical audit*

Clinical audit is a means of measuring the three types of control. It may focus on specific topics or may encompass the performance of several critical care units. A successful audit requires commitment from senior staff to ensure practice is defined, data are collected and change is effected where necessary. Regular audit meetings should follow a pre-defined timetable to ensure maximum staff attendance. Discussion of the topic being audited must lead to recommended changes in practice and these must be followed through after the meeting. Where change is suggested by audit, a further review is required to ensure such change has occurred.

Learning from mistakes is fundamental to the improvement of patient safety. Incident reporting systems are now widespread amongst critical care units to:

- Ensure action is taken to prevent similar incidents in the future.
- Fulfil legal duties to report certain kinds of accident, violent incidents, dangerous occurrences and occupational ill health.
- Ensure accurate information is collected to identify trends and take steps to prevent similar incidents from re-occurring.
- Provide evidence in pursuance of litigation claims, both for and against the hospital.
- Record incidents of particular interest for quality assurance, including the ability to demonstrate accident reductions as part of a risk-management strategy.

It is essential that confidentiality is maintained and disciplinary action is avoided, except where acts or omissions are malicious, criminal, or constitute gross or repeated misconduct. Incident-reporting systems require audit and analysis to establish areas where system improvement may be used to increase patient safety [41].

31.3.8 *Policies and procedures*

Policies are guidelines for behaviour and decision-making in the critical care unit. They enable the department to achieve its objectives. Procedures are actions prospectively determined to guide staff in defined situations. They outline steps that must be taken take to perform a task, and provide them with direction in the performance of their duties.

An example is an admission policy that would typically:

- Identify who has day-to-day responsibility to make admission decisions.
- Include a mechanism for reviewing difficult cases and difficult ethical decisions.
- Identify those who are too well or too sick to benefit from critical care admission (in the context of other facilities available locally).
- Identify priorities for admission during times of high utilisation of beds.
- Identify when and how to transfer patients to other units.
- Identify categories of patients who should or should not be admitted to critical care units, including conditions where admission is mandatory.
- Identify any age criteria by which admission is precluded.
- Clarify the links with local incident-management policies, contingency plans and triggers for the implementation of these plans.

For policies and procedures to be successful in their aim of supporting the department to achieve its objectives they must be consistent with the strategic plan. Policy development should be based on best evidence to ensure the best opportunity for its acceptance. For staff to comply with policies and procedures they must be accessible and communicated to all those affected.

31.4 Illustrative Case: Change Leadership in Action

As a result of a sedation audit, Dr Topmost, the director of critical care, discovers a higher numbers of breaches of the unit's sedation guidelines and a longer average time to extubation for patients admitted during Professor Wayward's duty weeks than during other consultants' duty weeks. Dr Topmost had previously set up a multidisciplinary team to review literature and construct the sedation guidelines which included sedation monitoring and daily sedation holds [42].

Dr Topmost asked Professor Wayward to meet with him to discuss the audit's findings. He decided to try to understand Professor Wayward's viewpoint rather than insisting he fell into line with his colleagues. Professor Wayward acknowledged the critical care team had accepted the guidelines as a group but he did not believe they were consistent with his training interpretation of the evidence. He was not in favour of sedation holds. Professor Wayward was not part of the original multidisciplinary team that produced the guideline.

In order to encourage his participation, Dr Topmost set Professor Wayward the objective of leading another multidisciplinary team and updating the sedation guideline after a critical appraisal of the latest evidence. Professor Wayward was also asked to ensure colleagues had an adequate chance to discuss the evidence before the new guideline was launched.

The review introduced new evidence to the guideline that supported some of Professor Wayward's viewpoint [43]. However, the new guideline focussed much more on adherence to the monitoring of sedation. Through a process of educational forums involving all his colleagues, the new guideline achieved comprehensive acceptance, and a subsequent audit showed all were in compliance with it.

References

[1] Morahan, P.S., Kasperbauer, D., McDade, S.A. *et al.* (1998). Training future leaders of academic medicine: internal programs at three academic health centers, *Acad Med*, **73**, 1159–1168.

[2] Mecklenburg, G.A. (2001). Career performance: how are we doing? *J Healthc Manag*, **46**, 8–13.

[3] Yukl, G. (2001). *Leadership in Organizations*, fifth edition, Prentice Hall, Upper Saddle River, New Jersey.

[4] Tichy, N.M. and Cohen, E. (1997). *The Leadership Engine: How Winning Companies Build Leaders at Every Level*, first edition, Harper Collins Publishers, New York.

[5] Collins, J. (2001). *Good to Great: Why Some Companies Make the Leap… and Others Don't*, Harper Business, New York.

[6] Shortell, S.M. and Kaluzny, A.D. (1996). 'Organization theory and health service management', in Shortell, S.M. and Kaluzny, A.D. (eds), *Essentials of Health Care Management*, Thompson Delmar Learning, New York, pp. 3–33.

[7] Starkweather, D.B. and Shropshire, D.G. (1994). 'Management Effectiveness', in Taylor, R.J. and Taylor, S.B. (eds), *The AUPHA Manual of Health Services Management*, Jones and Bartlett Learning, Burlington, MA, pp. 19–44.

[8] Likert, R. (1961). *New Patterns of Management*, McGraw-Hill Education, New York.
[9] Doyle, M.E. and Smith, M.K. (1999). *Born and Bred? Leadership, heart and informal education*, YMCA George Williams College/The Rank Foundation, London.
[10] Muir-Gray, J.A. (2001). *Evidence-based healthcare: How to Make Health Policy and Management Decisions*, second edition, Churchill Livingstone, New York.
[11] Berenholtz, S. and Pronovost, P.J. (2003). Barriers to translating evidence into practice, *Curr Opin Crit Care*, **9**, 321–325.
[12] Alexander, J.A. and Morlock, L.L. (1996). 'Power and politics in health services organizations', in Shortell, S.M. and Kaluzny, A.D. (eds), *Essentials of Health Care Management*, Thomson Delmar Learning, New York, pp. 256–288.
[13] Francis, D and Young, D. (1992). *Improving Work Groups: A Practical Manual for Team Building*, Pfeiffer, San Diego.
[14] Pronovost, P., Berenholtz, S., Dorman, T. *et al.* (2003). Improving communication in the ICU using daily goals, *J Crit Care*, **18**, 71–75.
[15] Higgins, J.M. (1991). T*he Management Challenge: An Introduction to Management*, Macmillan, New York.
[16] Pearce, J.A. and Robinson, R.B. (1989). *Management*, Random House, New York.
[17] Thorens, J.B., Kaelin, R.M., Jolliet, P. *et al.* (1995). Influence of the quality of nursing on the duration of weaning from mechanical ventilation in patients with chronic obstruction pulmonary disease, *Crit Care Med*, **23**, 1807–1815.
[18] Vicca, A.F. (1999). Nursing staff workload as a determinant of methecillin-resistant *Staphylococcus aureus* spread in an adult intensive therapy unit, *J Hosp Infect*, **43**, 109–113.
[19] Pronovost, P., Dang, G., Dorman, T. *et al.* (2001). Intensive care unit nurse staffing and the risk of complications after abdominal aortic surgery, *Eff Clin Pract*, **4**, 199–206.
[20] Studdert, D.M., Mello, M.M., Burns, J.P. *et al.* (2003). Conflict in the care of patients with prolonged stay in the ICU: types, sources, and predictors, *Intens Care Med*, **29**, 1489–1497.
[21] Key, M.K. (2000). A method for mediating conflict among different mindsets, *J Healthc Qual*, **22**, 4–8.
[22] Marcus, L. (1999). Renegotiating health care. Interview by Richard L. Reece, *Physician Exec*, **25**, 18–23.
[23] Donaldson, L. (1995). Management for doctors: conflict, power, negotiation, *BMJ*, **310**, 104–107.

[24] Aschenbrener, C.A. and Siders, C.T. (1999). Conflict management part 2, Managing low-to-mid intensity conflict in the health care setting, *Physician Exec*, **25**, 44–50.

[25] Rakich, J.S., Longest, B.B. and Darr, K. (1998). *Managing Health Services Organizations*, third edition, Health Professions Press, Baltimore.

[26] Camillus, J.C. (1986). *Strategic Planning and Management Control. Systems for Survival and Success*, Lexington Books, Lanham, MD.

[27] Pronovost, P.J., Angus, D.C., Dorman, T. *et al.* (2002). Physician staffing patterns and clinical outcomes in critically ill patients: a systematic review, *JAMA*, **288**, 2151–2162.

[28] Carson, S.S., Stocking, C. Podsadecki, T. *et al.* (1996). Effects of organizational change in the medical intensive care unit of a teaching hospital: a comparison of 'open' and 'closed' formats, *JAMA*, **276**, 322–328.

[29] Multz, A.S., Chalfin, D.B., Samson, I.M. *et al.* (1998). A "closed" medical intensive care unit (MICU) improves resource utilization when compared with an "open" MICU, *Am J Respir Crit Care Med*, **157**, 1468–1473.

[30] Ghorra, S., Reinert, S.E., Cioffi, W. *et al.* (1999). Analysis of the effect of conversion from open to closed surgical intensive care unit, *Ann Surg*, **229**, 163–171.

[31] Li, T.C., Phillips, M.C., Shaw, L. *et al.* (1984). On-site physician staffing in a community hospital intensive care unit. Impact on test and procedure use and on patient outcome, *JAMA*, **252**, 2023–2027.

[32] Reynolds, H.N., Haupt, M.T., Thill-Baharozian, M.C. *et al.* (1988). Impact of critical care physician staffing on patients with septic shock in a university hospital medical intensive care unit, *JAMA*, **260**, 3446–3450.

[33] Baldock, G., Foley, P. and Brett, S. (2001). The impact of organisational change on outcome in an intensive care unit in the United Kingdom, *Intens Care Med*, **27**, 865–872.

[34] Department of Health (1998). *A First Class Service — Quality in the New NHS*, Department of Health, London.

[35] Berwick, D.M. (1989). Continuous improvement as an ideal in health care, *N Engl J Med*, **320**, 53–56.

[36] Berenholtz, S.M., Dorman, T., Ngo, K., *et al.* (2002). Qualitative review of intensive care unit quality indicators, *J Crit Care*, **17**, 1–12.

[37] Donabedian, A. (1988). The quality of care – how can it be assessed? *JAMA*, **260**, 1743–1748.

[38] Webb, A.R. (2005). Is what you have or how you use it or what you achieve the more important determinant of quality? *J Crit Care*, **20**, 124–125.

[39] Suter, P., Armaganidis, A., Beaufils, F. *et al.* (1994). Predicting outcome in ICU patients, 2nd European consensus conference in intensive care medicine, *Intens Care Med*, **20**, 390–397.

[40] Shortell, S.M., Zimmerman, J.E., Rousseau, D.M. *et al.* (1994). The performance of intensive care units: does good management make a difference? *Med Care*, **32**, 508–525.

[41] Vincent, C.A. (2004). Analysis of clinical incidents: a window on the system not a search for root causes, *Qual Safety Health Care*, **13**, 242–243.

[42] Kress, J.P., Pohlman, A.S., O'Connor, M.F. *et al.* (2000). Daily interruption of sedative infusions in critically ill patients undergoing mechanical ventilation, *N Engl J Med*, **342**, 1471–1477.

[43] Mehta, S., Burry, L., Martinez, M. *et al.* (2008). A randomized trial of daily awakening in critically ill patients managed with a sedation protocol: a pilot trial, *Crit Care Med*, **36**, 2092–2099.

32

Evidence-Based Intensive Care

Sunil Grover and Carlos M. H. Gómez

32.1 Corticosteroids

Steroids in sepsis have been used for decades, the rationale being that a certain amount of anti-inflammatory activity is beneficial. After a short course of high-dose steroids was accepted [1] and subsequently rejected [2], attention focussed on longer courses of lower doses. These appeared to show reversal of shock [3] and improved mortality [4], especially in patients unable to mount a corticotropin response to pharmacological stimulation. Interestingly, in a more recent multinational trial by the Corticoid Steroid Therapy for Septic Shock (CORTICUS) group [5], hydrocortisone administration in septic shock did not improve survival in non-responders or in responders (to corticotropin) but did shorten the time to reversal of shock.

Steroids in the adult acute respiratory distress syndrome (ARDS) have also been explored extensively. There is a hypothesis that the anti-inflammatory effect of steroids may reduce progression of the early inflammatory to the late fibro-proliferative phase of the condition. Balanced against this is the risk of secondary infection with potentially catastrophic consequences. Methylprednisolone has been shown to improve oxygenation, lung compliance and ventilator and shock-free days, but not survival [6].

In practice, the decision to administer high-doses of steroids in ARDS is taken after careful consideration of the individual case, usually in a multidisciplinary environment, when conventional treatment is failing and there is good evidence that the patient is free from infection.

32.2 Activated Protein C

It has long been recognised that there is a strong interaction between the inflammatory and coagulation cascades in sepsis and many other conditions [7]. Many trials designed to investigate a putative beneficial impact of selective pharmacological modulation of the inflammatory response in severe sepsis failed to prove this hypothesis in heterogeneous populations of critically ill patients [8–10].

Given that in sepsis there exists an activation of the coagulation cascade in the direction of procoagulation, manifested by low levels of the fibrinolytic protein C [11], attention shifted towards restoring this balance by administering recombinant activated protein C (APC). After encouraging results in experimental studies [12], huge multinational efforts were focussed on the design and execution of several large trials, which showed increased survival in patients with severe sepsis who received recombinant APC but at the cost of increased life-threatening haemorrhage, in particular catastrophic intracranial bleeding [13]. This, together with changes in the study protocol and APC production from a new master cell bank during the initial trial, gave rise to some of the more intense controversy witnessed in the intensive care community in recent times [14–16].

Further large studies showed a beneficial impact of APC on outcome in particularly ill medical patients with severe sepsis and more than one end organ dysfunction [17,18]. In October 2011, APC was withdrawn from the market worldwide as the preliminary results of the Recombinant Protein C Worldwide Evaluation in Severe Sepsis (PROWESS)-SHOCK trial demonstrated no mortality reduction at 28 days (223 deaths out of 846 patients in the APC group versus 202 out of 834 in the placebo group), or at 90 days. The results have been published recently [19].

32.3 Insulin

Early clinical trials with glucose–insulin–potassium administration in acute myocardial infarction yielded promising results [20]. Landmark work from 2001 in 1,500, predominantly cardiac, surgical patients [21] drove many intensive care units to target quite rigid — and difficult to obtain — blood glucose values of 4.4–6.1 mmol/l. The beneficial effects of glucose–insulin treatment are thought to be caused by an increase in glucose transport into, and its utilisation within, the cell [22,23], with consequent improvement in cellular and mitochondrial function in many organs [24,25].

Despite early encouraging results, subsequent studies as well as clinical experience raised the possibility of serious hypoglycaemia [26], especially in unconscious non-diabetics and in units not experienced or staffed to monitor for hypoglycaemia, giving rise to further evaluations in more heterogeneous critically ill patients. In a single-centre medical study of 1,200 medical intensive care patients, tight glycaemic control did not improve hospital mortality although it reduced morbidity, in particular the incidence of acute renal failure [27]. More recently, a meta-analysis of 8,400 patients from 29 randomised control trials also showed no difference in hospital mortality or requirement for renal replacement with tight glucose control, but an increased incidence of hypoglycaemia [28]. In a subsequent multicentre randomised study of 6,100 patients, tight glucose control was associated with increased hospital mortality overall, as well as in medical and surgical patient subgroups, with more episodes of severe hypoglycaemia [29].

32.4 Albumin

Traditionally human albumin has been considered useful in critical illness due to its colloid and oncotic properties. However, its cost, lack of coagulation products, high sodium content and the potential for extravasation in the context of a capillary leak has raised well-founded doubts as to its actual indications.

In liver disease albumin administration as part of general resuscitation manoeuvers, including restoration of intravascular space, treatment of infection and reversal of splanchnic ischaemia with terlipressin, is thought to be advantageous.

There is no evidence to support liberal administration of albumin in acute haemorrhagic shock although, equally, there is no evidence of such administration causing harm. Indeed, such a study has not been conducted and would be difficult to undertake.

The Cochrane group meta-analysis (1,400 patients) raised the possibility of a harmful effect of albumin when administered in the context of general intensive care [30]. However, a larger (3,500 patients) meta-analysis in a more general population did not reveal a difference in mortality in patients resuscitated with albumin [31]. This uncertainty lead to a large randomised control trial in 7,000 general intensive care patients, in which similar outcomes were observed with or without albumin [32]. In critically ill patients without inflammation or ongoing sepsis, an albumin and furosemide strategy was associated with more rapid and successful weaning from ventilator support when compared with furosemide only [33].

32.5 Pulmonary Artery Catheterisation

Use of a pulmonary artery catheter (PAC) [34] and measurement of thermodilution cardiac output at the bedside [35] date back to the 1960s and was developed in intensive care units in the 1970s and 1980s [36,37], was the subject of much controversy in the 1990s [38] and more recently has been tested against a variety of so-called less invasive cardiac output monitoring techniques.

The usefulness of measuring pulmonary artery pressure other than in established pulmonary hypertension, high-risk cardiac anaesthesia, intensive care and peri-operative intensive care remains to be established [39].

Measuring cardiac output in critically ill patients and its pharmacological manipulation, either directly or by altering systemic vascular resistance, has also been controversial [40,41]. Survivors of critical illness were observed to have higher cardiac output and therefore oxygen delivery [42,43]. Pre-operative manipulation of these haemodynamic variables in high-risk surgical patients proved advantageous [44]. However, in mixed populations of critically ill patients, subsequent attempts to augment these values to those observed in survivors were not successful in improving outcome and, indeed, in some studies were harmful [45]. Others used mixed venous saturation as a surrogate marker of cardiac output and haemodynamic performance but were unsuccessful in establishing a clear benefit in patients treated to achieve target values [46]. Interestingly a similar approach using central venous catheters to guide goal-directed therapy in the emergency room was associated with significant improvement in survival [47].

In a large randomised series of patients with ARDS, indices of lung injury, other organ failures, intensive care stay and survival were similar in patients with and without PAC, but complications — in particular arrhythmias — were more frequent in the PAC group [48]. These findings were reproduced in the peri-operative setting [49]. In an equally large randomised study of a heterogeneous group of general intensive care patients, PAC-guided treatment was associated with a similar mortality rate, frequency of organ failures and length of hospital stay [50].

There is, therefore, no evidence pointing to improved (or worsened) survival directly attributable to pulmonary artery catheterisation. In addition there remains a long-running debate with respect to the advantages of haemodynamic manipulation guided by PAC and some indirect evidence of harm related to its use [51]. PAC use has declined markedly in the general intensive care setting, but less so in cardiopulmonary intensive care and anaesthesia, where it still enjoys perceived advantages, although not supported by rigorous evidence.

32.6 Selective Digestive Decontamination

Many infections in the critically ill are caused by community organisms carried by otherwise healthy individuals or by hospital organisms carried by patients. Due to failure of host defence and possibly mucosal translocation in severe illness these organisms can become pathogenic [52]. Attempts to reduce the prevalence and impact of these organisms by prophylactic selective oropharyngeal decontamination [53] and parenteral selective decontamination of the digestive tract (SDD) [54] quickly gained acceptance, in part supported by favourable evidence of reduction in infections — particularly hospital-acquired pneumonia but not mortality [55,56].

There have also been favourable effects on survival reported in some randomised studies [57–59] and meta-analyses [60,61].

Comparisons between the two regimens in a Dutch large multicentre investigation revealed a reduction in 28-day mortality (after adjustments for covariables) from both regimens relative to standard care, without an associated increase in antibiotic resistance [62].

However, the issue of potential increased selection of multi-resistant organisms remains unresolved, particularly given the huge worldwide variation in microbiological flora prevalent in different units, a feature of antibiotic policies generally but also of patient characteristics. In a single-centre five-year study involving 1,900 patients, methicillin-resistant *Staphylococcus aureus* (MRSA) and Gram-negative prevalence rates were similar, relative to a cohort of reference patients in other intensive care units not using SDD [63]. There was, however an increase in resistant enterococci and coagulase-negative staphylococci. Furthermore, close inspection of the data revealed that patients receiving SDD were sub-selected and that there were different and varying patient groups across the reference group (which was taken from a more mixed multicentre population). Others have found an increased selection of extended-spectrum-β-lactamase-producing organisms [64] and SDD in heterogeneous groups of critically ill patients where resistant pathogens are endemic has been associated with increased resistant *Enterobacteriaceae*, MRSA [65] and multidrug-resistant Gram-negative bacteria [66]. Of particular concern is some evidence of a large increase in the prevalence of MRSA when SDD was attempted in units where this pathogen was endemic [67].

In summary there appears to be evidence to support selective decontamination of the digestive tract in predominantly surgical units with low prevalence rates of drug-resistant organisms, but this has not gained widespread acceptance in practice. In units with a more heterogeneous mix of patients, published and anecdotal evidence of the selection of multi-resistant strains does not support SDD.

References

[1] Schumer, W. (1976). Steroids in the treatment of clinical septic shock, *Ann Surg*, **184**, 333–341.

[2] Sprung, C.L., Caralis, P.V., Marcial, E.H. *et al.* (1984). The effects of high dose corticosteroids in patients with septic shock: a prospective, controlled study, *N Engl J Med*, **311**, 1137–1143.

[3] Briegel, J., Forst, H., Haller, M. *et al.* (1999). Stress doses of hydrocortisone reverse hyperdynamic septic shock: a prospective, randomized, double-blind, single center study, *Crit Care Med*, **27**, 723–732.

[4] Annane, D., Sébille, V., Charpentier, C. *et al.* (2002). Effect of treatment with low doses of hydrocortisone and fludrocortisone on mortality in patients with septic shock, *JAMA*, **288**, 862–871.

[5] Sprung, C.L., Annane, D., Keh, D. *et al.* (2008). Hydrocortisone therapy for patients with septic shock, *N Engl J Med*, **358**, 111–124.

[6] Steinberg, K.P., Hudson, L.D., Goodman, R.B. *et al.* (2006). Efficacy and safety of corticosteroids for persistent acute respiratory distress syndrome, *N Engl J Med*, **354**, 1671–1674.

[7] Esmon, C.T., Taylor, F.B. and Snow, T.R. (1991). Inflammation and coagulation: linked processes potentially regulated through a common pathway mediated by protein C, *Thromb Haemost*, **66**, 160–165.

[8] Bone, R.C., Balk, R.A., Fein, A.M. *et al.* (1995). A second large controlled clinical study of E5, a monoclonal antibody to endotoxin: results of a prospective, multicenter, randomized, controlled trial, *Crit Care Med*, **23**, 994–1006.

[9] Reinhart, K., Menges, T., Gardlund, B. *et al.* (2001). Randomized, placebo-controlled trail of the anti-tumor necrosis factor antibody fragment afelimomab in hyperinflammatory response during severe sepsis: the RAMSES Study, *Crit Care Med*, **29**, 765–769.

[10] Fisher, C.J., Agosti, J.M., Opal, S.M. *et al.* (1996). Treatment of septic shock with the tumor necrosis factor receptor: Fc fusion protein. The soluble TNF Receptor Sepsis Study Group, *N Engl J Med*, **334**,1697–1702.

[11] Fourier, F., Chopin, C., Goudemand, J. *et al.* (1992). Septic shock, multiple organ failure and disseminated intravascular coagulation: compared patterns of antithrombin III, protein C and protein S deficiencies, *Chest*, **101**, 816–823.

[12] Taylor, F.B., Chang, A., Esmon, C.T. *et al.* (1987). Protein C prevents the coagulopathic and lethal effects of *Escherichia coli* infusion in the baboon, *J Clin Invest*, **79**, 918–925.

[13] Bernard, G.R., Vincent, J.L., Laterre, P.F. *et al.* (2001). Efficacy and safety of recombinant human activated protein C for severe sepsis, *N Engl J Med*, **344**, 699–709.

[14] Warren, H.S., Suffredini, A.F. and Munford, R.S. (2002). Risks and benefits of activated protein C treatment for severe sepsis, *N Engl J Med*, **347**, 1027–1030.

[15] Ely, E.W., Wesley, E., Laterre, P.F. *et al.* (2003). Drotrecogin alfa (activated) administration across clinically important subgroups of patients with severe sepsis, *Crit Care Med*, **31**, 12–19.

[16] Abraham, E., Laterre, P.F., Garg, R. *et al.* (2005). Drotrecogin alfa (activated) for adults with severe sepsis and a low risk of death, *N Engl J Med*, **353**, 1332–1341.

[17] Siegl, J.P. (2002). Assessing the use of activated protein C in the treatment of severe sepsis, *N Engl J Med*, **347**, 1030–1034.

[18] Manns, B.J., Lee, H., Doig, C.J. *et al.* (2002). An economic evaluation of activated protein, C. treatment for severe sepsis, *N Engl J Med*, **347**, 993–1000.

[19] Ranieri, V.M., Thompson, B.T. and Barie, P.S. (2012). Drotrecogin alfa (activated) in adults with septic shock, *N Engl J Med*, **366**, 2055–2064.

[20] Díaz, R., Paolasso, E.A., Piegas, L.S. *et al.* (1998). Metabolic modulation of acute myocardial infarction: the ECLA Glucose-Insulin-Potassium pilot trial, *Circulation*, **98**, 2227–2234.

[21] Van den Berghe, G., Wouters, P., Weekers, F. *et al.* (2001). Intensive insulin therapy in critically ill patients, *N Engl J Med*, **345**, 1359–1367.

[22] Evans, T.W. (2001). Hemodynamic and metabolic therapy in critically ill patients, *N Engl J Med*, **345**, 1417–1418.

[23] Stanley, A.W., Moraski, R.E., Russell, R.O. *et al.* (1975). Effects of glucose-insulin-potassium on myocardial substrate availability and utilisation in stable coronary artery disease: studies on myocardial carbohydrates, lipid and oxygen arterial-coronary sinus differences in patients with coronary artery disease, *Am J Cardiol*, **36**, 929–937.

[24] Vanhorebeek, I., De Vos, R., Mesotten, M. *et al.* (2005). Protection of hepatocyte mitochondrial ultrastructure and function by strict glucose control with insulin in critically ill patients, *Lancet*, **365**, 53–59.

[25] Langouche, L., Vanhorebeek, I., Vlasselaers, D. *et al.* (2005). Intensive insulin therapy protects the endothelium of critically ill patients, *J Clin Invest*, **115**, 2277–2286.

[26] Vriesendorp, T.M., DeVries, J.H., van Santen, S. *et al.* (2006). Evaluation of short-term consequences of hypoglycaemia in an intensive care unit, *Crit Care Med*, **34**, 2714–2718.

[27] Van den Berghe, G., Wilmer, A., Hermans, G. *et al.* (2006). Intensive insulin therapy in the medical ICU, *N Engl J Med*, **354**, 449–461.

[28] Wiener, R.S., Wiener, D.C., Larson, R.J. (2008). Benefits and risks of tight glucose control in critically ill adults, *JAMA*, **300**, 933–944.

[29] NICE-SUGAR Investigators, Finfer S., Chittock, D.R. *et al.* (2009). Intensive versus conventional glucose control in critically ill patients, *N Engl J Med*, **360**, 1283–1297.

[30] Cochrane Injuries Group Albumin Reviewers (1998). Human albumin administration in critically ill patients: systematic review of randomised trials, *BMJ*, **317**, 235–240.

[31] Wikes, M.M. and Navickis, R.J. (2001). Patient survival after human albumin administration: a meta-analysis of randomized, controlled trials, *Ann Intern Med*, **135**, 149–164.
[32] Finfer, S., Bellomo, R., Boyce, N. *et al.* (2004). Comparison of albumin and saline for fluid resuscitation in the intensive care unit, *N Engl J Med*, **350**, 2247–2256.
[33] Martin, G.S., Moss, M., Wheeler, A.P. *et al.* (2005). A randomized, controlled trial of frusemide with or without albumin in hypoproteinemic patients with acute lung injury, *Crit Care Med*, **33**, 1681–1687.
[34] Bradley, R.D. (1964). Diagnostic right heart catheterisation with miniature catheters in severely ill patients, *Lancet*, **2**, 941–942.
[35] Branthwaite, M.A. and Bradley, R.D. (1968). Measurement of cardiac output by thermodilution in man, *J Appl Phys*, **24**, 434–438.
[36] Swan, H.J.C., Ganz, W., Forrester, J. *et al.* (1970). Catheterization of the heart in man with use of a flow-directed balloon-tipped catheter, *N Engl J Med*, **283**, 447–451.
[37] Goldenheim, P.D. and Kazemi, H. (1984). Cardiopulmonary monitoring of critically ill patients, *N Engl J Med*, **311**, 776–780.
[38] Gimosair, Y. and Sprung, C.L. (1996). The Swan-Ganz catheter. Twenty five years of monitoring, *Crit Care Clin*, **12**, 771–776.
[39] Dalen, J.E. and Bone, R.C. (1996). Is it time to pull the pulmonary artery catheter? *JAMA*, **276**, 916–918.
[40] Gomez, C.M.H., and Palazzo, M.G. (1998). Pulmonary artery catheterisation in anaesthesia and intensive care, *Br J Anaesth*, **81**, 945–956.
[41] Hinds, C. and Watson, D. (1995). Manipulating hemodynamics and oxygen transport in critically ill patients, *N Engl J Med*, **333**, 1074–1075.
[42] Shoemaker, W., Montgomery, E., Kaplan, E. *et al.* (1973). Physiologic patterns in surviving and nonsurviving shock patients, *Arch Surg*, **106**, 630–636.
[43] Yu, M., Levy, M., Smith, P. *et al.* (1993). Effect of maximizing oxygen delivery on morbidity and mortality rates in critically ill patients: a prospective, randomized, controlled study, *Crit Care Med*, **21**, 830–838.
[44] Boyd, O., Grounds, R.M. and Bennett, E.D. (1993). A randomized clinical trial of the effect of deliberate perioperative increase of oxygen delivery on mortality in high risk surgical patients, *JAMA*, **270**, 2699–2707.
[45] Hayes, M.A., Timmins, A.C., Yau, E.H.S. *et al.* (1994). Elevation of systemic oxygen delivery in the treatment of critically ill patients, *N Engl J Med*, **330**, 1717–1722.
[46] Gattinoni, L., Brazzi, L., Pelosi, P. *et al.* (1995). A trial of goal-orientated hemodynamic therapy in critically ill patients, *N Engl J Med*, **333**, 1025–1032.

[47] Rivers, E., Nguyen, B., Havstad, S. *et al.* (2001). Early goal-directed therapy in the treatment of severe sepsis and septic shock, *N Engl J Med*, **345**, 1368–1377.

[48] National Heart, Lung, and Blood Institute Acute Respiratory Distress Syndrome (ARDS) Clinical Trials Network, Wheeler, A.P., Bernard, G.R. *et al.* (2006). Pulmonary artery versus central venous catheter to guide treatment of acute lung injury, *N Engl J Med*, **354**, 2213–2224.

[49] Sandham, J.D., Hull, R.D., Brant, R.F. *et al.* (2003). A randomized, controlled trial of the use of pulmonary-artery catheters in high-risk surgical patients, *N Engl J Med*, **348**, 5–14.

[50] Harvey, S., Harrison, D.A., Singer, M. *et al.* (2005). Assessment of the clinical effectiveness of pulmonary artery catheters in management of patients in intensive care (PAC-Man): a randomised controlled trial, *Lancet*, **366**, 472–477.

[51] Connors Jr, A.F., Speroff, T., Dawson, N.V. *et al.* (1996). The effectiveness of right heart catheterization in the initial care of critically ill patients, *JAMA*, **276**, 889–897.

[52] Vincent, J.L. (2003). Nosocomial infections in adult intensive care units, *Lancet*, **361**, 2068–2077.

[53] Bergmans, D.C., Bonten, M.J., Gaillard, C.A. *et al.* (2001). Prevention of ventilator-associated pneumonia by oral decontamination: a prospective, randomized, double-blind, placebo-controlled study, *Am J Respir Crit Care Med*, **164**, 382–388.

[54] Baxby, D., van Saene, H.K.F., Stoutenbeek, C.P. *et al.* (1996), Selective decontamination of the digestive tract: 13 years on, what it is and what it is not, *Intens Care Med*, **22**, 699–706.

[55] Stoutenbeek, C.P., van Saene, H.K.F., Miranda, D.R. *et al.* (1984). The effect of selective decontamination of the digestive tract on colonization and infection rate in multiple trauma patients, *Intens Care Med*, **10**, 185–192.

[56] Garrouste-Orgeas, M., Chevret, S., Arlet, G. *et al.* (1997). Oropharyngeal or gastric colonization and nosocomial pneumonia in adult intensive care unit patients: a prospective study based on genomic DNA analysis, *Am J Respir Crit Care Med*, **156**, 1647–1655.

[57] Krueger, W.A., Lenhart, F.P., Neeser, G. *et al.* (2002). Influence of combined intravenous and topical antibiotic prophylaxis on the incidence of infections, organ dysfunctions, and mortality in critically ill surgical patients: a prospective, stratified, randomized, double-blind, placebo-controlled clinical trial, *Am J Respir Crit Care Med*, **166**, 1029–1037.

[58] de Jonge, E., Schultz, M., Spanjaard, L. *et al.* (2003). Effects of selective decontamination of the digestive tract on mortality and acquisition of resistant bacteria in intensive care: a randomised controlled trial, *Lancet*, **362**, 1011–1016.

[59] de la Cal, M.A., Cerdá, E., Garcia-Hierro, P. *et al.* (2005). Survival benefit in critically ill burned patients receiving selective decontamination of the digestive tract: a randomized, placebo-controlled, double-blind trial, *Ann Surg*, **241**, 424–430.

[60] Van Nieuwenhoven, C.A., Buskens, E., van Tiel, F.H. *et al.* (2001). Relationship between methodological trial quality and the effects of selective digestive decontamination on pneumonia and mortality in critically ill patients, *JAMA*, **286**, 335–340.

[61] D'Amico, R., Pifferi, S., Leonetti, C. *et al.* (1998), Effectiveness of antibiotic prophylaxis in critically ill adult patients: systemic review of randomised controlled trials, *BMJ*, **316**, 1275–1285.

[62] De Smet, A.M.G.A., Kluytmans, J.A.J.W., Cooper, B.S. *et al.* (2009). Decontamination of the digestive tract and oropharynx in ICU patients, *N Engl J Med*, **360**, 20–31.

[63] Heininger, A., Meyer, E., Schwab, F. *et al.* (2006). Effects of long-term routine use of selective digestive decontamination on antimicrobial resistance, *Intens Care Med*, **32**, 1569–1576.

[64] Al Naiemi, N.N., Heddema, E.R., Bart, A. *et al.* (2006). Emergence of multidrug-resistant, Gram negative bacteria during selective decontamination of the digestive tract on an intensive care unit, *J Antimicrob Chemother*, **58**, 853–856.

[65] Verwaest, C., Verhaegen, J., Ferdinande, P. *et al.* (1997), Randomized, controlled trial of selective digestive decontamination in 600 mechanically ventilated patients in a multidisciplinary intensive care unit, *Crit Care Med*, **25**, 63–71.

[66] Misset, B., Kitzis, M.D., Mahe, P. *et al.* (1993). Bacteriological side effects of gut decontamination with polymyxin E, gentamicin, and amphotericin B, *Infect Control Hosp Epidemiol*, **14**, 62–64.

[67] Lingnau, W., Berger, J., Javorsky, F. *et al.* (1998). Changing bacterial ecology during a five year period of selective intestinal decontamination, *J Hosp Infect*, **39**, 195–206.

Index